Anatomy & Physiology
Made
Incredibly Easy!
Clear Useful
& Readable

Anatomy
and
Physiology
Review
&
Guide

To Accompany any Textbook of Anatomy or Physiology

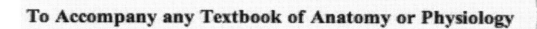

Anatomy and Physiology
Review & Guide
Made
Incredibily Easy !

To accompany any textbook of Anatomy or Physiology

Author

Hashim Khalil Erzouki   MD , PhD

Editorial

Dr. Hikmat Al Shaarbaf
Professor Internal Medicine
Dean Medical College
Baghdad Iraq

Dr Charles W. Schindler
Preclinical Pharmacology
NIDA INtramura Research

Desiger Mr. Zaid A. Al Mashhadani

Copyright

By

Hashim Khalil Erzouki MD PhD

September 2013

DEDICATION

To my dear parents who taught me the hard work, the love and the respect to the others. My wife Hind who gave me real support and wonderful care and kindness, to my growing kids, Hibba, Mona, Sara, Saadi, Ali and Basim for their patience and understanding throughout these past years, but most of all for their love, support and belief in me. My Two sons in law Hisham and Zaid my three beautiful grandchildren Lina, Layth and Lamees who certainly make my life brighter, happier and illuminated with light. To all students, readers, colleagues and my fellow workers: loves, respects and appreciations.

V I T A E

Hashim Khalil Erzouki was born in Iraq, 1945. In 1964, he graduated from High School. In 1964-1967 he attended Mosul - University in Iraq to study Medical Science. At 9 p.m., Day 9, Month 9, 1968, he left his native country to enrol in Sofia - University Medical College - Bulgaria. He graduated as a medical doctor in 1975 and for the next years practiced medicine in Europe, Africa and Asia. In 1983, he moved to the United States of America for the specific purpose of obtaining an advanced degree in cardiovascular physiology. Prior to Georgetown University, he attended Kaplan Educational Centre in Washington, D.C. to study clinical and medical basic science for approximately 2 years. In 1986 he enrolled in Graduate School at Georgetown University. 1989 awarded $18000 by American Heart Associations (AHA) for new findings on cocaine effects on cardio respiratory systems. Georgetown University gave me the great opportunity to teach a complete course of physiology to the minority students as Ph.D. requirements and thereby to learn the art of teaching. April 18 1991 graduated from Georgetown University. In 1992, I took a position with NIH. I become principle investigator for numerous research and design projects. The research experience taught me to read papers, understand methodologies, examine the results and draw my own conclusions as well as to raise new questions the author's had not examined. My philosophy is that you have to make time for what is important to you. Teaching is not only important, but it is my calling and I enjoy every minute of doing it. In my lifetime I have seen patients with many diverse heath care needs, assisted in several emergency situations, tutoring, teaching, and researching. I have had an excellent exposure to public health service and research institutes in the USA, Europe, Africa and Asia. Furthermore, I have coordinated several scientific conferences and have met numerous physicians, scientists, nurses and technicians. My experience influenced my development as scientist, a health care professional, teacher and person. My ultimate goal is to use my technical skills, medical and teaching expertise in designing Physiology and Medical books publication projects, which are relevant, easy, applicable, and important. I wish to expand my skills and build a solid foundation for a respected Medical Publications Program. In essence, any publication should technically centre and aims to improve the quality of learning and the quality of life.

A C K N O W L E D G E M E N T S

Only with the assistance and encouragement of numerous individuals was I able to complete this anatomy and physiology review guide, which considered as a basic foundation to my medical physiology book. To my two mentors, Dr. Hikmet Shear Baff and Dr. Charles Schindler whose knowledge and advices contributed immensely to my work and publications, go my deepest respect and appreciation. As exceptionally great professors and scientists they constantly followed my progress and development in science, and publications specially are the main editors in my textbook of Erzouki's Medical Physiology. To my best helper in designing this book Mr Zaid Ahmed Al-Mashhadani who works hard to make the book comes to its final shape.
Big smile, best wishes for all students and all readers. At the end there is a saying in my native language "He who teaches me a letter, has me for a slave". For all my teachers, who taught me more than a letter and more than a word, go my appreciation forever.

VI

Table of Contents

LIST OF CHAPTERS

CHAPTER ONE

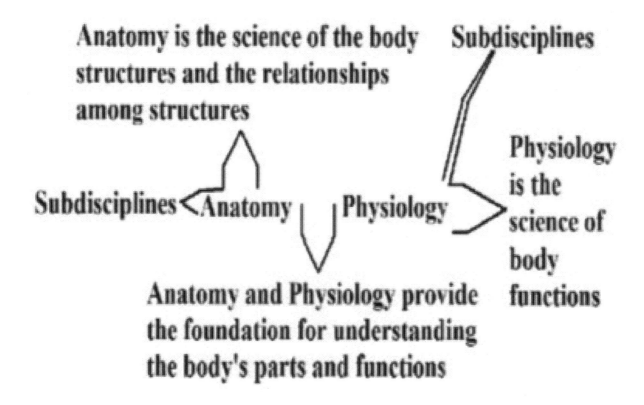

Anatomy is the science of the body structures and the relationships among structures

Subdisciplines

Subdisciplines ← Anatomy   Physiology →

Physiology is the science of body functions

Anatomy and Physiology provide the foundation for understanding the body's parts and functions

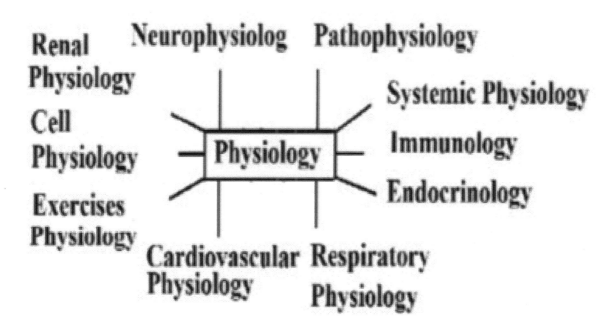

Renal Physiology

Neurophysiolog   Pathophysiology

Cell Physiology

Physiology

Systemic Physiology

Immunology

Exercises Physiology

Endocrinology

Cardiovascular Physiology   Respiratory Physiology

Hierarchy of Life Organization

Level of Organization	Explanation	Example
Atomic Level	Atoms are defined as the smallest unit of an element that still maintains the property of that element.	Carbon, Hydrogen, Oxygen
Molecular Level	Atoms combine to form molecules which can have entirely different properties than the atoms they contain.	Water, DNA, Carbohydrates
Cellular Level	Cells are the smallest unit of life. Cells are enclosed by a membrane or cell wall and in multicellular organisms often perform specific functions.	Muscle cell, Skin cell, Neuron
Tissue Level	Tissues are groups of cells with similar functions	Muscle, Epithelial, Connective
Organ Level	Organs are two or more types of tissues that work together to complete a specific task.	Heart, Liver, Stomach
Organ System Level	An organ system is group of organs that carries out more generalized set of functions.	Digestive System, Circulatory System
Organismal Level	An organism has several organ systems that function together.	Human

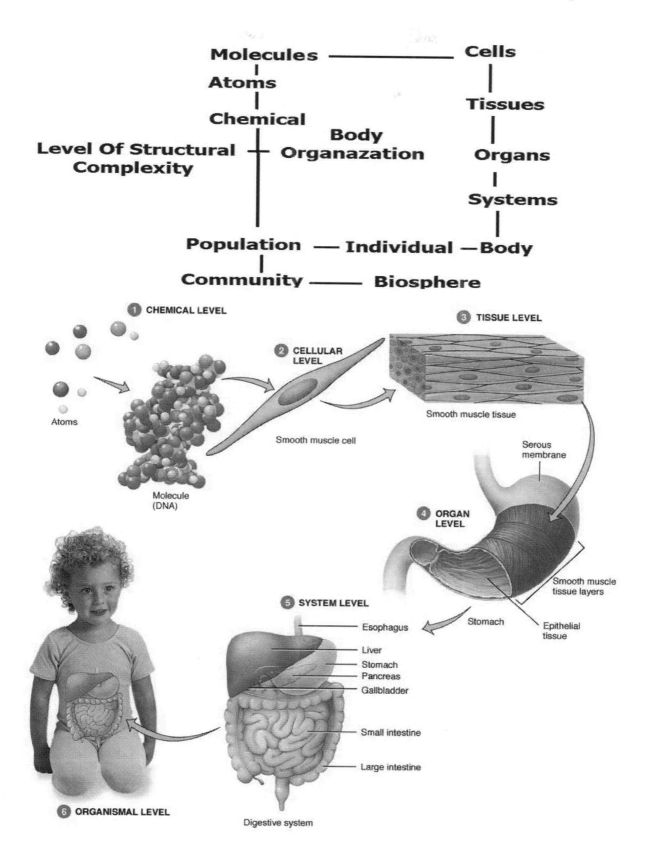

Molecules ——— Cells
| |
Atoms   Tissues
| |
Chemical   Organs
| |
Level Of Structural —+— Body   Systems
Complexity   Organazation
| |
Population —— Individual —Body
|
Community ——— Biosphere

① CHEMICAL LEVEL

② CELLULAR LEVEL

③ TISSUE LEVEL

Atoms

Molecule (DNA)

Smooth muscle cell

Smooth muscle tissue

Serous membrane

④ ORGAN LEVEL

Smooth muscle tissue layers

Stomach

Epithelial tissue

⑤ SYSTEM LEVEL

Esophagus
Liver
Stomach
Pancreas
Gallbladder
Small intestine
Large intestine

⑥ ORGANISMAL LEVEL

Digestive system

Level of Biological Organiztion

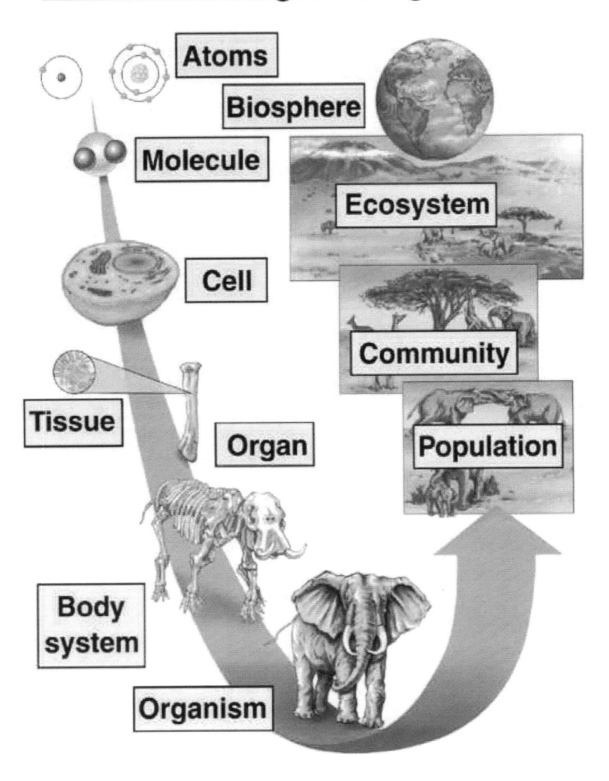

Organ systems	A group of organs that contribute to specific functions within the body. *Examples:* gastrointestinal system, nervous system
Organs	A group of tissues precisely arranged so that so they can work together to perform specific functions. *Examples:* liver, brain
Tissues	A group of cells with similar structure and function. There are only four types of tissues: epithelial tissue, connective tissue, muscle tissue, and nerve tissue.
Cells	The smallest living unit in the body. *Examples:* hepatocyte, neuron
Chemicals	Atoms or molecules that are the building blocks of all matter. *Examples:* oxygen, protein

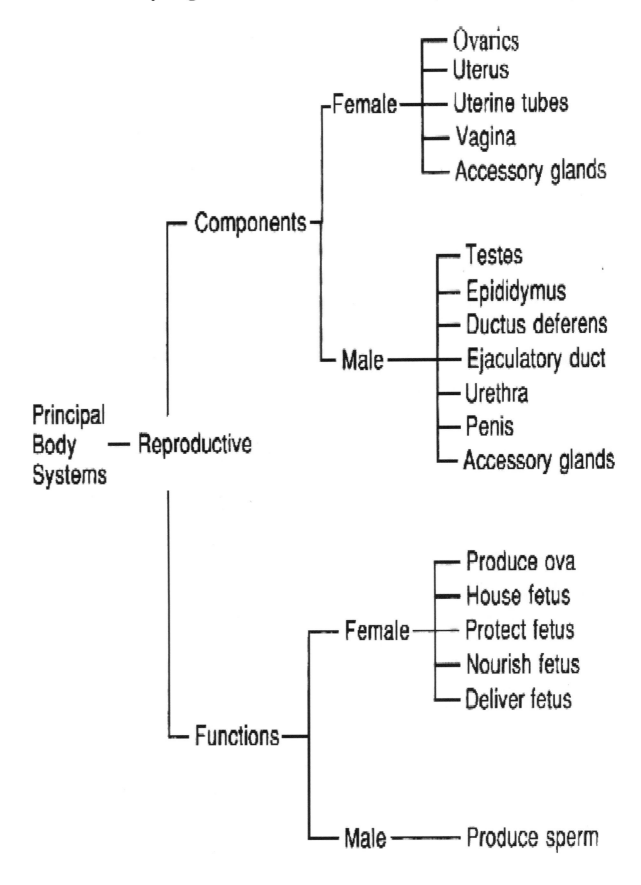

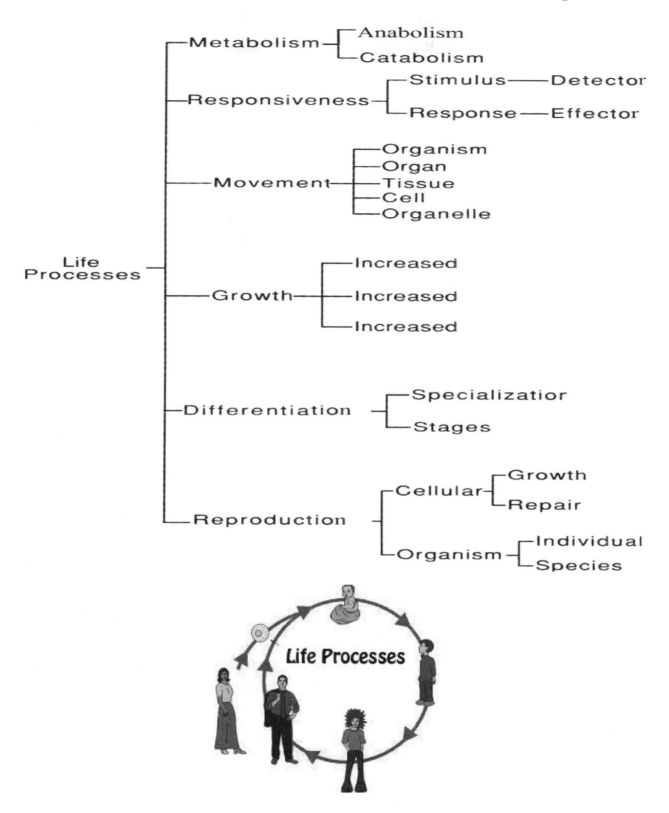

Life Processes

- Metabolism
  - Anabolism
  - Catabolism
- Responsiveness
  - Stimulus — Detector
  - Response — Effector
- Movement
  - Organism
  - Organ
  - Tissue
  - Cell
  - Organelle
- Growth
  - Increased
  - Increased
  - Increased
- Differentiation
  - Specializatior
  - Stages
- Reproduction
  - Cellular
    - Growth
    - Repair
  - Organism
    - Individual
    - Species

Life Processes

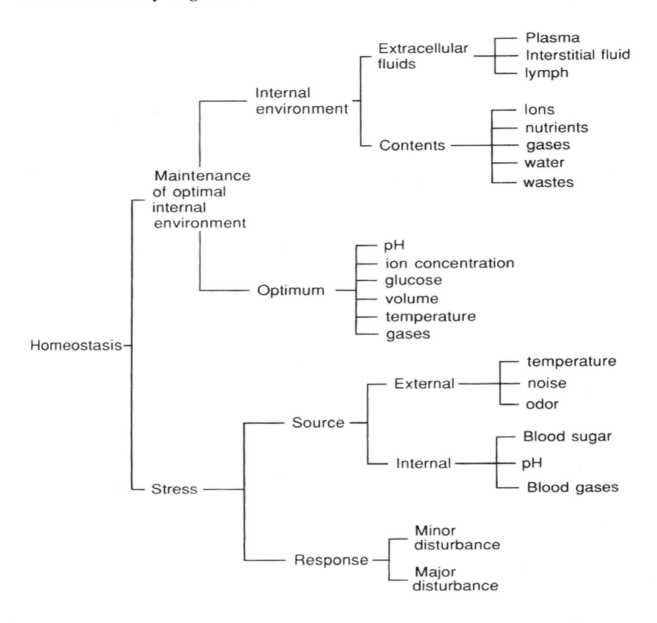

Homeostasis
- Maintenance of optimal internal environment
  - Internal environment
    - Extracellular fluids
      - Plasma
      - Interstitial fluid
      - lymph
    - Contents
      - Ions
      - nutrients
      - gases
      - water
      - wastes
  - Optimum
    - pH
    - ion concentration
    - glucose
    - volume
    - temperature
    - gases
- Stress
  - Source
    - External
      - temperature
      - noise
      - odor
    - Internal
      - Blood sugar
      - pH
      - Blood gases
  - Response
    - Minor disturbance
    - Major disturbance

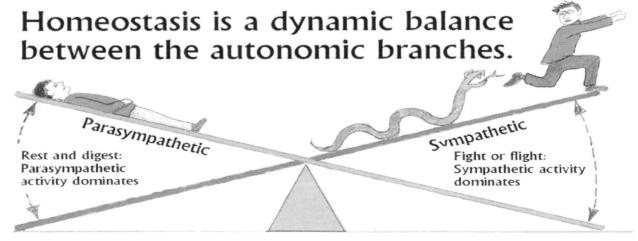

Homeostasis is a dynamic balance between the autonomic branches.

Parasympathetic

Rest and digest: Parasympathetic activity dominates

Sympathetic

Fight or flight: Sympathetic activity dominates

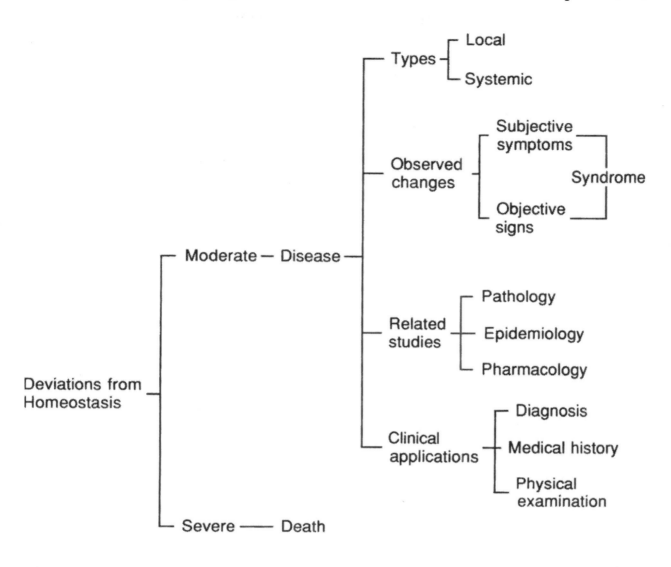

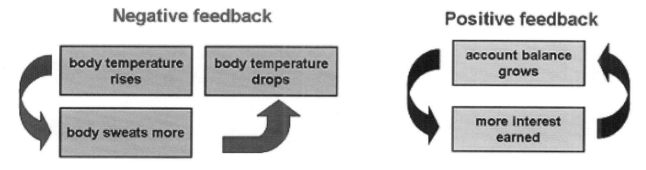

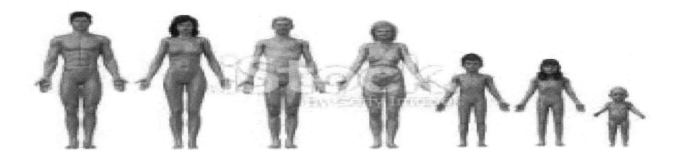

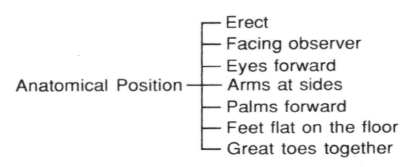

Anatomical Position
- Erect
- Facing observer
- Eyes forward
- Arms at sides
- Palms forward
- Feet flat on the floor
- Great toes together

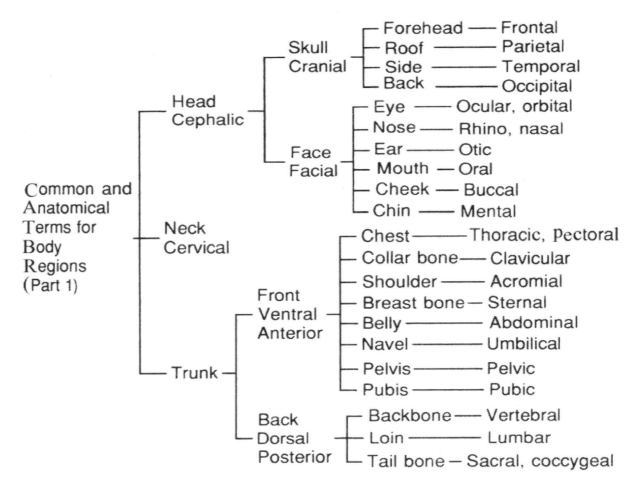

Common and Anatomical Terms for Body Regions (Part 1)

- Head Cephalic
  - Skull Cranial
    - Forehead — Frontal
    - Roof — Parietal
    - Side — Temporal
    - Back — Occipital
  - Face Facial
    - Eye — Ocular, orbital
    - Nose — Rhino, nasal
    - Ear — Otic
    - Mouth — Oral
    - Cheek — Buccal
    - Chin — Mental
- Neck Cervical
- Trunk
  - Front Ventral Anterior
    - Chest — Thoracic, Pectoral
    - Collar bone — Clavicular
    - Shoulder — Acromial
    - Breast bone — Sternal
    - Belly — Abdominal
    - Navel — Umbilical
    - Pelvis — Pelvic
    - Pubis — Pubic
  - Back Dorsal Posterior
    - Backbone — Vertebral
    - Loin — Lumbar
    - Tail bone — Sacral, coccygeal

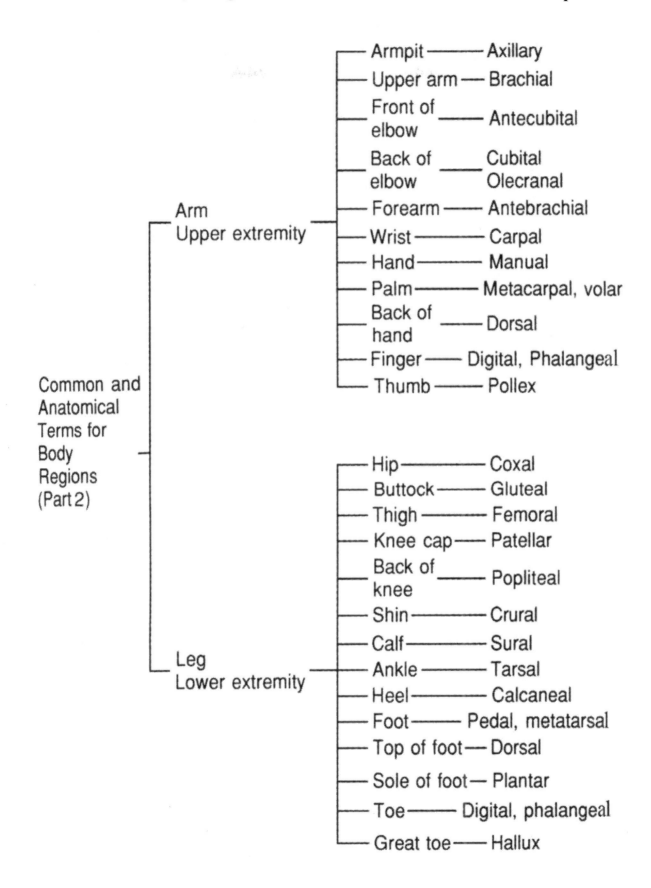

Common and
Anatomical
Terms for
Body
Regions
(Part 2)

Arm / Upper extremity

Common	Anatomical
Armpit	Axillary
Upper arm	Brachial
Front of elbow	Antecubital
Back of elbow	Cubital / Olecranal
Forearm	Antebrachial
Wrist	Carpal
Hand	Manual
Palm	Metacarpal, volar
Back of hand	Dorsal
Finger	Digital, Phalangeal
Thumb	Pollex

Leg / Lower extremity

Common	Anatomical
Hip	Coxal
Buttock	Gluteal
Thigh	Femoral
Knee cap	Patellar
Back of knee	Popliteal
Shin	Crural
Calf	Sural
Ankle	Tarsal
Heel	Calcaneal
Foot	Pedal, metatarsal
Top of foot	Dorsal
Sole of foot	Plantar
Toe	Digital, phalangeal
Great toe	Hallux

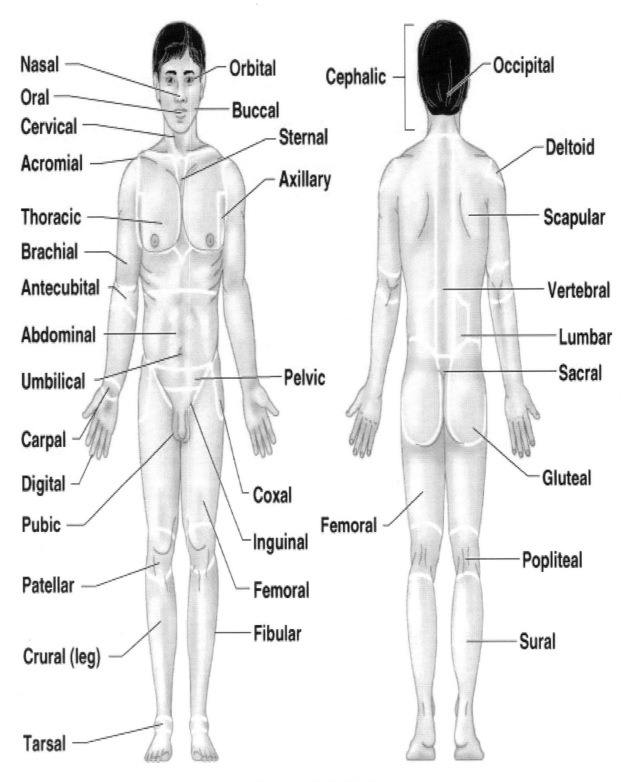

Nasal
Oral
Cervical
Acromial
Thoracic
Brachial
Antecubital
Abdominal
Umbilical
Carpal
Digital
Pubic
Patellar
Crural (leg)
Tarsal

Orbital
Buccal
Sternal
Axillary
Pelvic
Coxal
Inguinal
Femoral
Fibular

Cephalic
Occipital
Deltoid
Scapular
Vertebral
Lumbar
Sacral
Gluteal
Femoral
Popliteal
Sural

(a) Anterior BODY REGIONS **(b) Posterior**
SURFACE LABEL

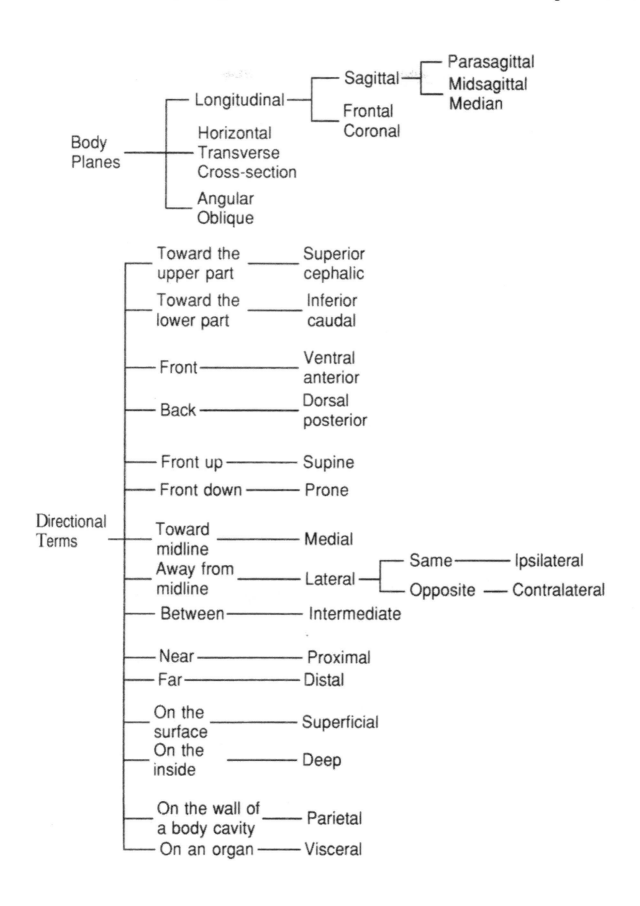

Body Planes
— Longitudinal — Sagittal — Parasagittal / Midsagittal / Median
— Frontal / Coronal
— Horizontal / Transverse / Cross-section
— Angular / Oblique

Directional Terms
— Toward the upper part — Superior / cephalic
— Toward the lower part — Inferior / caudal
— Front — Ventral / anterior
— Back — Dorsal / posterior
— Front up — Supine
— Front down — Prone
— Toward midline — Medial
— Away from midline — Lateral — Same — Ipsilateral
— Opposite — Contralateral
— Between — Intermediate
— Near — Proximal
— Far — Distal
— On the surface — Superficial
— On the inside — Deep
— On the wall of a body cavity — Parietal
— On an organ — Visceral

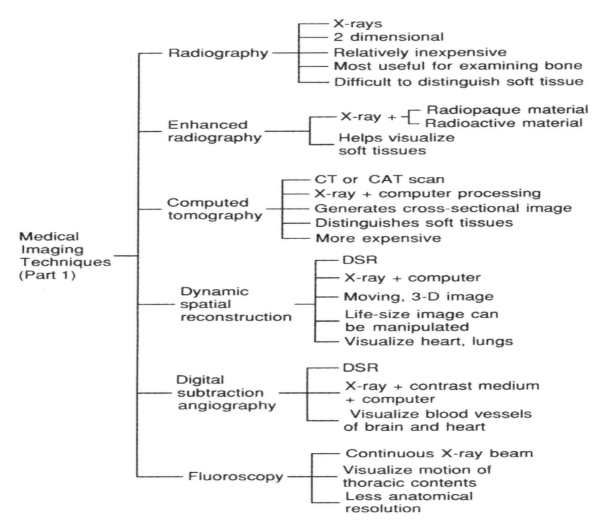

- **Medical Imaging Techniques (Part 1)**
  - **Radiography**
    - X-rays
    - 2 dimensional
    - Relatively inexpensive
    - Most useful for examining bone
    - Difficult to distinguish soft tissue
  - **Enhanced radiography**
    - X-ray +
      - Radiopaque material
      - Radioactive material
    - Helps visualize soft tissues
  - **Computed tomography**
    - CT or CAT scan
    - X-ray + computer processing
    - Generates cross-sectional image
    - Distinguishes soft tissues
    - More expensive
  - **Dynamic spatial reconstruction**
    - DSR
    - X-ray + computer
    - Moving, 3-D image
    - Life-size image can be manipulated
    - Visualize heart, lungs
  - **Digital subtraction angiography**
    - DSR
    - X-ray + contrast medium + computer
    - Visualize blood vessels of brain and heart
  - **Fluoroscopy**
    - Continuous X-ray beam
    - Visualize motion of thoracic contents
    - Less anatomical resolution

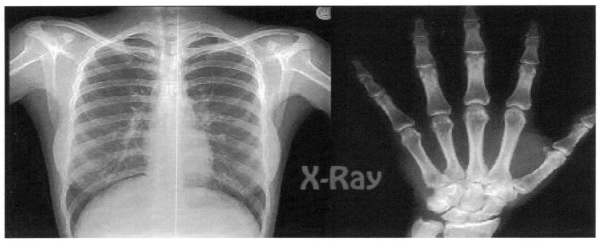

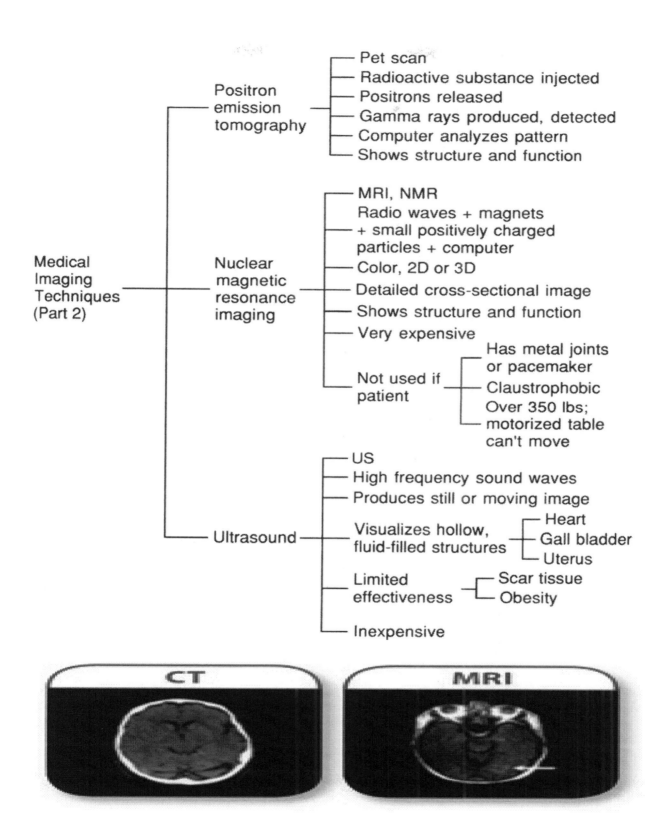

Medical Imaging Techniques (Part 2)

- Positron emission tomography
  - Pet scan
  - Radioactive substance injected
  - Positrons released
  - Gamma rays produced, detected
  - Computer analyzes pattern
  - Shows structure and function

- Nuclear magnetic resonance imaging
  - MRI, NMR
  - Radio waves + magnets + small positively charged particles + computer
  - Color, 2D or 3D
  - Detailed cross-sectional image
  - Shows structure and function
  - Very expensive
  - Not used if patient
    - Has metal joints or pacemaker
    - Claustrophobic
    - Over 350 lbs; motorized table can't move

- Ultrasound
  - US
  - High frequency sound waves
  - Produces still or moving image
  - Visualizes hollow, fluid-filled structures
    - Heart
    - Gall bladder
    - Uterus
  - Limited effectiveness
    - Scar tissue
    - Obesity
  - Inexpensive

CT

MRI

CHAPTER TWO

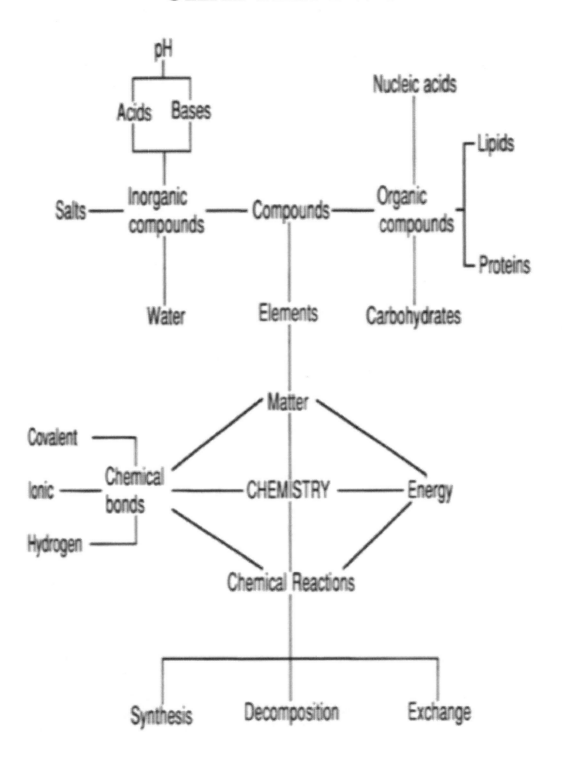

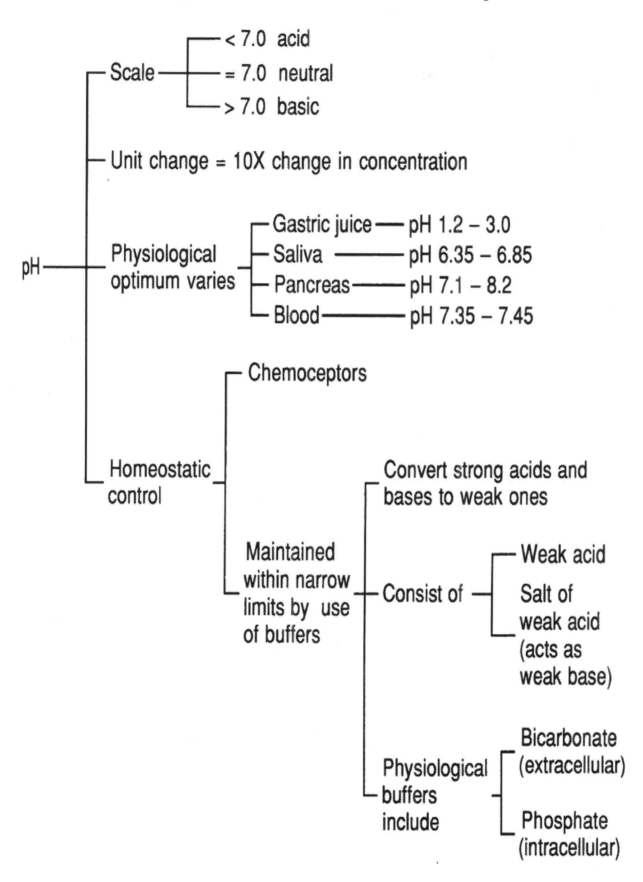

pH
- Scale
  - < 7.0 acid
  - = 7.0 neutral
  - > 7.0 basic
- Unit change = 10X change in concentration
- Physiological optimum varies
  - Gastric juice — pH 1.2 – 3.0
  - Saliva — pH 6.35 – 6.85
  - Pancreas — pH 7.1 – 8.2
  - Blood — pH 7.35 – 7.45
- Homeostatic control
  - Chemoceptors
  - Maintained within narrow limits by use of buffers
    - Convert strong acids and bases to weak ones
    - Consist of
      - Weak acid
      - Salt of weak acid (acts as weak base)
    - Physiological buffers include
      - Bicarbonate (extracellular)
      - Phosphate (intracellular)

Concentration of Hydrogen ions compared to distilled water	pH Chart List	Examples
10,000,000	pH 0	Battery acid
1,000,000	pH 1	Hydrochloric acid
100,000	pH 2	Lemon juice, vinegar
10,000	pH 3	Grapefruit, soft drink
1,000	pH 4	Tomato juice, acid rain
100	pH 5	Black coffee
10	pH 6	Urine, saliva
1	pH 7	"Pure" water
1/10	pH 8	Sea water
1/100	pH 9	Baking soda,
1/1,000	pH 10	Great Salt Lake
1/10,000	pH 11	Ammonia solution
1/100,000	pH 12	Soapy water
1/1,000,000	pH 13	Bleach
1/10,000,000	pH 14	Liquid drain cleaner

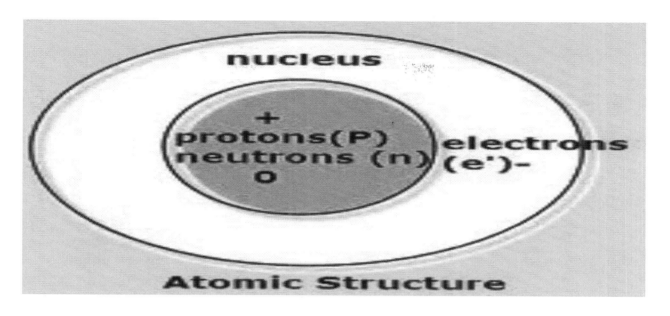

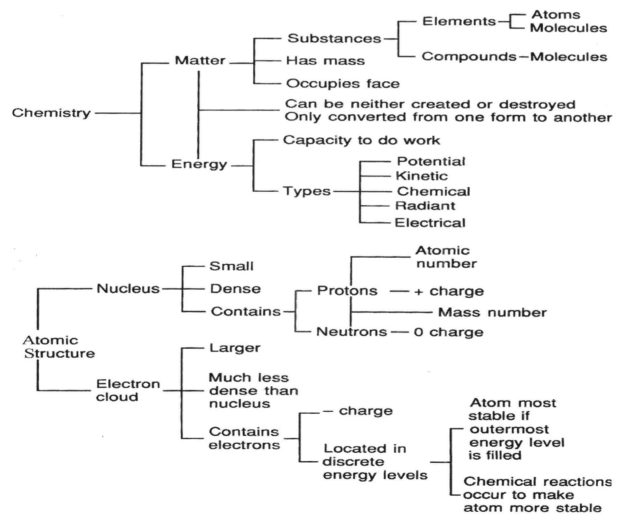

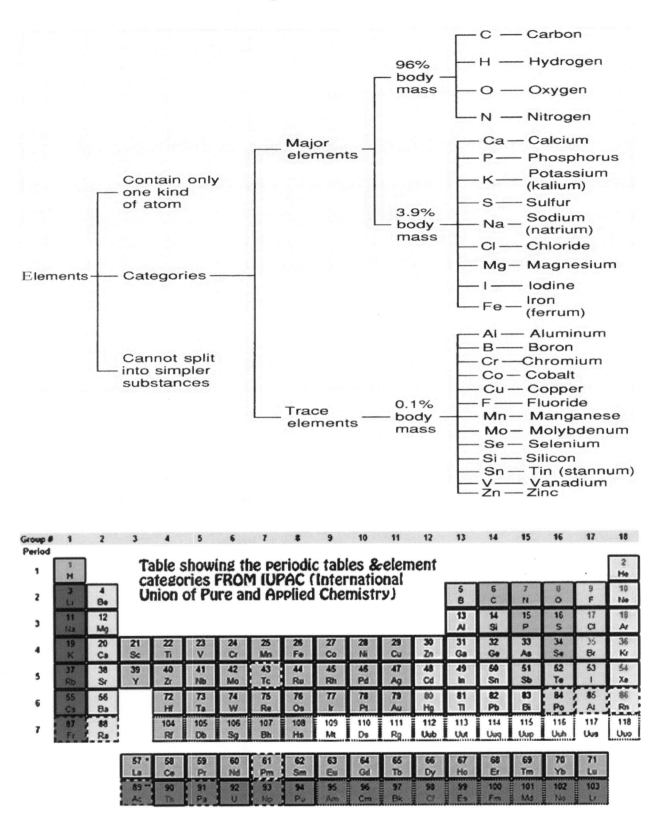

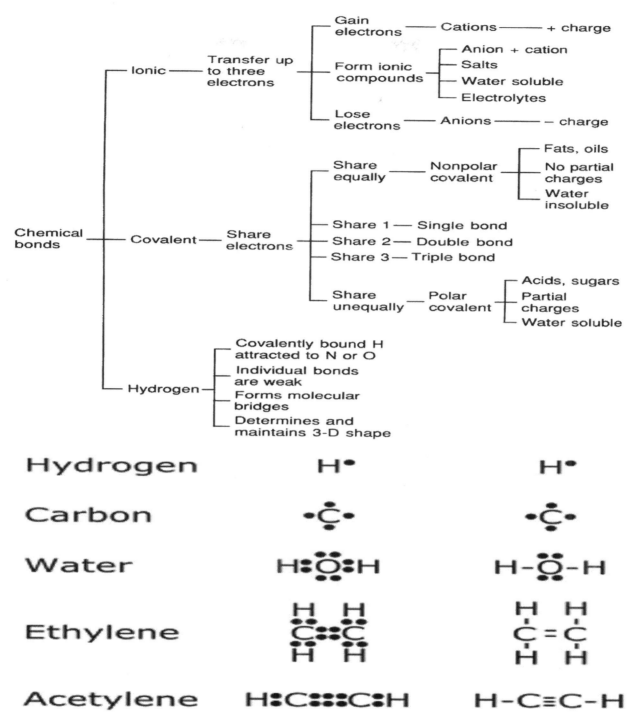

Examples of Lewis dot-style chemical bonds between carbon C, hydrogen H, and oxygen O. Lewis dot depictures represent an early attempt to describe chemical bonding and are still widely used today

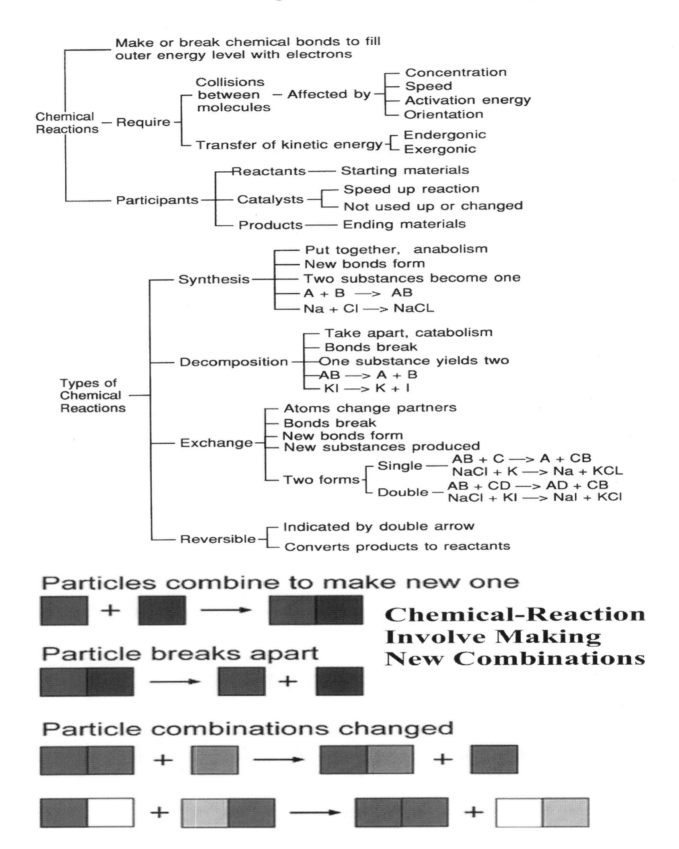

Chemical Reactions
— Make or break chemical bonds to fill outer energy level with electrons
— Require
  — Collisions between molecules — Affected by
    — Concentration
    — Speed
    — Activation energy
    — Orientation
  — Transfer of kinetic energy
    — Endergonic
    — Exergonic
— Participants
  — Reactants —— Starting materials
  — Catalysts
    — Speed up reaction
    — Not used up or changed
  — Products —— Ending materials

Types of Chemical Reactions
— Synthesis
  — Put together, anabolism
  — New bonds form
  — Two substances become one
  — A + B —> AB
  — Na + Cl —> NaCL
— Decomposition
  — Take apart, catabolism
  — Bonds break
  — One substance yields two
  — AB —> A + B
  — KI —> K + I
— Exchange
  — Atoms change partners
  — Bonds break
  — New bonds form
  — New substances produced
  — Two forms
    — Single
      AB + C —> A + CB
      NaCl + K —> Na + KCL
    — Double
      AB + CD —> AD + CB
      NaCl + KI —> NaI + KCl
— Reversible
  — Indicated by double arrow
  — Converts products to reactants

Particles combine to make new one

Particle breaks apart

Chemical-Reaction Involve Making New Combinations

Particle combinations changed

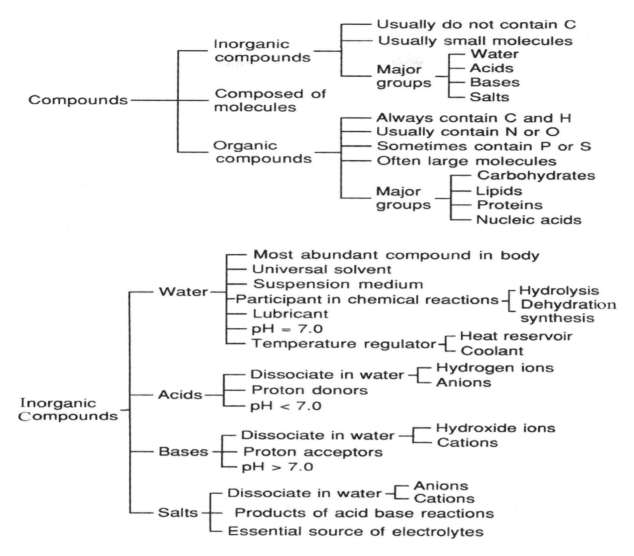

Compounds:

A compound is a substance formed when two or more elements are chemically joined. Water, salt, and sugar are examples of compounds. When the elements are joined, the atoms lose their individual properties and have different properties from the elements they are composed of. A chemical formula is used a quick way to show the composition of compounds. Letters, numbers, and symbols are used to represent elements and the number of elements in each compound.

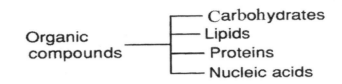

Organic compounds
— Carbohydrates
— Lipids
— Proteins
— Nucleic acids

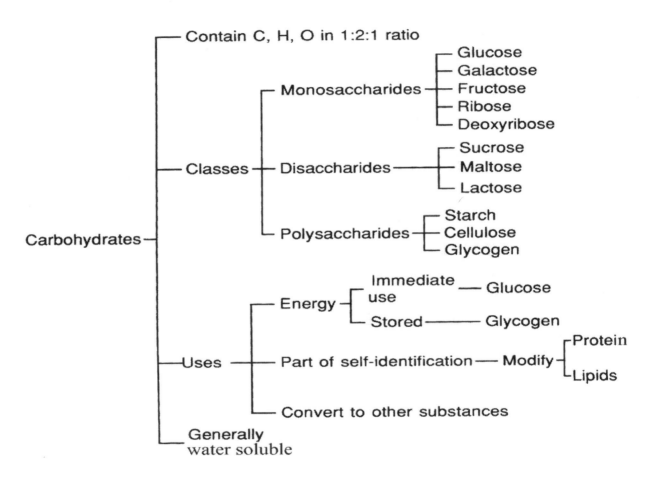

Carbohydrates
— Contain C, H, O in 1:2:1 ratio
— Classes
  — Monosaccharides
    — Glucose
    — Galactose
    — Fructose
    — Ribose
    — Deoxyribose
  — Disaccharides
    — Sucrose
    — Maltose
    — Lactose
  — Polysaccharides
    — Starch
    — Cellulose
    — Glycogen
— Uses
  — Energy
    — Immediate use — Glucose
    — Stored — Glycogen
  — Part of self-identification — Modify
    — Protein
    — Lipids
  — Convert to other substances
— Generally water soluble

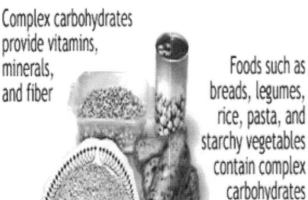

Complex carbohydrates provide vitamins, minerals, and fiber

Foods such as breads, legumes, rice, pasta, and starchy vegetables contain complex carbohydrates

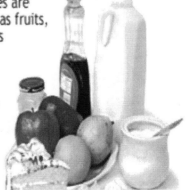

Simple carbohydrates are found in foods such as fruits, milk, and vegetables

Cake, candy, and other refined sugar products are simple sugars which also provide energy but lack vitamins, minerals, and fiber

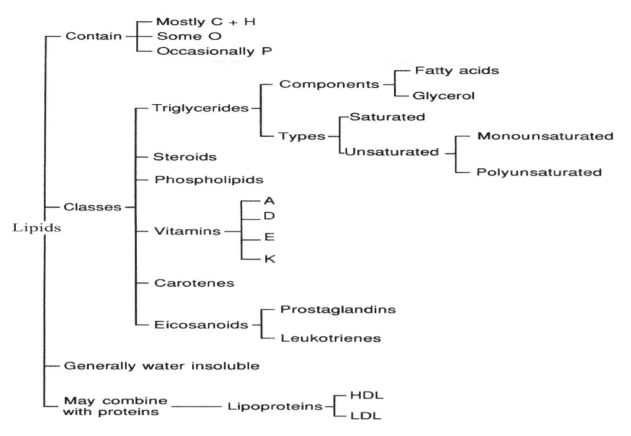

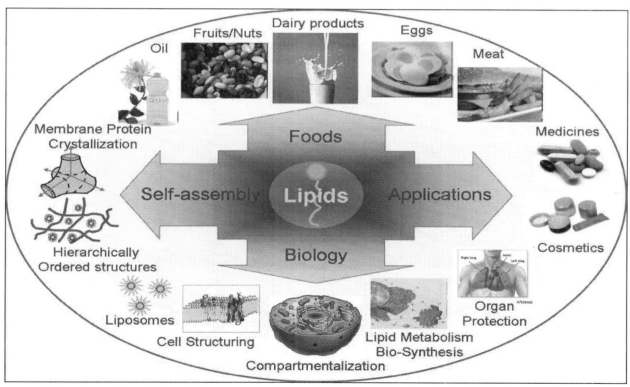

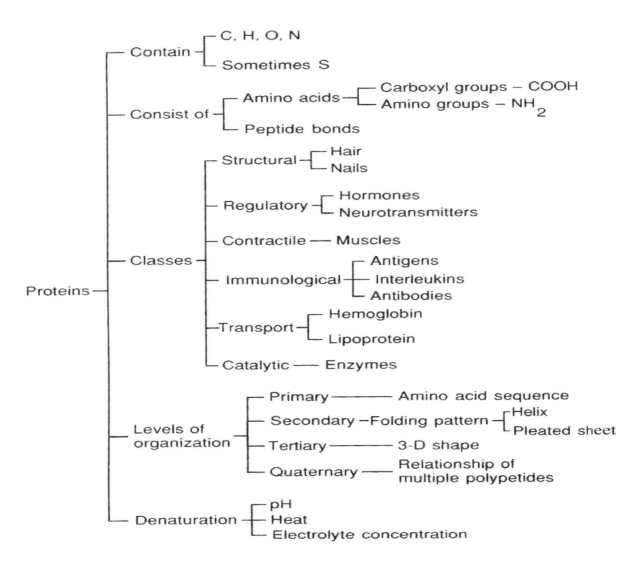

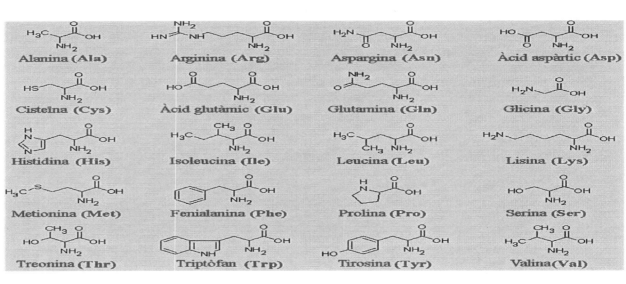

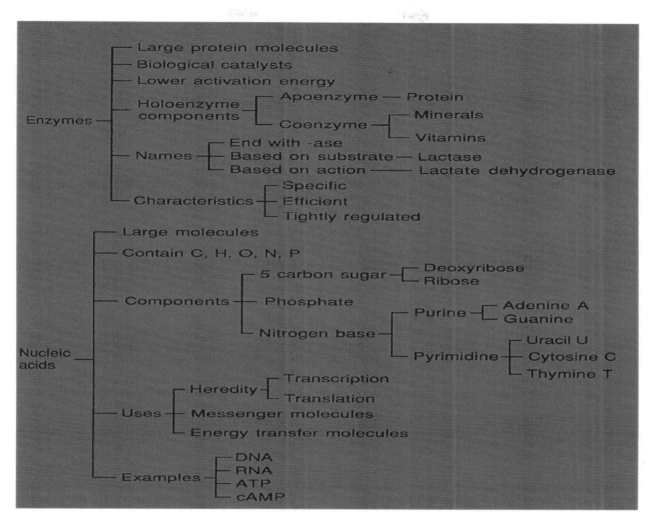

Enzymes
- Large protein molecules
- Biological catalysts
- Lower activation energy
- Holoenzyme components
  - Apoenzyme — Protein
  - Coenzyme
    - Minerals
    - Vitamins
- Names
  - End with -ase
  - Based on substrate — Lactase
  - Based on action — Lactate dehydrogenase
- Characteristics
  - Specific
  - Efficient
  - Tightly regulated

Nucleic acids
- Large molecules
- Contain C, H, O, N, P
- Components
  - 5 carbon sugar
    - Deoxyribose
    - Ribose
  - Phosphate
  - Nitrogen base
    - Purine
      - Adenine A
      - Guanine
    - Pyrimidine
      - Uracil U
      - Cytosine C
      - Thymine T
- Uses
  - Heredity
    - Transcription
    - Translation
  - Messenger molecules
  - Energy transfer molecules
- Examples
  - DNA
  - RNA
  - ATP
  - cAMP

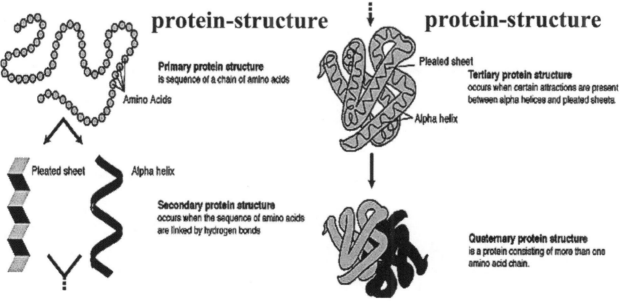

protein-structure   protein-structure

Primary protein structure is sequence of a chain of amino acids

Amino Acids

Pleated sheet

Alpha helix

Tertiary protein structure occurs when certain attractions are present between alpha helices and pleated sheets.

Secondary protein structure occurs when the sequence of amino acids are linked by hydrogen bonds

Quaternary protein structure is a protein consisting of more than one amino acid chain.

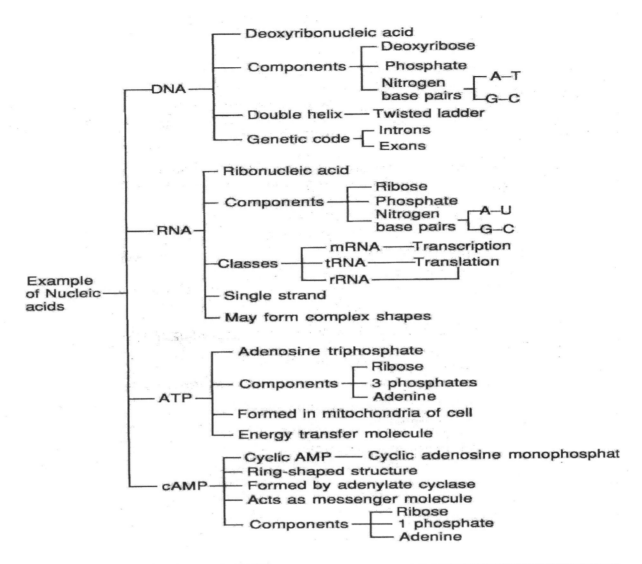

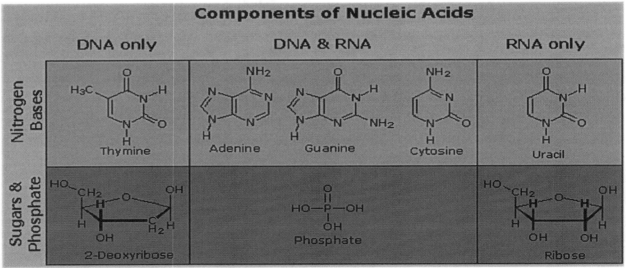

CHAPTER THREE

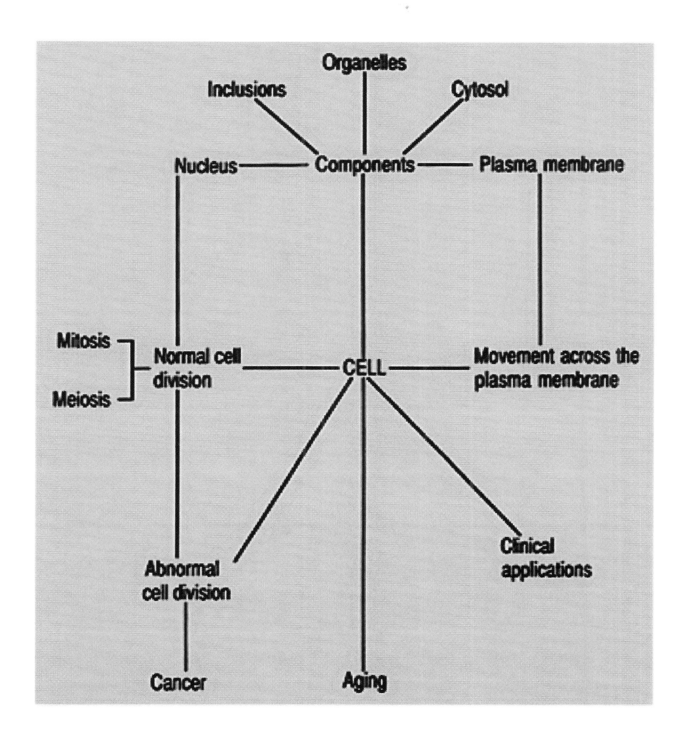

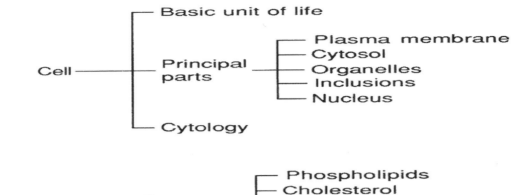

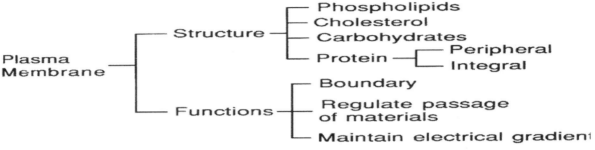

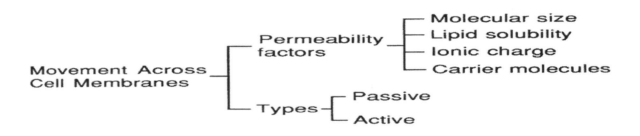

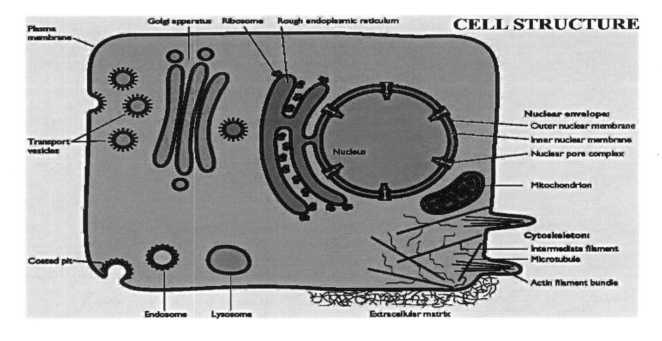

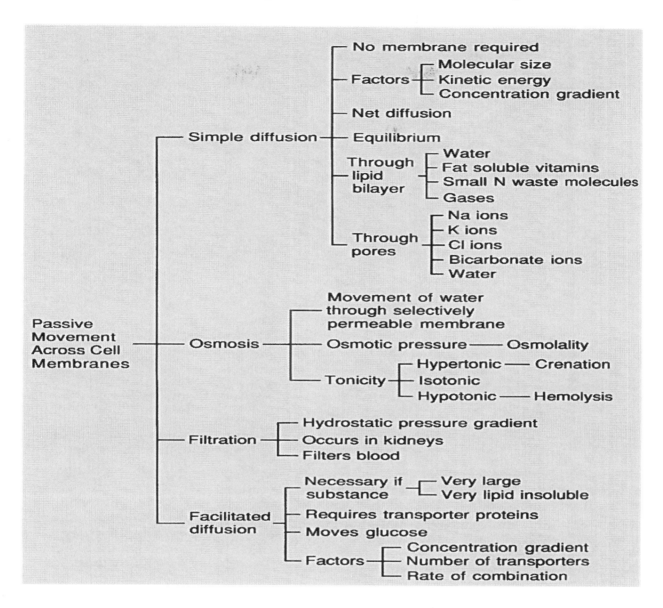

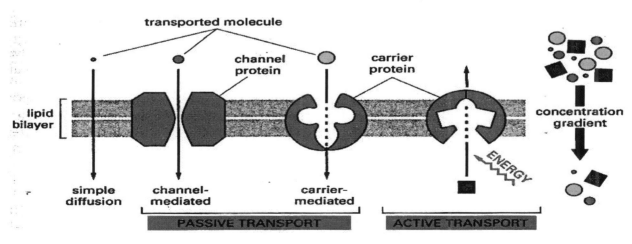

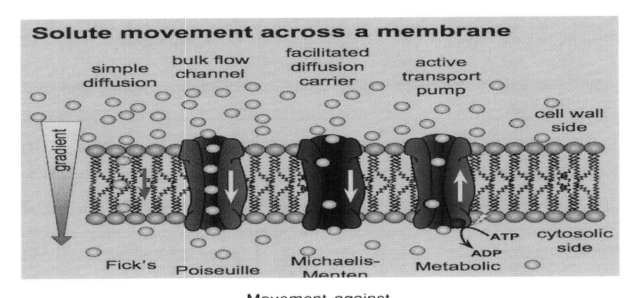

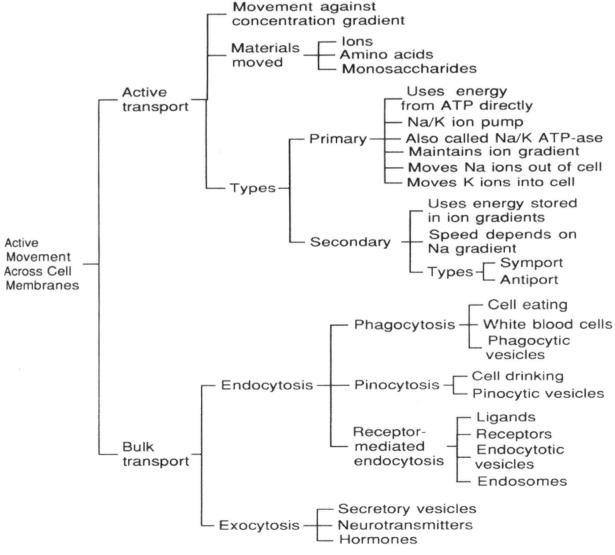

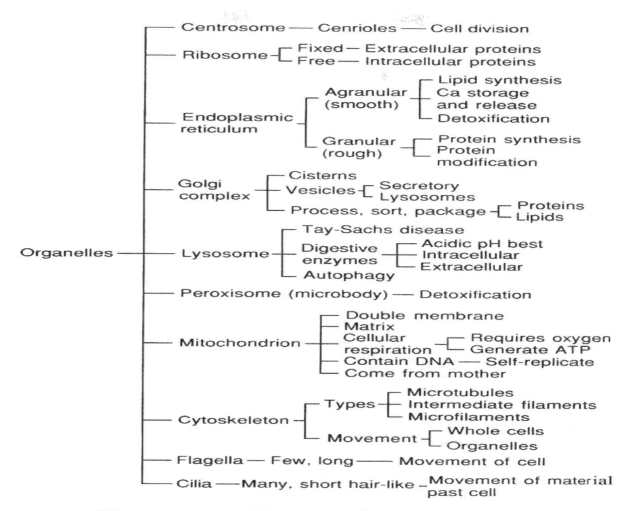

Organelles of the Cell

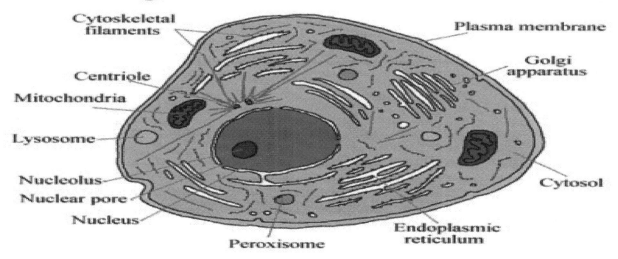

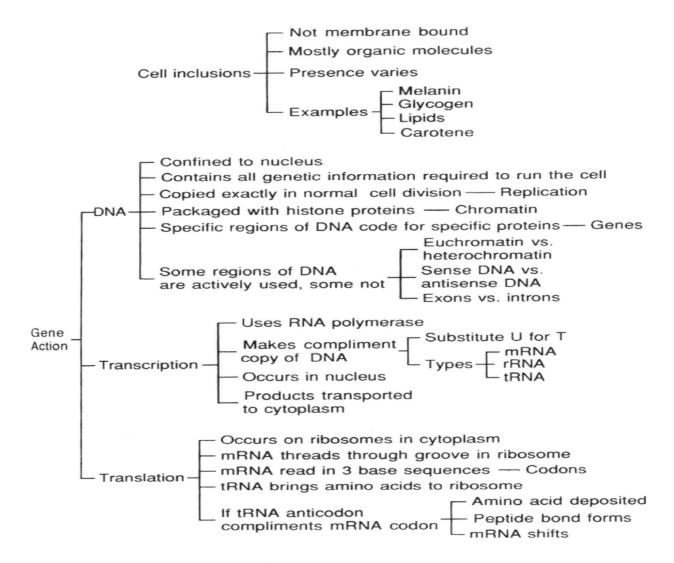

Gene

A segment of DNA, occupying a specific places on a chromosome that is the basic unit of heredity. Genes act by directing the production of RNA, which determines the synthesis of proteins that make up living matter and are the catalysts of all cellular processes. The proteins that are determined by genetic DNA result in specific physical traits, such as the shape of a plant leaf, the coloration of an animal's coat, or the texture of a person's hair. Different forms of genes, called alleles, determine how these traits are expressed in a given individual. Humans are thought to have about 35,000 genes, while bacteria have between 500 and 6,000.

Cell Cycle and Cell Division
- Cell cycle
  - Sequence of events in the life of a cell
  - Stages
    - G₁ — Gap 1 or Growth 1 ─┐
    - S — Synthesis ───────────┤ Interphase
    - G₂ — Gap 2 or Growth 2 ─┘
    - M — Mitosis
- Mitosis
  - Purpose
    - Replace damaged cells
    - Growth
  - Produces — 2 cells
    - Identical to original cell
    - Diploid
    - 46 chromosomes
      - 44 autosomes
      - X X or XY
  - Original cell no longer exists
  - Brief part of cell life cycle
  - Stages
    - Prophase
    - Metaphase
    - Anaphase
    - Telophase
- Meiosis
  - Produces
    - Gametes – Types
      - Sperm
      - Ovum
    - 4 cells
      - Different from original cell
      - Haploid
      - 23 chromosomes
        - 22 autosomes
        - X or Y
  - Occurs in two divisions
    - Meiosis I
      - Reduction division
      - Synapsis occurs
      - Crossing over occurs
      - Paired chromosomes separate
      - Chromosome number cut
      - Nondisjunction may occur
    - Meiosis II
      - Equatorial division
      - Sister chromatids separate

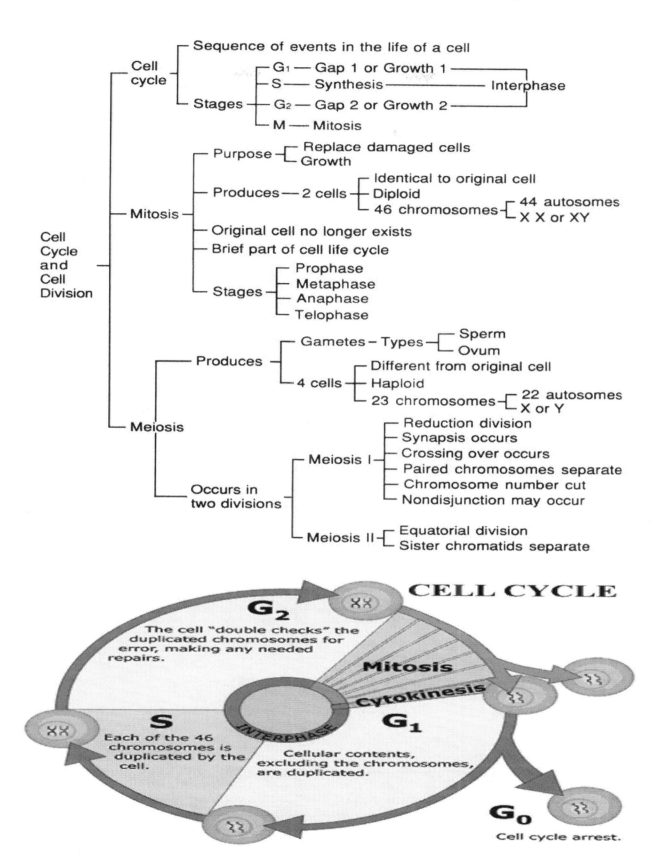

CELL CYCLE

G₂ — The cell "double checks" the duplicated chromosomes for error, making any needed repairs.

Mitosis
Cytokinesis

S — Each of the 46 chromosomes is duplicated by the cell.

INTERPHASE

G₁ — Cellular contents, excluding the chromosomes, are duplicated.

G₀ — Cell cycle arrest.

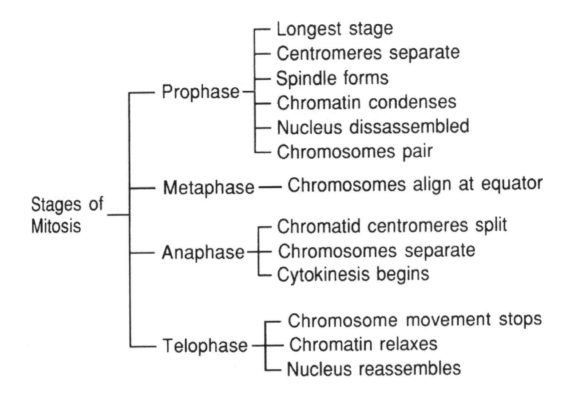

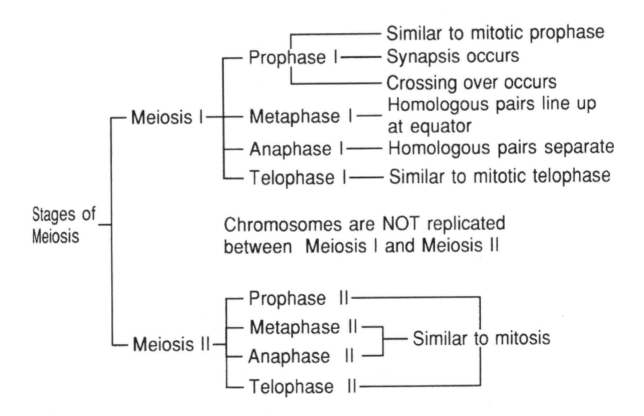

Do Now: compare these two, how are they similar? How are they different?

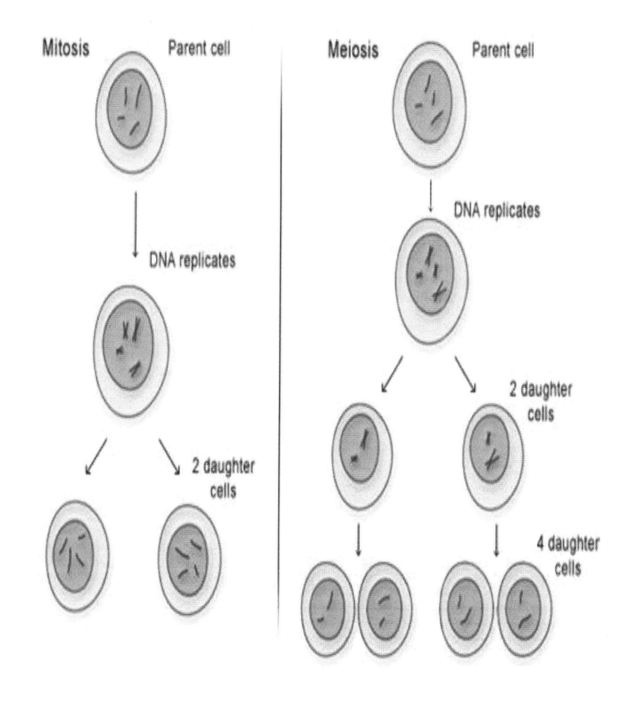

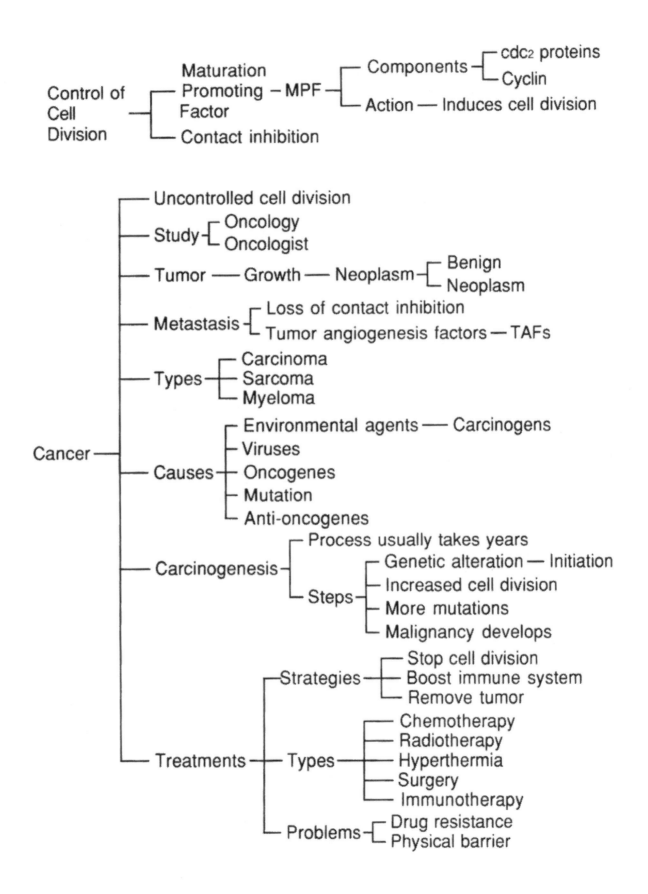

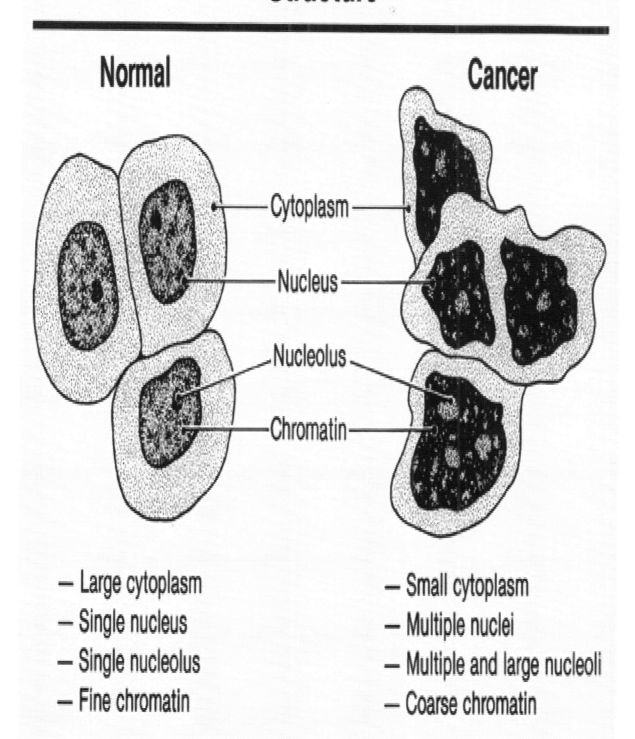

Normal and Cancer Cells
Structure

Normal   **Cancer**

Cytoplasm

Nucleus

Nucleolus

Chromatin

– Large cytoplasm   – Small cytoplasm
– Single nucleus   – Multiple nuclei
– Single nucleolus   – Multiple and large nucleoli
– Fine chromatin   – Coarse chromatin

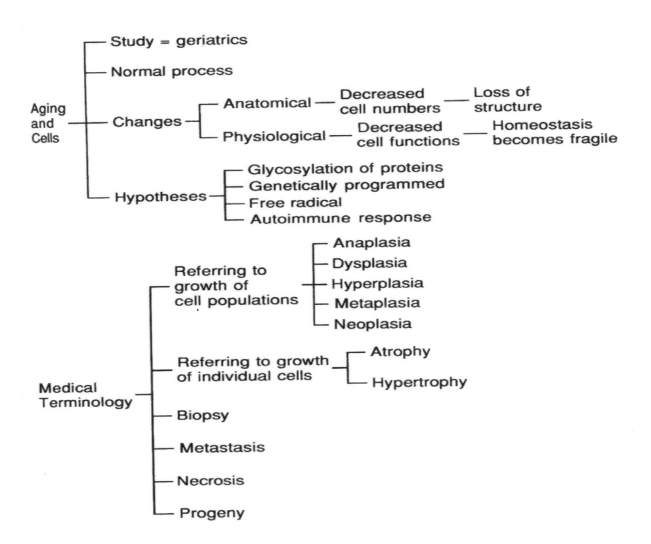

```
                  ┌── Study = geriatrics
                  │
                  ├── Normal process
                  │
                  │              ┌── Anatomical ── Decreased ── Loss of
Aging             │              │                 cell numbers   structure
and ──────────────┼── Changes ──┤
Cells             │              └── Physiological ── Decreased ── Homeostasis
                  │                                   cell functions  becomes fragile
                  │
                  │                 ┌── Glycosylation of proteins
                  │                 ├── Genetically programmed
                  └── Hypotheses ──┤── Free radical
                                    └── Autoimmune response
```

```
                                                      ┌── Anaplasia
                                                      │
                                 Referring to         ├── Dysplasia
                             ┌── growth of ───────────┤── Hyperplasia
                             │   cell populations     ├── Metaplasia
                             │                        └── Neoplasia
                             │
                             │   Referring to growth  ┌── Atrophy
                             ├── of individual cells ─┤
Medical                      │                        └── Hypertrophy
Terminology ─────────────────┤
                             ├── Biopsy
                             │
                             ├── Metastasis
                             │
                             ├── Necrosis
                             │
                             └── Progeny
```

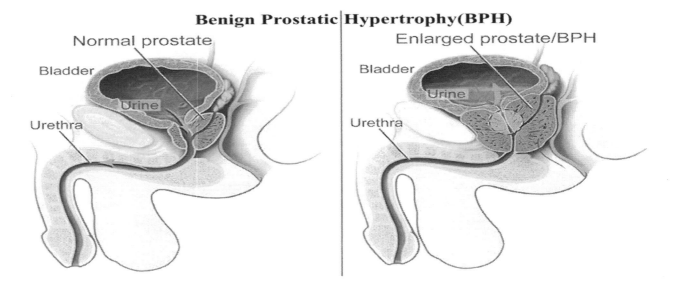

Benign Prostatic Hypertrophy(BPH)

Normal prostate   Enlarged prostate/BPH

Bladder   Bladder

Urine   Urine

Urethra   Urethra

CHAPTER FOUR

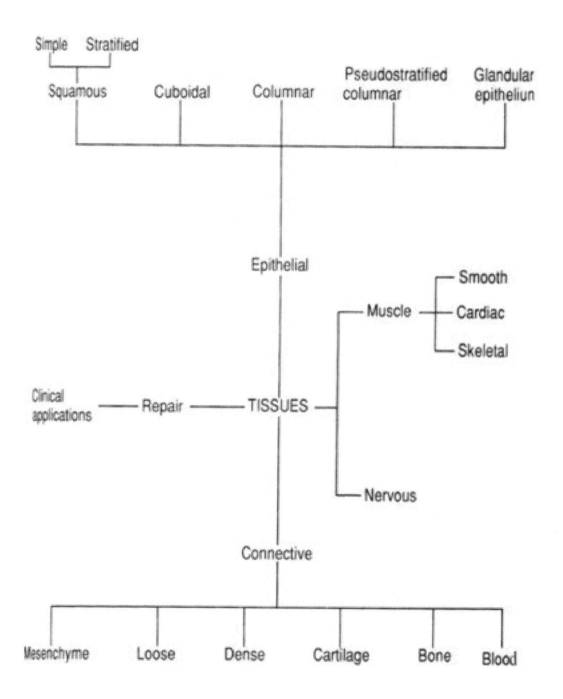

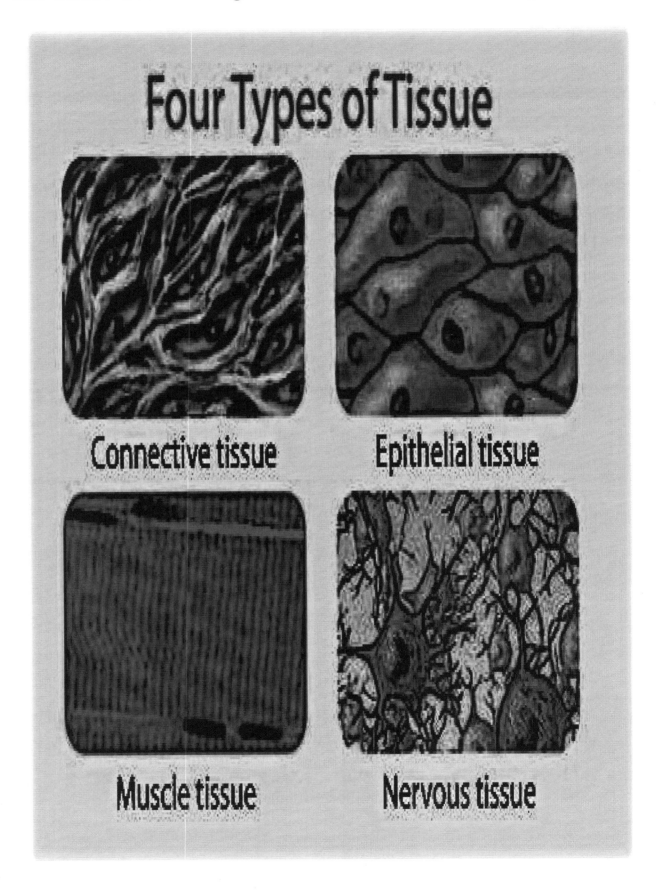

Four Types of Tissue

Connective tissue

Epithelial tissue

Muscle tissue

Nervous tissue

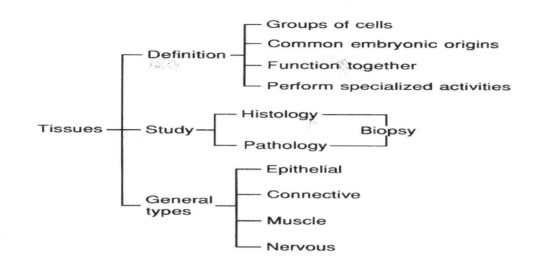

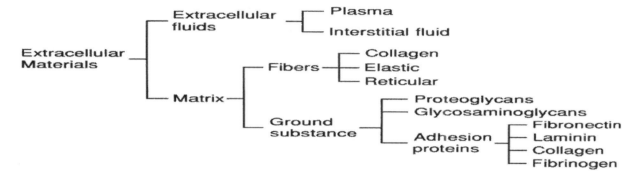

Illustration depicting extracellular matrix in relation to epithelium, endothelium and connective tissue

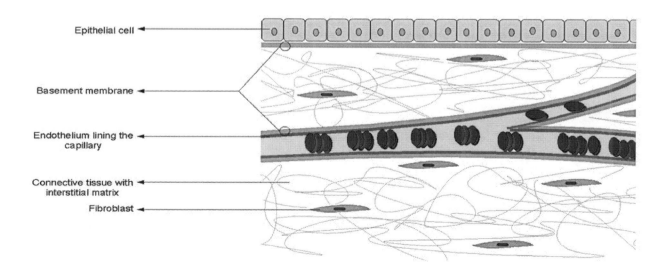

Characteristics of Tissues

Tissue	Function	Location	Distinguishing Features
Epithelial	Protection, secretion, absorption, excretion	Covers body surfaces, covers and lines internal organs, compose glands	Lacks blood vessels
Connective	Bind, support, protect, fill spaces, store fat, produce blood cells	Widely distributed throughout the body	Matrix between cells, good blood supply
Muscle	Movement	Attached to bones, in the walls of hollow internal organs, heart	Contractile
Nervous	Transmit impulses for coordination, regulation, integration, and sensory reception	Brain, spinal cord, nerves	Cells connect to each other and other body parts

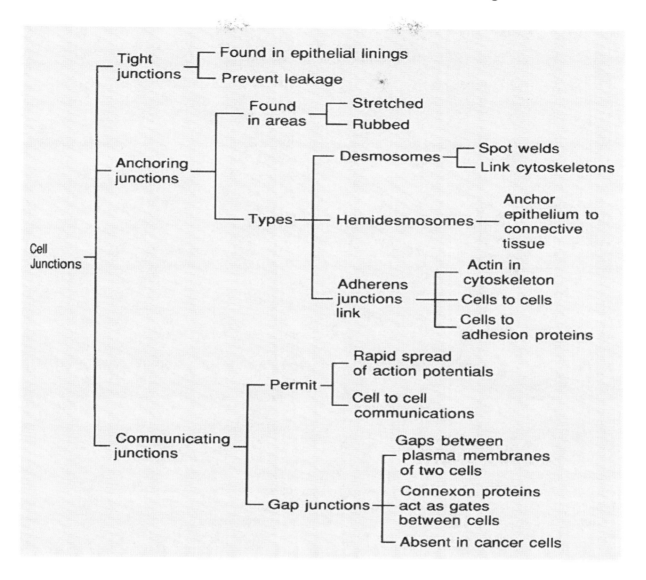

Cell Junctions
- Tight junctions
  - Found in epithelial linings
  - Prevent leakage
- Anchoring junctions
  - Found in areas
    - Stretched
    - Rubbed
  - Types
    - Desmosomes
      - Spot welds
      - Link cytoskeletons
    - Hemidesmosomes — Anchor epithelium to connective tissue
    - Adherens junctions link
      - Actin in cytoskeleton
      - Cells to cells
      - Cells to adhesion proteins
- Communicating junctions
  - Permit
    - Rapid spread of action potentials
    - Cell to cell communications
  - Gap junctions
    - Gaps between plasma membranes of two cells
    - Connexon proteins act as gates between cells
    - Absent in cancer cells

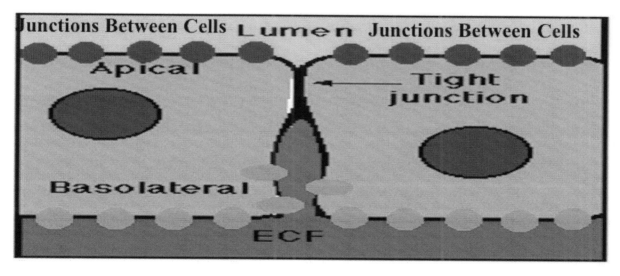

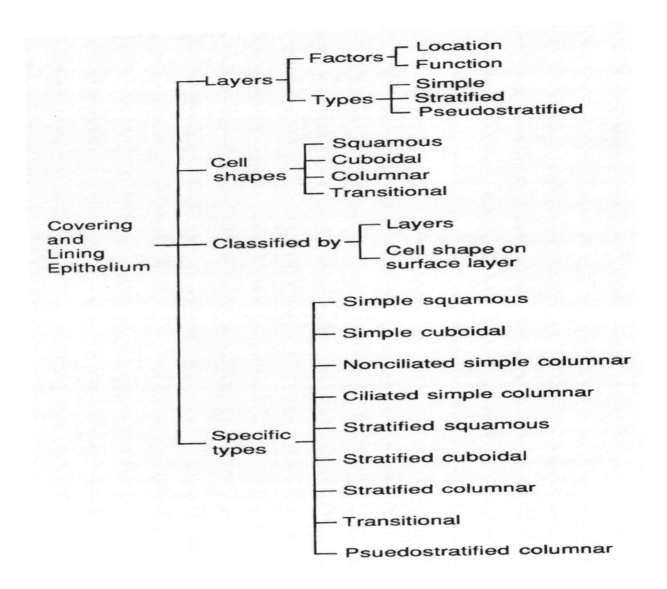

Covering and Lining Epithelium
- Layers
  - Factors
    - Location
    - Function
  - Types
    - Simple
    - Stratified
    - Pseudostratified
- Cell shapes
  - Squamous
  - Cuboidal
  - Columnar
  - Transitional
- Classified by
  - Layers
  - Cell shape on surface layer
- Specific types
  - Simple squamous
  - Simple cuboidal
  - Nonciliated simple columnar
  - Ciliated simple columnar
  - Stratified squamous
  - Stratified cuboidal
  - Stratified columnar
  - Transitional
  - Psuedostratified columnar

Types of Epithelium

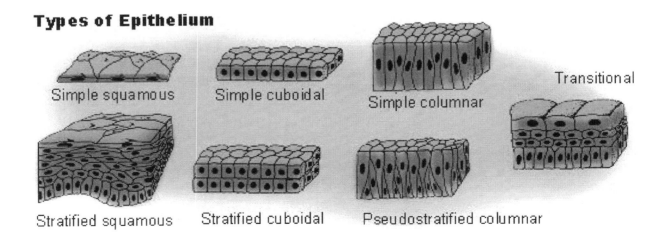

Simple squamous　　Simple cuboidal　　Simple columnar　　Transitional

Stratified squamous　　Stratified cuboidal　　Pseudostratified columnar

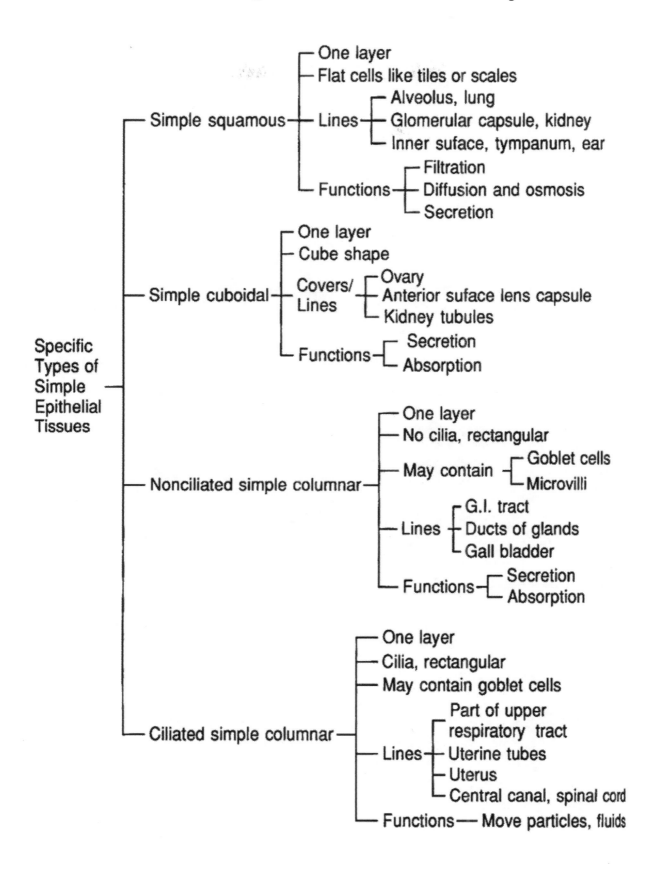

Epithelial Types

Simple Squamous
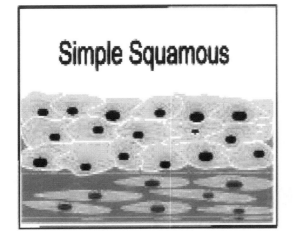

Simple Cuboidal
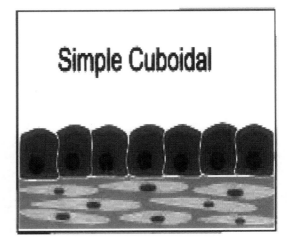

Simple Columnar
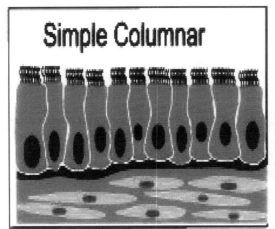

Stratified Squamous
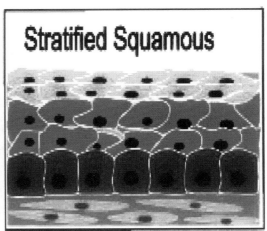

Pseudostratified Columnar
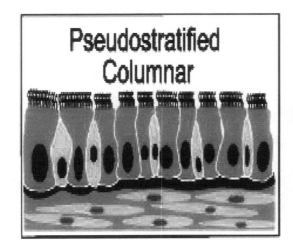

Transitional
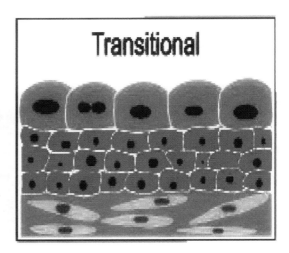

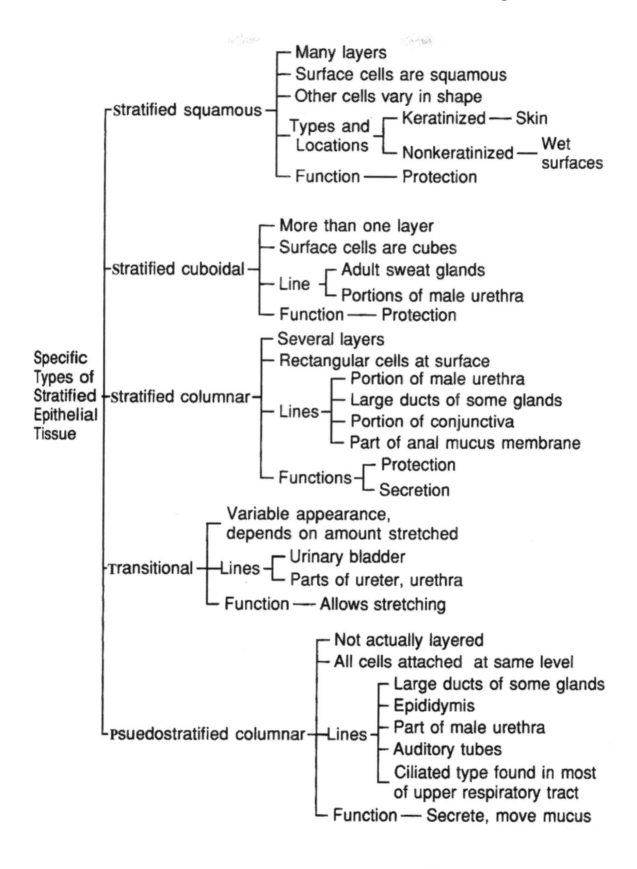

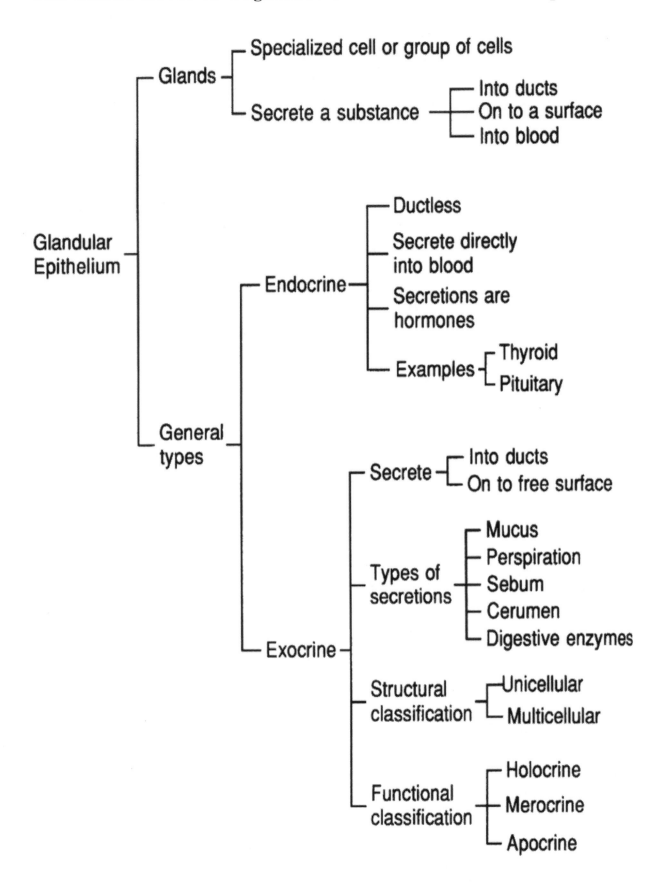

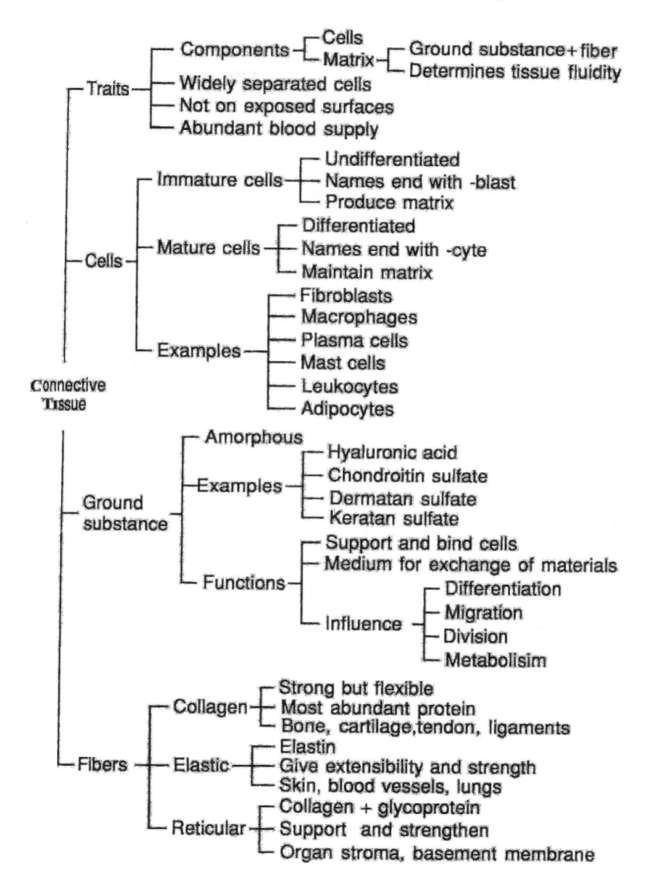

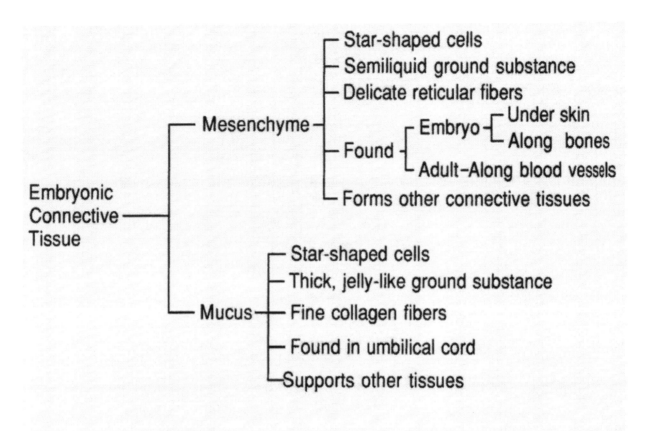

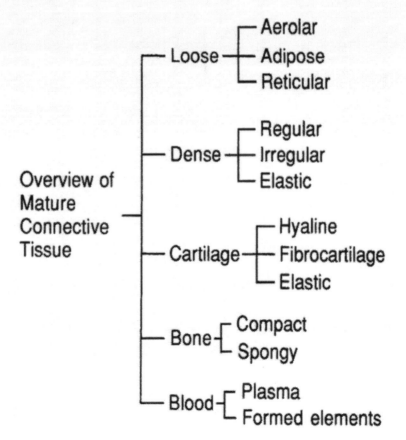

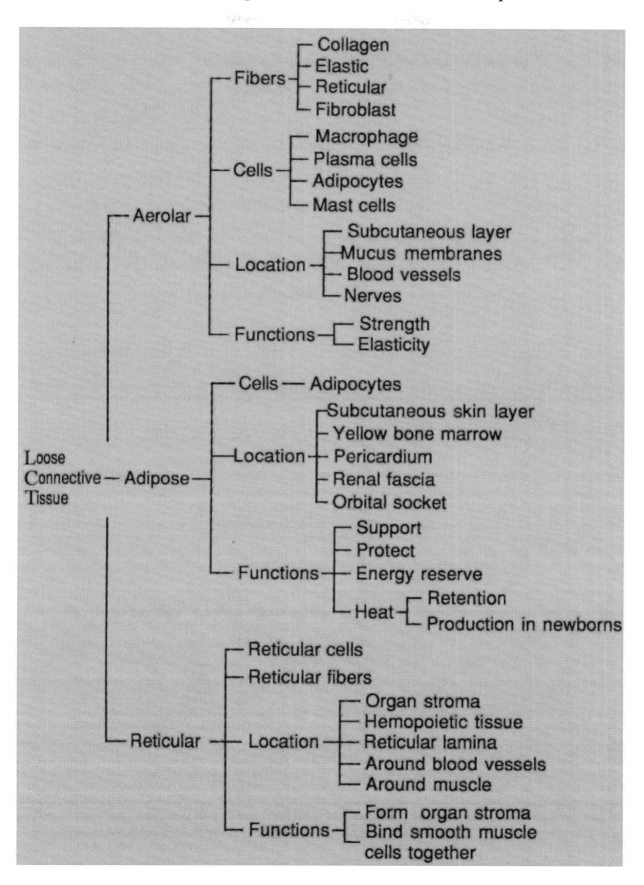

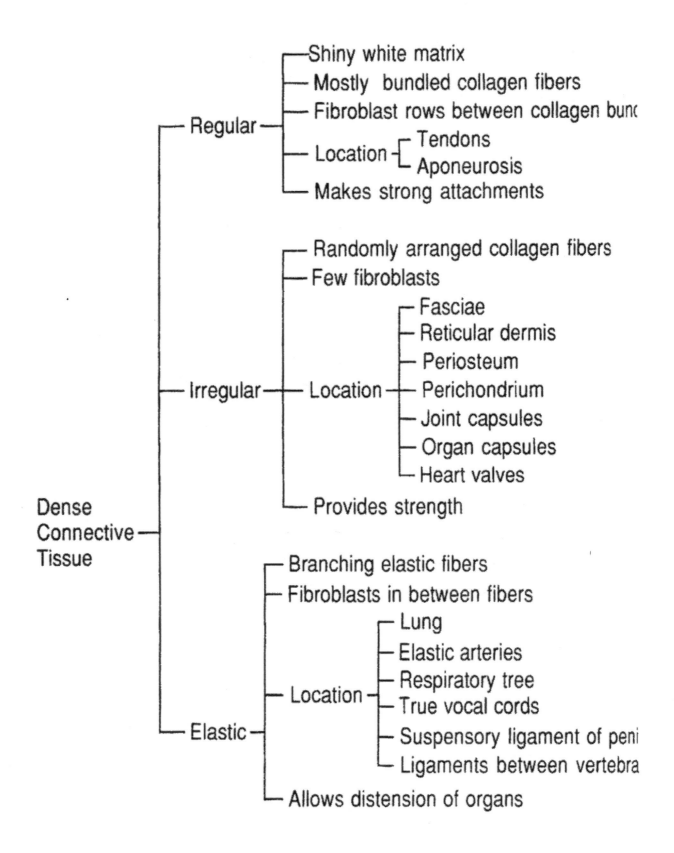

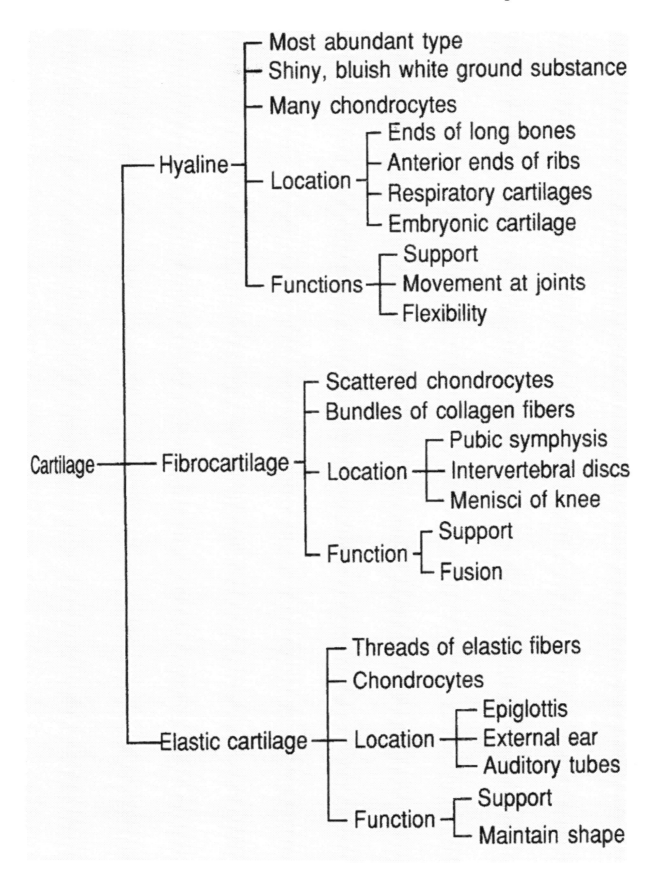

Cartilage
- Hyaline
  - Most abundant type
  - Shiny, bluish white ground substance
  - Many chondrocytes
  - Location
    - Ends of long bones
    - Anterior ends of ribs
    - Respiratory cartilages
    - Embryonic cartilage
  - Functions
    - Support
    - Movement at joints
    - Flexibility
- Fibrocartilage
  - Scattered chondrocytes
  - Bundles of collagen fibers
  - Location
    - Pubic symphysis
    - Intervertebral discs
    - Menisci of knee
  - Function
    - Support
    - Fusion
- Elastic cartilage
  - Threads of elastic fibers
  - Chondrocytes
  - Location
    - Epiglottis
    - External ear
    - Auditory tubes
  - Function
    - Support
    - Maintain shape

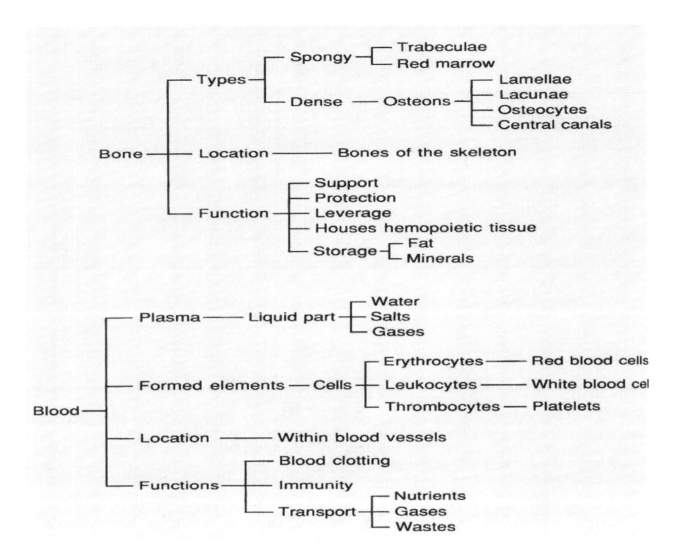

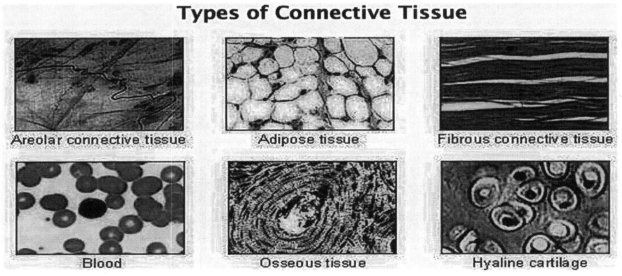

Types of Connective Tissue

Areolar connective tissue

Adipose tissue

Fibrous connective tissue

Blood

Osseous tissue

Hyaline cartilage

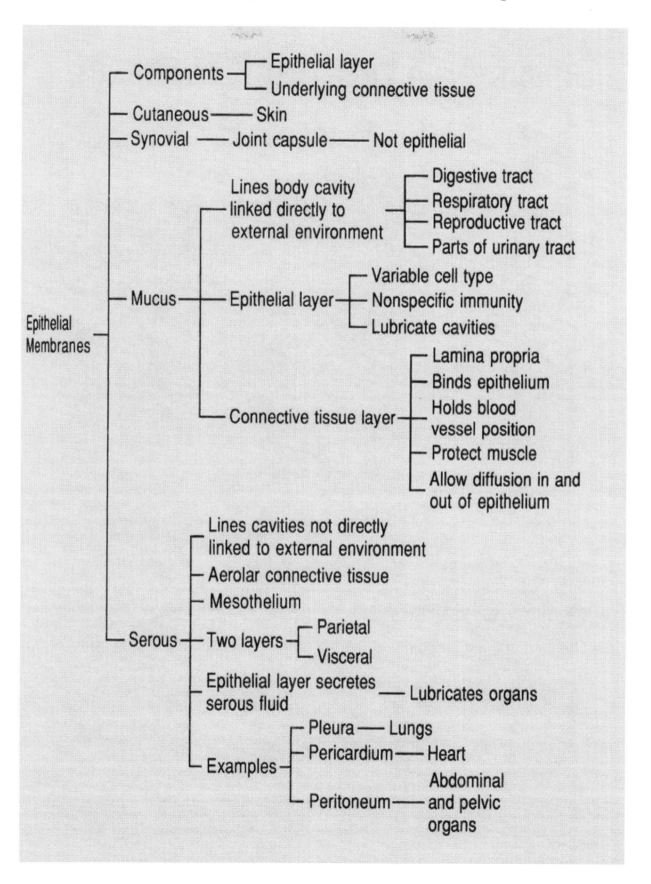

DIFFERENT TYPES OF CELLS TIEEUE

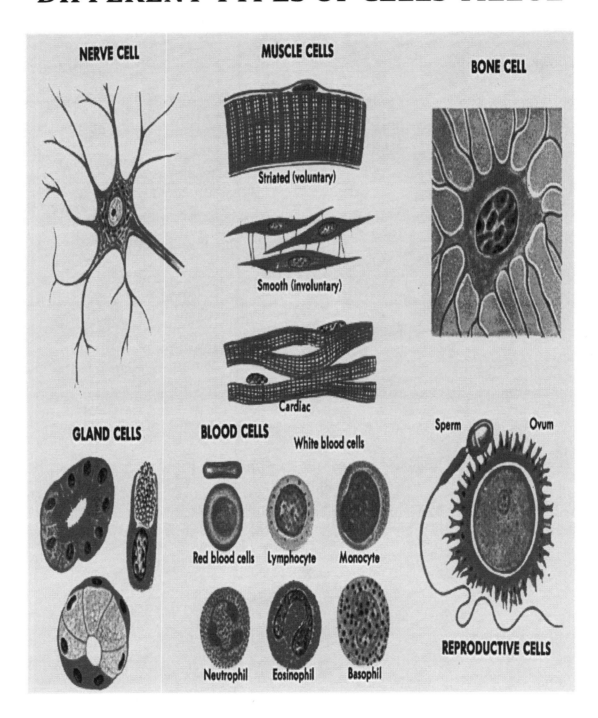

NERVE CELL

MUSCLE CELLS

BONE CELL

Striated (voluntary)

Smooth (involuntary)

Cardiac

GLAND CELLS

BLOOD CELLS

White blood cells

Sperm   Ovum

Red blood cells   Lymphocyte   Monocyte

Neutrophil   Eosinophil   Basophil

REPRODUCTIVE CELLS

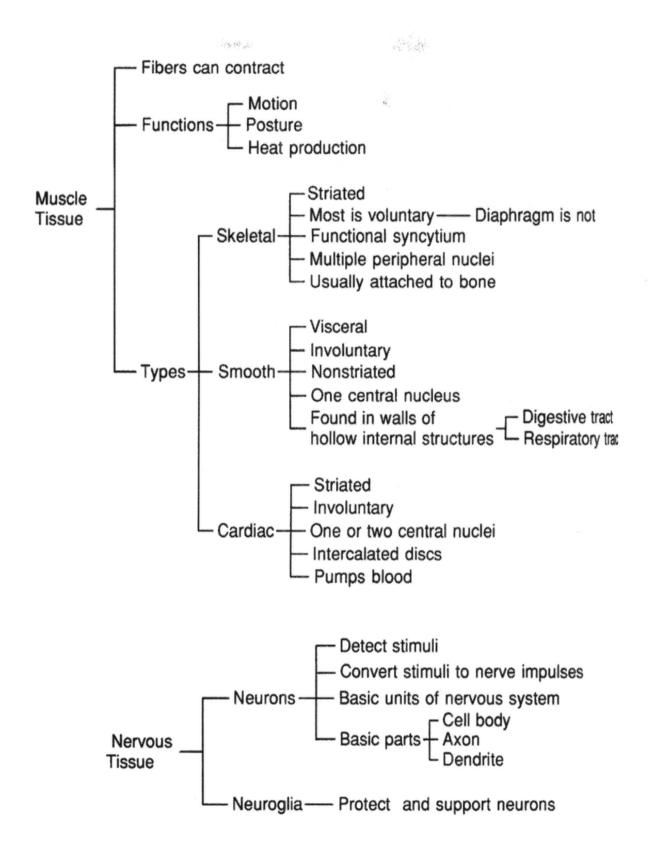

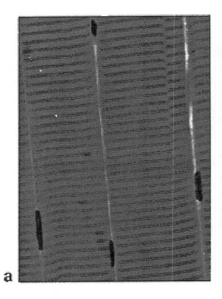

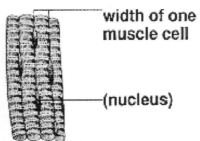

width of one
muscle cell

(nucleus)

TYPE: Skeletal muscle

DESCRIPTION: Long, striated cells with multiple nuclei

COMMON LOCATIONS: In skeletal muscles

FUNCTION: Contraction for voluntary movements

a

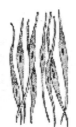

(cells teased apart for clarity here)

TYPE: Smooth muscle

DESCRIPTION: Long, spindle-shaped cells, each with a single nucleus

COMMON LOCATIONS: In hollow organs (e.g., stomach)

FUNCTION: Propulsion of substances along internal passageways

b

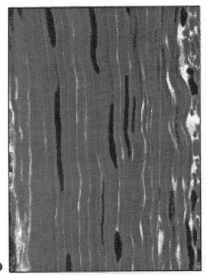

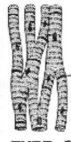

junction between adjacent cells

TYPE: Cardiac muscle

DESCRIPTION: Branching, striated cells fused at plasma membranes

COMMON LOCATIONS: Wall of heart

FUNCTION: Pumping of blood in the circulatory system

c

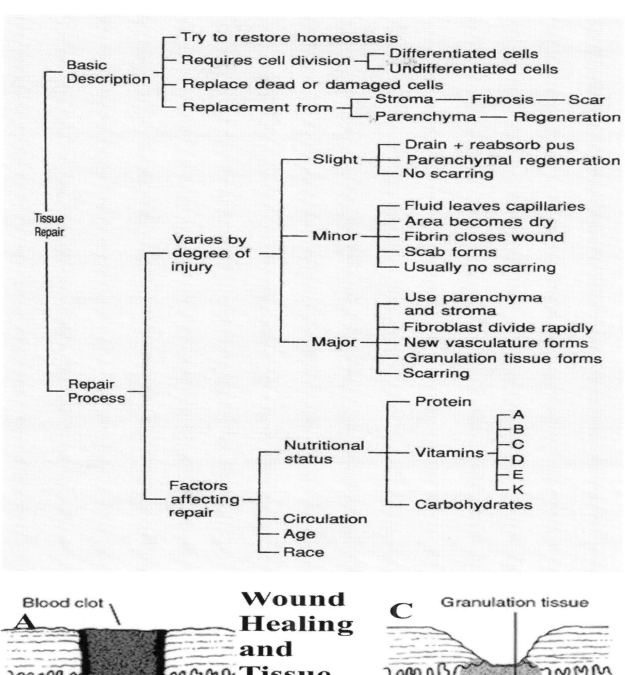

Tissue Repair

- Basic Description
  - Try to restore homeostasis
  - Requires cell division
    - Differentiated cells
    - Undifferentiated cells
  - Replace dead or damaged cells
  - Replacement from
    - Stroma — Fibrosis — Scar
    - Parenchyma — Regeneration
- Repair Process
  - Varies by degree of injury
    - Slight
      - Drain + reabsorb pus
      - Parenchymal regeneration
      - No scarring
    - Minor
      - Fluid leaves capillaries
      - Area becomes dry
      - Fibrin closes wound
      - Scab forms
      - Usually no scarring
    - Major
      - Use parenchyma and stroma
      - Fibroblast divide rapidly
      - New vasculature forms
      - Granulation tissue forms
      - Scarring
  - Factors affecting repair
    - Nutritional status
      - Protein
      - Vitamins
        - A
        - B
        - C
        - D
        - E
        - K
      - Carbohydrates
    - Circulation
    - Age
    - Race

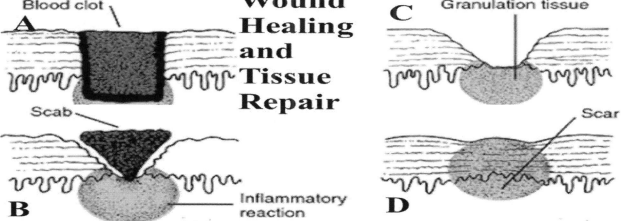

Wound Healing and Tissue Repair

A — Blood clot

B — Scab / Inflammatory reaction

C — Granulation tissue

D — Scar

CHAPTER FIVE

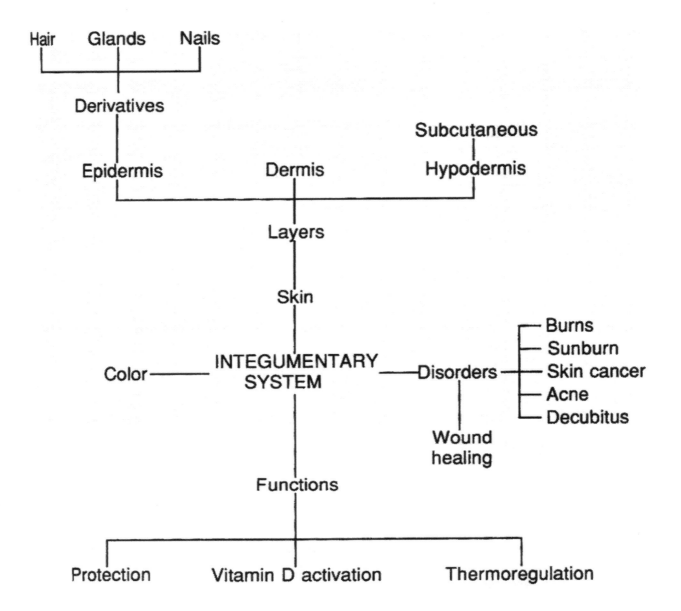

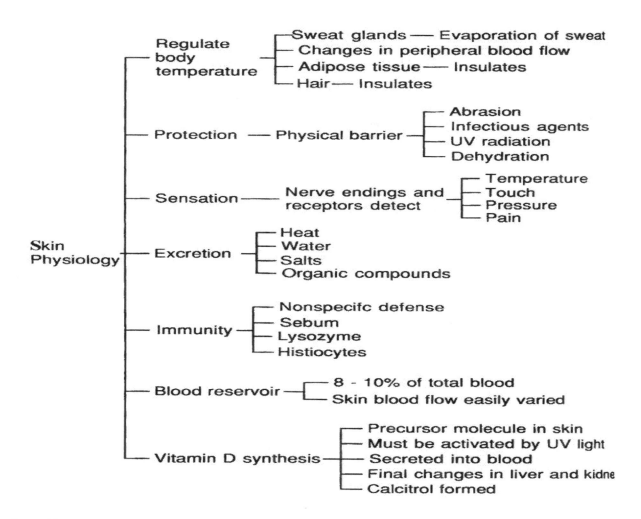

Anatomy and physiology of Human Cross section skin

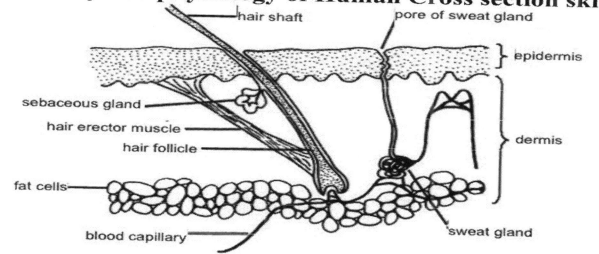

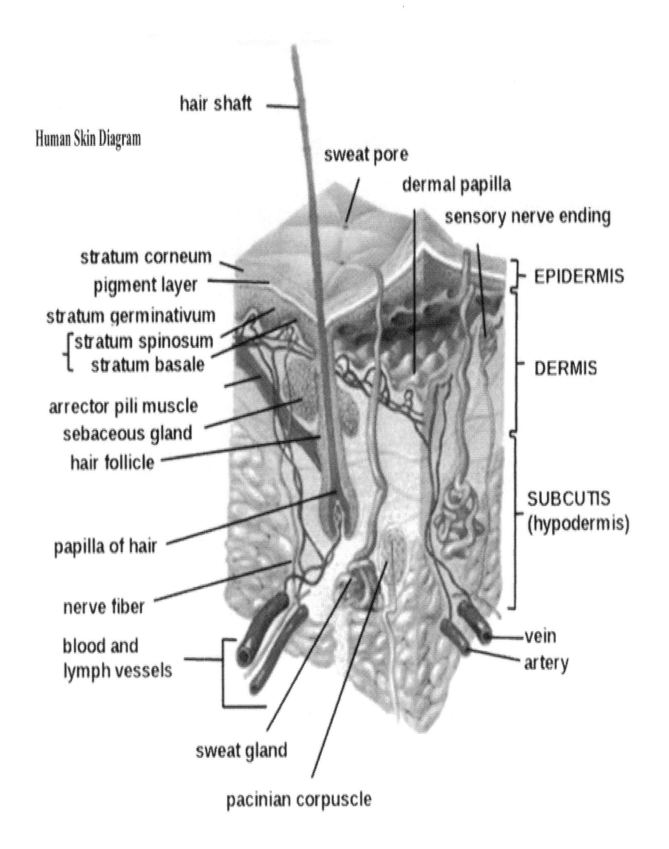

Human Skin Diagram

hair shaft

sweat pore

dermal papilla

sensory nerve ending

EPIDERMIS

stratum corneum

pigment layer

stratum germinativum

{ stratum spinosum

stratum basale

DERMIS

arrector pili muscle

sebaceous gland

hair follicle

SUBCUTIS
(hypodermis)

papilla of hair

nerve fiber

vein

blood and
lymph vessels

artery

sweat gland

pacinian corpuscle

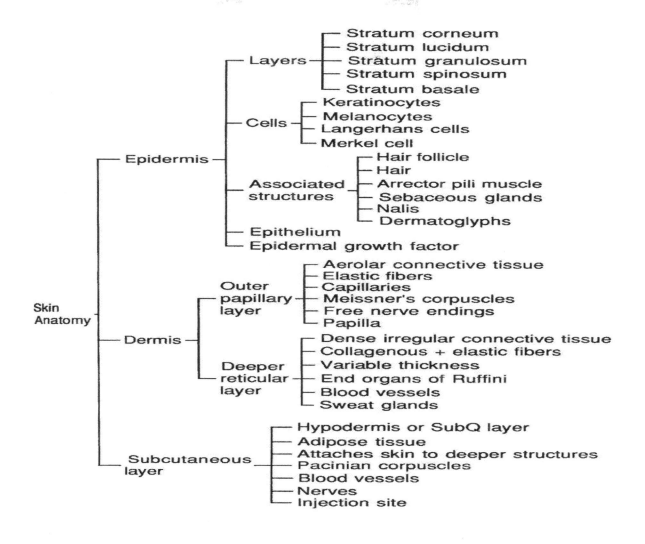

Skin Anatomy
- Epidermis
  - Layers
    - Stratum corneum
    - Stratum lucidum
    - Stratum granulosum
    - Stratum spinosum
    - Stratum basale
  - Cells
    - Keratinocytes
    - Melanocytes
    - Langerhans cells
    - Merkel cell
  - Associated structures
    - Hair follicle
    - Hair
    - Arrector pili muscle
    - Sebaceous glands
    - Nalis
    - Dermatoglyphs
  - Epithelium
  - Epidermal growth factor
- Dermis
  - Outer papillary layer
    - Aerolar connective tissue
    - Elastic fibers
    - Capillaries
    - Meissner's corpuscles
    - Free nerve endings
    - Papilla
  - Deeper reticular layer
    - Dense irregular connective tissue
    - Collagenous + elastic fibers
    - Variable thickness
    - End organs of Ruffini
    - Blood vessels
    - Sweat glands
- Subcutaneous layer
  - Hypodermis or SubQ layer
  - Adipose tissue
  - Attaches skin to deeper structures
  - Pacinian corpuscles
  - Blood vessels
  - Nerves
  - Injection site

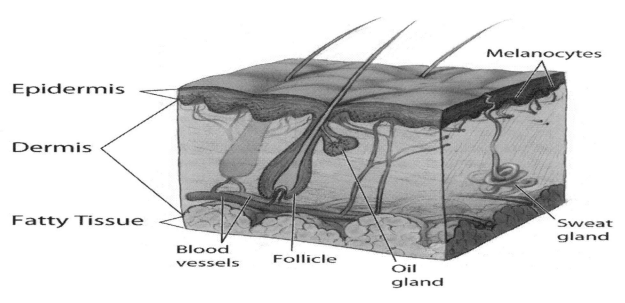

Epidermis

Dermis

Fatty Tissue

Melanocytes

Sweat gland

Blood vessels

Follicle

Oil gland

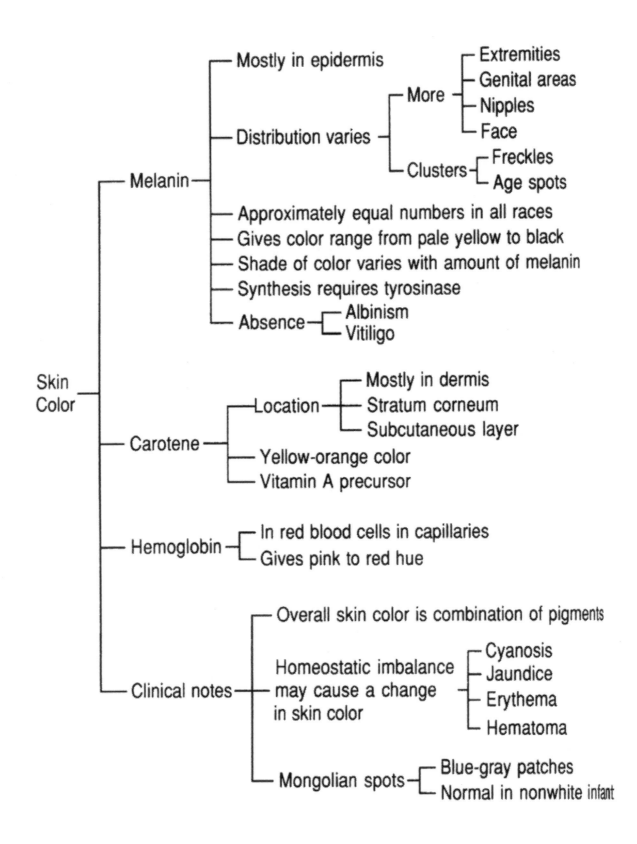

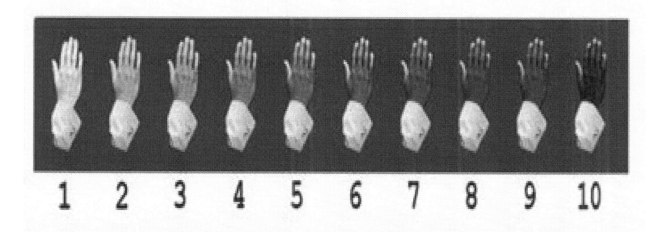

Skin color scale used by researchers
Scale of Skin Color Darkness

1 2 3 4 5 6 7 8 9 10

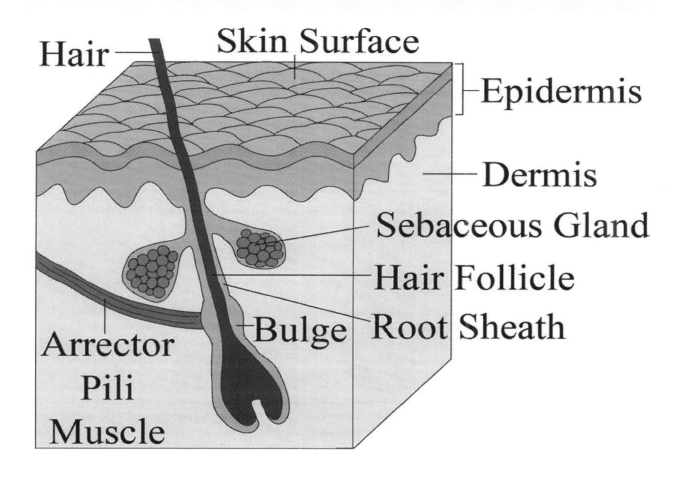

Hair — Skin Surface
Epidermis
Dermis
Sebaceous Gland
Hair Follicle
Bulge Root Sheath
Arrector Pili Muscle

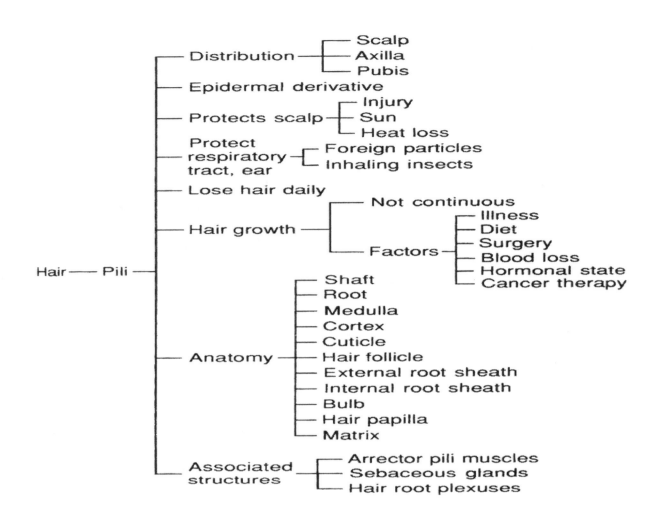

Hair — Pili

- Distribution
  - Scalp
  - Axilla
  - Pubis
- Epidermal derivative
- Protects scalp
  - Injury
  - Sun
  - Heat loss
- Protect respiratory tract, ear
  - Foreign particles
  - Inhaling insects
- Lose hair daily
- Hair growth
  - Not continuous
  - Factors
    - Illness
    - Diet
    - Surgery
    - Blood loss
    - Hormonal state
    - Cancer therapy
- Anatomy
  - Shaft
  - Root
  - Medulla
  - Cortex
  - Cuticle
  - Hair follicle
  - External root sheath
  - Internal root sheath
  - Bulb
  - Hair papilla
  - Matrix
- Associated structures
  - Arrector pili muscles
  - Sebaceous glands
  - Hair root plexuses

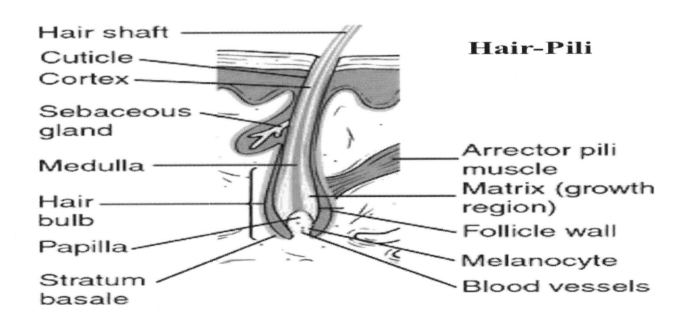

Hair-Pili

Hair shaft
Cuticle
Cortex
Sebaceous gland
Medulla
Hair bulb
Papilla
Stratum basale

Arrector pili muscle
Matrix (growth region)
Follicle wall
Melanocyte
Blood vessels

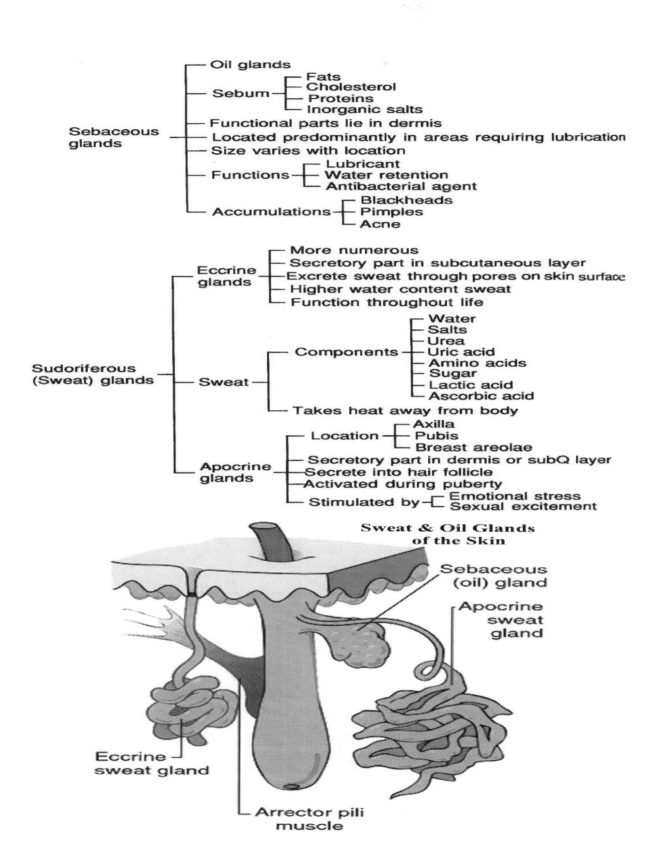

Sebaceous glands
— Oil glands
— Sebum — Fats
        — Cholesterol
        — Proteins
        — Inorganic salts
— Functional parts lie in dermis
— Located predominantly in areas requiring lubrication
— Size varies with location
— Functions — Lubricant
            — Water retention
            — Antibacterial agent
— Accumulations — Blackheads
                — Pimples
                — Acne

Sudoriferous (Sweat) glands
— Eccrine glands
    — More numerous
    — Secretory part in subcutaneous layer
    — Excrete sweat through pores on skin surface
    — Higher water content sweat
    — Function throughout life
— Sweat
    — Components — Water
                — Salts
                — Urea
                — Uric acid
                — Amino acids
                — Sugar
                — Lactic acid
                — Ascorbic acid
    — Takes heat away from body
— Apocrine glands
    — Location — Axilla
              — Pubis
              — Breast areolae
    — Secretory part in dermis or subQ layer
    — Secrete into hair follicle
    — Activated during puberty
    — Stimulated by — Emotional stress
                    — Sexual excitement

Sweat & Oil Glands of the Skin

Sebaceous (oil) gland

Apocrine sweat gland

Eccrine sweat gland

Arrector pili muscle

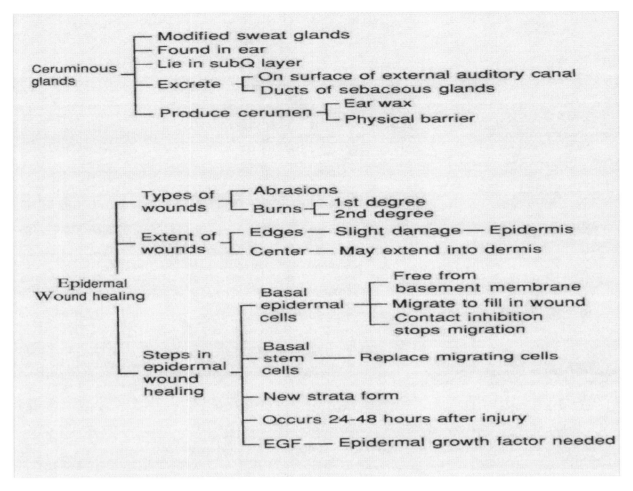

Ceruminous glands
— Modified sweat glands
— Found in ear
— Lie in subQ layer
— Excrete
  — On surface of external auditory canal
  — Ducts of sebaceous glands
— Produce cerumen
  — Ear wax
  — Physical barrier

Epidermal Wound healing

Types of wounds
— Abrasions
— Burns
  — 1st degree
  — 2nd degree

Extent of wounds
— Edges — Slight damage — Epidermis
— Center — May extend into dermis

Steps in epidermal wound healing

Basal epidermal cells
— Free from basement membrane
— Migrate to fill in wound
— Contact inhibition stops migration

Basal stem cells — Replace migrating cells

New strata form

Occurs 24-48 hours after injury

EGF — Epidermal growth factor needed

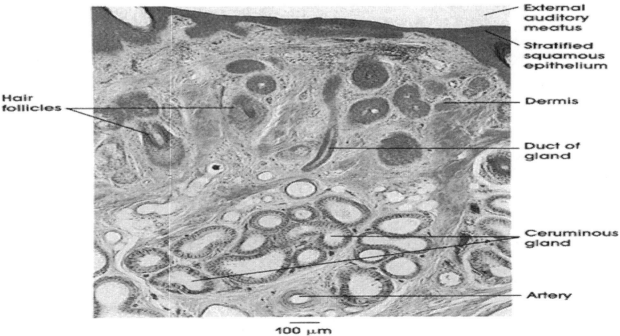

Hair follicles

External auditory meatus

Stratified squamous epithelium

Dermis

Duct of gland

Ceruminous gland

Artery

100 μm

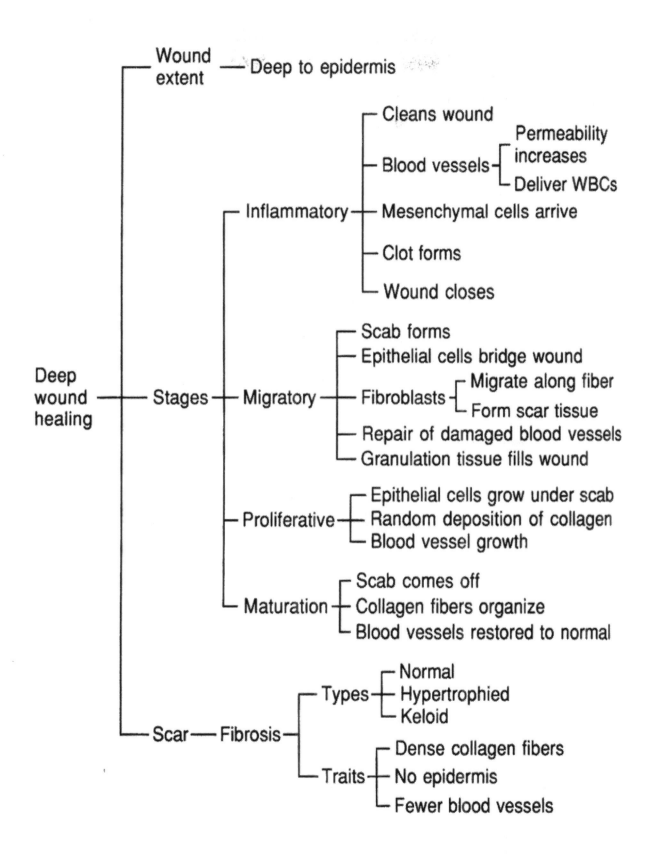

Deep wound healing
- Wound extent — Deep to epidermis
- Stages
  - Inflammatory
    - Cleans wound
    - Blood vessels
      - Permeability increases
      - Deliver WBCs
    - Mesenchymal cells arrive
    - Clot forms
    - Wound closes
  - Migratory
    - Scab forms
    - Epithelial cells bridge wound
    - Fibroblasts
      - Migrate along fiber
      - Form scar tissue
    - Repair of damaged blood vessels
    - Granulation tissue fills wound
  - Proliferative
    - Epithelial cells grow under scab
    - Random deposition of collagen
    - Blood vessel growth
  - Maturation
    - Scab comes off
    - Collagen fibers organize
    - Blood vessels restored to normal
- Scar — Fibrosis
  - Types
    - Normal
    - Hypertrophied
    - Keloid
  - Traits
    - Dense collagen fibers
    - No epidermis
    - Fewer blood vessels

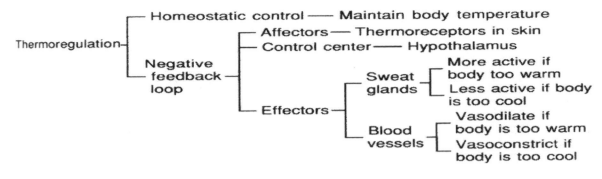

Thermoregulation
- Homeostatic control — Maintain body temperature
- Negative feedback loop
  - Affectors — Thermoreceptors in skin
  - Control center — Hypothalamus
  - Effectors
    - Sweat glands
      - More active if body too warm
      - Less active if body is too cool
    - Blood vessels
      - Vasodilate if body is too warm
      - Vasoconstrict if body is too cool

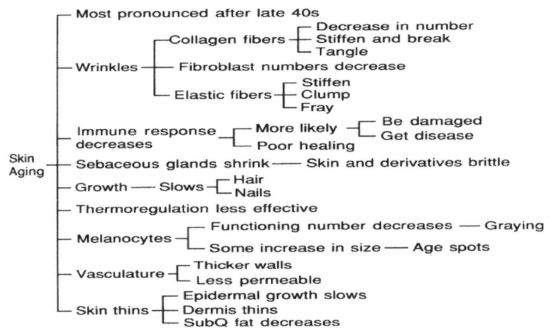

Skin Aging
- Most pronounced after late 40s
- Wrinkles
  - Collagen fibers
    - Decrease in number
    - Stiffen and break
    - Tangle
  - Fibroblast numbers decrease
  - Elastic fibers
    - Stiffen
    - Clump
    - Fray
- Immune response decreases
  - More likely
    - Be damaged
    - Get disease
  - Poor healing
- Sebaceous glands shrink — Skin and derivatives brittle
- Growth — Slows
  - Hair
  - Nails
- Thermoregulation less effective
- Melanocytes
  - Functioning number decreases — Graying
  - Some increase in size — Age spots
- Vasculature
  - Thicker walls
  - Less permeable
- Skin thins
  - Epidermal growth slows
  - Dermis thins
  - SubQ fat decreases

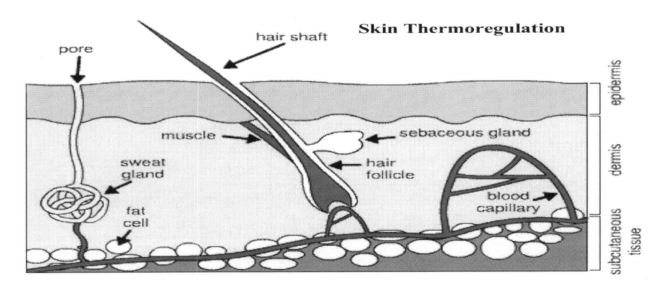

Skin Thermoregulation

pore
hair shaft
muscle
sweat gland
fat cell
sebaceous gland
hair follicle
blood capillary
epidermis
dermis
subcutaneous tissue

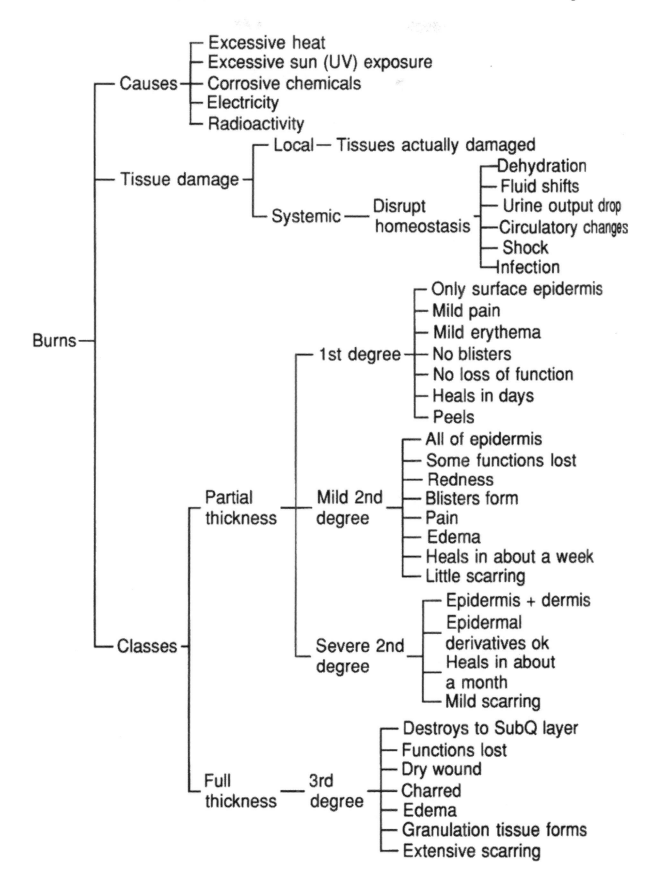

Burns
- Causes
  - Excessive heat
  - Excessive sun (UV) exposure
  - Corrosive chemicals
  - Electricity
  - Radioactivity
- Tissue damage
  - Local — Tissues actually damaged
  - Systemic — Disrupt homeostasis
    - Dehydration
    - Fluid shifts
    - Urine output drop
    - Circulatory changes
    - Shock
    - Infection
- Classes
  - Partial thickness
    - 1st degree
      - Only surface epidermis
      - Mild pain
      - Mild erythema
      - No blisters
      - No loss of function
      - Heals in days
      - Peels
    - Mild 2nd degree
      - All of epidermis
      - Some functions lost
      - Redness
      - Blisters form
      - Pain
      - Edema
      - Heals in about a week
      - Little scarring
    - Severe 2nd degree
      - Epidermis + dermis
      - Epidermal derivatives ok
      - Heals in about a month
      - Mild scarring
  - Full thickness
    - 3rd degree
      - Destroys to SubQ layer
      - Functions lost
      - Dry wound
      - Charred
      - Edema
      - Granulation tissue forms
      - Extensive scarring

Different degrees of burns and the effects on the skin

Epidermis

Dermis

Subcutaneous

Muscle

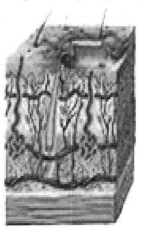

Superficial
(first degree)
burn

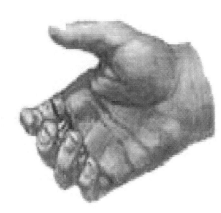

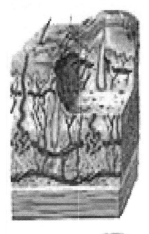

Partial thickness
(second degree)
burn

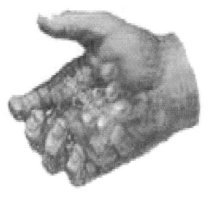

Full thickness
(third degree)
burn

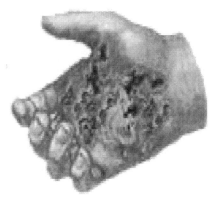

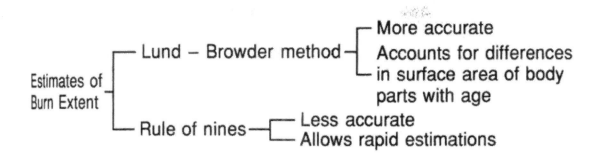

Estimates of Burn Extent
- Lund – Browder method
  - More accurate
  - Accounts for differences in surface area of body parts with age
- Rule of nines
  - Less accurate
  - Allows rapid estimations

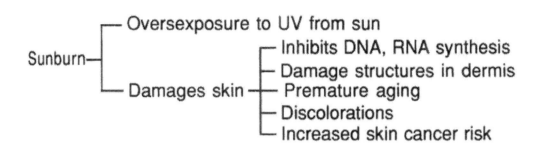

Sunburn
- Oversexposure to UV from sun
- Damages skin
  - Inhibits DNA, RNA synthesis
  - Damage structures in dermis
  - Premature aging
  - Discolorations
  - Increased skin cancer risk

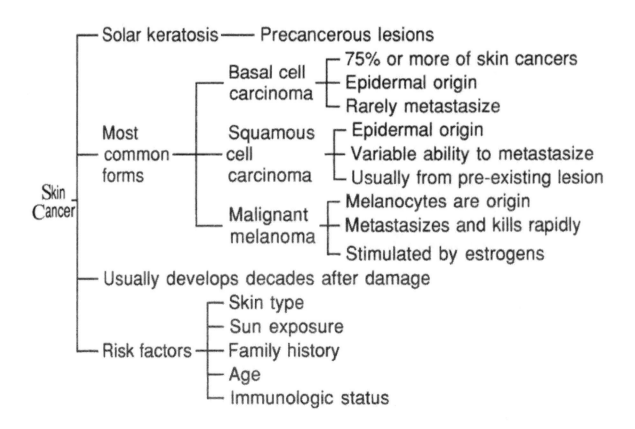

Skin Cancer
- Solar keratosis —— Precancerous lesions
- Most common forms
  - Basal cell carcinoma
    - 75% or more of skin cancers
    - Epidermal origin
    - Rarely metastasize
  - Squamous cell carcinoma
    - Epidermal origin
    - Variable ability to metastasize
    - Usually from pre-existing lesion
  - Malignant melanoma
    - Melanocytes are origin
    - Metastasizes and kills rapidly
    - Stimulated by estrogens
- Usually develops decades after damage
- Risk factors
  - Skin type
  - Sun exposure
  - Family history
  - Age
  - Immunologic status

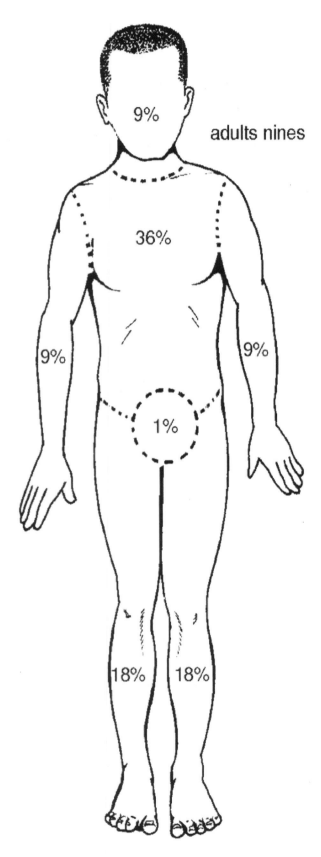

THE RULES OF NINES AND SEVENS

adults nines

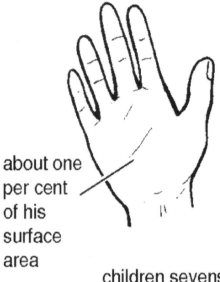

about one per cent of his surface area

children sevens

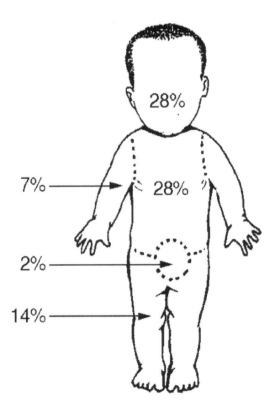

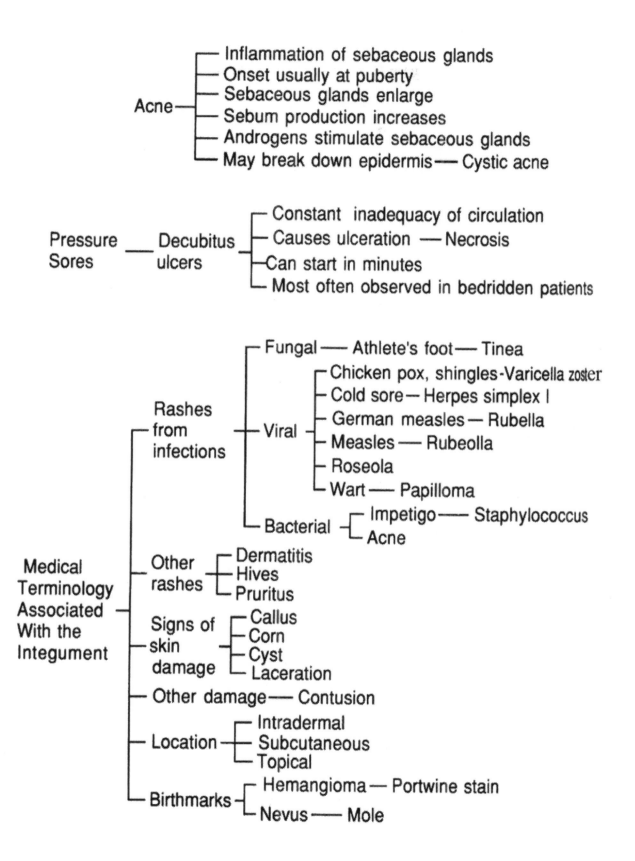

Acne
— Inflammation of sebaceous glands
— Onset usually at puberty
— Sebaceous glands enlarge
— Sebum production increases
— Androgens stimulate sebaceous glands
— May break down epidermis — Cystic acne

Pressure Sores — Decubitus ulcers
— Constant inadequacy of circulation
— Causes ulceration — Necrosis
— Can start in minutes
— Most often observed in bedridden patients

Medical Terminology Associated With the Integument

Rashes from infections
— Fungal — Athlete's foot — Tinea
— Viral
  — Chicken pox, shingles-Varicella zoster
  — Cold sore — Herpes simplex I
  — German measles — Rubella
  — Measles — Rubeolla
  — Roseola
  — Wart — Papilloma
— Bacterial
  — Impetigo — Staphylococcus
  — Acne

Other rashes
— Dermatitis
— Hives
— Pruritus

Signs of skin damage
— Callus
— Corn
— Cyst
— Laceration

Other damage — Contusion

Location
— Intradermal
— Subcutaneous
— Topical

Birthmarks
— Hemangioma — Portwine stain
— Nevus — Mole

CHAPTER SIX

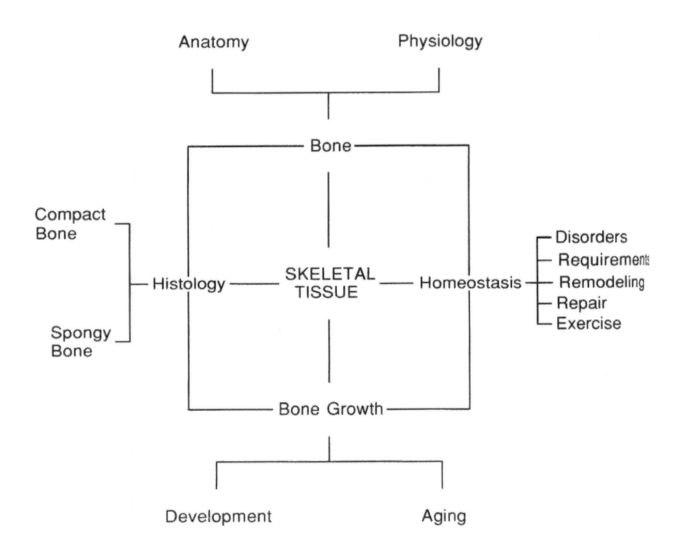

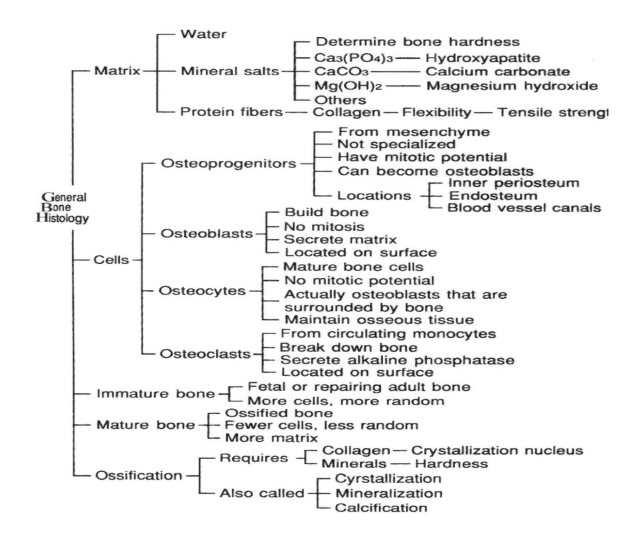

General Bone Histology

- Matrix
  - Water
  - Mineral salts
    - Determine bone hardness
    - Ca₃(PO₄)₃ — Hydroxyapatite
    - CaCO₃ — Calcium carbonate
    - Mg(OH)₂ — Magnesium hydroxide
    - Others
  - Protein fibers — Collagen — Flexibility — Tensile strengt

- Cells
  - Osteoprogenitors
    - From mesenchyme
    - Not specialized
    - Have mitotic potential
    - Can become osteoblasts
    - Locations
      - Inner periosteum
      - Endosteum
      - Blood vessel canals
  - Osteoblasts
    - Build bone
    - No mitosis
    - Secrete matrix
    - Located on surface
  - Osteocytes
    - Mature bone cells
    - No mitotic potential
    - Actually osteoblasts that are surrounded by bone
    - Maintain osseous tissue
  - Osteoclasts
    - From circulating monocytes
    - Break down bone
    - Secrete alkaline phosphatase
    - Located on surface

- Immature bone
  - Fetal or repairing adult bone
  - More cells, more random

- Mature bone
  - Ossified bone
  - Fewer cells, less random
  - More matrix

- Ossification
  - Requires
    - Collagen — Crystallization nucleus
    - Minerals — Hardness
  - Also called
    - Cyrstallization
    - Mineralization
    - Calcification

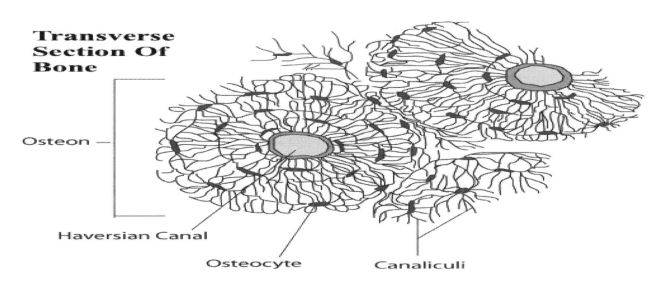

Transverse Section Of Bone

Osteon

Haversian Canal

Osteocyte

Canaliculi

Cancellous Bone (Spongy Bone)

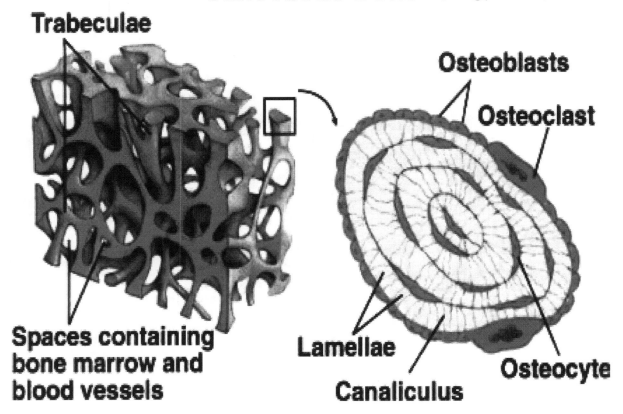

Trabeculae

Osteoblasts

Osteoclast

Spaces containing bone marrow and blood vessels

Lamellae

Canaliculus

Osteocyte

Compact Bone & Spongy (Cancellous Bone)

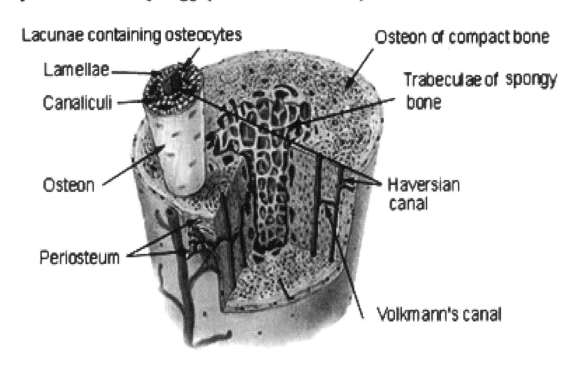

Lacunae containing osteocytes

Lamellae

Canaliculi

Osteon

Periosteum

Osteon of compact bone

Trabeculae of spongy bone

Haversian canal

Volkmann's canal

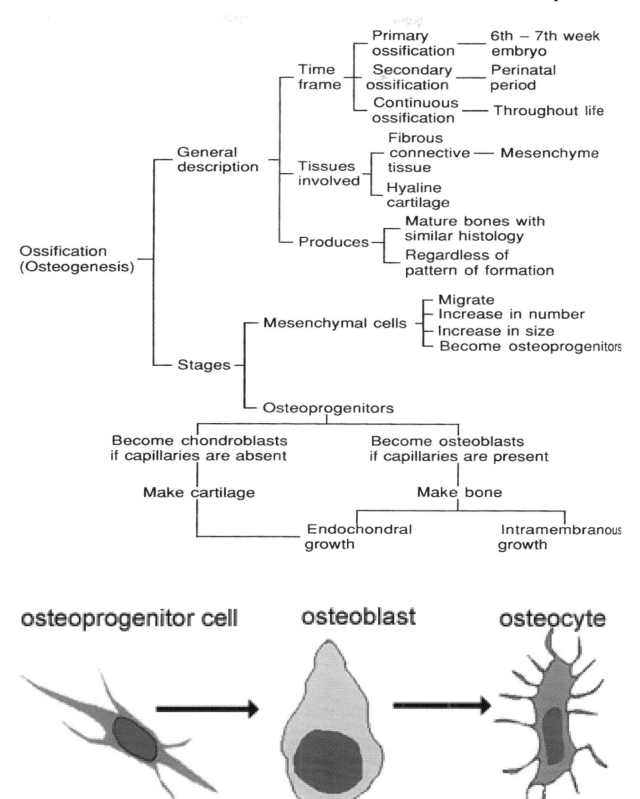

Ossification (Osteogenesis)

General description
- Time frame
  - Primary ossification — 6th – 7th week embryo
  - Secondary ossification — Perinatal period
  - Continuous ossification — Throughout life
- Tissues involved
  - Fibrous connective tissue — Mesenchyme
  - Hyaline cartilage
- Produces
  - Mature bones with similar histology
  - Regardless of pattern of formation

Stages
- Mesenchymal cells
  - Migrate
  - Increase in number
  - Increase in size
  - Become osteoprogenitors
- Osteoprogenitors
  - Become chondroblasts if capillaries are absent
    - Make cartilage
    - Endochondral growth
  - Become osteoblasts if capillaries are present
    - Make bone
    - Intramembranous growth

osteoprogenitor cell → osteoblast → osteocyte

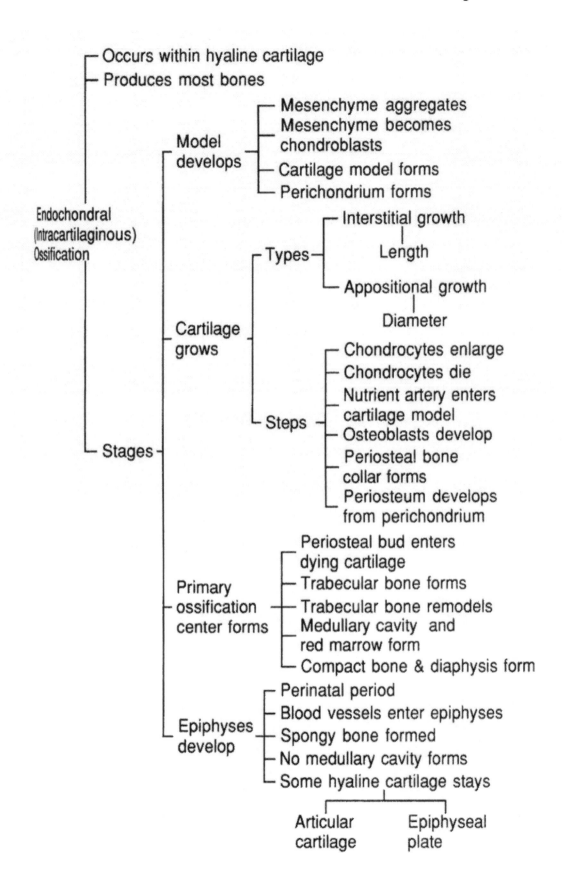

- Occurs within hyaline cartilage
- Produces most bones

Endochondral (Intracartilaginous) Ossification

Stages

Model develops
- Mesenchyme aggregates
- Mesenchyme becomes chondroblasts
- Cartilage model forms
- Perichondrium forms

Cartilage grows
- Types
  - Interstitial growth
    - Length
  - Appositional growth
    - Diameter
- Steps
  - Chondrocytes enlarge
  - Chondrocytes die
  - Nutrient artery enters cartilage model
  - Osteoblasts develop
  - Periosteal bone collar forms
  - Periosteum develops from perichondrium

Primary ossification center forms
- Periosteal bud enters dying cartilage
- Trabecular bone forms
- Trabecular bone remodels
- Medullary cavity and red marrow form
- Compact bone & diaphysis form

Epiphyses develop
- Perinatal period
- Blood vessels enter epiphyses
- Spongy bone formed
- No medullary cavity forms
- Some hyaline cartilage stays
  - Articular cartilage
  - Epiphyseal plate

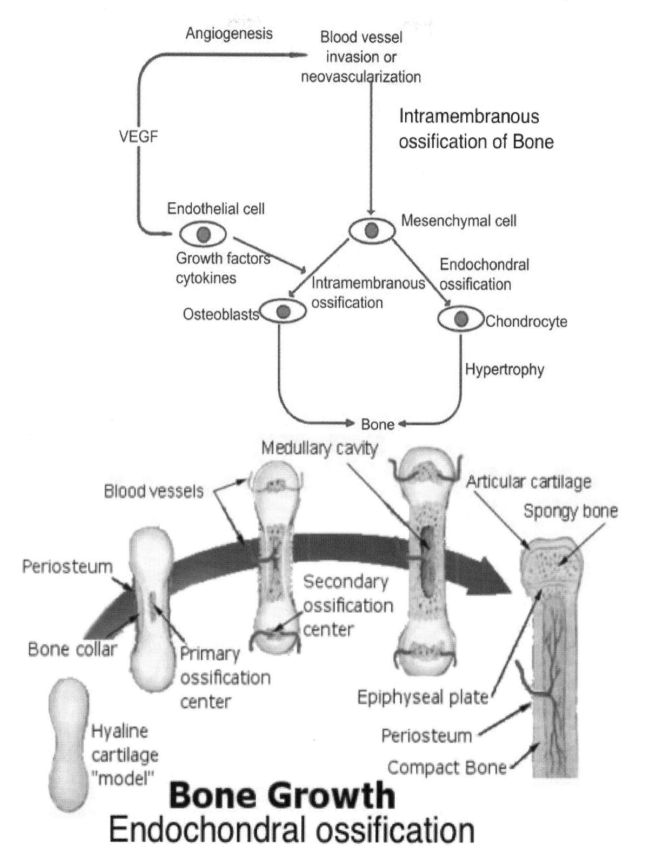

Angiogenesis → Blood vessel invasion or neovascularization

Intramembranous ossification of Bone

VEGF

Endothelial cell

Mesenchymal cell

Growth factors cytokines

Endochondral ossification

Osteoblasts   Intramembranous ossification   Chondrocyte

Hypertrophy

Bone

Medullary cavity

Blood vessels

Articular cartilage

Spongy bone

Periosteum

Secondary ossification center

Bone collar   Primary ossification center

Epiphyseal plate

Periosteum

Compact Bone

Hyaline cartilage "model"

Bone Growth
Endochondral ossification

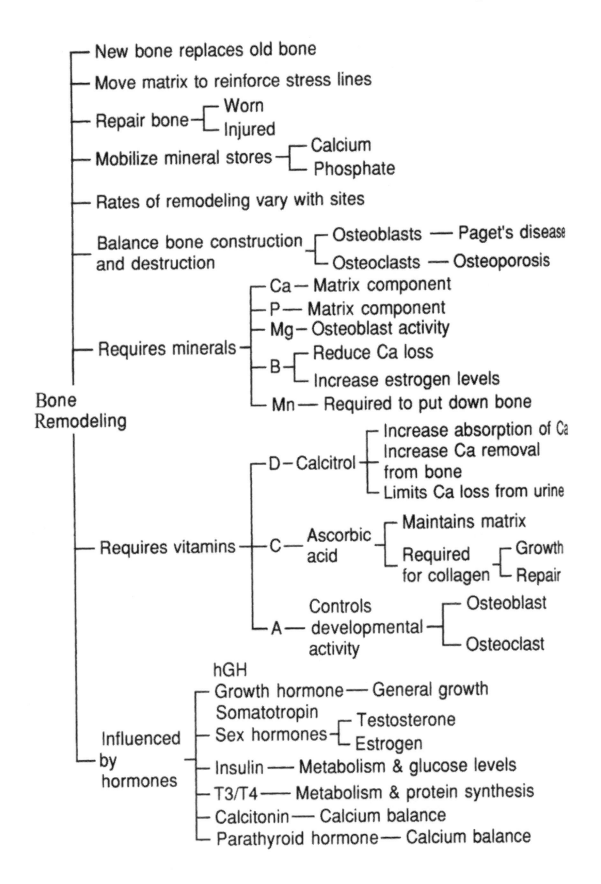

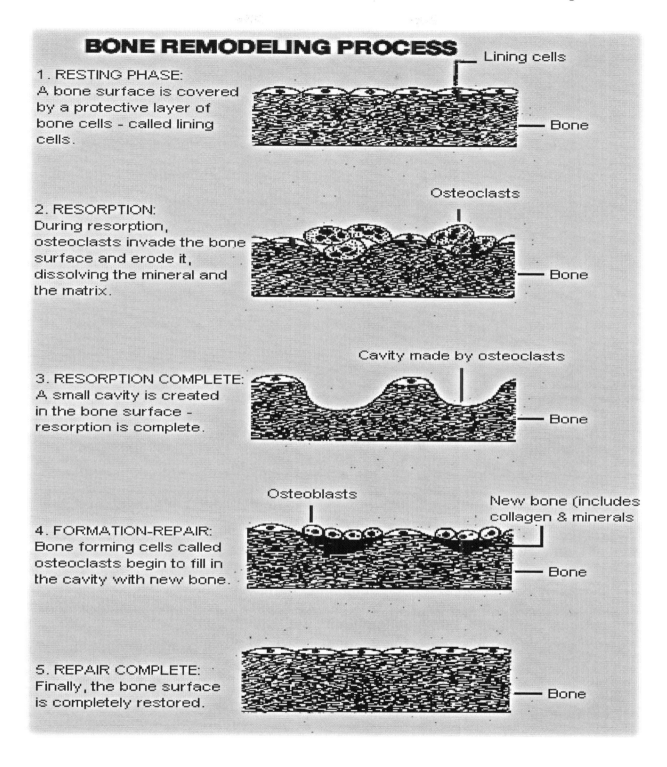

BONE REMODELING PROCESS

1. RESTING PHASE:
A bone surface is covered by a protective layer of bone cells - called lining cells.

Lining cells

Bone

2. RESORPTION:
During resorption, osteoclasts invade the bone surface and erode it, dissolving the mineral and the matrix.

Osteoclasts

Bone

3. RESORPTION COMPLETE:
A small cavity is created in the bone surface - resorption is complete.

Cavity made by osteoclasts

Bone

4. FORMATION-REPAIR:
Bone forming cells called osteoclasts begin to fill in the cavity with new bone.

Osteoblasts

New bone (includes collagen & minerals

Bone

5. REPAIR COMPLETE:
Finally, the bone surface is completely restored.

Bone

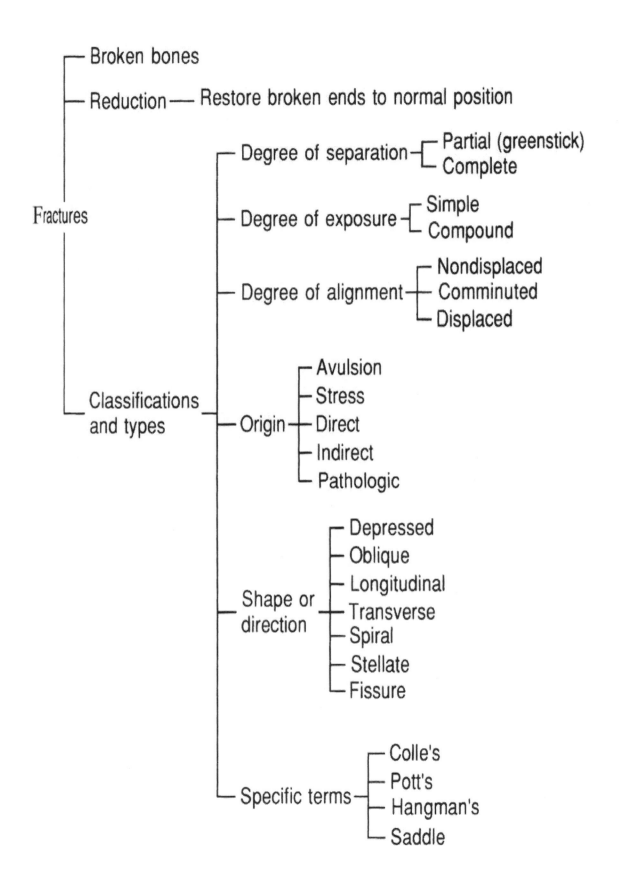

Fractures
- Broken bones
- Reduction — Restore broken ends to normal position
- Classifications and types
  - Degree of separation
    - Partial (greenstick)
    - Complete
  - Degree of exposure
    - Simple
    - Compound
  - Degree of alignment
    - Nondisplaced
    - Comminuted
    - Displaced
  - Origin
    - Avulsion
    - Stress
    - Direct
    - Indirect
    - Pathologic
  - Shape or direction
    - Depressed
    - Oblique
    - Longitudinal
    - Transverse
    - Spiral
    - Stellate
    - Fissure
  - Specific terms
    - Colle's
    - Pott's
    - Hangman's
    - Saddle

CLASSIFICATION OF FRACTURES

SIMPLE (CLOSED)

- Skin is not broken
- Requires cast

COMPOUND (OPEN)

- Bone has broken through the skin
- Increased chance of infections, which can be life-threatening.
- Requires surgery, hospitalization and IV antibiotic

Types of Fractures

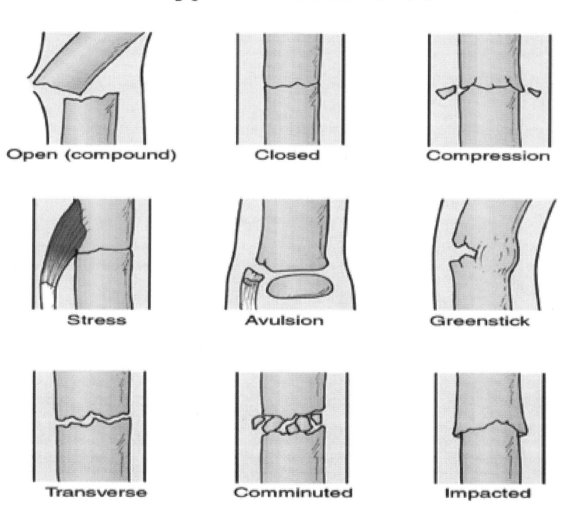

Open (compound)	Closed	Compression
Stress	Avulsion	Greenstick
Transverse	Comminuted	Impacted

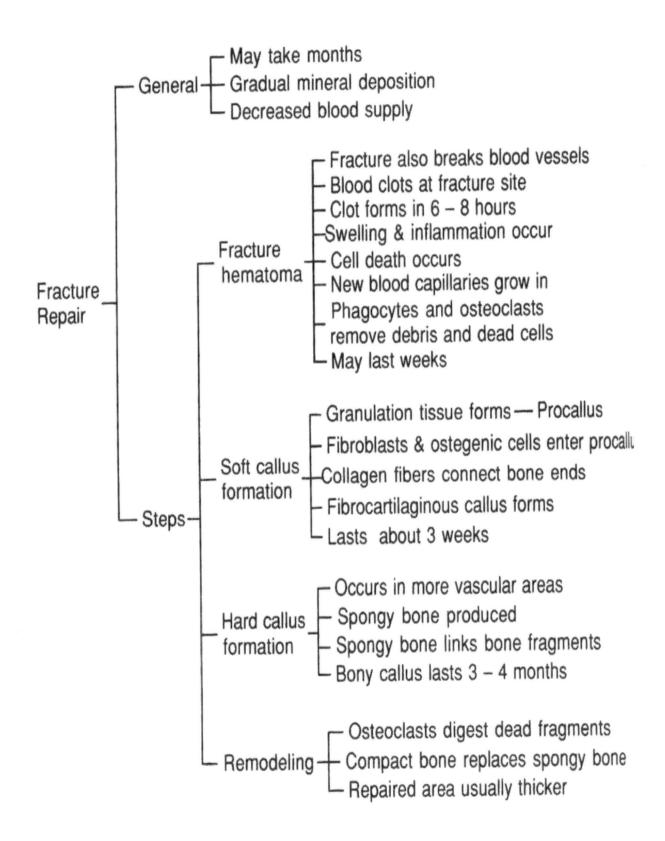

Fracture Repair
- General
  - May take months
  - Gradual mineral deposition
  - Decreased blood supply
- Steps
  - Fracture hematoma
    - Fracture also breaks blood vessels
    - Blood clots at fracture site
    - Clot forms in 6 – 8 hours
    - Swelling & inflammation occur
    - Cell death occurs
    - New blood capillaries grow in
    - Phagocytes and osteoclasts remove debris and dead cells
    - May last weeks
  - Soft callus formation
    - Granulation tissue forms — Procallus
    - Fibroblasts & ostegenic cells enter procallu
    - Collagen fibers connect bone ends
    - Fibrocartilaginous callus forms
    - Lasts about 3 weeks
  - Hard callus formation
    - Occurs in more vascular areas
    - Spongy bone produced
    - Spongy bone links bone fragments
    - Bony callus lasts 3 – 4 months
  - Remodeling
    - Osteoclasts digest dead fragments
    - Compact bone replaces spongy bone
    - Repaired area usually thicker

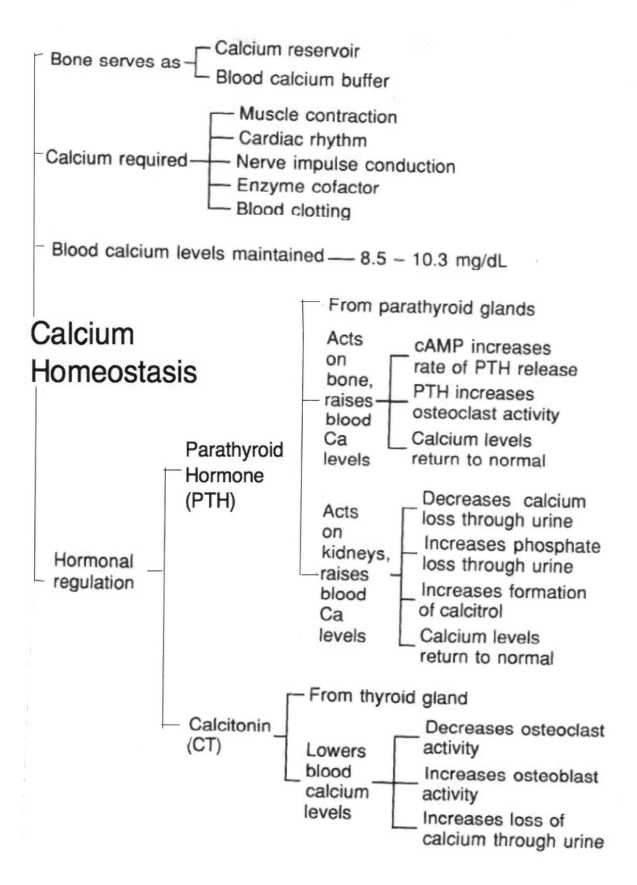

Bone serves as
- Calcium reservoir
- Blood calcium buffer

Calcium required
- Muscle contraction
- Cardiac rhythm
- Nerve impulse conduction
- Enzyme cofactor
- Blood clotting

Blood calcium levels maintained — 8.5 – 10.3 mg/dL

Calcium Homeostasis

Hormonal regulation

Parathyroid Hormone (PTH)
- From parathyroid glands
- Acts on bone, raises blood Ca levels
  - cAMP increases rate of PTH release
  - PTH increases osteoclast activity
  - Calcium levels return to normal
- Acts on kidneys, raises blood Ca levels
  - Decreases calcium loss through urine
  - Increases phosphate loss through urine
  - Increases formation of calcitrol
  - Calcium levels return to normal

Calcitonin (CT)
- From thyroid gland
- Lowers blood calcium levels
  - Decreases osteoclast activity
  - Increases osteoblast activity
  - Increases loss of calcium through urine

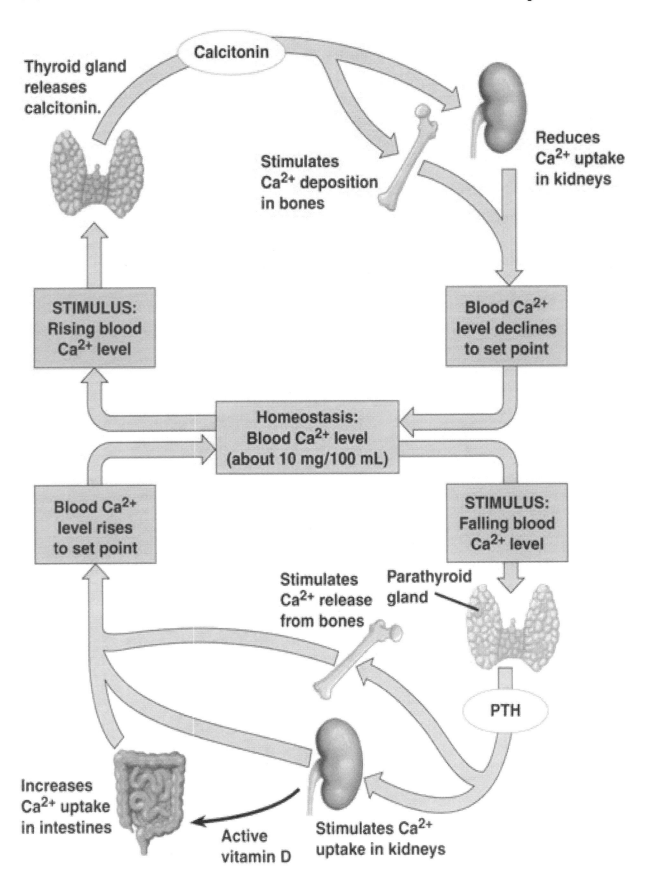

Thyroid gland releases calcitonin.

Calcitonin

Stimulates Ca^{2+} deposition in bones

Reduces Ca^{2+} uptake in kidneys

STIMULUS: Rising blood Ca^{2+} level

Blood Ca^{2+} level declines to set point

Homeostasis: Blood Ca^{2+} level (about 10 mg/100 mL)

Blood Ca^{2+} level rises to set point

STIMULUS: Falling blood Ca^{2+} level

Stimulates Ca^{2+} release from bones

Parathyroid gland

PTH

Increases Ca^{2+} uptake in intestines

Active vitamin D

Stimulates Ca^{2+} uptake in kidneys

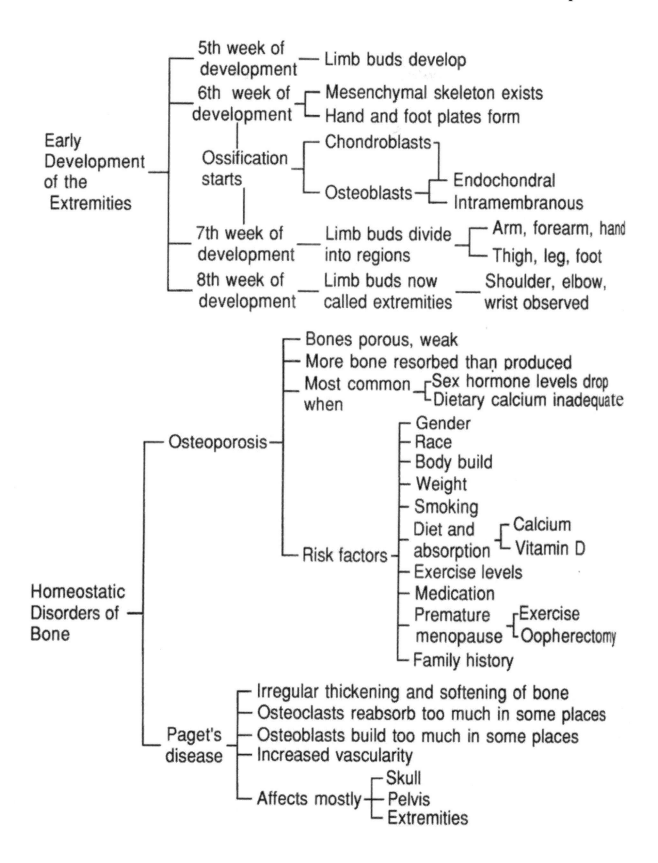

Early Development of the Extremities
- 5th week of development — Limb buds develop
- 6th week of development
  - Mesenchymal skeleton exists
  - Hand and foot plates form
- Ossification starts
  - Chondroblasts
  - Osteoblasts
    - Endochondral
    - Intramembranous
- 7th week of development — Limb buds divide into regions
  - Arm, forearm, hand
  - Thigh, leg, foot
- 8th week of development — Limb buds now called extremities — Shoulder, elbow, wrist observed

Homeostatic Disorders of Bone
- Osteoporosis
  - Bones porous, weak
  - More bone resorbed than produced
  - Most common when
    - Sex hormone levels drop
    - Dietary calcium inadequate
  - Risk factors
    - Gender
    - Race
    - Body build
    - Weight
    - Smoking
    - Diet and absorption
      - Calcium
      - Vitamin D
    - Exercise levels
    - Medication
    - Premature menopause
      - Exercise
      - Oopherectomy
    - Family history
- Paget's disease
  - Irregular thickening and softening of bone
  - Osteoclasts reabsorb too much in some places
  - Osteoblasts build too much in some places
  - Increased vascularity
  - Affects mostly
    - Skull
    - Pelvis
    - Extremities

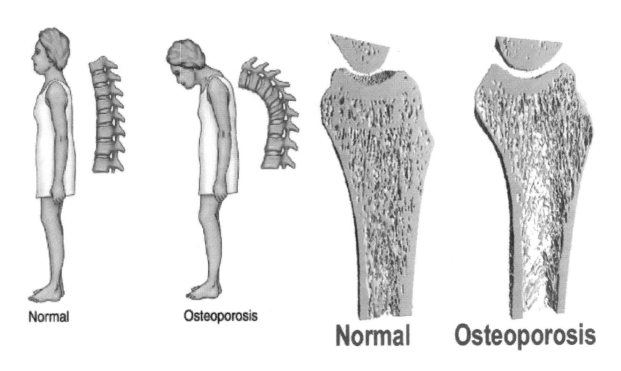

Normal   Osteoporosis

Normal   **Osteoporosis**

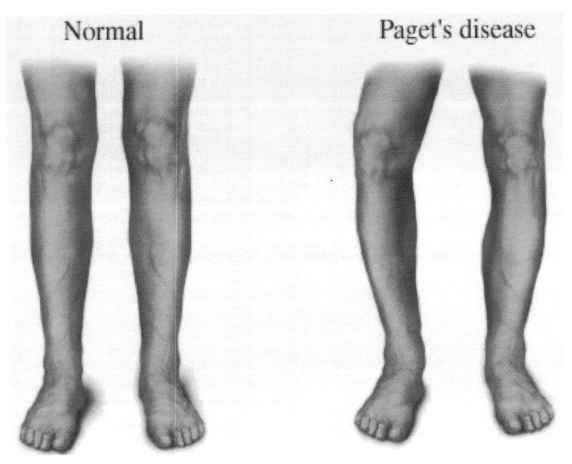

Normal   Paget's disease

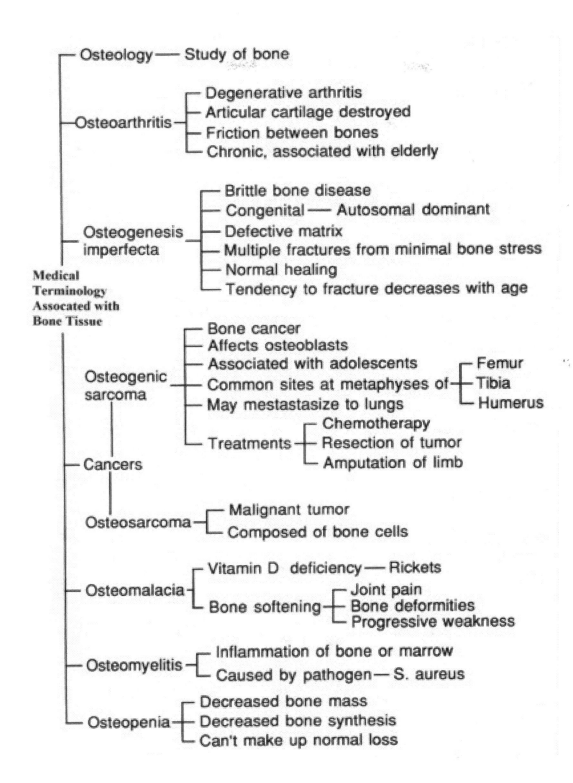

Medical Terminology Associated with Bone Tissue

- Osteology — Study of bone
- Osteoarthritis
  - Degenerative arthritis
  - Articular cartilage destroyed
  - Friction between bones
  - Chronic, associated with elderly
- Osteogenesis imperfecta
  - Brittle bone disease
  - Congenital — Autosomal dominant
  - Defective matrix
  - Multiple fractures from minimal bone stress
  - Normal healing
  - Tendency to fracture decreases with age
- Cancers
  - Osteogenic sarcoma
    - Bone cancer
    - Affects osteoblasts
    - Associated with adolescents
    - Common sites at metaphyses of
      - Femur
      - Tibia
      - Humerus
    - May mestastasize to lungs
    - Treatments
      - Chemotherapy
      - Resection of tumor
      - Amputation of limb
  - Osteosarcoma
    - Malignant tumor
    - Composed of bone cells
- Osteomalacia
  - Vitamin D deficiency — Rickets
  - Bone softening
    - Joint pain
    - Bone deformities
    - Progressive weakness
- Osteomyelitis
  - Inflammation of bone or marrow
  - Caused by pathogen — S. aureus
- Osteopenia
  - Decreased bone mass
  - Decreased bone synthesis
  - Can't make up normal loss

Paget's Disease

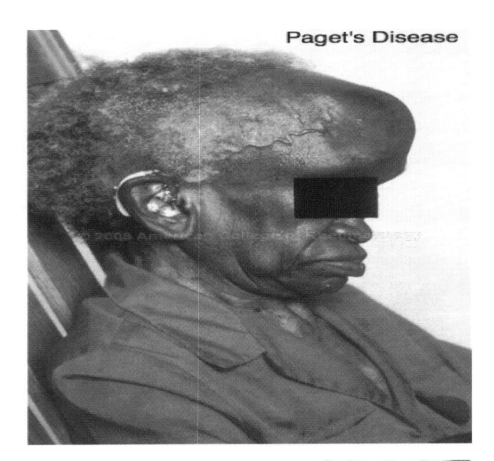

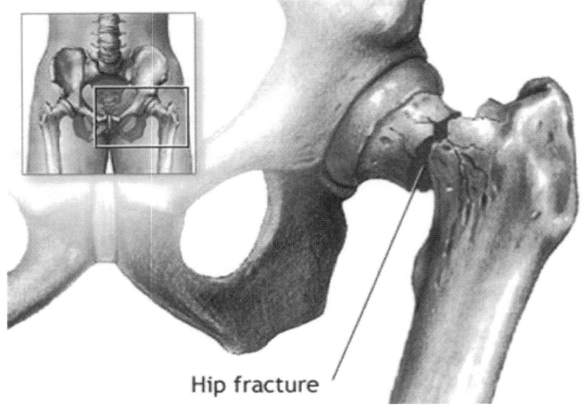

Hip fracture

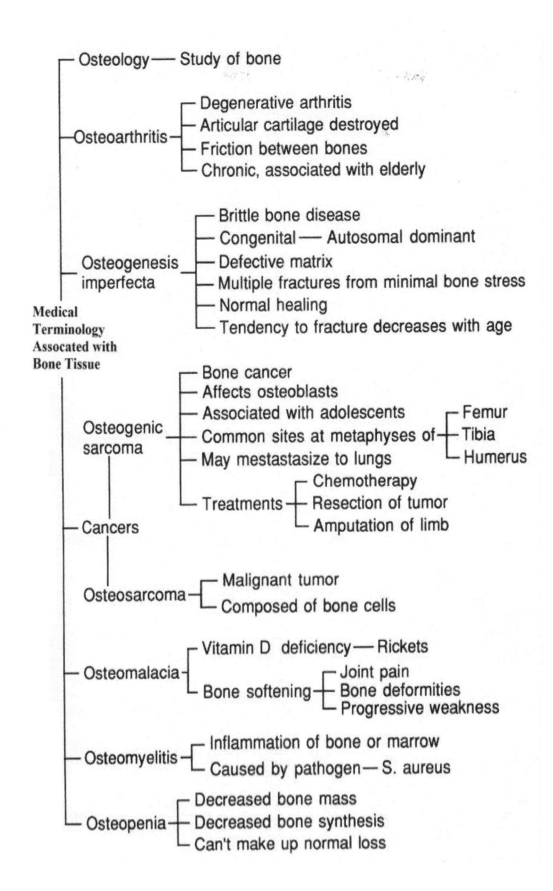

Osteology —— Study of bone

Osteoarthritis
- Degenerative arthritis
- Articular cartilage destroyed
- Friction between bones
- Chronic, associated with elderly

Osteogenesis imperfecta
- Brittle bone disease
- Congenital —— Autosomal dominant
- Defective matrix
- Multiple fractures from minimal bone stress
- Normal healing
- Tendency to fracture decreases with age

Medical Terminology Assocated with Bone Tissue

Cancers

Osteogenic sarcoma
- Bone cancer
- Affects osteoblasts
- Associated with adolescents
- Common sites at metaphyses of
  - Femur
  - Tibia
  - Humerus
- May mestastasize to lungs
- Treatments
  - Chemotherapy
  - Resection of tumor
  - Amputation of limb

Osteosarcoma
- Malignant tumor
- Composed of bone cells

Osteomalacia
- Vitamin D deficiency —— Rickets
- Bone softening
  - Joint pain
  - Bone deformities
  - Progressive weakness

Osteomyelitis
- Inflammation of bone or marrow
- Caused by pathogen —— S. aureus

Osteopenia
- Decreased bone mass
- Decreased bone synthesis
- Can't make up normal loss

CHAPTER SEVEN

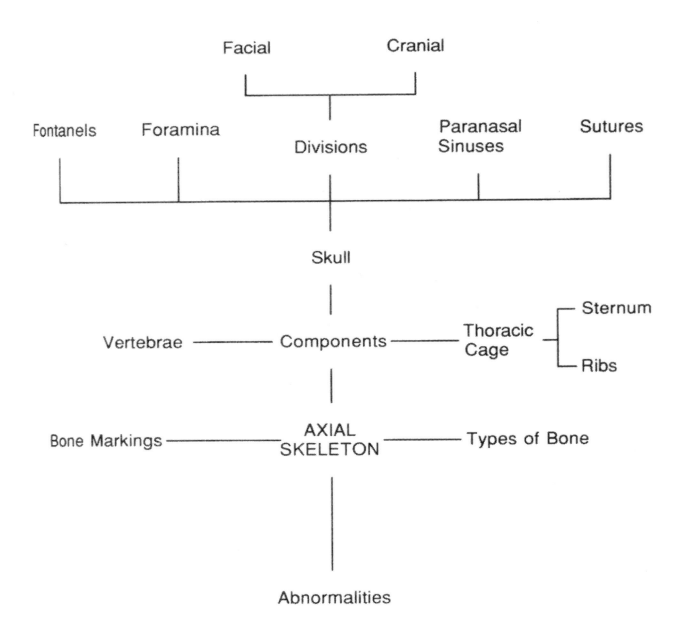

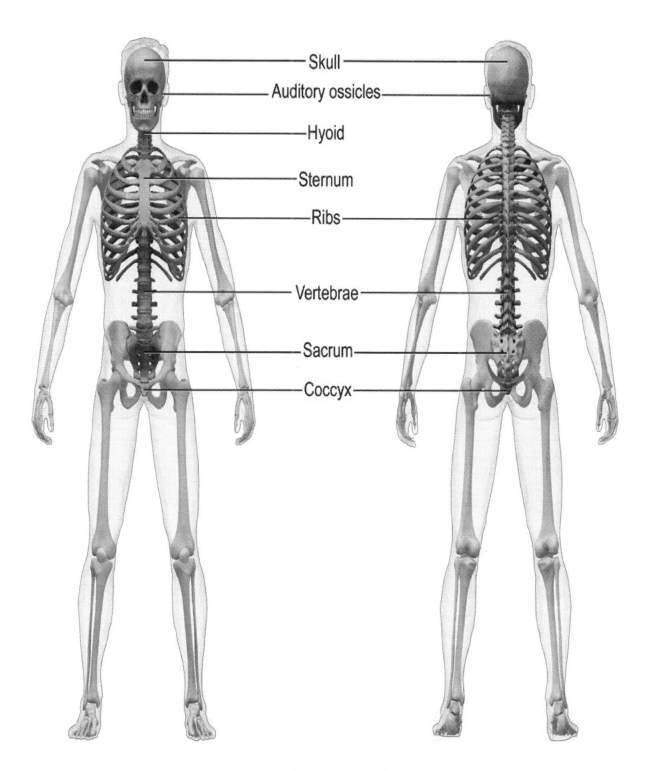

Skull

Auditory ossicles

Hyoid

Sternum

Ribs

Vertebrae

Sacrum

Coccyx

The Axial Skeleton

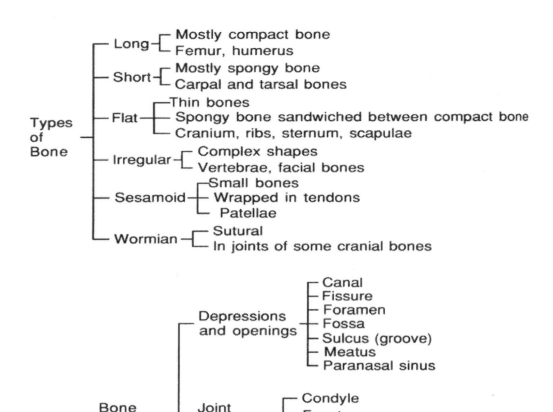

Types
of
Bone
- Long — Mostly compact bone
  - Femur, humerus
- Short — Mostly spongy bone
  - Carpal and tarsal bones
- Flat — Thin bones
  - Spongy bone sandwiched between compact bone
  - Cranium, ribs, sternum, scapulae
- Irregular — Complex shapes
  - Vertebrae, facial bones
- Sesamoid — Small bones
  - Wrapped in tendons
  - Patellae
- Wormian — Sutural
  - In joints of some cranial bones

Bone Markings
- Depressions and openings
  - Canal
  - Fissure
  - Foramen
  - Fossa
  - Sulcus (groove)
  - Meatus
  - Paranasal sinus
- Joint processes
  - Condyle
  - Facet
  - Head
- Attachment processes
  - Crest
  - Epicondyle
  - Line
  - Spine
  - Trochanter
  - Tubercle
  - Tuberosity

Types of Bones
The skeleton has more than 200 bones divided into four major groups.

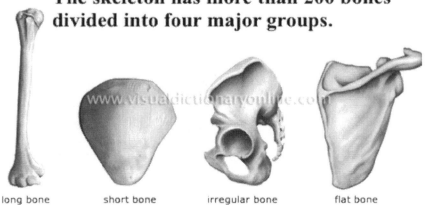

long bone   short bone   irregular bone   flat bone

Bone Markings

NAME OF BONE MARKING	DESCRIPTION
PROJECTIONS THAT ARE SITES OF MUSCLE AND LIGAMENT ATTACHMENT	
Tuberosity (too"bĕ-ros'ĭ-te)	Large rounded projection; may be roughened
Crest	Narrow ridge of bone; usually prominent
Trochanter (tro-kan'ter)	Very large, blunt, irregularly shaped process (the only examples are on the femur)
Line	Narrow ridge of bone; less prominent than a crest
Tubercle (too'ber-kl)	Small rounded projection or process
Epicondyle (ep"ĭ-kon'dĭl)	Raised area on or above a condyle
Spine	Sharp, slender, often pointed projection
Process	Any bony prominence
PROJECTIONS THAT HELP TO FORM JOINTS	
Head	Bony expansion carried on a narrow neck
Facet	Smooth, nearly flat articular surface
Condyle (kon'dĭl)	Rounded articular projection
Ramus (ra'mus)	Armlike bar of bone
DEPRESSIONS AND OPENINGS ALLOWING BLOOD VESSELS AND NERVES TO PASS	
Meatus (me-a'tus)	Canal-like passageway
Sinus	Cavity within a bone, filled with air and lined with mucous membrane
Fossa (fos'ah)	Shallow, basinlike depression in a bone, often serving as an articular surface
Groove	Furrow
Fissure	Narrow, slitlike opening
Foramen (fo-ra'men)	Round or oval opening through a bone

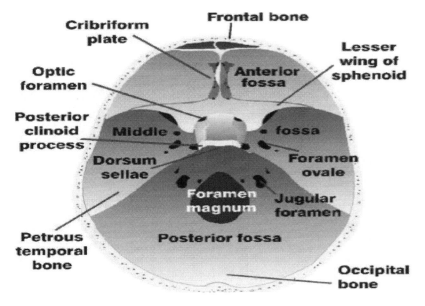

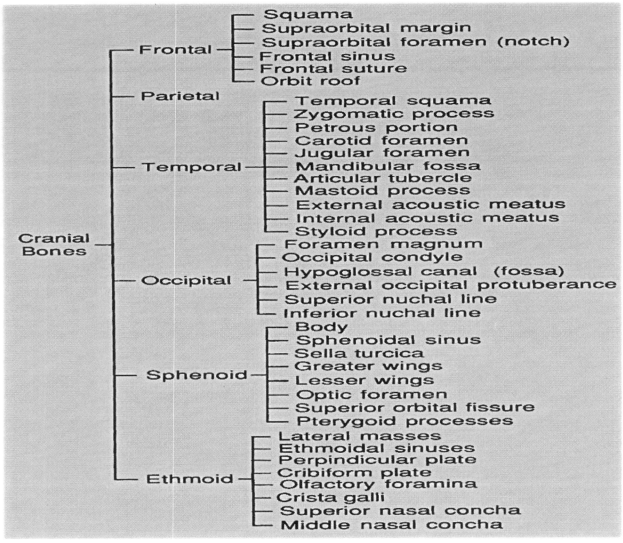

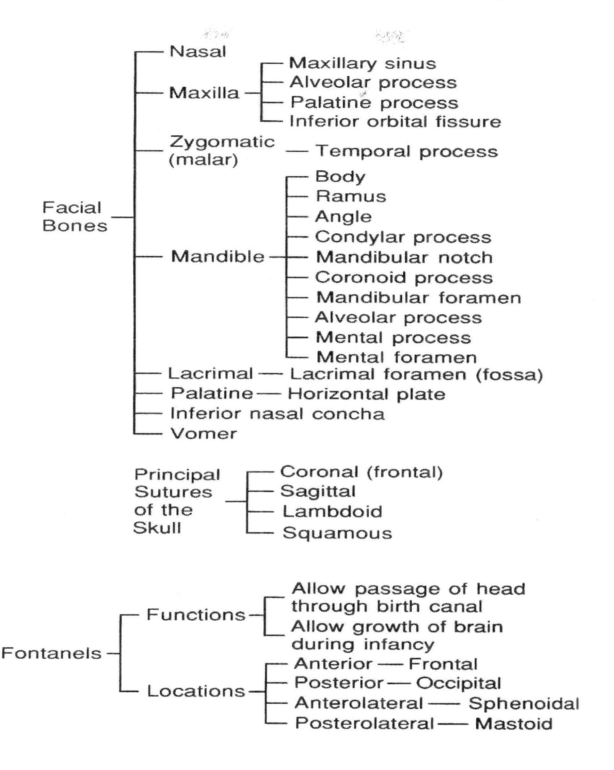

Facial Bones
- Nasal
- Maxilla
  - Maxillary sinus
  - Alveolar process
  - Palatine process
  - Inferior orbital fissure
- Zygomatic (malar)
  - Temporal process
- Mandible
  - Body
  - Ramus
  - Angle
  - Condylar process
  - Mandibular notch
  - Coronoid process
  - Mandibular foramen
  - Alveolar process
  - Mental process
  - Mental foramen
- Lacrimal — Lacrimal foramen (fossa)
- Palatine — Horizontal plate
- Inferior nasal concha
- Vomer

Principal Sutures of the Skull
- Coronal (frontal)
- Sagittal
- Lambdoid
- Squamous

Fontanels
- Functions
  - Allow passage of head through birth canal
  - Allow growth of brain during infancy
- Locations
  - Anterior — Frontal
  - Posterior — Occipital
  - Anterolateral — Sphenoidal
  - Posterolateral — Mastoid

Bones and structures of the adult human skull
22 bones (8 cranial; 14 facial)

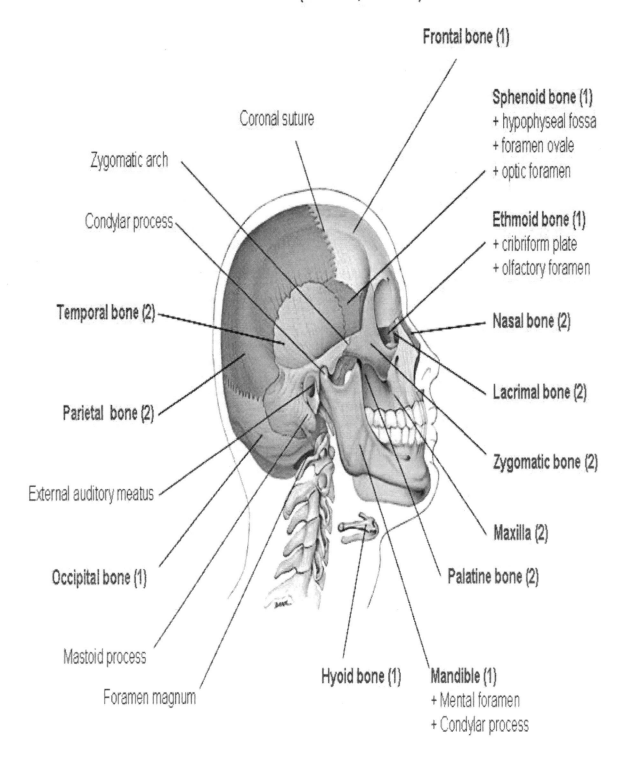

Frontal bone (1)

Sphenoid bone (1)
+ hypophyseal fossa
+ foramen ovale
+ optic foramen

Ethmoid bone (1)
+ cribriform plate
+ olfactory foramen

Coronal suture

Zygomatic arch

Condylar process

Nasal bone (2)

Temporal bone (2)

Lacrimal bone (2)

Parietal bone (2)

Zygomatic bone (2)

External auditory meatus

Maxilla (2)

Occipital bone (1)

Palatine bone (2)

Mastoid process

Hyoid bone (1)   Mandible (1)
+ Mental foramen
+ Condylar process

Foramen magnum

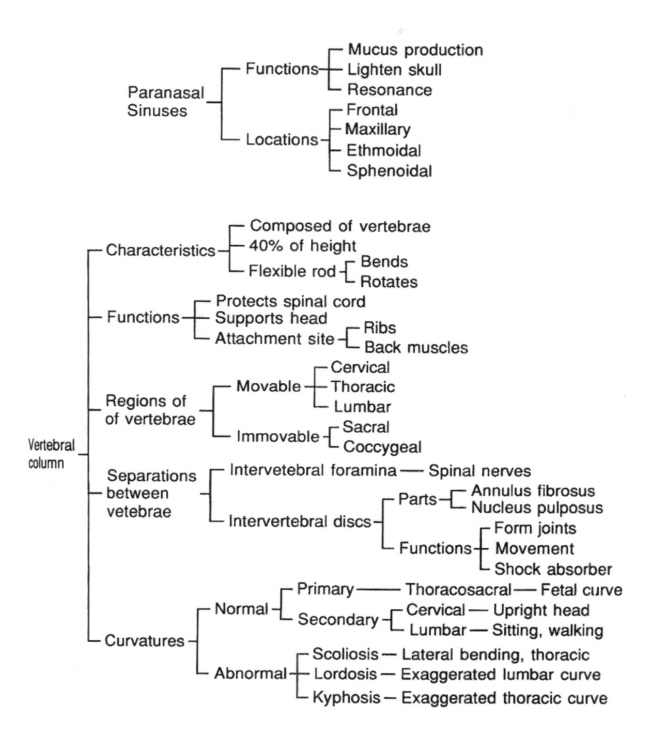

Paranasal Sinuses
- Functions
  - Mucus production
  - Lighten skull
  - Resonance
- Locations
  - Frontal
  - Maxillary
  - Ethmoidal
  - Sphenoidal

Vertebral column
- Characteristics
  - Composed of vertebrae
  - 40% of height
  - Flexible rod
    - Bends
    - Rotates
- Functions
  - Protects spinal cord
  - Supports head
  - Attachment site
    - Ribs
    - Back muscles
- Regions of of vertebrae
  - Movable
    - Cervical
    - Thoracic
    - Lumbar
  - Immovable
    - Sacral
    - Coccygeal
- Separations between vetebrae
  - Intervetebral foramina — Spinal nerves
  - Intervertebral discs
    - Parts
      - Annulus fibrosus
      - Nucleus pulposus
    - Functions
      - Form joints
      - Movement
      - Shock absorber
- Curvatures
  - Normal
    - Primary —— Thoracosacral — Fetal curve
    - Secondary
      - Cervical — Upright head
      - Lumbar — Sitting, walking
  - Abnormal
    - Scoliosis — Lateral bending, thoracic
    - Lordosis — Exaggerated lumbar curve
    - Kyphosis — Exaggerated thoracic curve

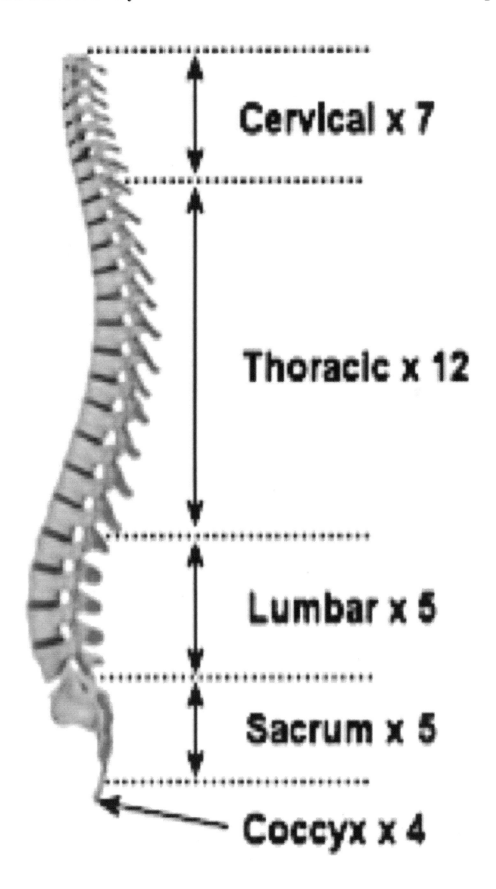

Cervical x 7

Thoracic x 12

Lumbar x 5

Sacrum x 5

Coccyx x 4

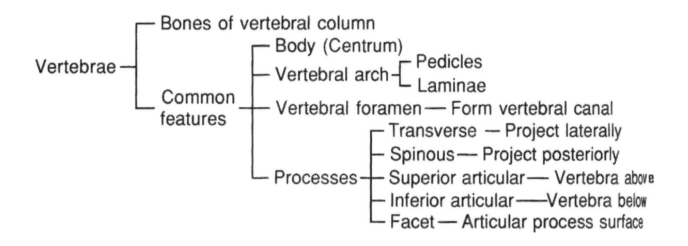

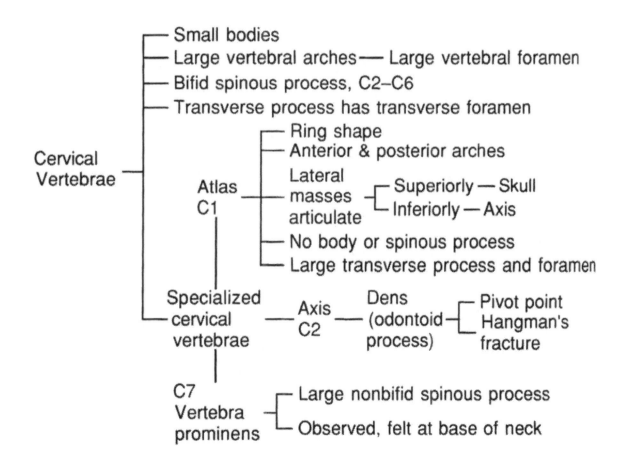

Cervical Vertebrae

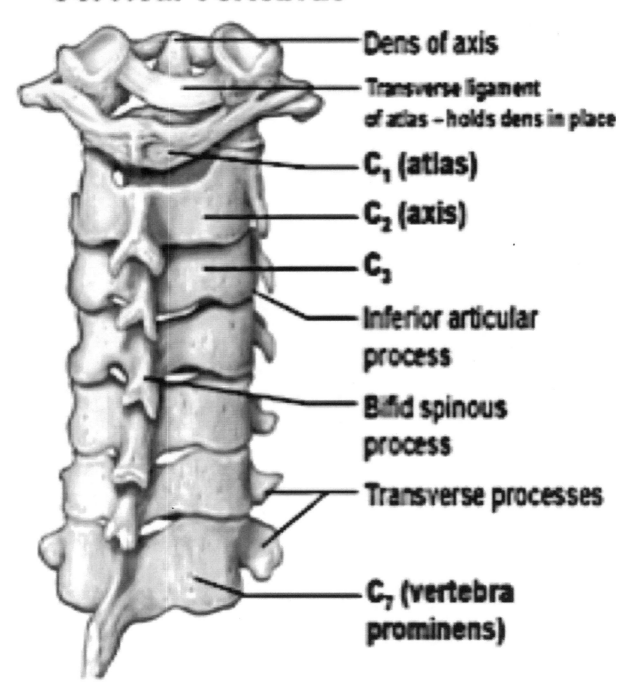

- Dens of axis
- Transverse ligament of atlas – holds dens in place
- C₁ (atlas)
- C₂ (axis)
- C₃
- Inferior articular process
- Bifid spinous process
- Transverse processes
- C₇ (vertebra prominens)

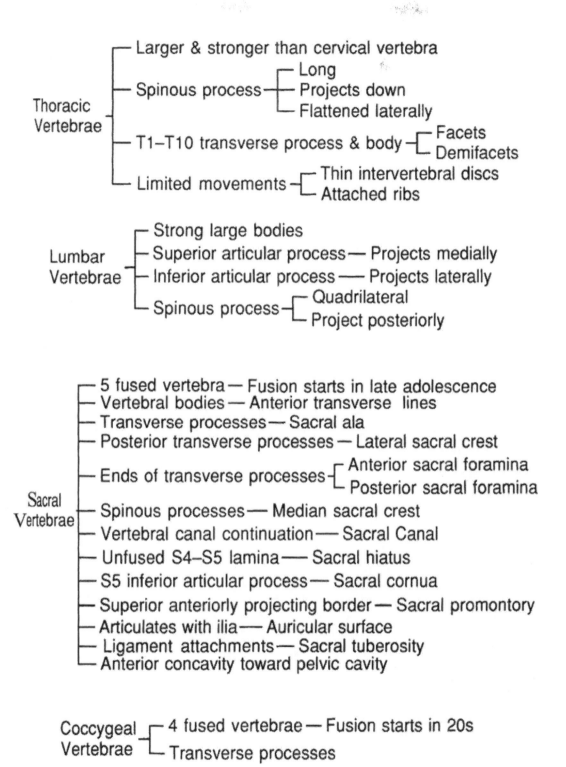

Thoracic Vertebrae
- Larger & stronger than cervical vertebra
- Spinous process
  - Long
  - Projects down
  - Flattened laterally
- T1–T10 transverse process & body
  - Facets
  - Demifacets
- Limited movements
  - Thin intervertebral discs
  - Attached ribs

Lumbar Vertebrae
- Strong large bodies
- Superior articular process — Projects medially
- Inferior articular process — Projects laterally
- Spinous process
  - Quadrilateral
  - Project posteriorly

Sacral Vertebrae
- 5 fused vertebra — Fusion starts in late adolescence
- Vertebral bodies — Anterior transverse lines
- Transverse processes — Sacral ala
- Posterior transverse processes — Lateral sacral crest
- Ends of transverse processes
  - Anterior sacral foramina
  - Posterior sacral foramina
- Spinous processes — Median sacral crest
- Vertebral canal continuation — Sacral Canal
- Unfused S4–S5 lamina — Sacral hiatus
- S5 inferior articular process — Sacral cornua
- Superior anteriorly projecting border — Sacral promontory
- Articulates with ilia — Auricular surface
- Ligament attachments — Sacral tuberosity
- Anterior concavity toward pelvic cavity

Coccygeal Vertebrae
- 4 fused vertebrae — Fusion starts in 20s
- Transverse processes

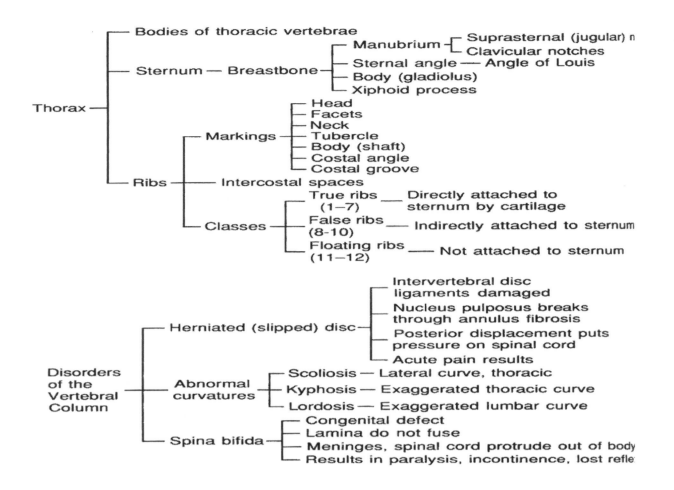

```
Thorax ─┬─ Bodies of thoracic vertebrae
        │
        ├─ Sternum ── Breastbone ─┬─ Manubrium ─┬─ Suprasternal (jugular) n
        │                         │             └─ Clavicular notches
        │                         ├─ Sternal angle ── Angle of Louis
        │                         ├─ Body (gladiolus)
        │                         └─ Xiphoid process
        │
        └─ Ribs ─┬─ Markings ─┬─ Head
                 │            ├─ Facets
                 │            ├─ Neck
                 │            ├─ Tubercle
                 │            ├─ Body (shaft)
                 │            ├─ Costal angle
                 │            └─ Costal groove
                 │
                 ├─ Intercostal spaces
                 │
                 └─ Classes ─┬─ True ribs (1–7) ── Directly attached to sternum by cartilage
                             ├─ False ribs (8-10) ── Indirectly attached to sternum
                             └─ Floating ribs (11–12) ── Not attached to sternum
```

```
Disorders
of the        ─┬─ Herniated (slipped) disc ─┬─ Intervertebral disc ligaments damaged
Vertebral      │                            ├─ Nucleus pulposus breaks through annulus fibrosis
Column         │                            ├─ Posterior displacement puts pressure on spinal cord
               │                            └─ Acute pain results
               │
               ├─ Abnormal curvatures ─┬─ Scoliosis ── Lateral curve, thoracic
               │                       ├─ Kyphosis ── Exaggerated thoracic curve
               │                       └─ Lordosis ── Exaggerated lumbar curve
               │
               └─ Spina bifida ─┬─ Congenital defect
                                ├─ Lamina do not fuse
                                ├─ Meninges, spinal cord protrude out of body
                                └─ Results in paralysis, incontinence, lost refle
```

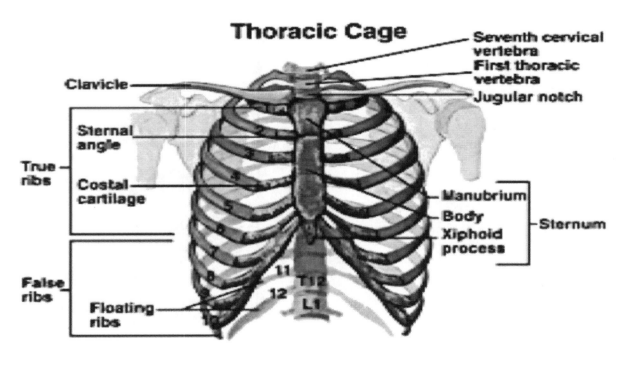

Thoracic Cage

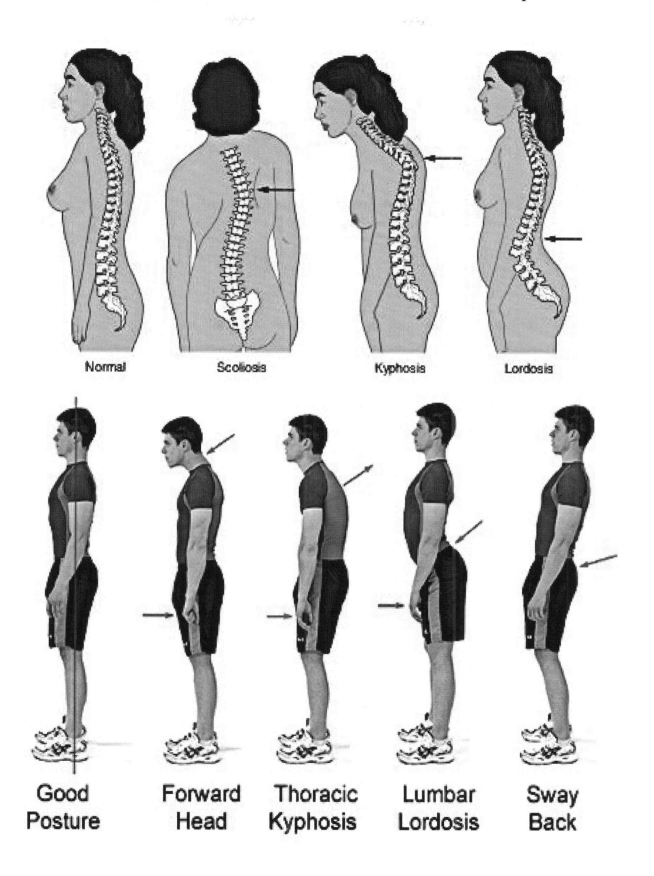

Normal   Scoliosis   Kyphosis   Lordosis

| Good Posture | Forward Head | Thoracic Kyphosis | Lumbar Lordosis | Sway Back |

CHAPTER EIGHT

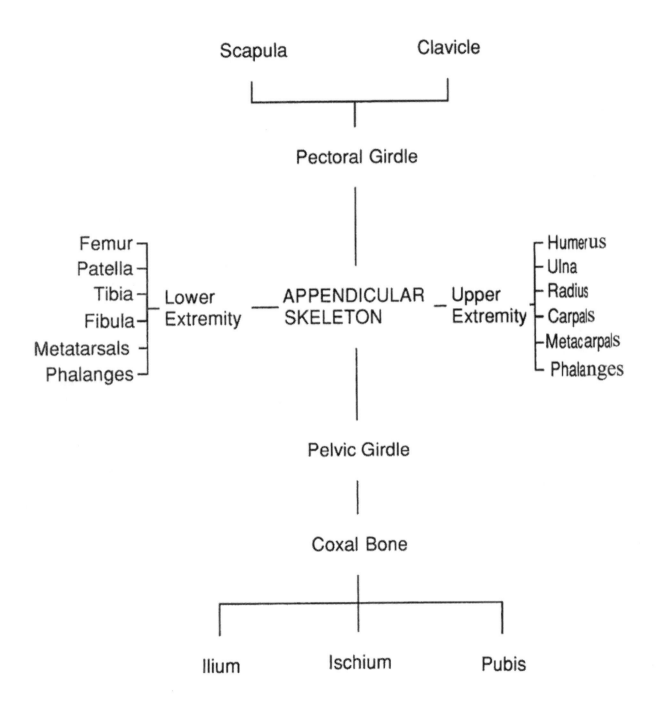

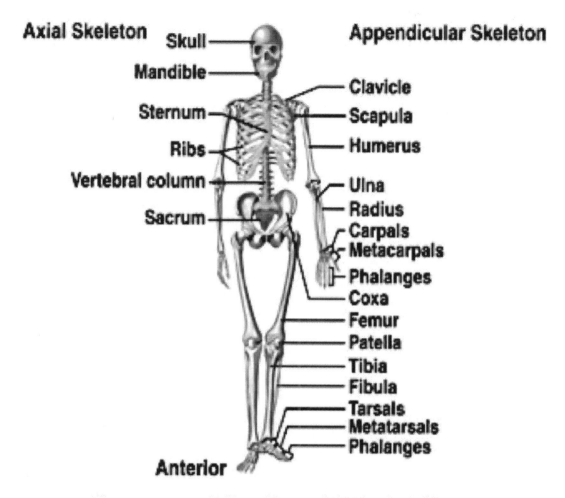

Axial Skeleton · Skull · Appendicular Skeleton
Mandible
Sternum — Clavicle
Ribs — Scapula
Vertebral column — Humerus
Sacrum — Ulna
— Radius
— Carpals
— Metacarpals
— Phalanges
— Coxa
— Femur
— Patella
— Tibia
— Fibula
— Tarsals
— Metatarsals
— Phalanges
Anterior

Appendicular Skeleton

Upper Extremity
* Humerus
* Radius
* Ulna
* Carpals
  - Metacarpals
  - Phalanges

Lower Extremity
Femur
Patella
Tibia
Fibula
Tarsals
　　Metatarsals
　　Phalanges

Pectoral Girdles
* Clavicle
* Scapula

Pelvic Girdles
Os Coxae (Innominate bone)
—Ilium　　& Pubis
—Ischium

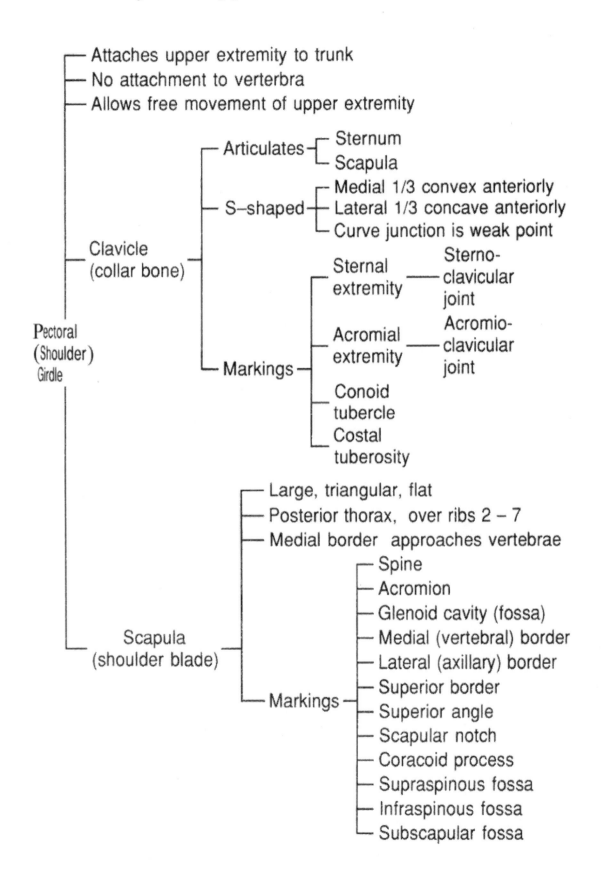

Pectoral (Shoulder) Girdle
— Attaches upper extremity to trunk
— No attachment to verterbra
— Allows free movement of upper extremity

Clavicle (collar bone)
- Articulates
  - Sternum
  - Scapula
- S–shaped
  - Medial 1/3 convex anteriorly
  - Lateral 1/3 concave anteriorly
  - Curve junction is weak point
- Markings
  - Sternal extremity — Sterno-clavicular joint
  - Acromial extremity — Acromio-clavicular joint
  - Conoid tubercle
  - Costal tuberosity

Scapula (shoulder blade)
- Large, triangular, flat
- Posterior thorax, over ribs 2 – 7
- Medial border approaches vertebrae
- Markings
  - Spine
  - Acromion
  - Glenoid cavity (fossa)
  - Medial (vertebral) border
  - Lateral (axillary) border
  - Superior border
  - Superior angle
  - Scapular notch
  - Coracoid process
  - Supraspinous fossa
  - Infraspinous fossa
  - Subscapular fossa

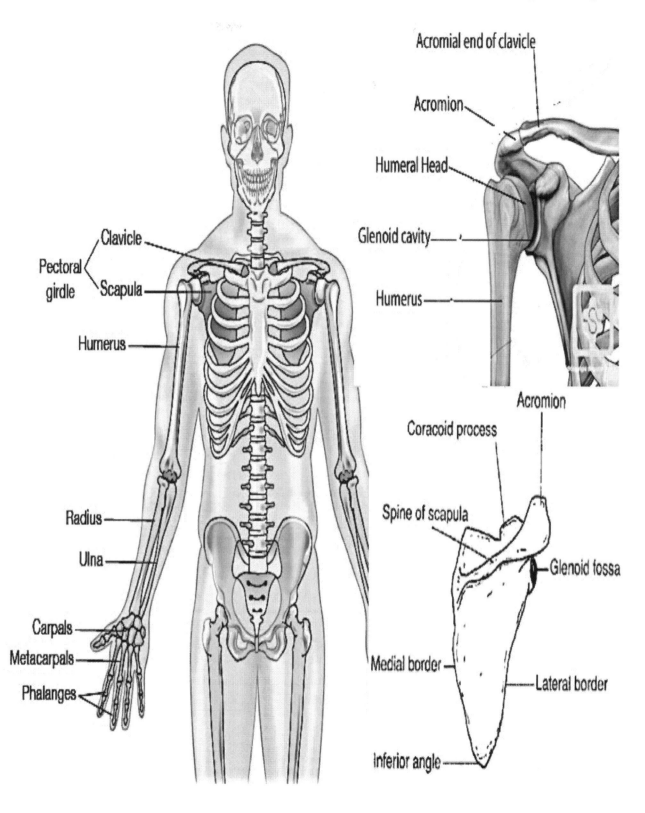

Acromial end of clavicle

Acromion

Humeral Head

Glenoid cavity

Humerus

Clavicle

Pectoral girdle

Scapula

Humerus

Radius

Ulna

Carpals

Metacarpals

Phalanges

Coracoid process

Acromion

Spine of scapula

Glenoid fossa

Medial border

Lateral border

Inferior angle

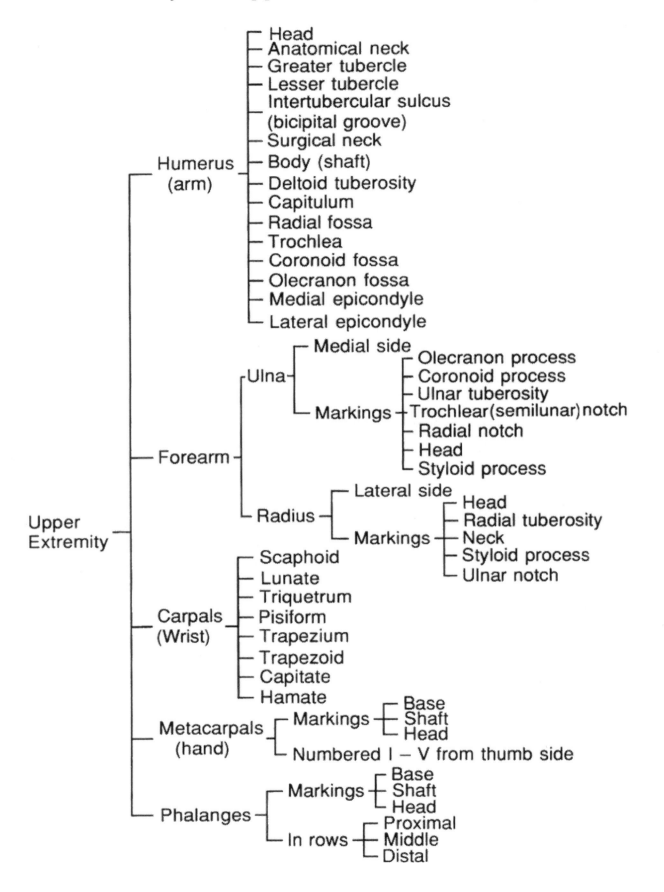

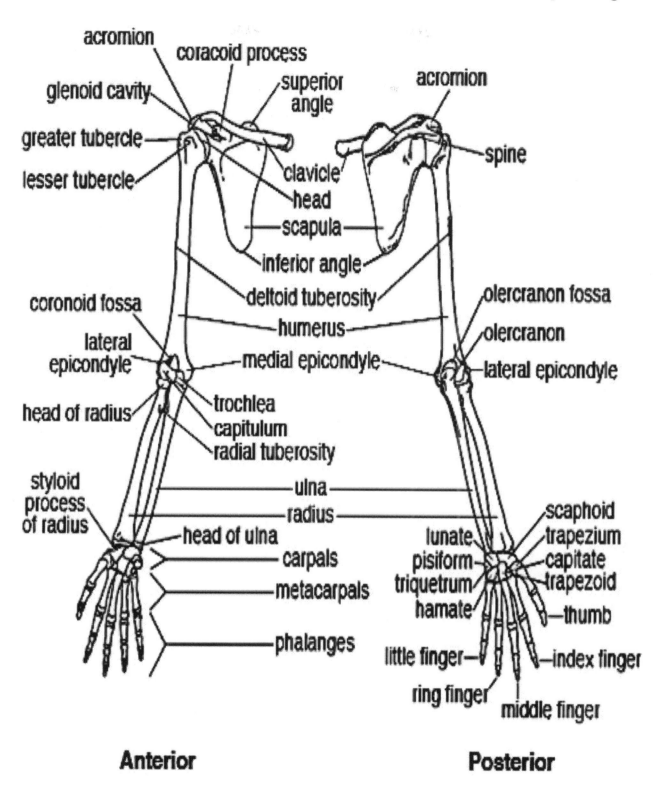

acromion

coracoid process

glenoid cavity

superior angle

greater tubercle

lesser tubercle

clavicle

head

scapula

acromion

spine

inferior angle

deltoid tuberosity

coronoid fossa

humerus

olercranon fossa

olercranon

lateral epicondyle

medial epicondyle

lateral epicondyle

head of radius

trochlea

capitulum

radial tuberosity

styloid process of radius

ulna

radius

head of ulna

carpals

metacarpals

phalanges

scaphoid

trapezium

lunate

capitate

pisiform

trapezoid

triquetrum

hamate

thumb

little finger

index finger

ring finger

middle finger

Anterior   **Posterior**

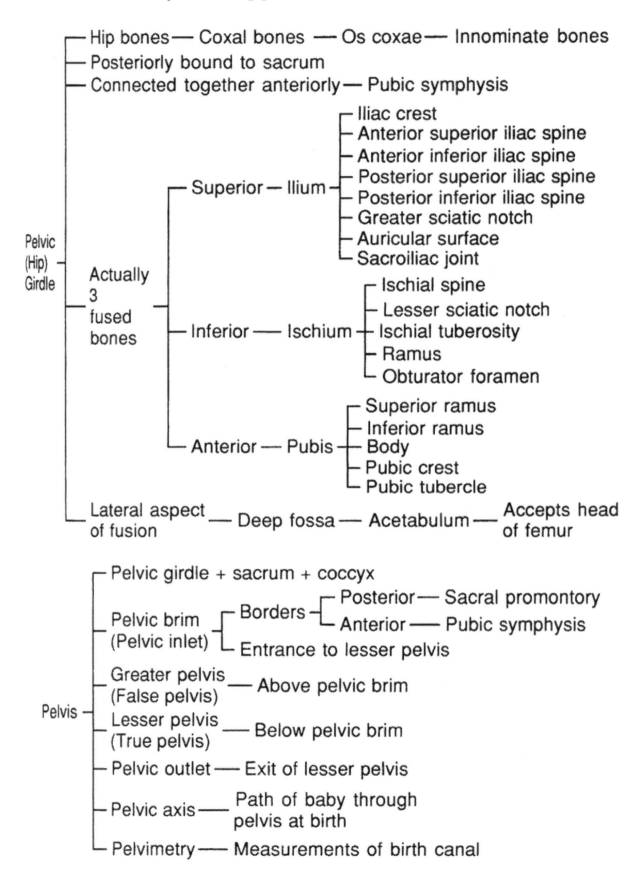

- Pelvic (Hip) Girdle
  - Hip bones — Coxal bones — Os coxae — Innominate bones
  - Posteriorly bound to sacrum
  - Connected together anteriorly — Pubic symphysis
  - Actually 3 fused bones
    - Superior — Ilium
      - Iliac crest
      - Anterior superior iliac spine
      - Anterior inferior iliac spine
      - Posterior superior iliac spine
      - Posterior inferior iliac spine
      - Greater sciatic notch
      - Auricular surface
      - Sacroiliac joint
    - Inferior — Ischium
      - Ischial spine
      - Lesser sciatic notch
      - Ischial tuberosity
      - Ramus
      - Obturator foramen
    - Anterior — Pubis
      - Superior ramus
      - Inferior ramus
      - Body
      - Pubic crest
      - Pubic tubercle
  - Lateral aspect of fusion — Deep fossa — Acetabulum — Accepts head of femur

- Pelvis
  - Pelvic girdle + sacrum + coccyx
  - Pelvic brim (Pelvic inlet)
    - Borders
      - Posterior — Sacral promontory
      - Anterior — Pubic symphysis
    - Entrance to lesser pelvis
  - Greater pelvis (False pelvis) — Above pelvic brim
  - Lesser pelvis (True pelvis) — Below pelvic brim
  - Pelvic outlet — Exit of lesser pelvis
  - Pelvic axis — Path of baby through pelvis at birth
  - Pelvimetry — Measurements of birth canal

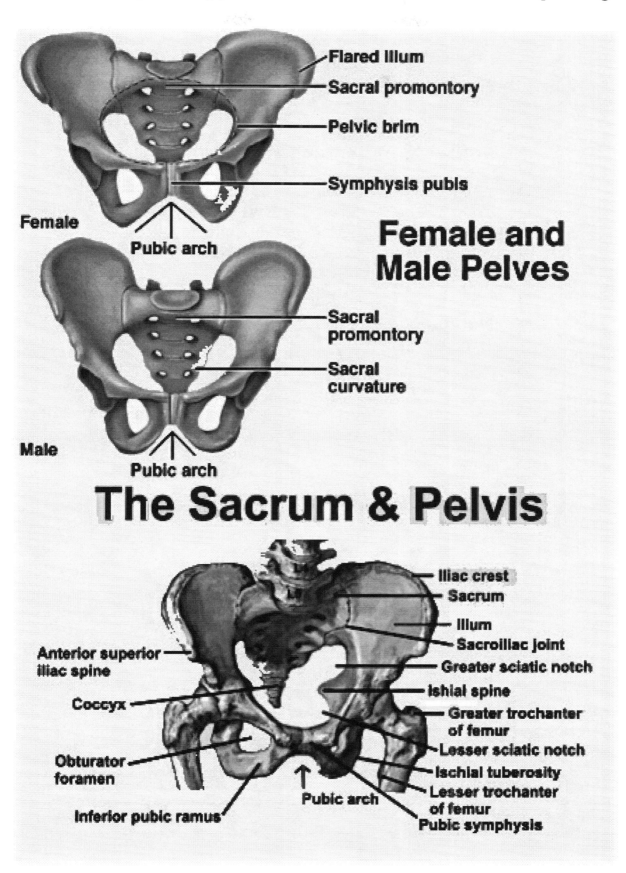

Flared Ilium
Sacral promontory
Pelvic brim
Symphysis pubis

Female

Pubic arch

Female and Male Pelves

Sacral promontory
Sacral curvature

Male

Pubic arch

The Sacrum & Pelvis

Iliac crest
Sacrum
Ilium
Sacroiliac joint
Greater sciatic notch
Ischial spine
Greater trochanter of femur
Lesser sciatic notch
Ischial tuberosity
Lesser trochanter of femur
Pubic symphysis

Anterior superior iliac spine
Coccyx
Obturator foramen
Inferior pubic ramus
Pubic arch

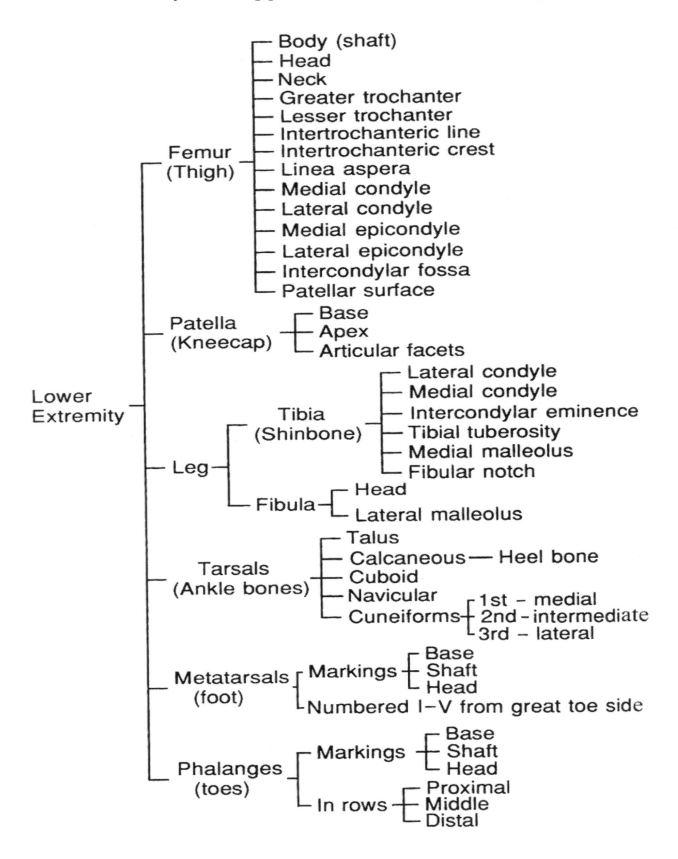

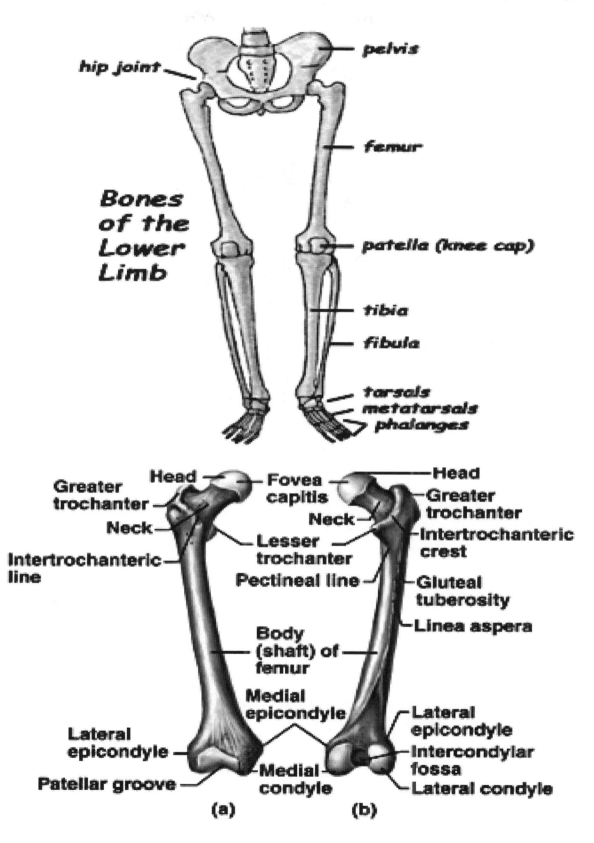

hip joint

pelvis

Bones
of the
Lower
Limb

femur

patella (knee cap)

tibia

fibula

tarsals
metatarsals
phalanges

Greater
trochanter

Head

Fovea
capitis

Head

Greater
trochanter

Neck

Neck

Intertrochanteric
crest

Intertrochanteric
line

Lesser
trochanter

Pectineal line

Gluteal
tuberosity

Linea aspera

Body
(shaft) of
femur

Medial
epicondyle

Lateral
epicondyle

Patellar groove

Medial
condyle

(a)

Lateral
epicondyle

Intercondylar
fossa

Lateral condyle

(b)

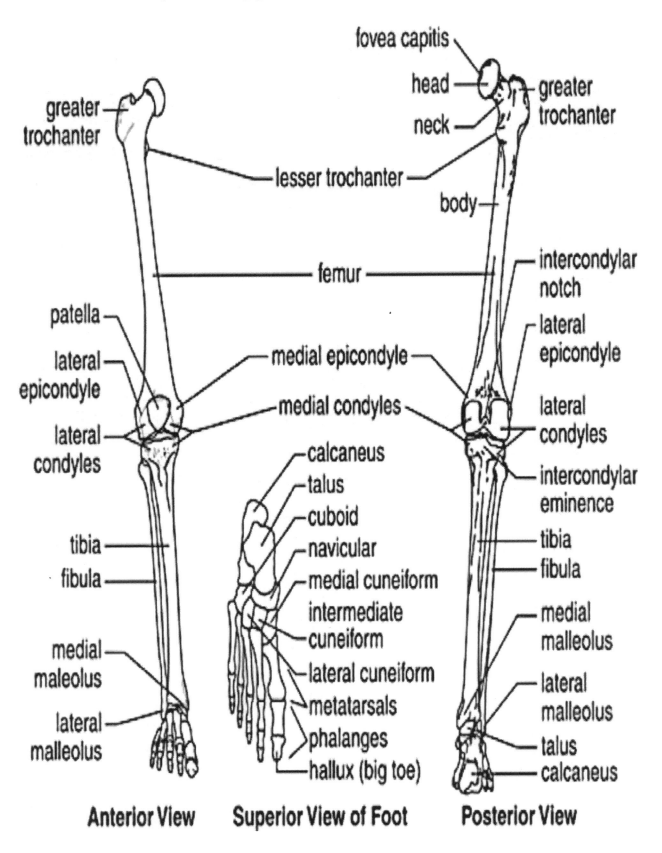

fovea capitis

head

greater trochanter

neck

greater trochanter

lesser trochanter

body

femur

intercondylar notch

patella

lateral epicondyle

lateral epicondyle

medial epicondyle

lateral condyles

lateral condyles

medial condyles

calcaneus

intercondylar eminence

talus

cuboid

tibia

navicular

fibula

tibia

medial cuneiform

fibula

intermediate cuneiform

medial maleolus

lateral cuneiform

medial maleolus

lateral malleolus

metatarsals

lateral malleolus

phalanges

talus

hallux (big toe)

calcaneus

Anterior View   Superior View of Foot   Posterior View

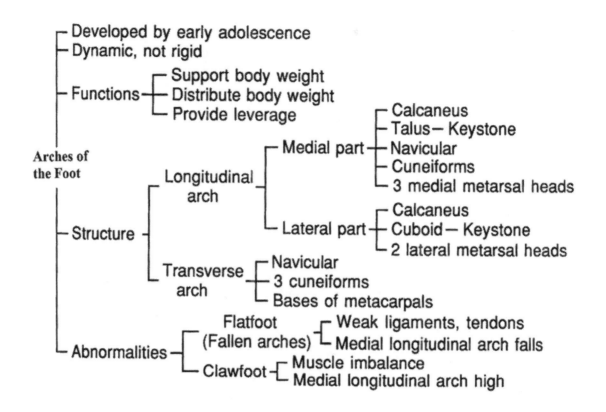

Arches of the Foot
- Developed by early adolescence
- Dynamic, not rigid
- Functions
  - Support body weight
  - Distribute body weight
  - Provide leverage
- Structure
  - Longitudinal arch
    - Medial part
      - Calcaneus
      - Talus — Keystone
      - Navicular
      - Cuneiforms
      - 3 medial metarsal heads
    - Lateral part
      - Calcaneus
      - Cuboid — Keystone
      - 2 lateral metarsal heads
  - Transverse arch
    - Navicular
    - 3 cuneiforms
    - Bases of metacarpals
- Abnormalities
  - Flatfoot (Fallen arches)
    - Weak ligaments, tendons
    - Medial longitudinal arch falls
  - Clawfoot
    - Muscle imbalance
    - Medial longitudinal arch high

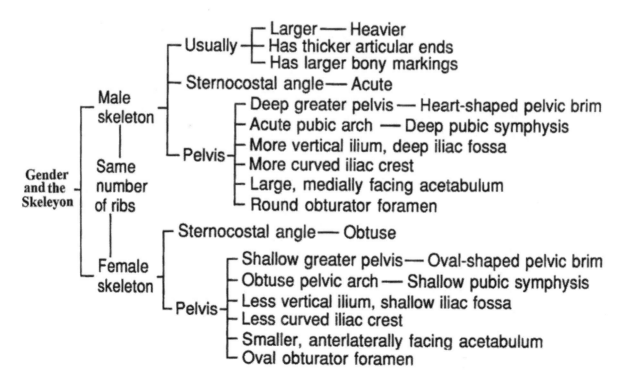

Gender and the Skeleyon
- Male skeleton
  - Usually
    - Larger — Heavier
    - Has thicker articular ends
    - Has larger bony markings
  - Sternocostal angle — Acute
  - Pelvis
    - Deep greater pelvis — Heart-shaped pelvic brim
    - Acute pubic arch — Deep pubic symphysis
    - More vertical ilium, deep iliac fossa
    - More curved iliac crest
    - Large, medially facing acetabulum
    - Round obturator foramen
- Same number of ribs
- Female skeleton
  - Sternocostal angle — Obtuse
  - Pelvis
    - Shallow greater pelvis — Oval-shaped pelvic brim
    - Obtuse pelvic arch — Shallow pubic symphysis
    - Less vertical ilium, shallow iliac fossa
    - Less curved iliac crest
    - Smaller, anterlaterally facing acetabulum
    - Oval obturator foramen

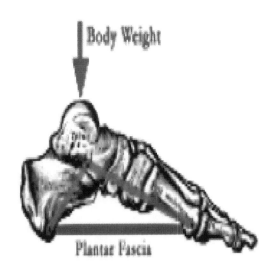

Body Weight

Plantar Fascia

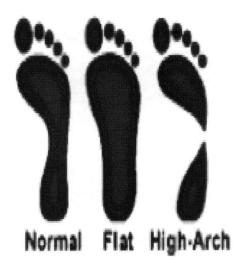

Normal   Flat   High-Arch

Quick Test for Weak Arch Muscles

Step 1

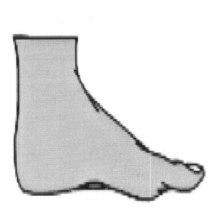

Start with your foot lifted off the ground

Step 2

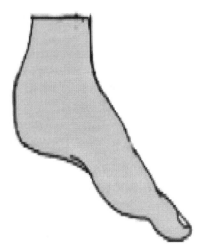

Point your foot down

Step 3

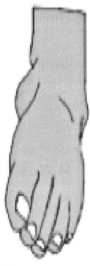

Turn your foot inward

CHAPTER NINE

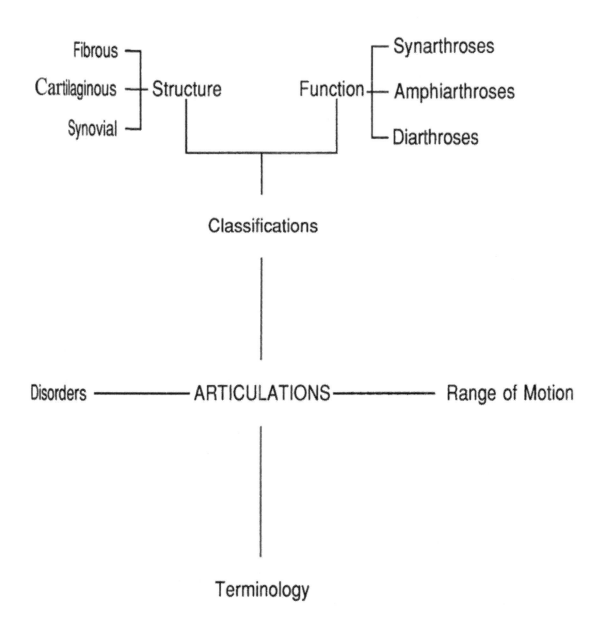

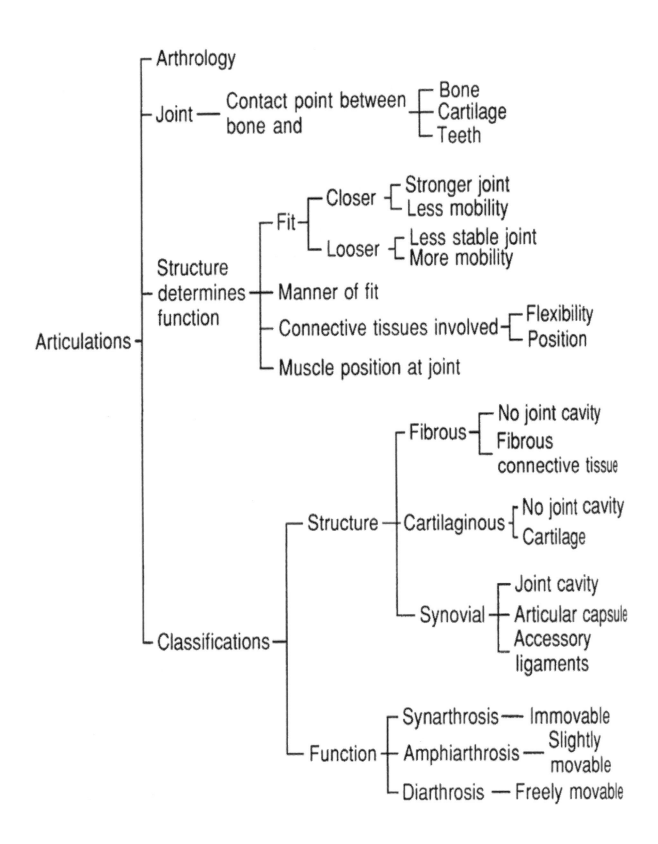

Types of Human Joints

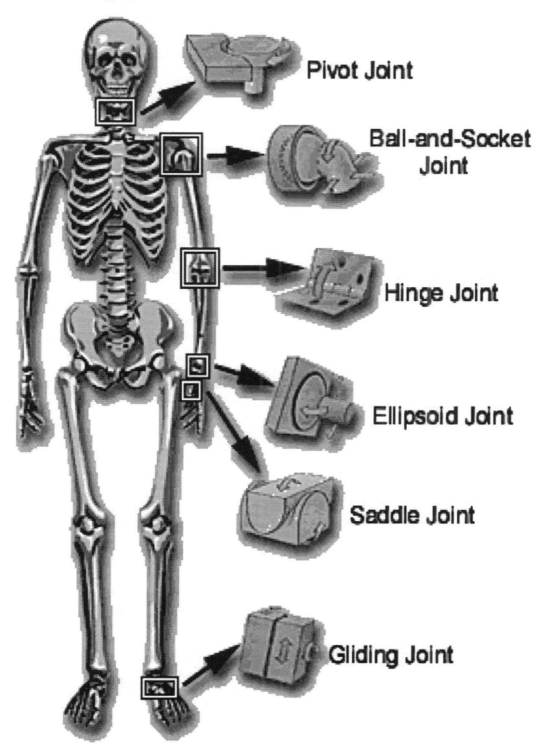

Pivot Joint

Ball-and-Socket Joint

Hinge Joint

Ellipsoid Joint

Saddle Joint

Gliding Joint

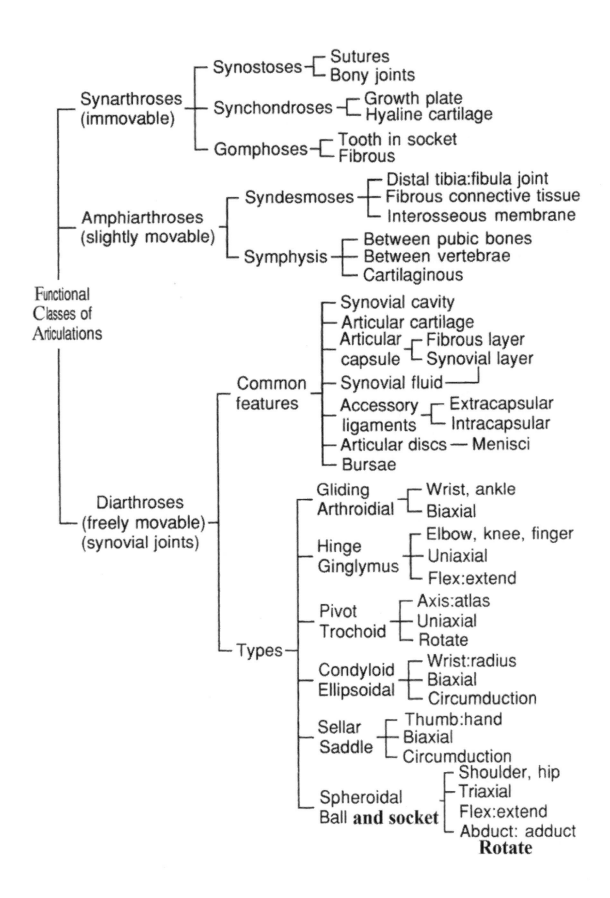

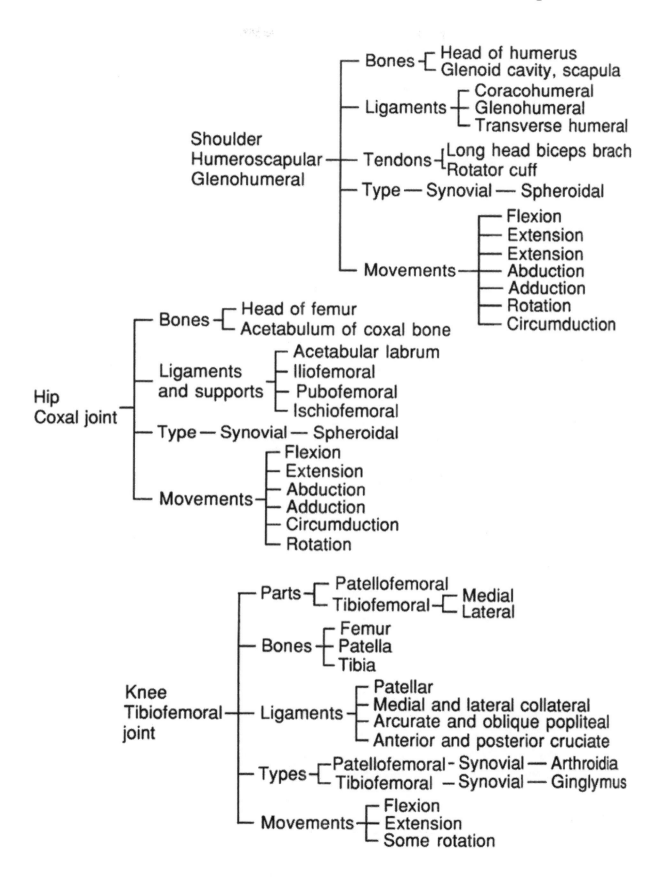

Shoulder
Humeroscapular
Glenohumeral

- Bones
  - Head of humerus
  - Glenoid cavity, scapula
- Ligaments
  - Coracohumeral
  - Glenohumeral
  - Transverse humeral
- Tendons
  - Long head biceps brach
  - Rotator cuff
- Type — Synovial — Spheroidal
- Movements
  - Flexion
  - Extension
  - Extension
  - Abduction
  - Adduction
  - Rotation
  - Circumduction

Hip
Coxal joint

- Bones
  - Head of femur
  - Acetabulum of coxal bone
- Ligaments and supports
  - Acetabular labrum
  - Iliofemoral
  - Pubofemoral
  - Ischiofemoral
- Type — Synovial — Spheroidal
- Movements
  - Flexion
  - Extension
  - Abduction
  - Adduction
  - Circumduction
  - Rotation

Knee
Tibiofemoral
joint

- Parts
  - Patellofemoral
  - Tibiofemoral
    - Medial
    - Lateral
- Bones
  - Femur
  - Patella
  - Tibia
- Ligaments
  - Patellar
  - Medial and lateral collateral
  - Arcurate and oblique popliteal
  - Anterior and posterior cruciate
- Types
  - Patellofemoral - Synovial — Arthroidia
  - Tibiofemoral - Synovial — Ginglymus
- Movements
  - Flexion
  - Extension
  - Some rotation

Types of Joints

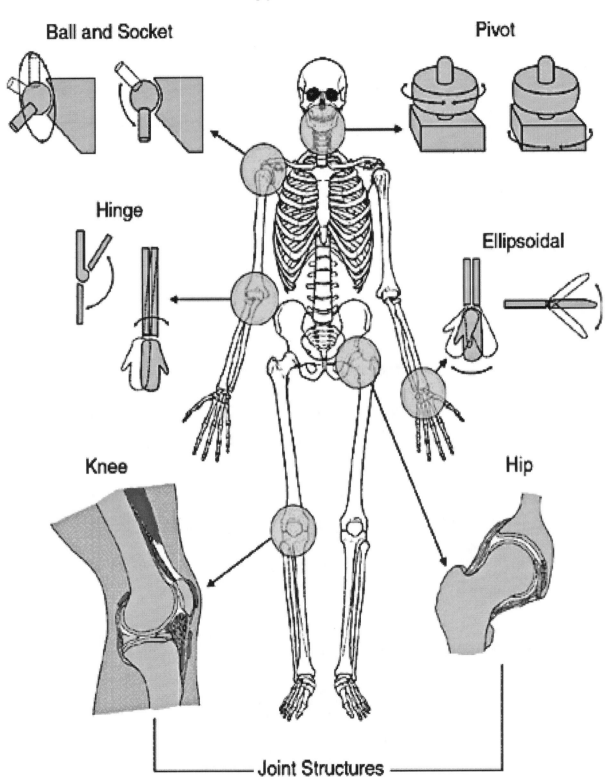

Ball and Socket

Pivot

Hinge

Ellipsoidal

Knee

Hip

Joint Structures

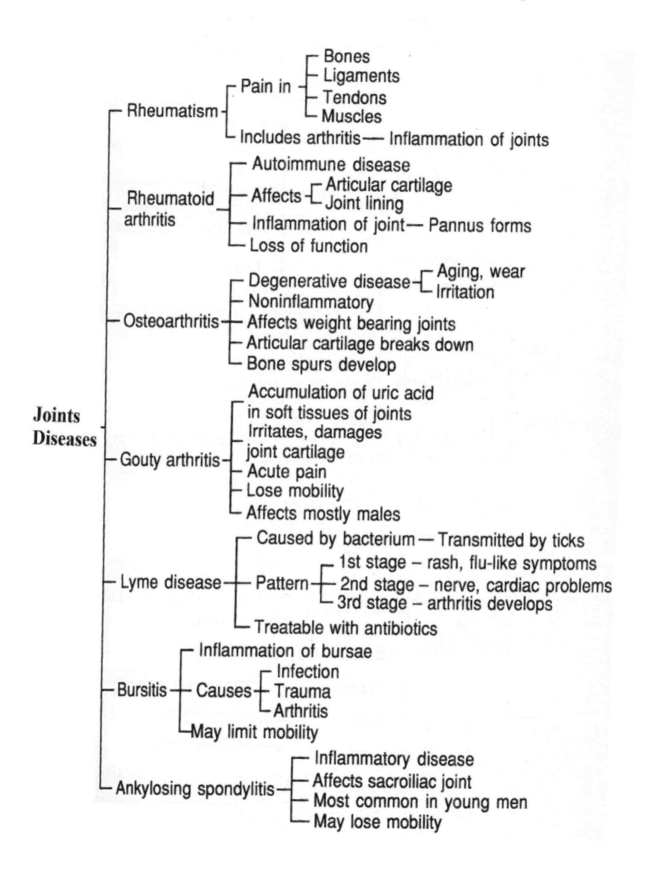

Rheumatoid Arthritis Joint

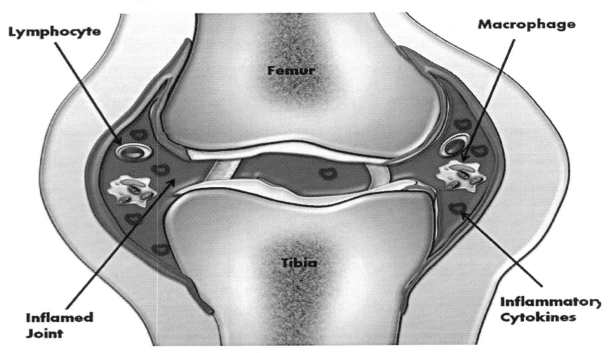

Lymphocyte

Macrophage

Femur

Tibia

Inflamed Joint

Inflammatory Cytokines

In Rheumatoid Arthritis, joints are inflamed due to immune reactions which results swelling, pain and loss of function. This inflamed condition can cause joint destruction and deformity.

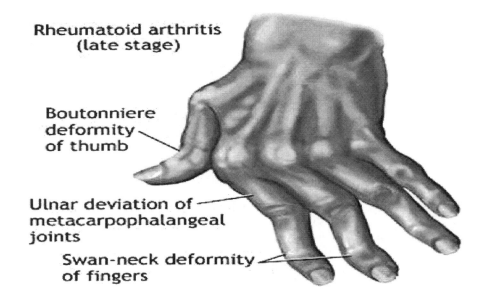

Rheumatoid arthritis (late stage)

Boutonniere deformity of thumb

Ulnar deviation of metacarpophalangeal joints

Swan-neck deformity of fingers

Polyarthritis

- This is the most confusing of the major criteria and probably leads to more diagnostic errors than any of the other manifestations. Rheumatic arthritis is more common in older children.
- The arthritis develops acutely (hours to overnight).
- The arthritis is migratory and affects several different large joints: the elbows, knees, ankles, and wrists. It rarely occurs in the fingers, toes, or spine.
- The involved joints are red, hot, and swollen.
- The involved joints are so acutely inflamed, swollen and tender that even a mere touch or the weight of a bed sheet over the joint causes unbearable pain.
- Movement of the joint is extremely painful.

Jones criteria for the diagnosis of acute rheumatic fever.

Diagnosis requires two major manifestations or one major and two minor manifestations along with evidence of preceding *Streptococcus pyogenes* infection. The presence of chorea or carditis may not require the addition of evidence of preceding *S. pyogenes* infection. Patients for whom a recurrent episode is being assessed may require only one major or several minor manifestations along with evidence of preceding *S. pyogenes* infection. Evidence of preceding *S. pyogenes* infection may include a positive throat swab or a raised or rising antistreptolysin O titer.

Major manifestations	Minor manifestations
• Carditis	• Arthralgia
• Polyarthritis	• Fever
• Chorea	• Elevated ESR or CRP
• Erythema marginatum	• EKG evidence of a prolonged PR interval
• Subcutaneous nodules	

Polyarthris in Rheumatic Fever

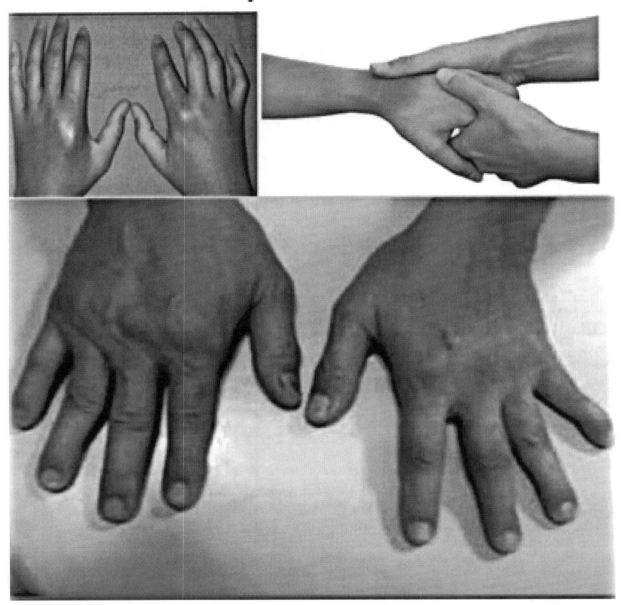

Polyarthris in Rheumatic Fever

AFFECTING LARGE JOINTS

ARTHRITIS IS MYGRATORY

PROMPT RESPONSE TO ANTIINFLAMMTORY THERAPY

SUBSIDES WITHOUT RESIDUAL DEFORMITY

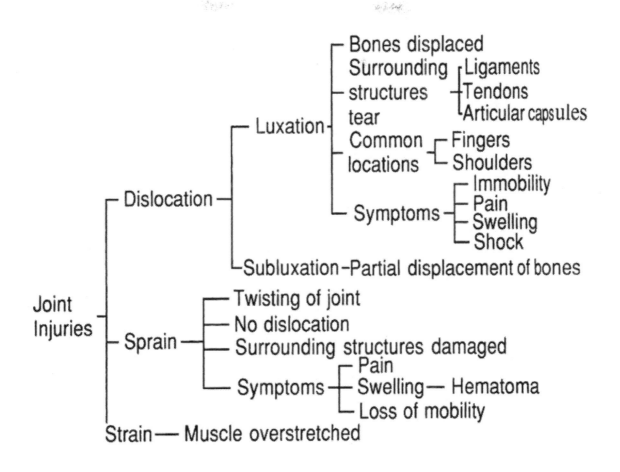

Joint Injuries
- Dislocation
  - Luxation
    - Bones displaced
    - Surrounding structures tear
      - Ligaments
      - Tendons
      - Articular capsules
    - Common locations
      - Fingers
      - Shoulders
    - Symptoms
      - Immobility
      - Pain
      - Swelling
      - Shock
  - Subluxation – Partial displacement of bones
- Sprain
  - Twisting of joint
  - No dislocation
  - Surrounding structures damaged
  - Symptoms
    - Pain
    - Swelling — Hematoma
    - Loss of mobility
- Strain — Muscle overstretched

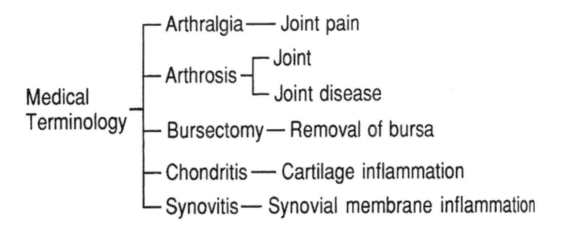

Medical Terminology
- Arthralgia — Joint pain
- Arthrosis
  - Joint
  - Joint disease
- Bursectomy — Removal of bursa
- Chondritis — Cartilage inflammation
- Synovitis — Synovial membrane inflammation

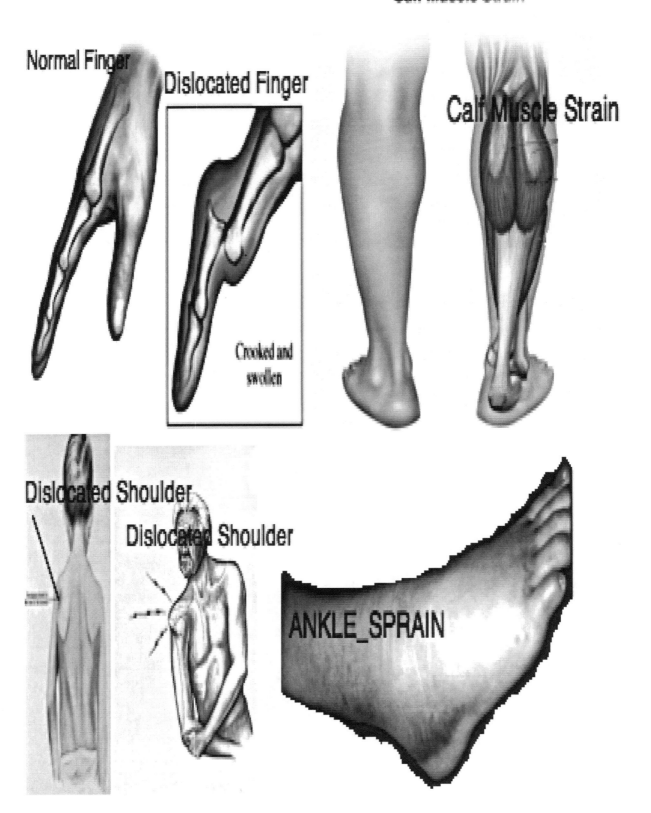

CHAPTER TEN

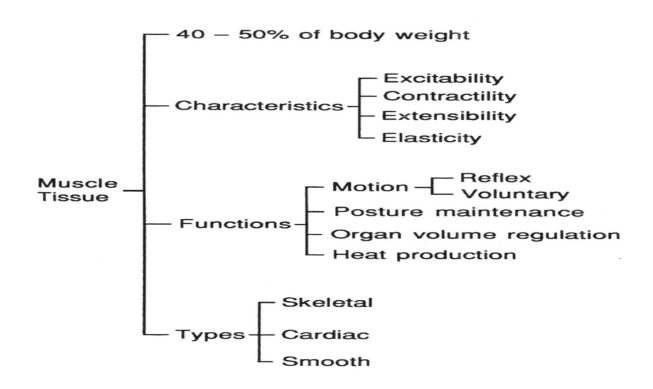

Muscle Tissue
- 40 — 50% of body weight
- Characteristics
  - Excitability
  - Contractility
  - Extensibility
  - Elasticity
- Functions
  - Motion
    - Reflex
    - Voluntary
  - Posture maintenance
  - Organ volume regulation
  - Heat production
- Types
  - Skeletal
  - Cardiac
  - Smooth

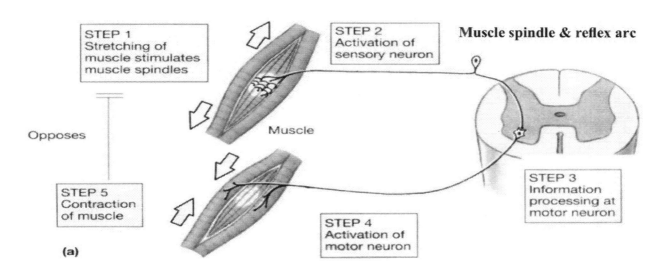

Muscle spindle & reflex arc

STEP 1
Stretching of muscle stimulates muscle spindles

STEP 2
Activation of sensory neuron

STEP 3
Information processing at motor neuron

STEP 4
Activation of motor neuron

STEP 5
Contraction of muscle

Opposes

Muscle

(a)

Muscle tissue are three types:

(1) 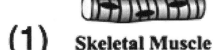 **Skeletal Muscle**

(2) 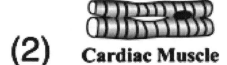 **Cardiac Muscle**

(3) 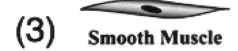 **Smooth Muscle**

Muscle tissue is composed of cells that have the special ability to shorten or contract in order to produce movement of the body parts. The tissue is highly cellular and is well supplied with blood vessels. The cells are long and slender so they are sometimes called muscle fibers, and these are usually arranged in bundles or layers that are surrounded by connective tissue. Actin and myosin are contractile proteins in muscle tissue.

Muscle tissue can be categorized into skeletal muscle tissue, smooth muscle tissue, and cardiac muscle tissue.

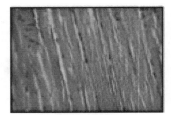 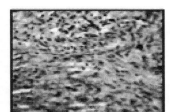 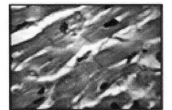

Skeletal muscle   Smooth muscle   Cardiac muscle

Skeletal muscle fibers are cylindrical, multinucleated, striated, and under voluntary control. Smooth muscle cells are spindle shaped, have a single, centrally located nucleus, and lack striations. They are called involuntary muscles. Cardiac muscle has branching fibers, one nucleus per cell, striations, and intercalated disks. Its contraction is not under voluntary control.

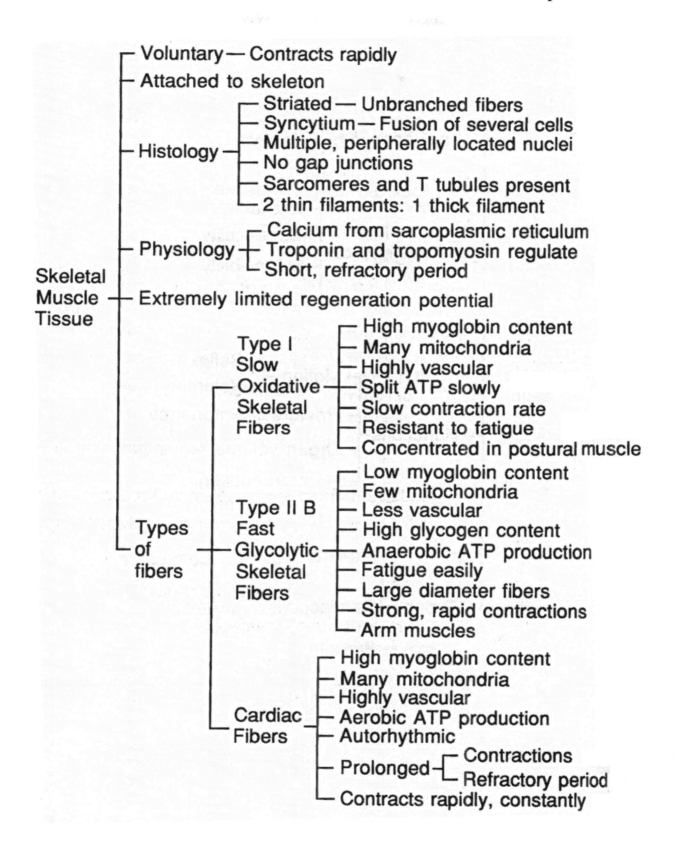

Skeletal Muscle Tissue
- Voluntary — Contracts rapidly
- Attached to skeleton
- Histology
  - Striated — Unbranched fibers
  - Syncytium — Fusion of several cells
  - Multiple, peripherally located nuclei
  - No gap junctions
  - Sarcomeres and T tubules present
  - 2 thin filaments: 1 thick filament
- Physiology
  - Calcium from sarcoplasmic reticulum
  - Troponin and tropomyosin regulate
  - Short, refractory period
- Extremely limited regeneration potential
- Types of fibers
  - Type I Slow Oxidative Skeletal Fibers
    - High myoglobin content
    - Many mitochondria
    - Highly vascular
    - Split ATP slowly
    - Slow contraction rate
    - Resistant to fatigue
    - Concentrated in postural muscle
  - Type II B Fast Glycolytic Skeletal Fibers
    - Low myoglobin content
    - Few mitochondria
    - Less vascular
    - High glycogen content
    - Anaerobic ATP production
    - Fatigue easily
    - Large diameter fibers
    - Strong, rapid contractions
    - Arm muscles
  - Cardiac Fibers
    - High myoglobin content
    - Many mitochondria
    - Highly vascular
    - Aerobic ATP production
    - Autorhythmic
    - Prolonged
      - Contractions
      - Refractory period
    - Contracts rapidly, constantly

Skeletal Muscle

Skeletal muscle cells are long multi-nucleated cylinders, separated by connective tissue. Each independent cell is stimulated by a branch from a motor neuron

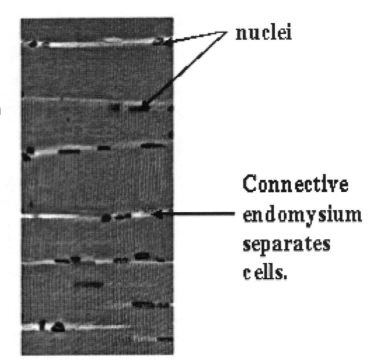

nuclei

Connective endomysium separates cells.

Structure of the Skeletal Muscle

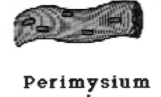

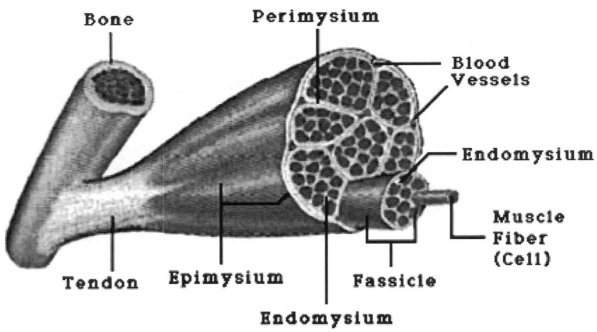

Bone

Perimysium

Blood Vessels

Endomysium

Muscle Fiber (Cell)

Tendon   Epimysium   Fassicle

Endomysium

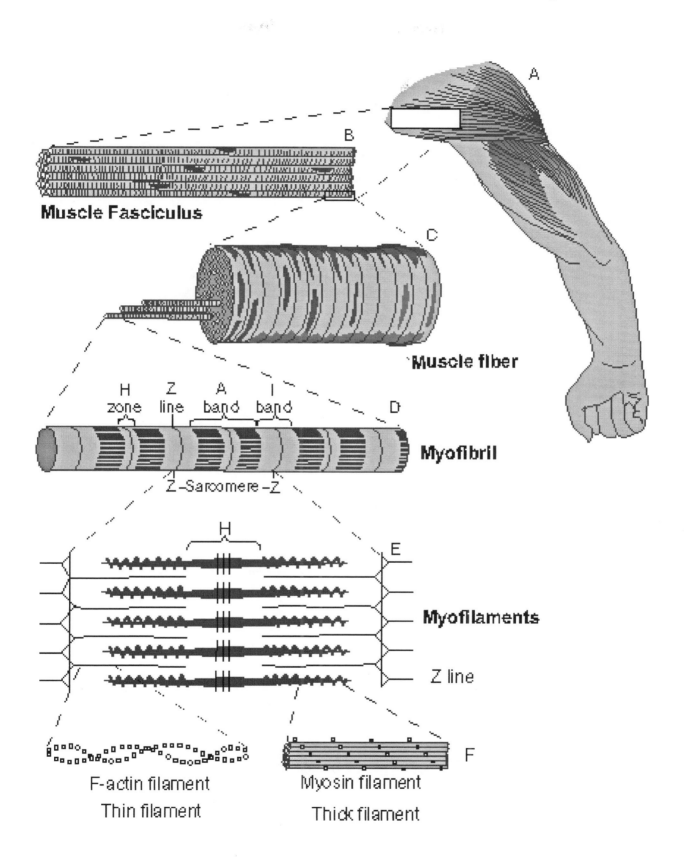

A

B
Muscle Fasciculus

C
Muscle fiber

H   Z   A   I
zone   line   band   band   D

Myofibril

Z–Sarcomere–Z

H

E

Myofilaments

Z line

F-actin filament
Thin filament

Myosin filament   F
Thick filament

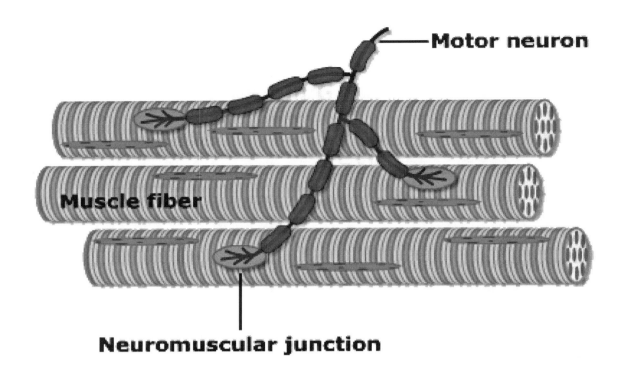

Motor neuron

Muscle fiber

Neuromuscular junction

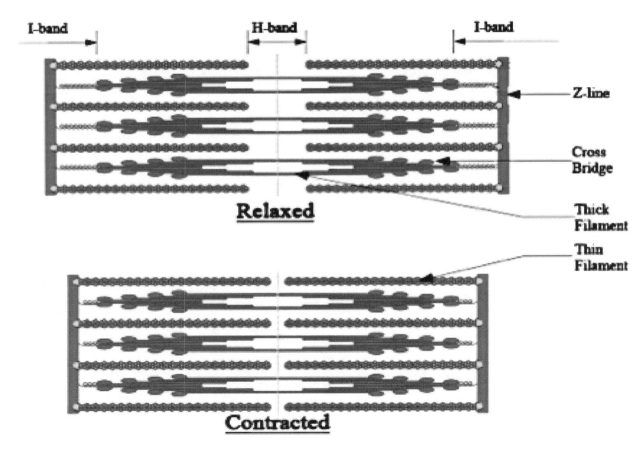

I-band

H-band

I-band

Z-line

Cross Bridge

Thick Filament

Thin Filament

Relaxed

Contracted

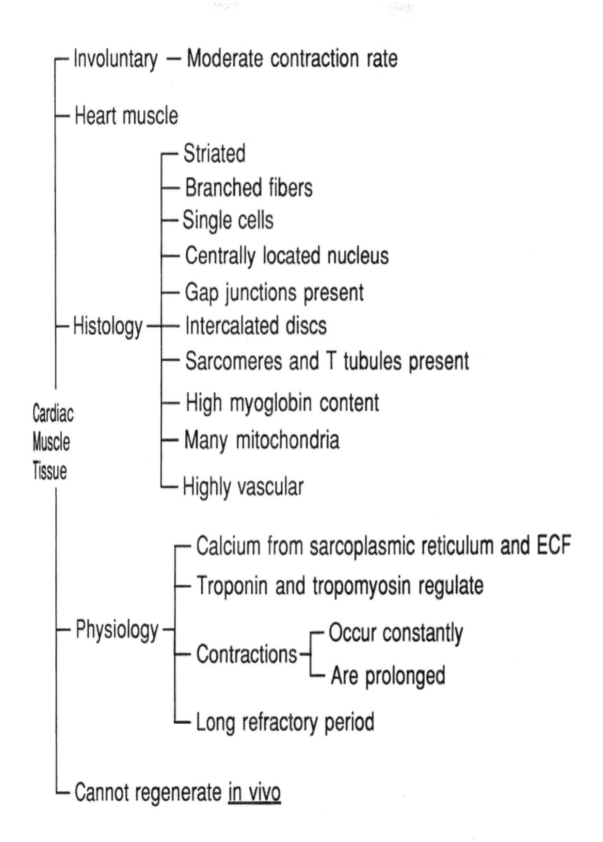

Cardiac Muscle Tissue

- Involuntary — Moderate contraction rate
- Heart muscle
- Histology
  - Striated
  - Branched fibers
  - Single cells
  - Centrally located nucleus
  - Gap junctions present
  - Intercalated discs
  - Sarcomeres and T tubules present
  - High myoglobin content
  - Many mitochondria
  - Highly vascular
- Physiology
  - Calcium from sarcoplasmic reticulum and ECF
  - Troponin and tropomyosin regulate
  - Contractions
    - Occur constantly
    - Are prolonged
  - Long refractory period
- Cannot regenerate _in vivo_

Cardiac Muscle Structure

Intercalated disks are anchoring structures containing gap junctions

Cardiac muscle cells are faintly striated, branching, mononucleated cells, which connect by means of intercalated disks to form a functional network.

The action potential travels through all cells connected together forming a functional <u>syncytium</u> in which cells function as a unit.

nucleus

Cardiac Muscle Cells (Myocytes)

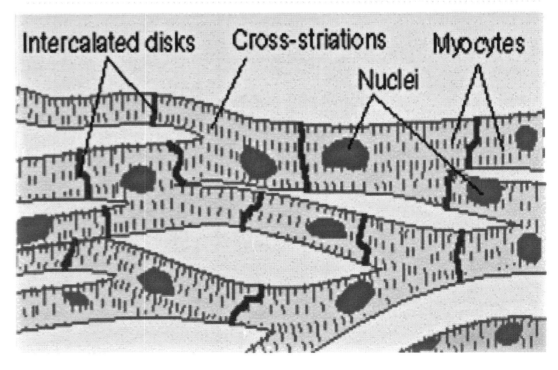

Intercalated disks   Cross-striations   Myocytes   Nuclei

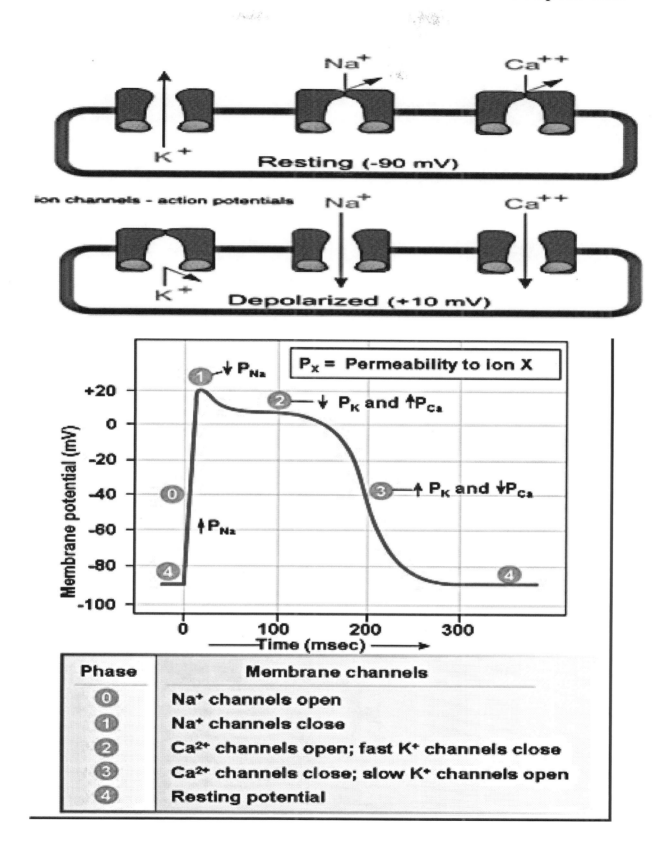

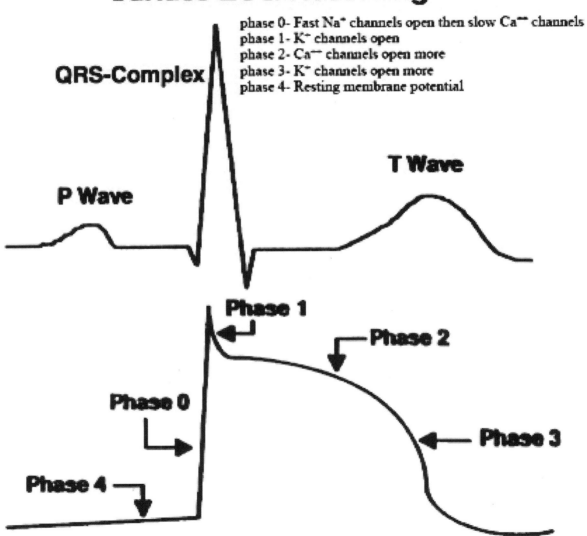

Intracellular
Na⁺ 10 mM
K⁺ 150 mM
Ca⁺⁺ 10⁻⁷ mM
Negatively charged proteins – large
Chloride – low concentration

Extracellular
Na⁺ 140 mM
K⁺ 4 mM
Ca⁺⁺ 2 mM
Chloride – high conc.

Surface ECG Recording

phase 0- Fast Na⁺ channels open then slow Ca⁺⁺ channels
phase 1- K⁺ channels open
phase 2- Ca⁺⁺ channels open more
phase 3- K⁺ channels open more
phase 4- Resting membrane potential

QRS-Complex

P Wave

T Wave

Phase 1

Phase 2

Phase 0

Phase 3

Phase 4

Ventricular Muscle Cell Action Potential

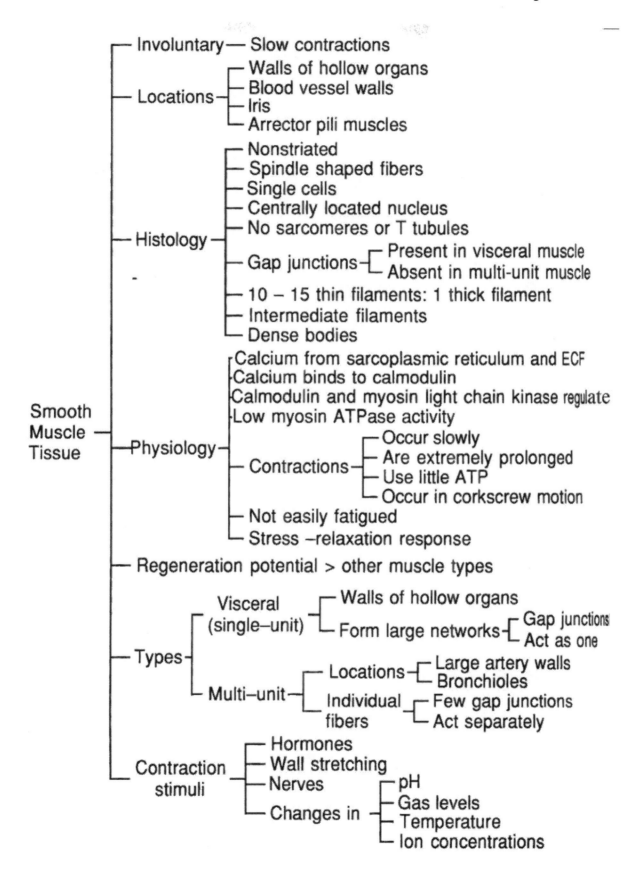

Smooth Muscle Tissue
- Involuntary — Slow contractions
- Locations
  - Walls of hollow organs
  - Blood vessel walls
  - Iris
  - Arrector pili muscles
- Histology
  - Nonstriated
  - Spindle shaped fibers
  - Single cells
  - Centrally located nucleus
  - No sarcomeres or T tubules
  - Gap junctions
    - Present in visceral muscle
    - Absent in multi-unit muscle
  - 10 – 15 thin filaments: 1 thick filament
  - Intermediate filaments
  - Dense bodies
- Physiology
  - Calcium from sarcoplasmic reticulum and ECF
  - Calcium binds to calmodulin
  - Calmodulin and myosin light chain kinase regulate
  - Low myosin ATPase activity
  - Contractions
    - Occur slowly
    - Are extremely prolonged
    - Use little ATP
    - Occur in corkscrew motion
  - Not easily fatigued
  - Stress –relaxation response
- Regeneration potential > other muscle types
- Types
  - Visceral (single–unit)
    - Walls of hollow organs
    - Form large networks
      - Gap junctions
      - Act as one
  - Multi–unit
    - Locations
      - Large artery walls
      - Bronchioles
    - Individual fibers
      - Few gap junctions
      - Act separately
- Contraction stimuli
  - Hormones
  - Wall stretching
  - Nerves
  - Changes in
    - pH
    - Gas levels
    - Temperature
    - Ion concentrations

Smooth Muscle Arrangement in the Gut

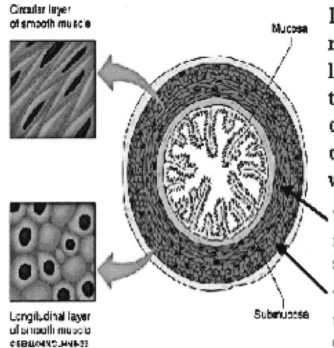

Circular layer
of smooth muscle

Mucosa

Longitudinal layer
of smooth muscle

Submucosa

In the intestine smooth muscle forms two distinct layers, one running along, the other running around the organ. Together these layers cause wave-like peristalsis which propels the contents.

The circular layer runs around the intestine and its contraction causes segmentation

The longitudinal layer runs along the intestine; it causes wave-like contractions.

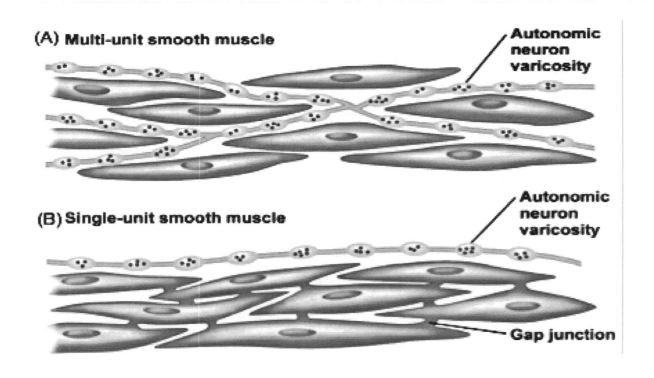

(A) Multi-unit smooth muscle

Autonomic neuron varicosity

(B) Single-unit smooth muscle

Autonomic neuron varicosity

Gap junction

Mechanism of smooth muscle contraction

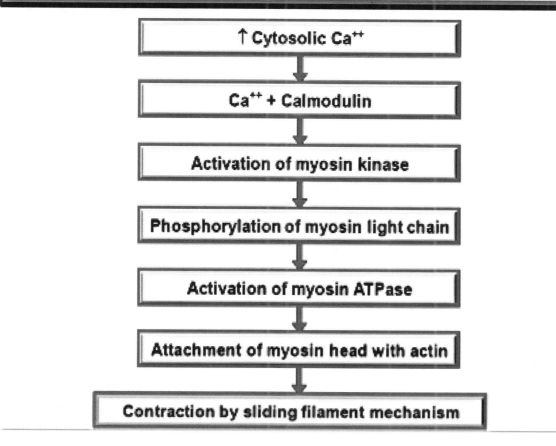

↑ Cytosolic Ca⁺⁺

↓

Ca⁺⁺ + Calmodulin

↓

Activation of myosin kinase

↓

Phosphorylation of myosin light chain

↓

Activation of myosin ATPase

↓

Attachment of myosin head with actin

↓

Contraction by sliding filament mechanism

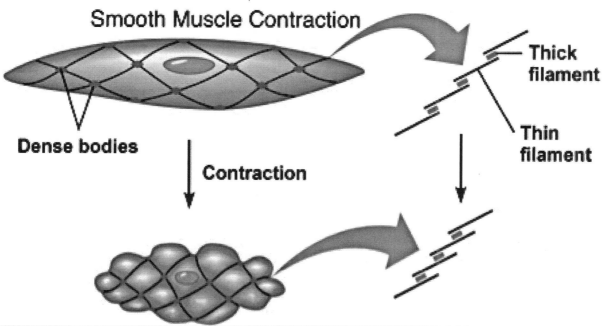

Smooth Muscle Contraction

Thick filament

Thin filament

Dense bodies

Contraction

The Neuromuscular Junction

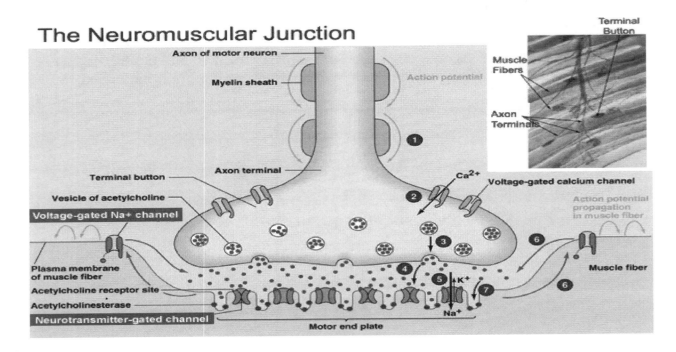

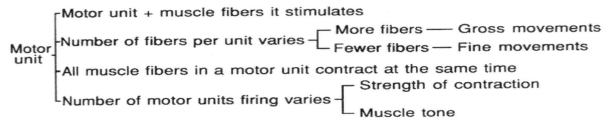

Motor unit
- Motor unit + muscle fibers it stimulates
- Number of fibers per unit varies
  - More fibers —— Gross movements
  - Fewer fibers —— Fine movements
- All muscle fibers in a motor unit contract at the same time
- Number of motor units firing varies
  - Strength of contraction
  - Muscle tone

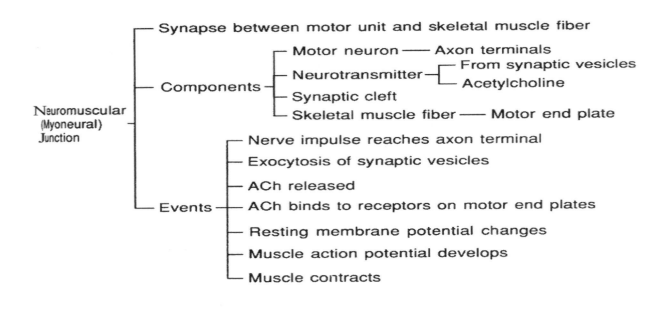

Neuromuscular (Myoneural) Junction
- Synapse between motor unit and skeletal muscle fiber
- Components
  - Motor neuron —— Axon terminals
  - Neurotransmitter
    - From synaptic vesicles
    - Acetylcholine
  - Synaptic cleft
  - Skeletal muscle fiber —— Motor end plate
- Events
  - Nerve impulse reaches axon terminal
  - Exocytosis of synaptic vesicles
  - ACh released
  - ACh binds to receptors on motor end plates
  - Resting membrane potential changes
  - Muscle action potential develops
  - Muscle contracts

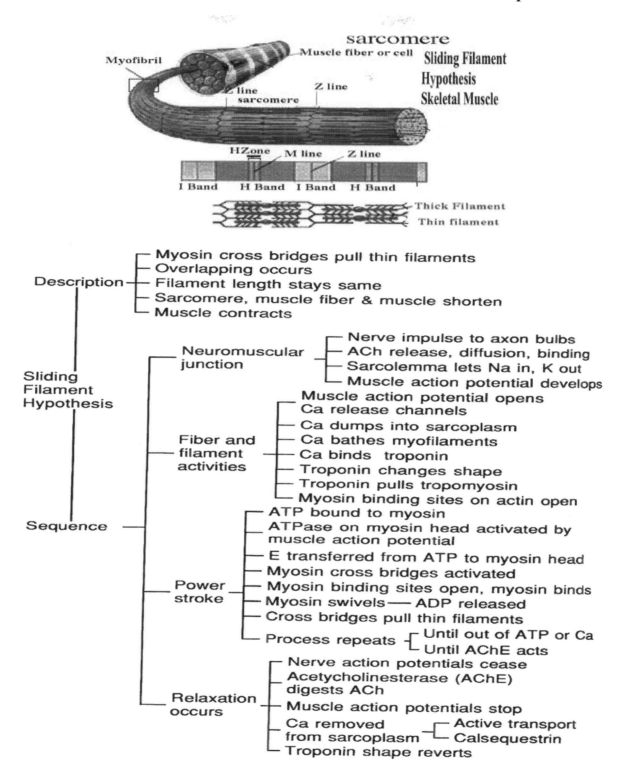

Sliding Filament Hypothesis Skeletal Muscle

Description
- Myosin cross bridges pull thin filaments
- Overlapping occurs
- Filament length stays same
- Sarcomere, muscle fiber & muscle shorten
- Muscle contracts

Sliding Filament Hypothesis

Sequence

Neuromuscular junction
- Nerve impulse to axon bulbs
- ACh release, diffusion, binding
- Sarcolemma lets Na in, K out
- Muscle action potential develops

Fiber and filament activities
- Muscle action potential opens Ca release channels
- Ca dumps into sarcoplasm
- Ca bathes myofilaments
- Ca binds troponin
- Troponin changes shape
- Troponin pulls tropomyosin
- Myosin binding sites on actin open

Power stroke
- ATP bound to myosin
- ATPase on myosin head activated by muscle action potential
- E transferred from ATP to myosin head
- Myosin cross bridges activated
- Myosin binding sites open, myosin binds
- Myosin swivels —— ADP released
- Cross bridges pull thin filaments
- Process repeats
  - Until out of ATP or Ca
  - Until AChE acts

Relaxation occurs
- Nerve action potentials cease
- Acetycholinesterase (AChE) digests ACh
- Muscle action potentials stop
- Ca removed from sarcoplasm
  - Active transport
  - Calsequestrin
- Troponin shape reverts

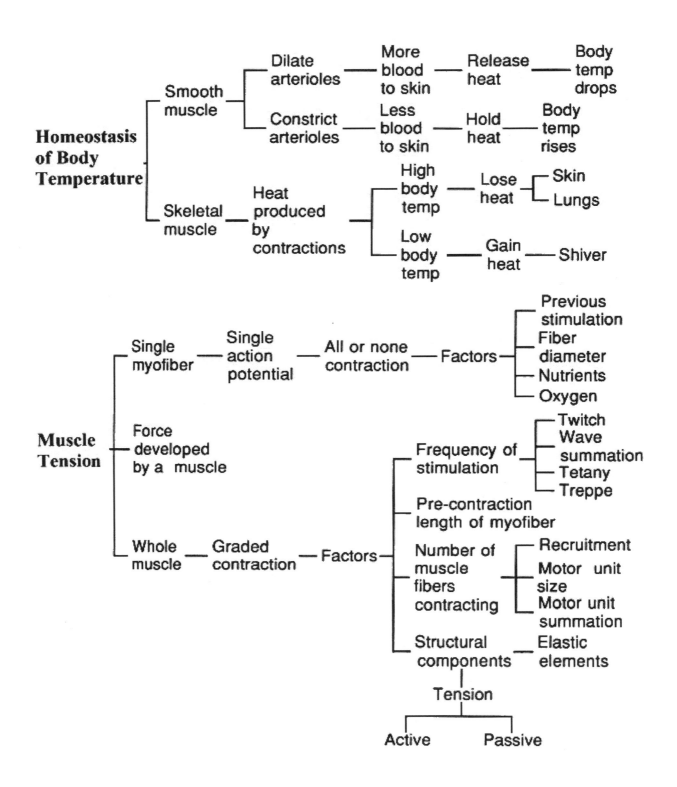

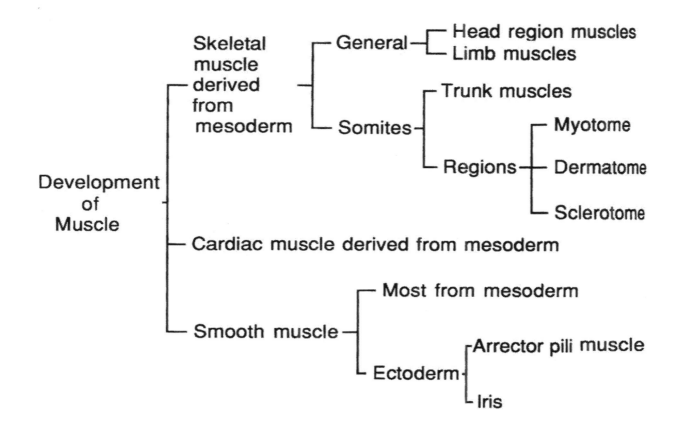

Development of Muscle
- Skeletal muscle derived from mesoderm
  - General
    - Head region muscles
    - Limb muscles
  - Somites
    - Trunk muscles
    - Regions
      - Myotome
      - Dermatome
      - Sclerotome
- Cardiac muscle derived from mesoderm
- Smooth muscle
  - Most from mesoderm
  - Ectoderm
    - Arrector pili muscle
    - Iris

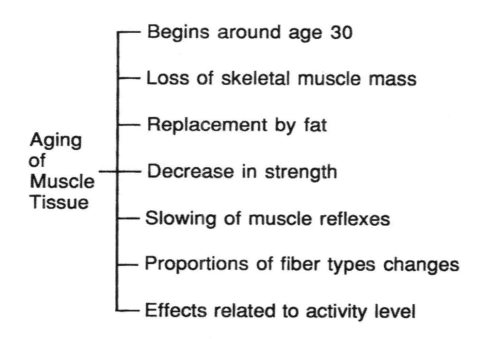

Aging of Muscle Tissue
- Begins around age 30
- Loss of skeletal muscle mass
- Replacement by fat
- Decrease in strength
- Slowing of muscle reflexes
- Proportions of fiber types changes
- Effects related to activity level

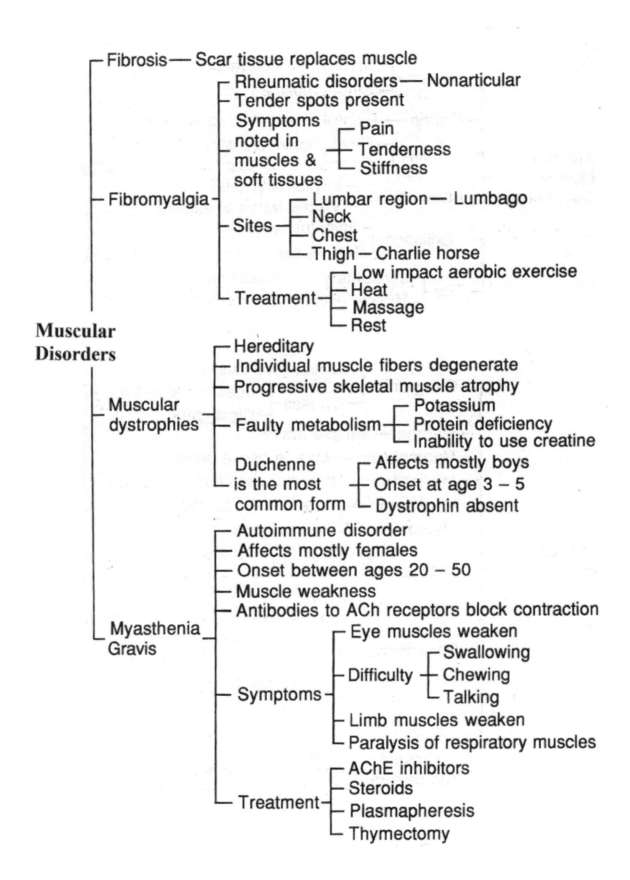

Muscular Disorders

- Fibrosis — Scar tissue replaces muscle
- Fibromyalgia
  - Rheumatic disorders — Nonarticular
  - Tender spots present
  - Symptoms noted in muscles & soft tissues
    - Pain
    - Tenderness
    - Stiffness
  - Sites
    - Lumbar region — Lumbago
    - Neck
    - Chest
    - Thigh — Charlie horse
  - Treatment
    - Low impact aerobic exercise
    - Heat
    - Massage
    - Rest
- Muscular dystrophies
  - Hereditary
  - Individual muscle fibers degenerate
  - Progressive skeletal muscle atrophy
  - Faulty metabolism
    - Potassium
    - Protein deficiency
    - Inability to use creatine
  - Duchenne is the most common form
    - Affects mostly boys
    - Onset at age 3 – 5
    - Dystrophin absent
- Myasthenia Gravis
  - Autoimmune disorder
  - Affects mostly females
  - Onset between ages 20 – 50
  - Muscle weakness
  - Antibodies to ACh receptors block contraction
  - Symptoms
    - Eye muscles weaken
    - Difficulty
      - Swallowing
      - Chewing
      - Talking
    - Limb muscles weaken
    - Paralysis of respiratory muscles
  - Treatment
    - AChE inhibitors
    - Steroids
    - Plasmapheresis
    - Thymectomy

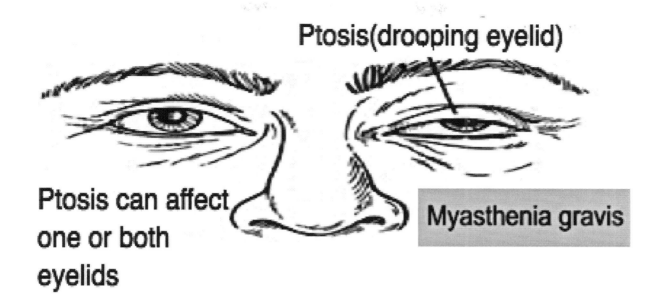

Ptosis(drooping eyelid)

Ptosis can affect one or both eyelids

Myasthenia gravis

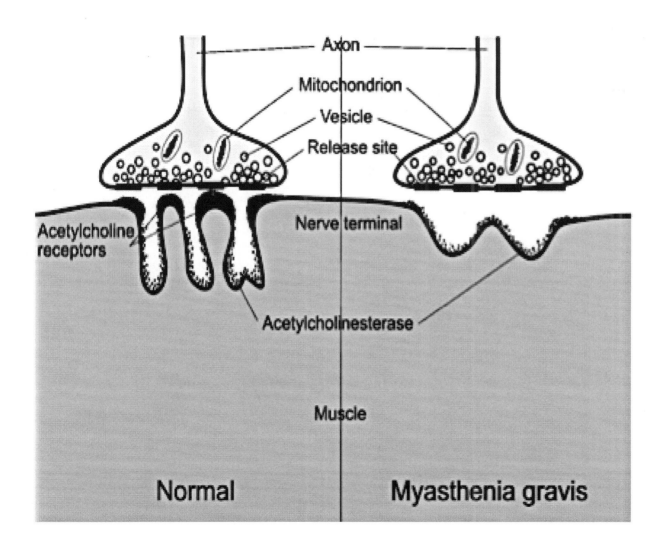

Axon

Mitochondrion

Vesicle

Release site

Nerve terminal

Acetylcholine receptors

Acetylcholinesterase

Muscle

Normal   Myasthenia gravis

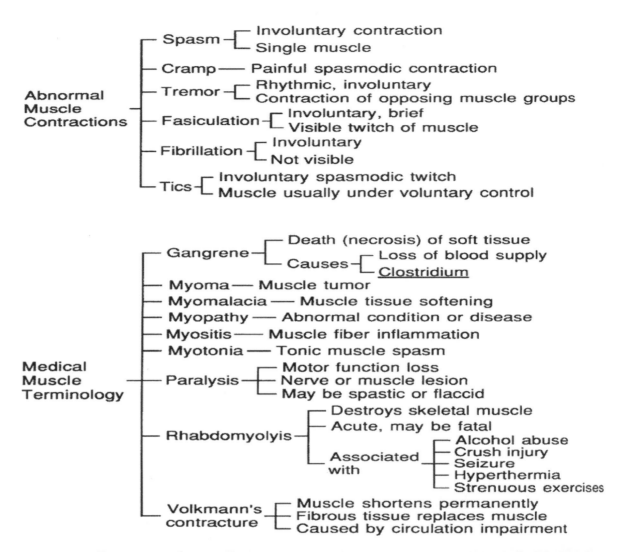

Abnormal Muscle Contractions
- Spasm
  - Involuntary contraction
  - Single muscle
- Cramp — Painful spasmodic contraction
- Tremor
  - Rhythmic, involuntary
  - Contraction of opposing muscle groups
- Fasiculation
  - Involuntary, brief
  - Visible twitch of muscle
- Fibrillation
  - Involuntary
  - Not visible
- Tics
  - Involuntary spasmodic twitch
  - Muscle usually under voluntary control

Medical Muscle Terminology
- Gangrene
  - Death (necrosis) of soft tissue
  - Causes
    - Loss of blood supply
    - Clostridium
- Myoma — Muscle tumor
- Myomalacia — Muscle tissue softening
- Myopathy — Abnormal condition or disease
- Myositis — Muscle fiber inflammation
- Myotonia — Tonic muscle spasm
- Paralysis
  - Motor function loss
  - Nerve or muscle lesion
  - May be spastic or flaccid
- Rhabdomyolyis
  - Destroys skeletal muscle
  - Acute, may be fatal
  - Associated with
    - Alcohol abuse
    - Crush injury
    - Seizure
    - Hyperthermia
    - Strenuous exercises
- Volkmann's contracture
  - Muscle shortens permanently
  - Fibrous tissue replaces muscle
  - Caused by circulation impairment

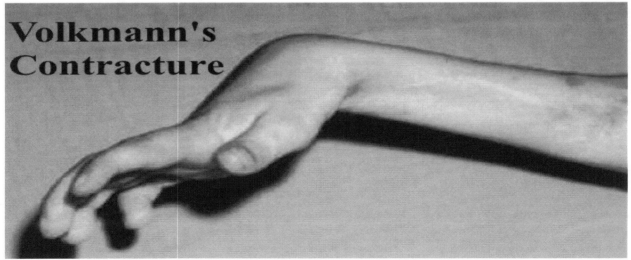

Volkmann's Contracture

CHAPTER ELEVEN

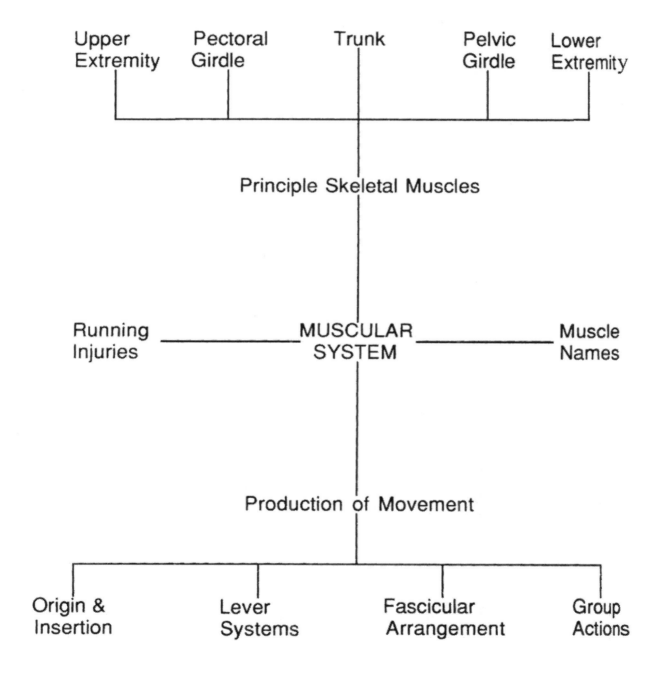

Upper Extremity   Pectoral Girdle   Trunk   Pelvic Girdle   Lower Extremity

Principle Skeletal Muscles

Running Injuries ———— MUSCULAR SYSTEM ———— Muscle Names

Production of Movement

Origin & Insertion   Lever Systems   Fascicular Arrangement   Group Actions

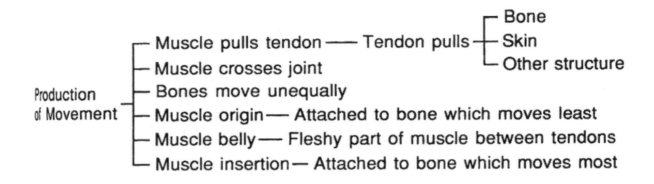

Production of Movement
- Muscle pulls tendon — Tendon pulls
  - Bone
  - Skin
  - Other structure
- Muscle crosses joint
- Bones move unequally
- Muscle origin — Attached to bone which moves least
- Muscle belly — Fleshy part of muscle between tendons
- Muscle insertion — Attached to bone which moves most

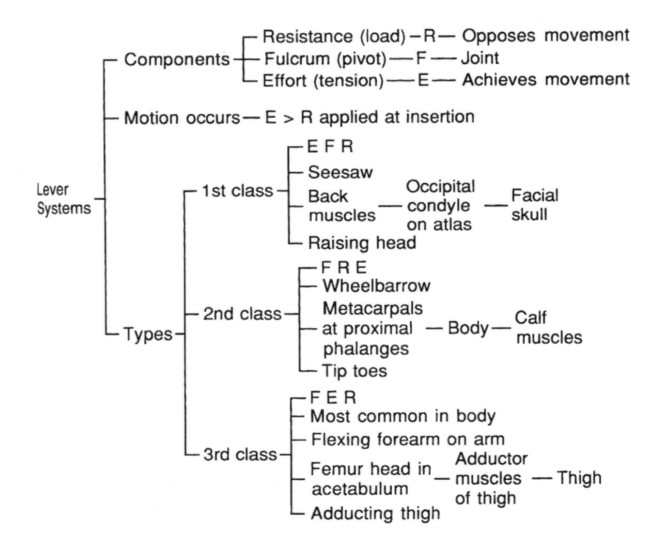

Lever Systems
- Components
  - Resistance (load) — R — Opposes movement
  - Fulcrum (pivot) — F — Joint
  - Effort (tension) — E — Achieves movement
- Motion occurs — E > R applied at insertion
- Types
  - 1st class
    - E F R
    - Seesaw
    - Back muscles — Occipital condyle on atlas — Facial skull
    - Raising head
  - 2nd class
    - F R E
    - Wheelbarrow
    - Metacarpals at proximal phalanges — Body — Calf muscles
    - Tip toes
  - 3rd class
    - F E R
    - Most common in body
    - Flexing forearm on arm
    - Femur head in acetabulum — Adductor muscles of thigh — Thigh
    - Adducting thigh

Bones, ligaments, and muscles are the structures that form levers in the body to create human movement. Levers are typically labeled as first class, second class, or third class. All three types are found in the body, but most levers in the human body are third class.

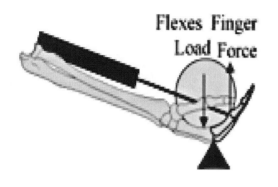

Power or Open Grip

This grip is stable and strong, but is slow and lacks flexibility.

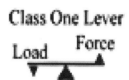

Class One Lever

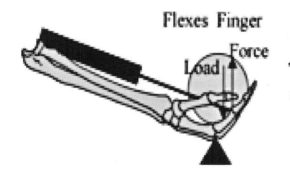

Open Grip

This grip is stable and strong, but is slow and lacks flexibility.

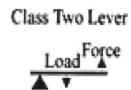

Class Two Lever

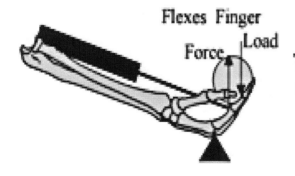

Pinch Grip

This grip provides quick and precise movements, but lacks strength.

Class Three Lever

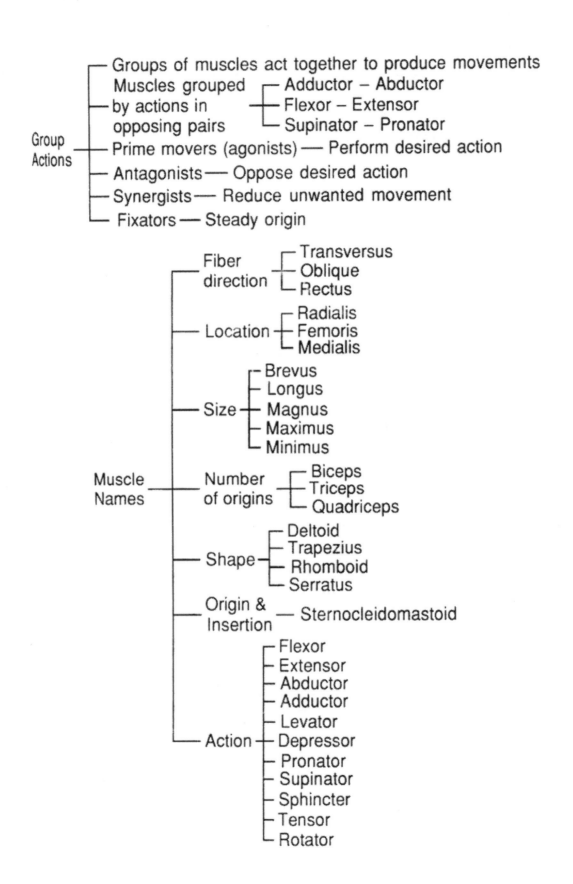

Group Actions
- Groups of muscles act together to produce movements
- Muscles grouped by actions in opposing pairs
  - Adductor – Abductor
  - Flexor – Extensor
  - Supinator – Pronator
- Prime movers (agonists) — Perform desired action
- Antagonists — Oppose desired action
- Synergists — Reduce unwanted movement
- Fixators — Steady origin

Muscle Names
- Fiber direction
  - Transversus
  - Oblique
  - Rectus
- Location
  - Radialis
  - Femoris
  - Medialis
- Size
  - Brevus
  - Longus
  - Magnus
  - Maximus
  - Minimus
- Number of origins
  - Biceps
  - Triceps
  - Quadriceps
- Shape
  - Deltoid
  - Trapezius
  - Rhomboid
  - Serratus
- Origin & Insertion
  - Sternocleidomastoid
- Action
  - Flexor
  - Extensor
  - Abductor
  - Adductor
  - Levator
  - Depressor
  - Pronator
  - Supinator
  - Sphincter
  - Tensor
  - Rotator

Muscles of Facial Expression

- Pulls scalp forward —— Frontalis
- Pulls scalp backward —— Occipitalis
- Raises eyebrows —— Frontalis
- Pulls eyebrow down —— Corrugator supercilli
- Wrinkles forehead —— Frontalis
- Closes eye —— Orbicularis oculi
- Elevates upper eyelid —— Levator palpebrae superioris
- Puckers lips —— Orbicularis oris
- Raises upper lip —— Levator labii superioris
- Depresses lower lip —— Depressor labii inferioris
- Pulls corner of mouth up, out —— Zygomaticus major
- Pulls lower lips and chin down —— Mentalis
- Pulls outer lower lip down, back —— Platysma
- Lowers mandible —— Platysma
- Pulls corners of mouth laterally —— Risorius
- Compresses cheeks —— Buccinator

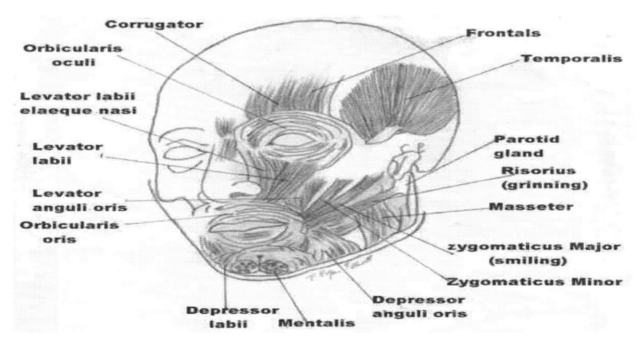

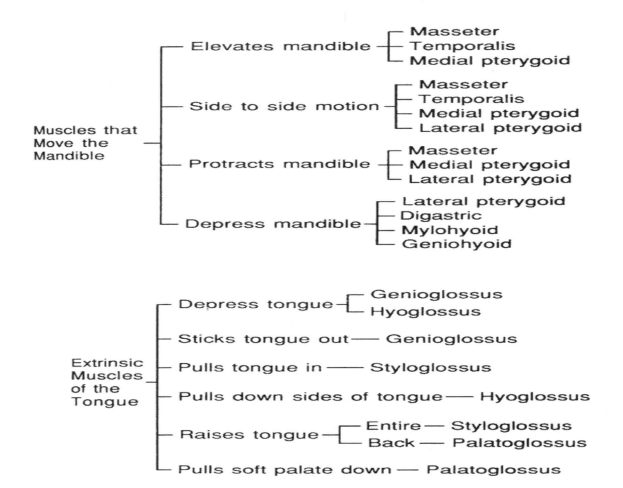

Muscles that Move the Mandible
- Elevates mandible
  - **Masseter**
  - Temporalis
  - Medial pterygoid
- Side to side motion
  - **Masseter**
  - Temporalis
  - **Medial pterygoid**
  - Lateral pterygoid
- Protracts mandible
  - **Masseter**
  - Medial pterygoid
  - Lateral pterygoid
- Depress mandible
  - Lateral pterygoid
  - Digastric
  - **Mylohyoid**
  - Geniohyoid

Extrinsic Muscles of the Tongue
- Depress tongue
  - Genioglossus
  - Hyoglossus
- Sticks tongue out —— Genioglossus
- Pulls tongue in —— Styloglossus
- Pulls down sides of tongue —— Hyoglossus
- Raises tongue
  - Entire — Styloglossus
  - Back — Palatoglossus
- Pulls soft palate down — Palatoglossus

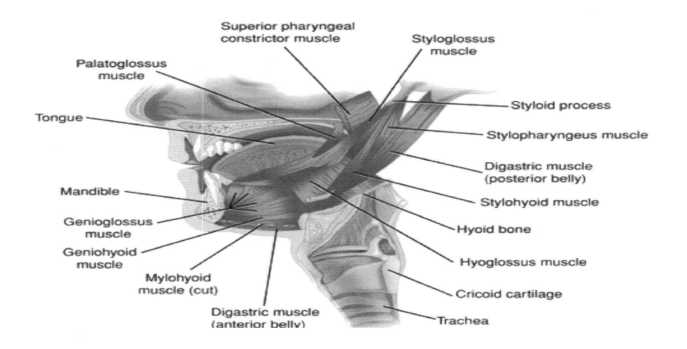

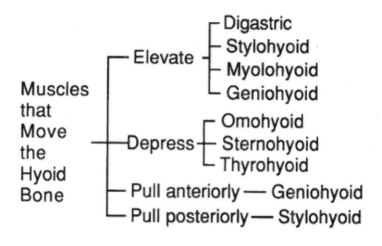

Muscles that Move the Hyoid Bone
- Elevate
  - Digastric
  - Stylohyoid
  - Myolohyoid
  - Geniohyoid
- Depress
  - Omohyoid
  - Sternohyoid
  - Thyrohyoid
- Pull anteriorly — Geniohyoid
- Pull posteriorly — Stylohyoid

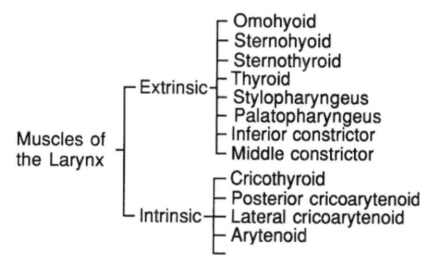

Muscles of the Larynx
- Extrinsic
  - Omohyoid
  - Sternohyoid
  - Sternothyroid
  - Thyroid
  - Stylopharyngeus
  - Palatopharyngeus
  - Inferior constrictor
  - Middle constrictor
- Intrinsic
  - Cricothyroid
  - Posterior cricoarytenoid
  - Lateral cricoarytenoid
  - Arytenoid

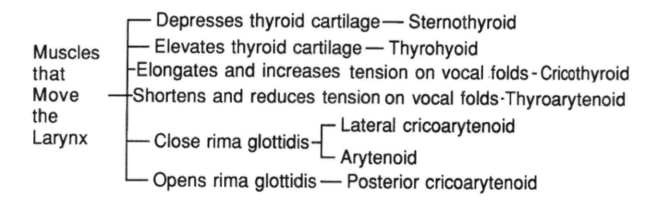

Muscles that Move the Larynx
- Depresses thyroid cartilage — Sternothyroid
- Elevates thyroid cartilage — Thyrohyoid
- Elongates and increases tension on vocal folds - Cricothyroid
- Shortens and reduces tension on vocal folds - Thyroarytenoid
- Close rima glottidis
  - Lateral cricoarytenoid
  - Arytenoid
- Opens rima glottidis — Posterior cricoarytenoid

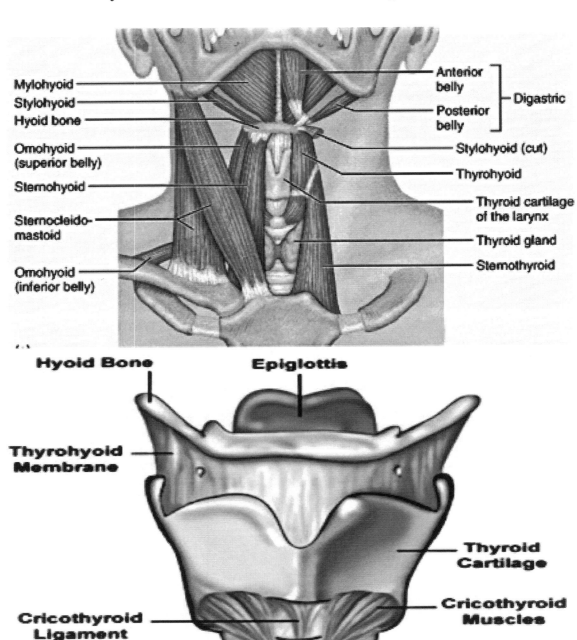

Mylohyoid
Stylohyoid
Hyoid bone
Omohyoid (superior belly)
Sternohyoid
Sternocleido-mastoid
Omohyoid (inferior belly)

Anterior belly
Posterior belly
Digastric
Stylohyoid (cut)
Thyrohyoid
Thyroid cartilage of the larynx
Thyroid gland
Sternothyroid

Hyoid Bone
Epiglottis
Thyrohyoid Membrane
Thyroid Cartilage
Cricothyroid Muscles
Cricothyroid Ligament
Cricoid Cartilage
Trachea

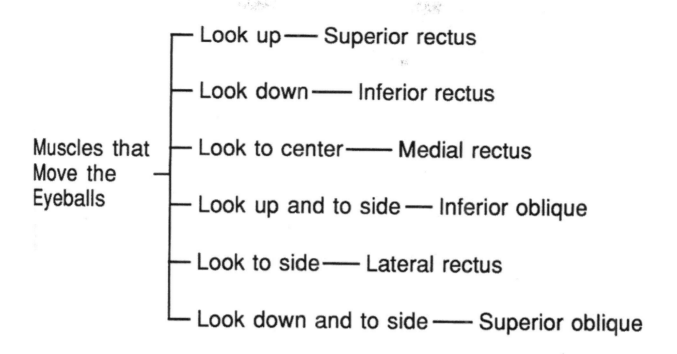

Muscles that Move the Eyeballs
- Look up —— Superior rectus
- Look down —— Inferior rectus
- Look to center —— Medial rectus
- Look up and to side — Inferior oblique
- Look to side —— Lateral rectus
- Look down and to side —— Superior oblique

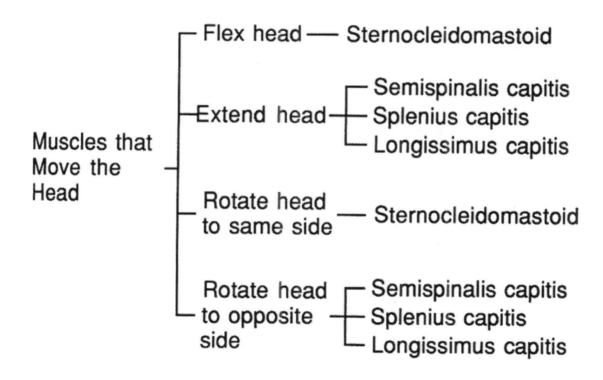

Muscles that Move the Head
- Flex head — Sternocleidomastoid
- Extend head
  - Semispinalis capitis
  - Splenius capitis
  - Longissimus capitis
- Rotate head to same side — Sternocleidomastoid
- Rotate head to opposite side
  - Semispinalis capitis
  - Splenius capitis
  - Longissimus capitis

Extrinsic Eye Muscles

- Medial rectus moves the eye towards the nose
- Lateral rectus moves the eye away from the nose
- Superior rectus moves the eye up
- Inferior rectus moves the eye down
- Superior oblique rotates the eye so that the top of the eye moves towards the nose.
- Inferior oblique rotates the eye so that the top of the eye moves away from the nose

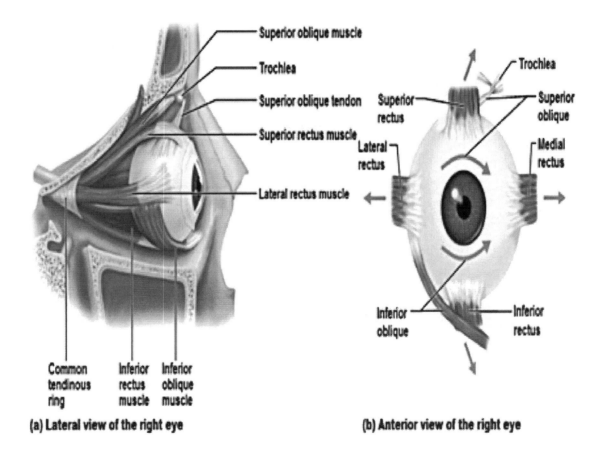

(a) Lateral view of the right eye

(b) Anterior view of the right eye

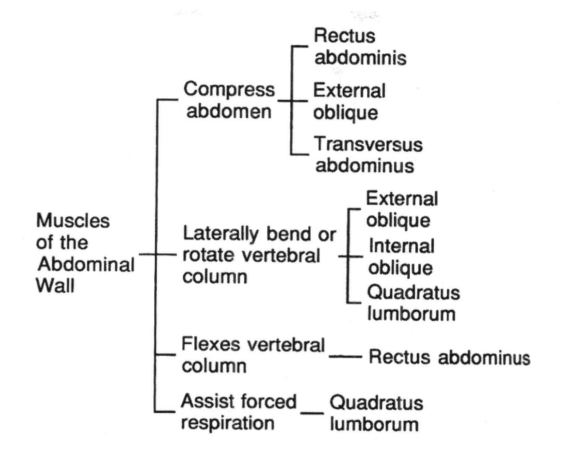

Muscles of the Abdominal Wall
- Compress abdomen
  - Rectus abdominis
  - External oblique
  - Transversus abdominus
- Laterally bend or rotate vertebral column
  - External oblique
  - Internal oblique
  - Quadratus lumborum
- Flexes vertebral column
  - Rectus abdominus
- Assist forced respiration
  - Quadratus lumborum

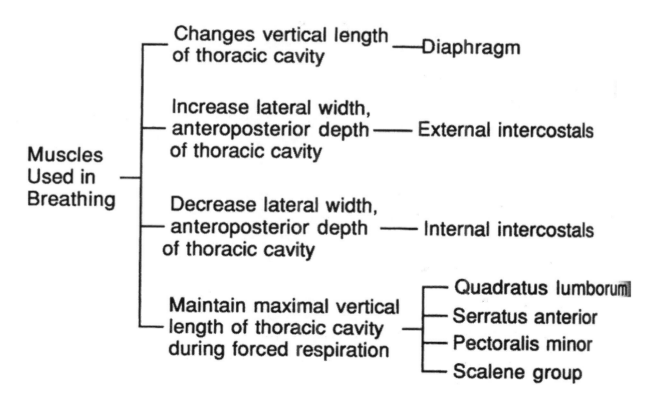

Muscles Used in Breathing
- Changes vertical length of thoracic cavity
  - Diaphragm
- Increase lateral width, anteroposterior depth of thoracic cavity
  - External intercostals
- Decrease lateral width, anteroposterior depth of thoracic cavity
  - Internal intercostals
- Maintain maximal vertical length of thoracic cavity during forced respiration
  - Quadratus lumborum
  - Serratus anterior
  - Pectoralis minor
  - Scalene group

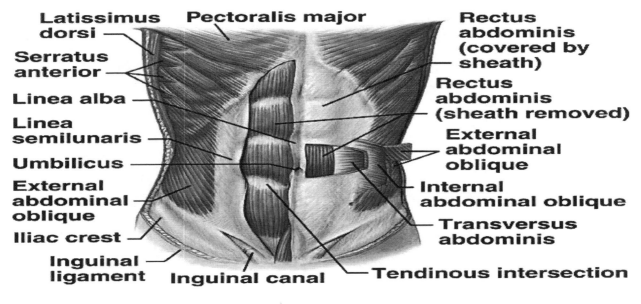

Latissimus dorsi
Pectoralis major
Rectus abdominis (covered by sheath)
Serratus anterior
Linea alba
Rectus abdominis (sheath removed)
Linea semilunaris
External abdominal oblique
Umbilicus
External abdominal oblique
Internal abdominal oblique
Iliac crest
Transversus abdominis
Inguinal ligament
Inguinal canal
Tendinous intersection

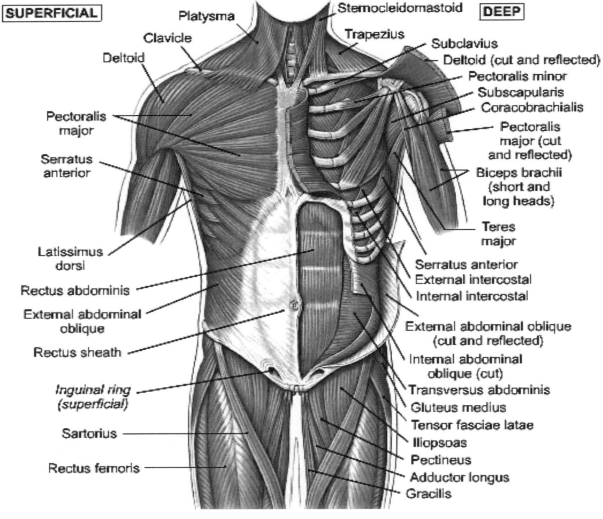

SUPERFICIAL
Platysma
Stemocleidomastoid
DEEP
Clavicle
Trapezius
Deltoid
Subclavius
Deltoid (cut and reflected)
Pectoralis minor
Subscapularis
Coracobrachialis
Pectoralis major
Pectoralis major (cut and reflected)
Serratus anterior
Biceps brachii (short and long heads)
Teres major
Latissimus dorsi
Serratus anterior
External intercostal
Internal intercostal
Rectus abdominis
External abdominal oblique
External abdominal oblique (cut and reflected)
Rectus sheath
Internal abdominal oblique (cut)
Transversus abdominis
Inguinal ring (superficial)
Gluteus medius
Tensor fasciae latae
Sartorius
Iliopsoas
Pectineus
Rectus femoris
Adductor longus
Gracilis

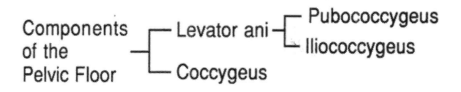

Components of the Pelvic Floor — Levator ani — Pubococcygeus / Iliococcygeus — Coccygeus

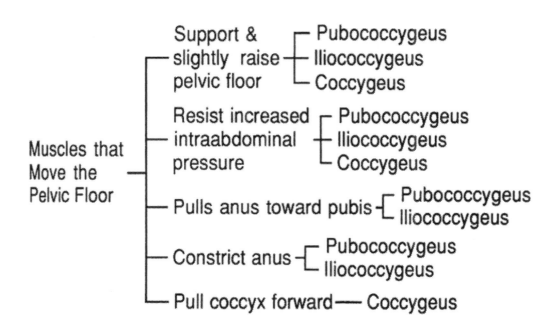

Muscles that Move the Pelvic Floor:
- Support & slightly raise pelvic floor — Pubococcygeus / Iliococcygeus / Coccygeus
- Resist increased intraabdominal pressure — Pubococcygeus / Iliococcygeus / Coccygeus
- Pulls anus toward pubis — Pubococcygeus / Iliococcygeus
- Constrict anus — Pubococcygeus / Iliococcygeus
- Pull coccyx forward — Coccygeus

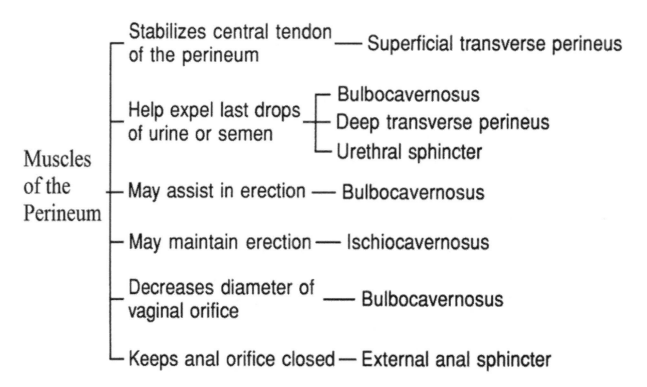

Muscles of the Perineum:
- Stabilizes central tendon of the perineum — Superficial transverse perineus
- Help expel last drops of urine or semen — Bulbocavernosus / Deep transverse perineus / Urethral sphincter
- May assist in erection — Bulbocavernosus
- May maintain erection — Ischiocavernosus
- Decreases diameter of vaginal orifice — Bulbocavernosus
- Keeps anal orifice closed — External anal sphincter

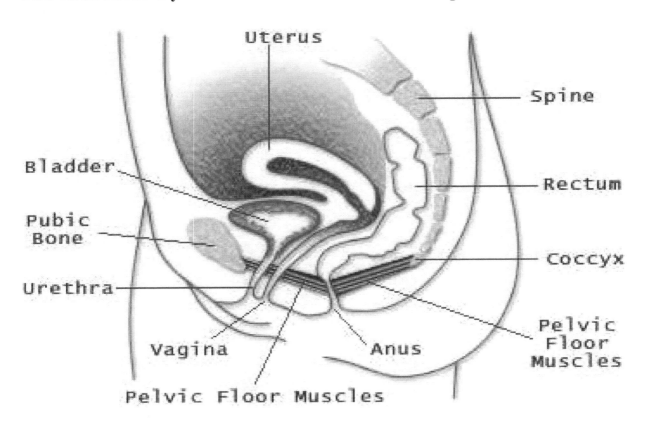

Uterus

Spine

Bladder

Rectum

Pubic Bone

Coccyx

Urethra

Pelvic Floor Muscles

Vagina

Anus

Pelvic Floor Muscles

Picture of Pelvic Floor Muscles

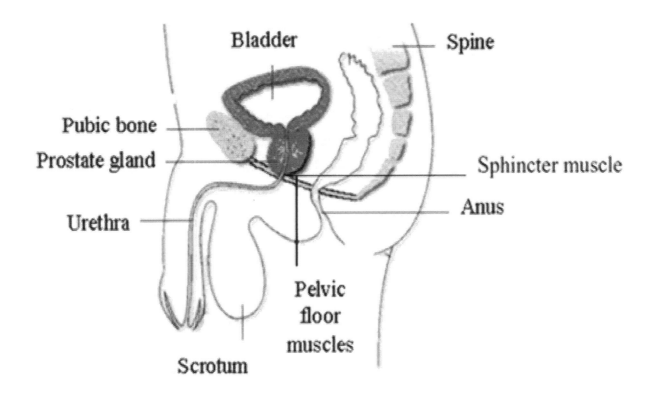

Bladder

Spine

Pubic bone

Prostate gland

Sphincter muscle

Anus

Urethra

Pelvic floor muscles

Scrotum

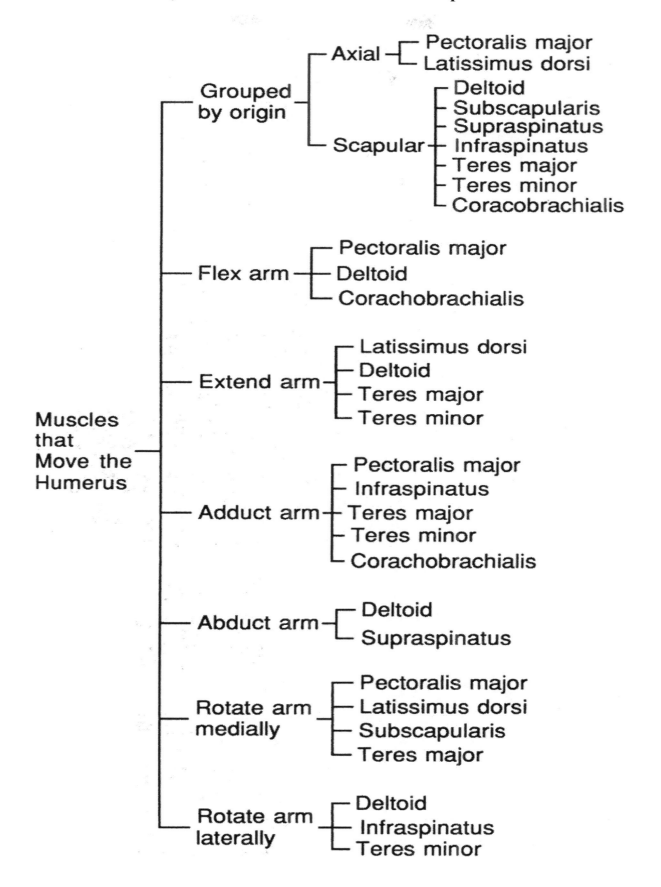

Muscles that Move the Humerus

- Grouped by origin
  - Axial
    - Pectoralis major
    - Latissimus dorsi
  - Scapular
    - Deltoid
    - Subscapularis
    - Supraspinatus
    - Infraspinatus
    - Teres major
    - Teres minor
    - Coracobrachialis
- Flex arm
  - Pectoralis major
  - Deltoid
  - Corachobrachialis
- Extend arm
  - Latissimus dorsi
  - Deltoid
  - Teres major
  - Teres minor
- Adduct arm
  - Pectoralis major
  - Infraspinatus
  - Teres major
  - Teres minor
  - Corachobrachialis
- Abduct arm
  - Deltoid
  - Supraspinatus
- Rotate arm medially
  - Pectoralis major
  - Latissimus dorsi
  - Subscapularis
  - Teres major
- Rotate arm laterally
  - Deltoid
  - Infraspinatus
  - Teres minor

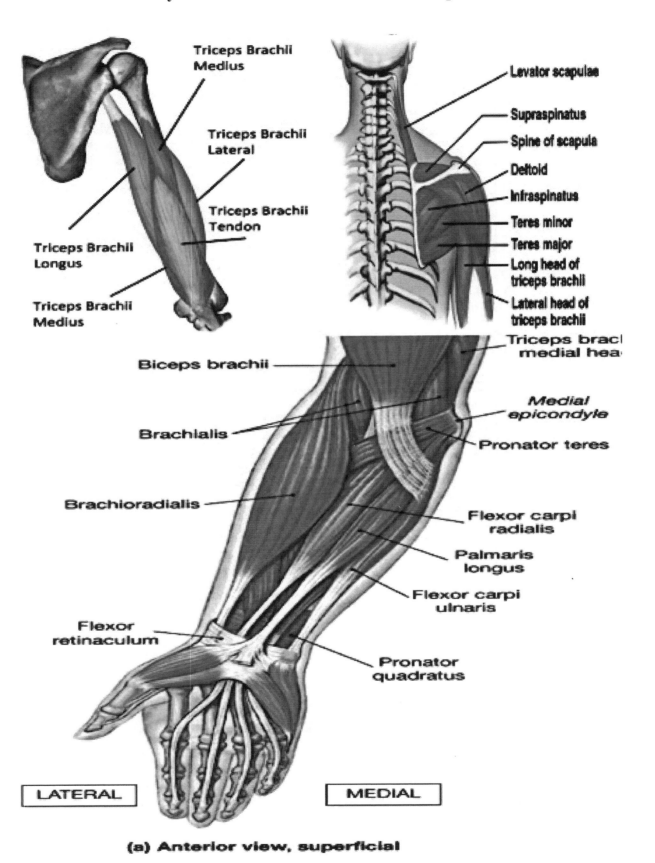

Triceps Brachii Medius

Triceps Brachii Lateral

Triceps Brachii Tendon

Triceps Brachii Longus

Triceps Brachii Medius

Levator scapulae

Supraspinatus

Spine of scapula

Deltoid

Infraspinatus

Teres minor

Teres major

Long head of triceps brachii

Lateral head of triceps brachii

Triceps brachii medial head

Medial epicondyle

Pronator teres

Biceps brachii

Brachialis

Brachioradialis

Flexor carpi radialis

Palmaris longus

Flexor carpi ulnaris

Flexor retinaculum

Pronator quadratus

LATERAL

MEDIAL

(a) Anterior view, superficial

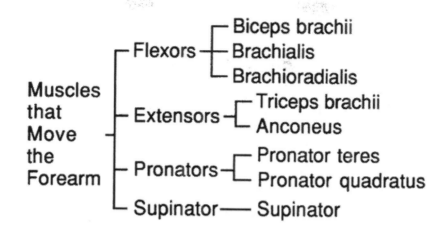

Muscles that Move the Forearm
- Flexors
  - Biceps brachii
  - Brachialis
  - Brachioradialis
- Extensors
  - Triceps brachii
  - Anconeus
- Pronators
  - Pronator teres
  - Pronator quadratus
- Supinator
  - Supinator

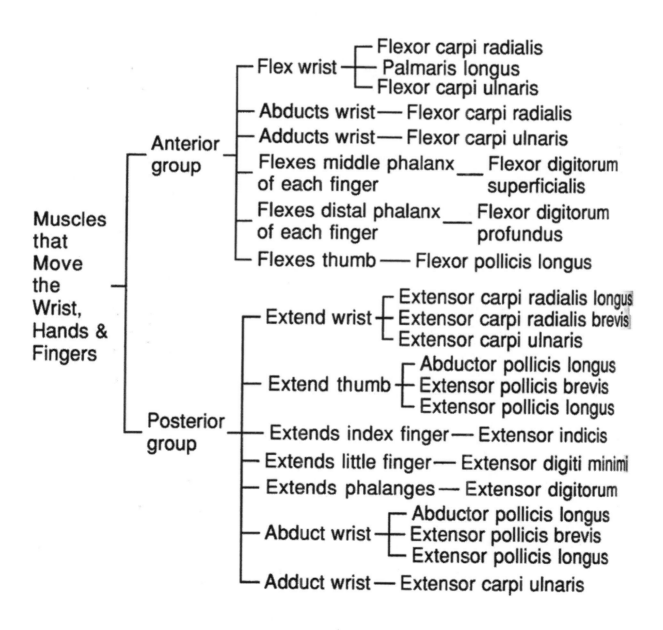

Muscles that Move the Wrist, Hands & Fingers
- Anterior group
  - Flex wrist
    - Flexor carpi radialis
    - Palmaris longus
    - Flexor carpi ulnaris
  - Abducts wrist — Flexor carpi radialis
  - Adducts wrist — Flexor carpi ulnaris
  - Flexes middle phalanx of each finger — Flexor digitorum superficialis
  - Flexes distal phalanx of each finger — Flexor digitorum profundus
  - Flexes thumb — Flexor pollicis longus
- Posterior group
  - Extend wrist
    - Extensor carpi radialis longus
    - Extensor carpi radialis brevis
    - Extensor carpi ulnaris
  - Extend thumb
    - Abductor pollicis longus
    - Extensor pollicis brevis
    - Extensor pollicis longus
  - Extends index finger — Extensor indicis
  - Extends little finger — Extensor digiti minimi
  - Extends phalanges — Extensor digitorum
  - Abduct wrist
    - Abductor pollicis longus
    - Extensor pollicis brevis
    - Extensor pollicis longus
  - Adduct wrist — Extensor carpi ulnaris

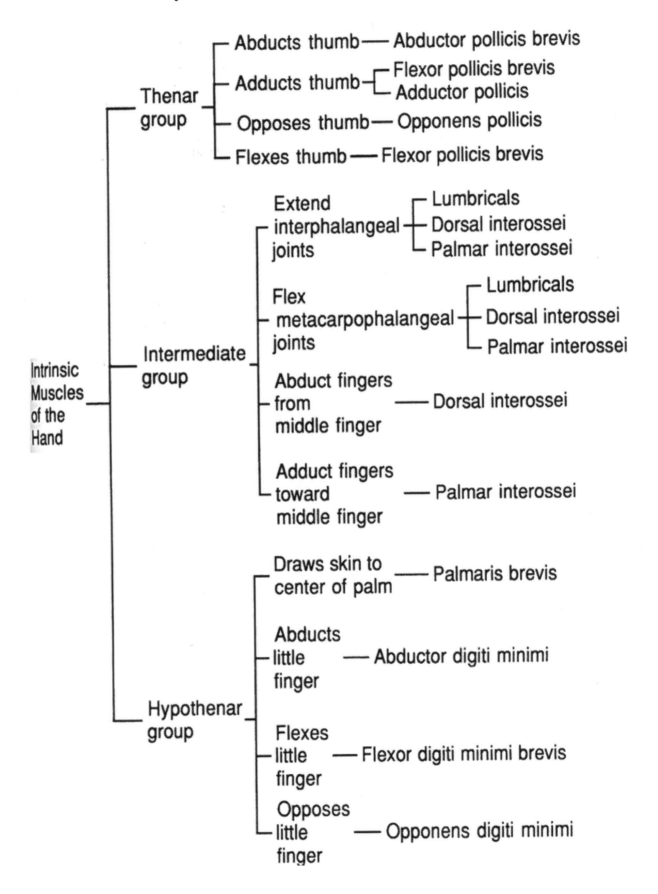

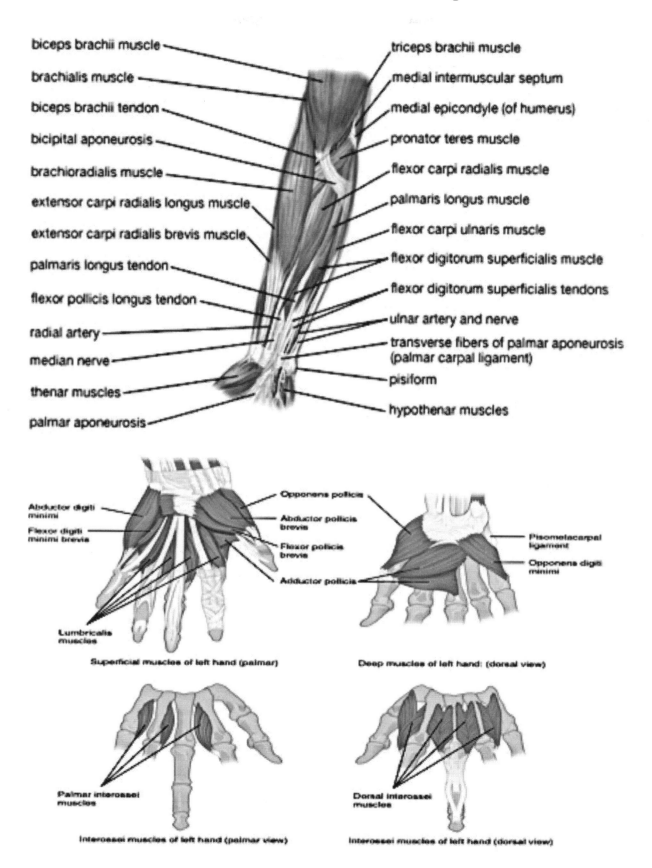

biceps brachii muscle
brachialis muscle
biceps brachii tendon
bicipital aponeurosis
brachioradialis muscle
extensor carpi radialis longus muscle
extensor carpi radialis brevis muscle
palmaris longus tendon
flexor pollicis longus tendon
radial artery
median nerve
thenar muscles
palmar aponeurosis

triceps brachii muscle
medial intermuscular septum
medial epicondyle (of humerus)
pronator teres muscle
flexor carpi radialis muscle
palmaris longus muscle
flexor carpi ulnaris muscle
flexor digitorum superficialis muscle
flexor digitorum superficialis tendons
ulnar artery and nerve
transverse fibers of palmar aponeurosis
(palmar carpal ligament)
pisiform
hypothenar muscles

Abductor digiti minimi
Flexor digiti minimi brevis
Lumbricalis muscles

Opponens pollicis
Abductor pollicis brevis
Flexor pollicis brevis
Adductor pollicis

Superficial muscles of left hand (palmar)

Pisometacarpal ligament
Opponens digiti minimi

Deep muscles of left hand: (dorsal view)

Palmar interossei muscles

Interossei muscles of left hand (palmar view)

Dorsal interossei muscles

Interossei muscles of left hand (dorsal view)

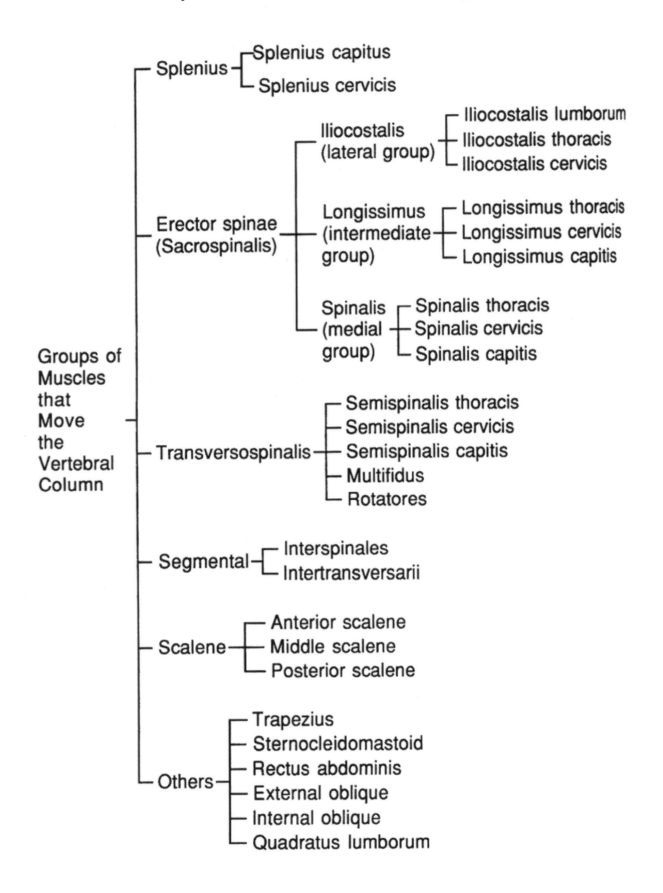

Groups of
Muscles
that
Move
the
Vertebral
Column

- Splenius
  - Splenius capitus
  - Splenius cervicis

- Erector spinae (Sacrospinalis)
  - Iliocostalis (lateral group)
    - Iliocostalis lumborum
    - Iliocostalis thoracis
    - Iliocostalis cervicis
  - Longissimus (intermediate group)
    - Longissimus thoracis
    - Longissimus cervicis
    - Longissimus capitis
  - Spinalis (medial group)
    - Spinalis thoracis
    - Spinalis cervicis
    - Spinalis capitis

- Transversospinalis
  - Semispinalis thoracis
  - Semispinalis cervicis
  - Semispinalis capitis
  - Multifidus
  - Rotatores

- Segmental
  - Interspinales
  - Intertransversarii

- Scalene
  - Anterior scalene
  - Middle scalene
  - Posterior scalene

- Others
  - Trapezius
  - Sternocleidomastoid
  - Rectus abdominis
  - External oblique
  - Internal oblique
  - Quadratus lumborum

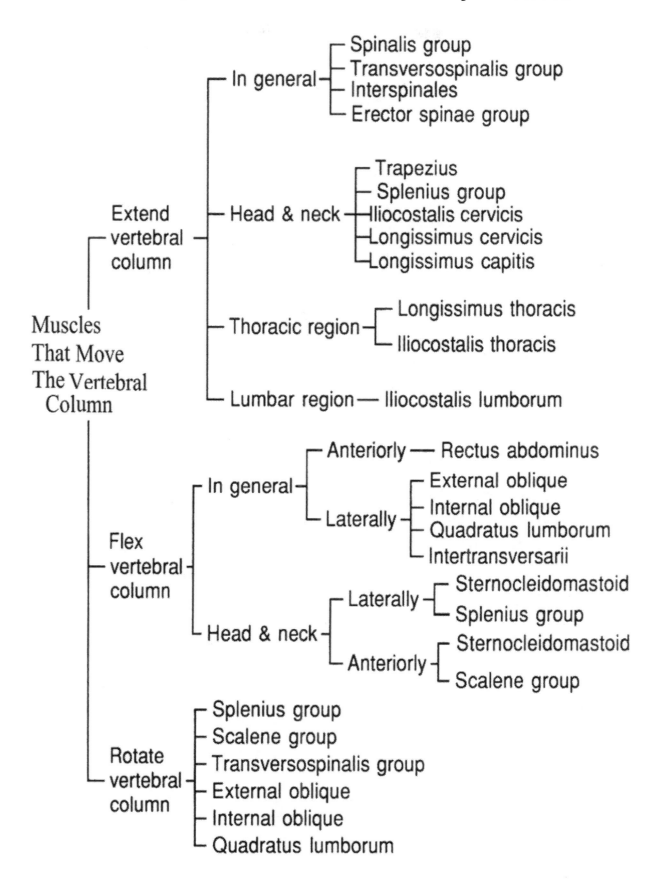

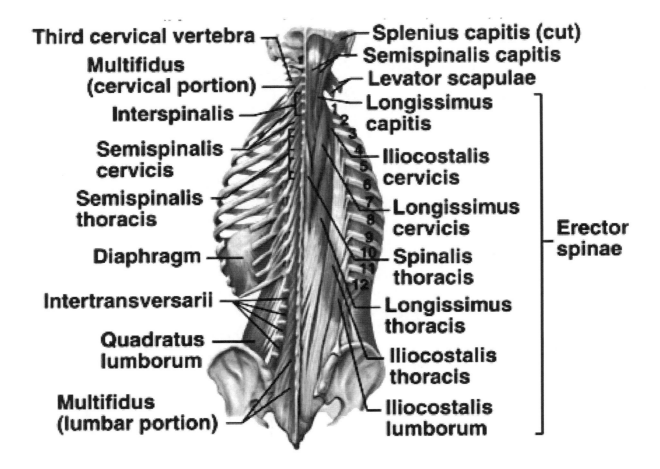

Third cervical vertebra

Multifidus (cervical portion)

Interspinalis

Semispinalis cervicis

Semispinalis thoracis

Diaphragm

Intertransversarii

Quadratus lumborum

Multifidus (lumbar portion)

Splenius capitis (cut)

Semispinalis capitis

Levator scapulae

Longissimus capitis

Iliocostalis cervicis

Longissimus cervicis

Spinalis thoracis

Longissimus thoracis

Iliocostalis thoracis

Iliocostalis lumborum

Erector spinae

1 2 3 4 5 6 7 8 9 10 11 12

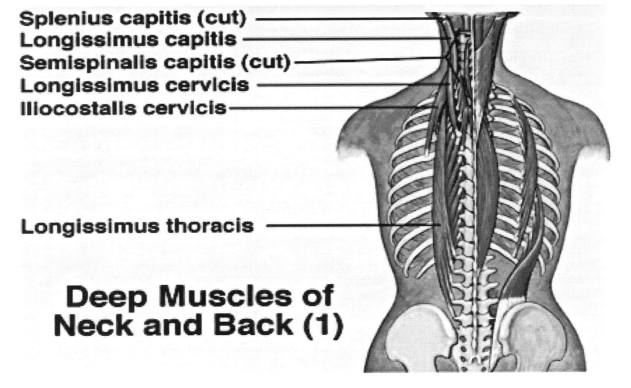

Splenius capitis (cut)

Longissimus capitis

Semispinalis capitis (cut)

Longissimus cervicis

Iliocostalis cervicis

Longissimus thoracis

Deep Muscles of Neck and Back (1)

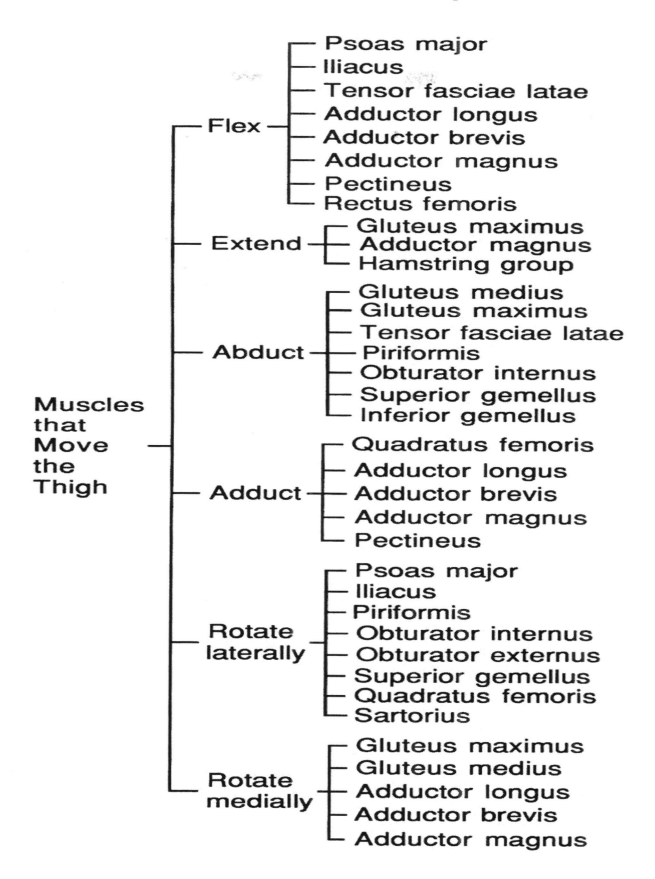

Muscles that Move the Thigh

- Flex
  - Psoas major
  - Iliacus
  - Tensor fasciae latae
  - Adductor longus
  - Adductor brevis
  - Adductor magnus
  - Pectineus
  - Rectus femoris
- Extend
  - Gluteus maximus
  - Adductor magnus
  - Hamstring group
- Abduct
  - Gluteus medius
  - Gluteus maximus
  - Tensor fasciae latae
  - Piriformis
  - Obturator internus
  - Superior gemellus
  - Inferior gemellus
- Adduct
  - Quadratus femoris
  - Adductor longus
  - Adductor brevis
  - Adductor magnus
  - Pectineus
- Rotate laterally
  - Psoas major
  - Iliacus
  - Piriformis
  - Obturator internus
  - Obturator externus
  - Superior gemellus
  - Quadratus femoris
  - Sartorius
- Rotate medially
  - Gluteus maximus
  - Gluteus medius
  - Adductor longus
  - Adductor brevis
  - Adductor magnus

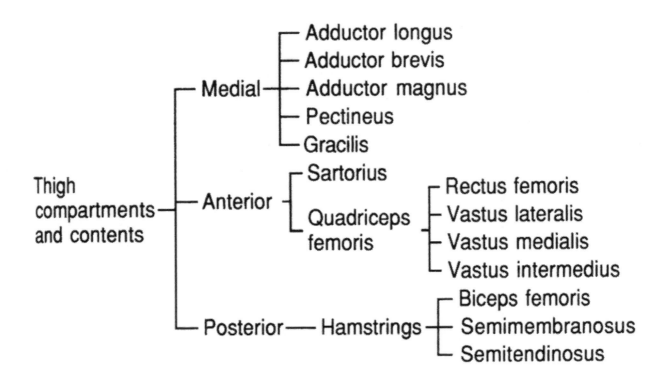

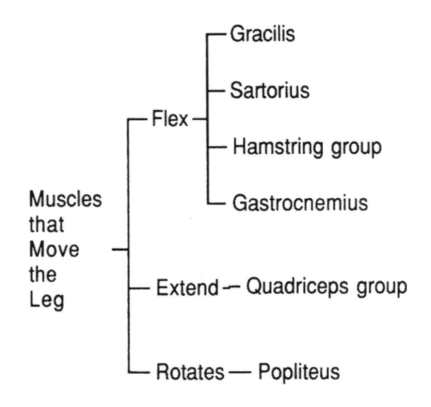

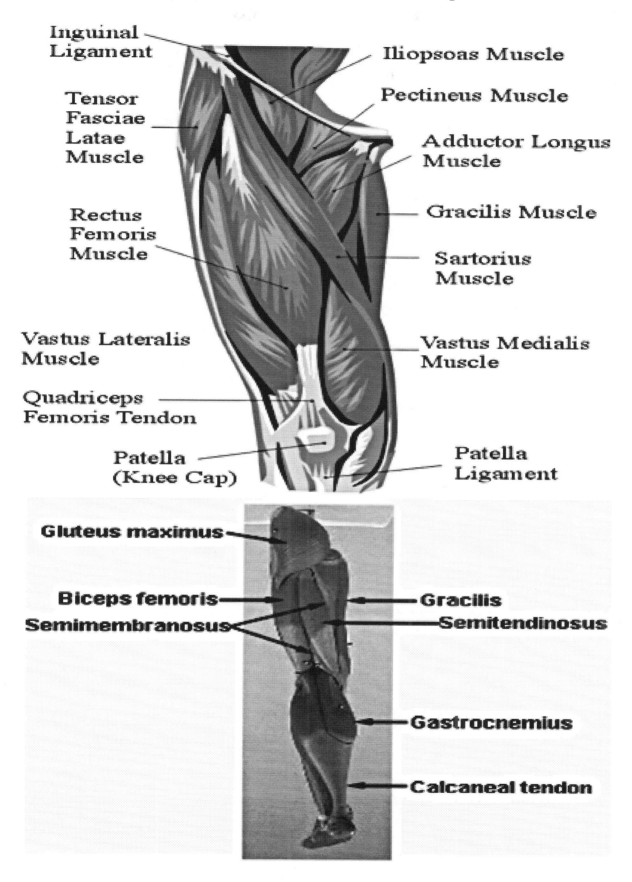

Inguinal Ligament

Tensor Fasciae Latae Muscle

Rectus Femoris Muscle

Vastus Lateralis Muscle

Quadriceps Femoris Tendon

Patella (Knee Cap)

Iliopsoas Muscle

Pectineus Muscle

Adductor Longus Muscle

Gracilis Muscle

Sartorius Muscle

Vastus Medialis Muscle

Patella Ligament

Gluteus maximus

Biceps femoris

Semimembranosus

Gracilis

Semitendinosus

Gastrocnemius

Calcaneal tendon

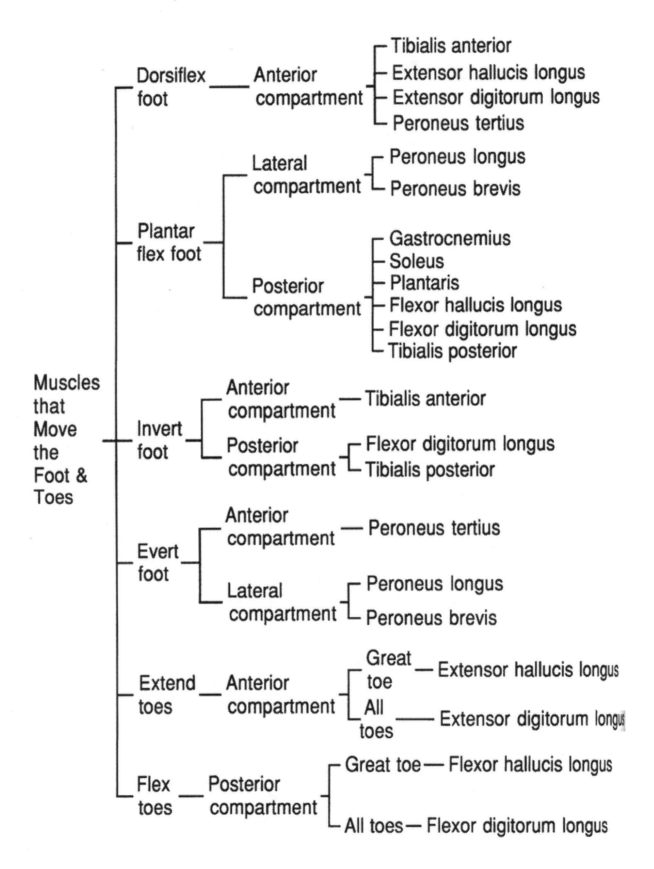

Muscles that Move the Foot & Toes

- Dorsiflex foot — Anterior compartment
  - Tibialis anterior
  - Extensor hallucis longus
  - Extensor digitorum longus
  - Peroneus tertius
- Plantar flex foot
  - Lateral compartment
    - Peroneus longus
    - Peroneus brevis
  - Posterior compartment
    - Gastrocnemius
    - Soleus
    - Plantaris
    - Flexor hallucis longus
    - Flexor digitorum longus
    - Tibialis posterior
- Invert foot
  - Anterior compartment
    - Tibialis anterior
  - Posterior compartment
    - Flexor digitorum longus
    - Tibialis posterior
- Evert foot
  - Anterior compartment
    - Peroneus tertius
  - Lateral compartment
    - Peroneus longus
    - Peroneus brevis
- Extend toes — Anterior compartment
  - Great toe — Extensor hallucis longus
  - All toes — Extensor digitorum longus
- Flex toes — Posterior compartment
  - Great toe — Flexor hallucis longus
  - All toes — Flexor digitorum longus

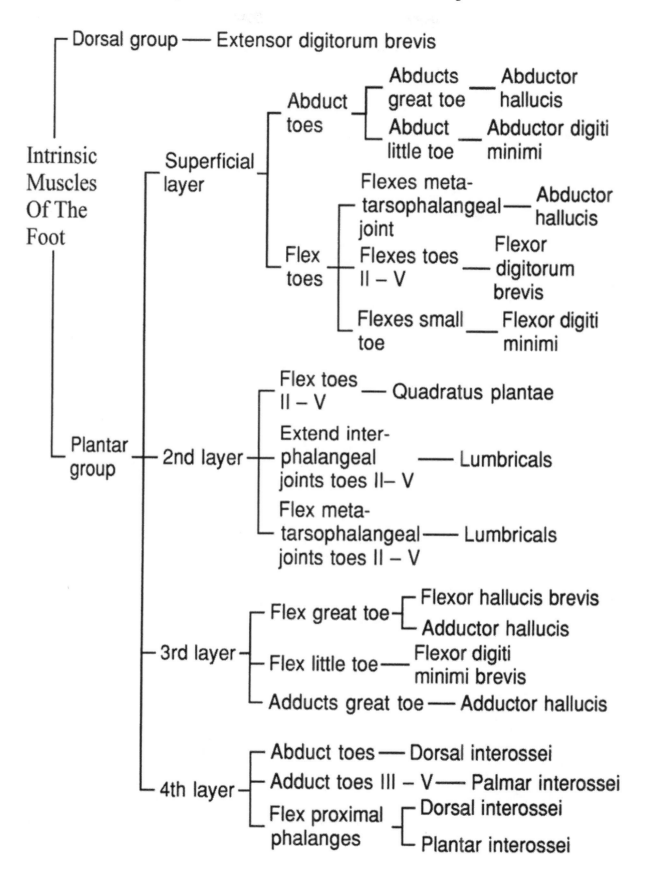

Dorsal group —— Extensor digitorum brevis

Intrinsic Muscles Of The Foot

Superficial layer
- Abduct toes
  - Abducts great toe —— Abductor hallucis
  - Abduct little toe —— Abductor digiti minimi
- Flex toes
  - Flexes meta-tarsophalangeal joint —— Abductor hallucis
  - Flexes toes II – V —— Flexor digitorum brevis
  - Flexes small toe —— Flexor digiti minimi

Plantar group

2nd layer
- Flex toes II – V —— Quadratus plantae
- Extend inter-phalangeal joints toes II– V —— Lumbricals
- Flex meta-tarsophalangeal joints toes II – V —— Lumbricals

3rd layer
- Flex great toe
  - Flexor hallucis brevis
  - Adductor hallucis
- Flex little toe —— Flexor digiti minimi brevis
- Adducts great toe —— Adductor hallucis

4th layer
- Abduct toes —— Dorsal interossei
- Adduct toes III – V —— Palmar interossei
- Flex proximal phalanges
  - Dorsal interossei
  - Plantar interossei

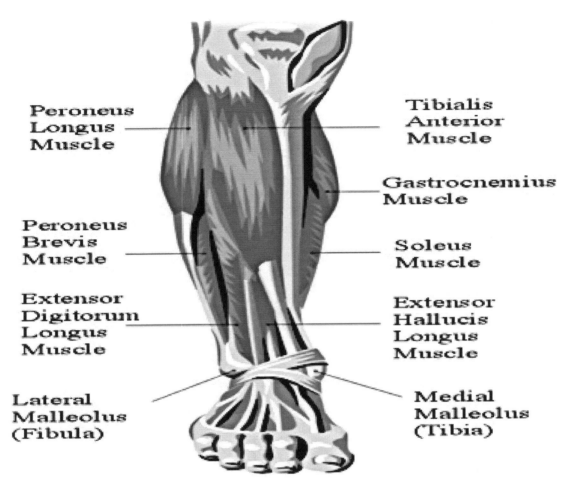

Peroneus Longus Muscle

Peroneus Brevis Muscle

Extensor Digitorum Longus Muscle

Lateral Malleolus (Fibula)

Tibialis Anterior Muscle

Gastrocnemius Muscle

Soleus Muscle

Extensor Hallucis Longus Muscle

Medial Malleolus (Tibia)

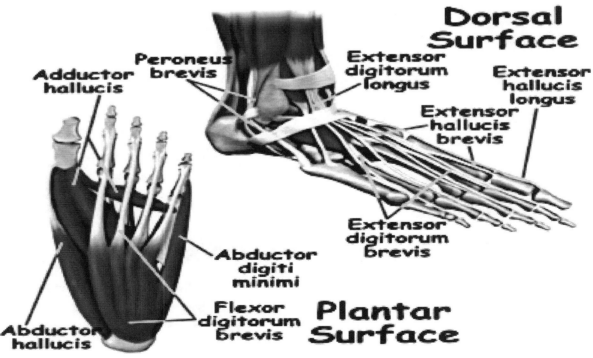

Dorsal Surface

Adductor hallucis

Peroneus brevis

Extensor digitorum longus

Extensor hallucis longus

Extensor hallucis brevis

Extensor digitorum brevis

Abductor digiti minimi

Flexor digitorum brevis

Plantar Surface

Abductor hallucis

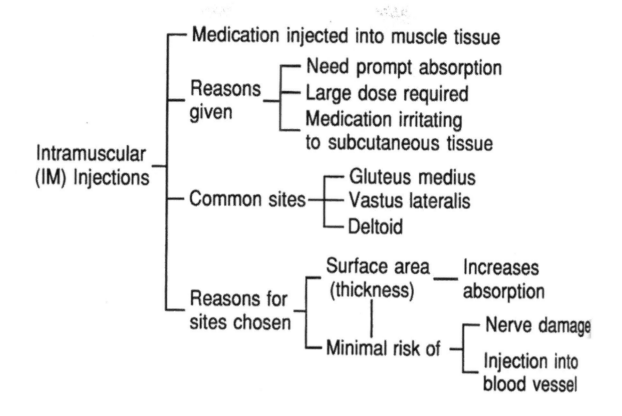

Intramuscular (IM) Injections
- Medication injected into muscle tissue
- Reasons given
  - Need prompt absorption
  - Large dose required
  - Medication irritating to subcutaneous tissue
- Common sites
  - Gluteus medius
  - Vastus lateralis
  - Deltoid
- Reasons for sites chosen
  - Surface area (thickness) — Increases absorption
  - Minimal risk of
    - Nerve damage
    - Injection into blood vessel

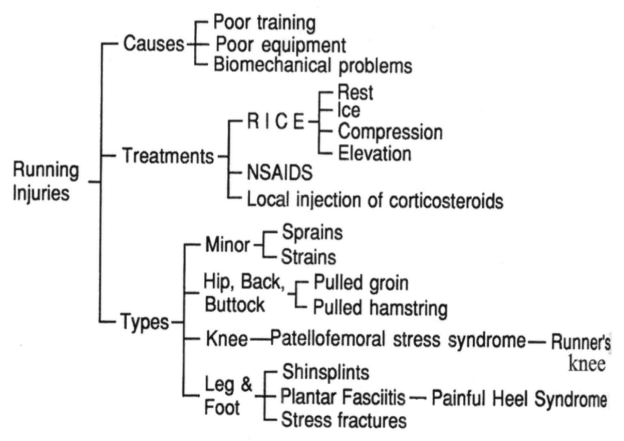

Running Injuries
- Causes
  - Poor training
  - Poor equipment
  - Biomechanical problems
- Treatments
  - R I C E
    - Rest
    - Ice
    - Compression
    - Elevation
  - NSAIDS
  - Local injection of corticosteroids
- Types
  - Minor
    - Sprains
    - Strains
  - Hip, Back, Buttock
    - Pulled groin
    - Pulled hamstring
  - Knee — Patellofemoral stress syndrome — Runner's knee
  - Leg & Foot
    - Shinsplints
    - Plantar Fasciitis — Painful Heel Syndrome
    - Stress fractures

How to Give an Intramuscular Shot

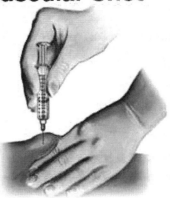

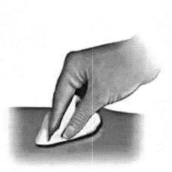

1. Use an alcohol swab to clean the skin where you will give the shot.

2. Hold the muscle firmly and insert the needle into the muscle at a 90° angle (straight up and down) with a quick firm motion.

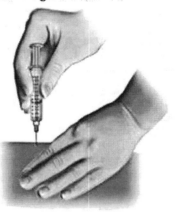

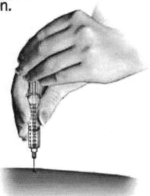

3. After you insert the needle completely, release your grasp of the muscle.

4. Gently pull back on the plunger of the syringe to check for blood. (If blood appears when you pull back on the plunger, withdraw the needle and syringe and gently press the alcohol swab on the injection site. Start over with a fresh needle.)

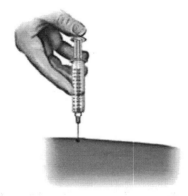

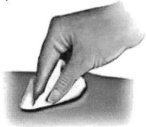

5. If no blood appears, inject all of the solution by gently and steadily pushing down the plunger.

6. Withdraw the needle and syringe and press an alcohol swab gently on the spot where the shot was given.

CHAPTER TWELVE

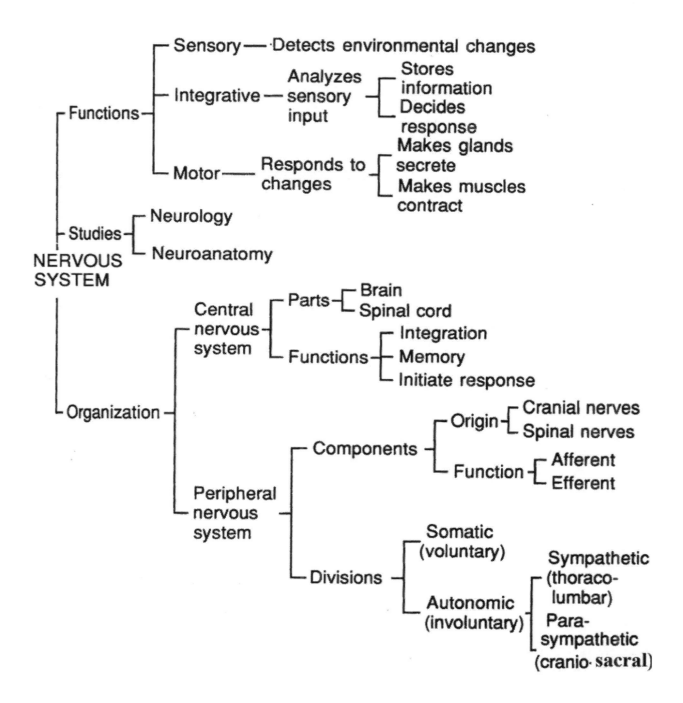

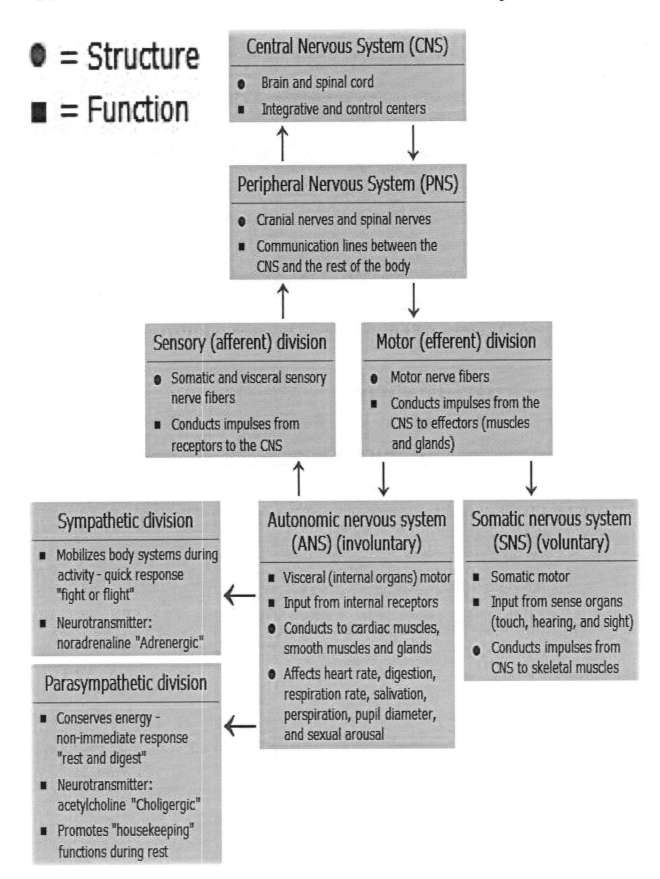

● = Structure

■ = Function

Central Nervous System (CNS)
- ● Brain and spinal cord
- ■ Integrative and control centers

Peripheral Nervous System (PNS)
- ● Cranial nerves and spinal nerves
- ■ Communication lines between the CNS and the rest of the body

Sensory (afferent) division
- ● Somatic and visceral sensory nerve fibers
- ■ Conducts impulses from receptors to the CNS

Motor (efferent) division
- ● Motor nerve fibers
- ■ Conducts impulses from the CNS to effectors (muscles and glands)

Sympathetic division
- ■ Mobilizes body systems during activity - quick response "fight or flight"
- ■ Neurotransmitter: noradrenaline "Adrenergic"

Parasympathetic division
- ■ Conserves energy - non-immediate response "rest and digest"
- ■ Neurotransmitter: acetylcholine "Choligergic"
- ■ Promotes "housekeeping" functions during rest

Autonomic nervous system (ANS) (involuntary)
- ■ Visceral (internal organs) motor
- ■ Input from internal receptors
- ● Conducts to cardiac muscles, smooth muscles and glands
- ● Affects heart rate, digestion, respiration rate, salivation, perspiration, pupil diameter, and sexual arousal

Somatic nervous system (SNS) (voluntary)
- ■ Somatic motor
- ■ Input from sense organs (touch, hearing, and sight)
- ● Conducts impulses from CNS to skeletal muscles

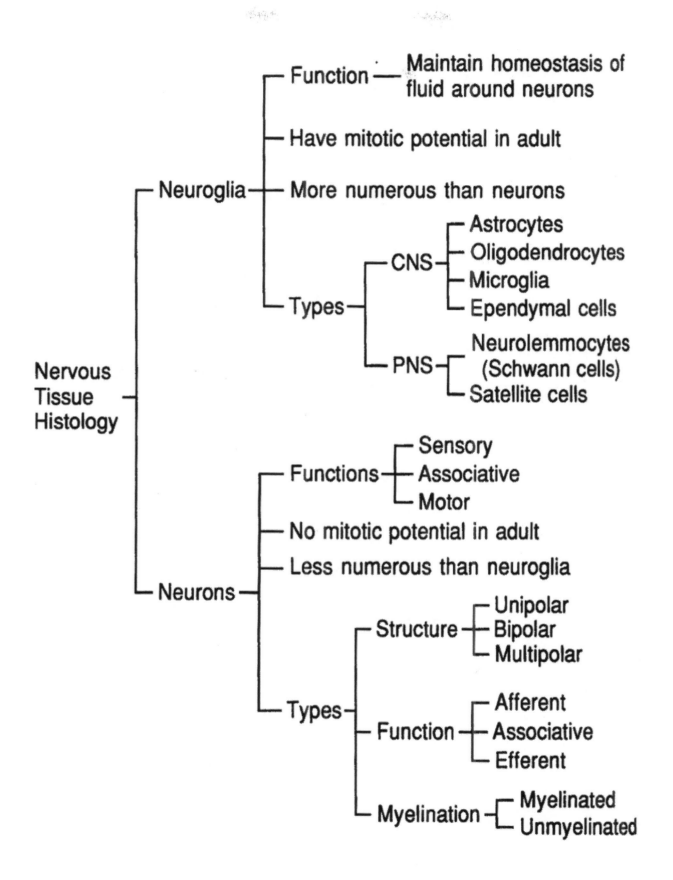

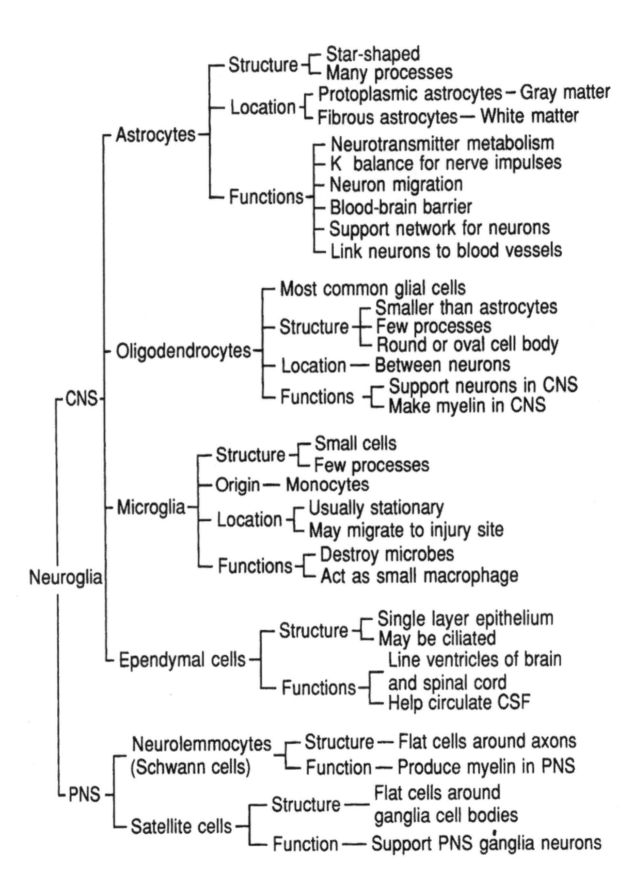

Neuroglia
- CNS
  - Astrocytes
    - Structure
      - Star-shaped
      - Many processes
    - Location
      - Protoplasmic astrocytes – Gray matter
      - Fibrous astrocytes – White matter
    - Functions
      - Neurotransmitter metabolism
      - K balance for nerve impulses
      - Neuron migration
      - Blood-brain barrier
      - Support network for neurons
      - Link neurons to blood vessels
  - Oligodendrocytes
    - Most common glial cells
    - Structure
      - Smaller than astrocytes
      - Few processes
      - Round or oval cell body
    - Location – Between neurons
    - Functions
      - Support neurons in CNS
      - Make myelin in CNS
  - Microglia
    - Structure
      - Small cells
      - Few processes
    - Origin – Monocytes
    - Location
      - Usually stationary
      - May migrate to injury site
    - Functions
      - Destroy microbes
      - Act as small macrophage
  - Ependymal cells
    - Structure
      - Single layer epithelium
      - May be ciliated
    - Functions
      - Line ventricles of brain and spinal cord
      - Help circulate CSF
- PNS
  - Neurolemmocytes (Schwann cells)
    - Structure – Flat cells around axons
    - Function – Produce myelin in PNS
  - Satellite cells
    - Structure – Flat cells around ganglia cell bodies
    - Function – Support PNS ganglia neurons

CNS Neuroglial Cells
Greatly outnumber neurons in the CNS
Scattered throughout NS to Support neurons

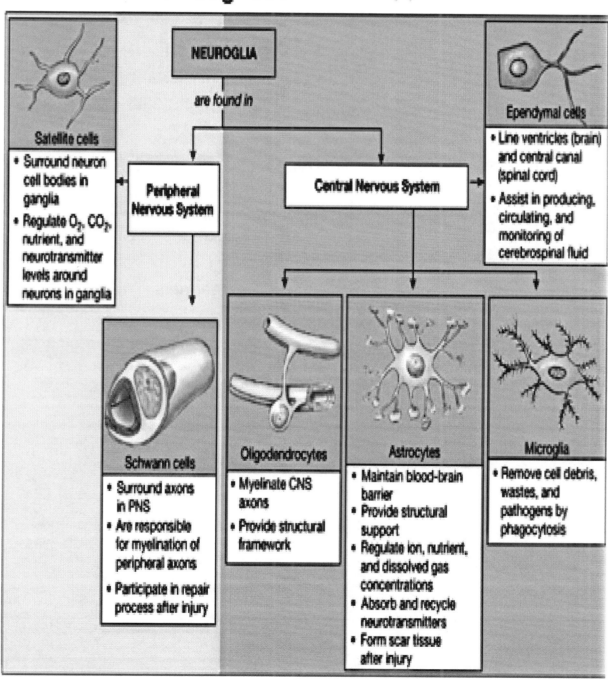

Satellite cells
- Surround neuron cell bodies in ganglia
- Regulate O_2, CO_2, nutrient, and neurotransmitter levels around neurons in ganglia

NEUROGLIA

are found in

Peripheral Nervous System

Central Nervous System

Ependymal cells
- Line ventricles (brain) and central canal (spinal cord)
- Assist in producing, circulating, and monitoring of cerebrospinal fluid

Schwann cells
- Surround axons in PNS
- Are responsible for myelination of peripheral axons
- Participate in repair process after injury

Oligodendrocytes
- Myelinate CNS axons
- Provide structural framework

Astrocytes
- Maintain blood-brain barrier
- Provide structural support
- Regulate ion, nutrient, and dissolved gas concentrations
- Absorb and recycle neurotransmitters
- Form scar tissue after injury

Microglia
- Remove cell debris, wastes, and pathogens by phagocytosis

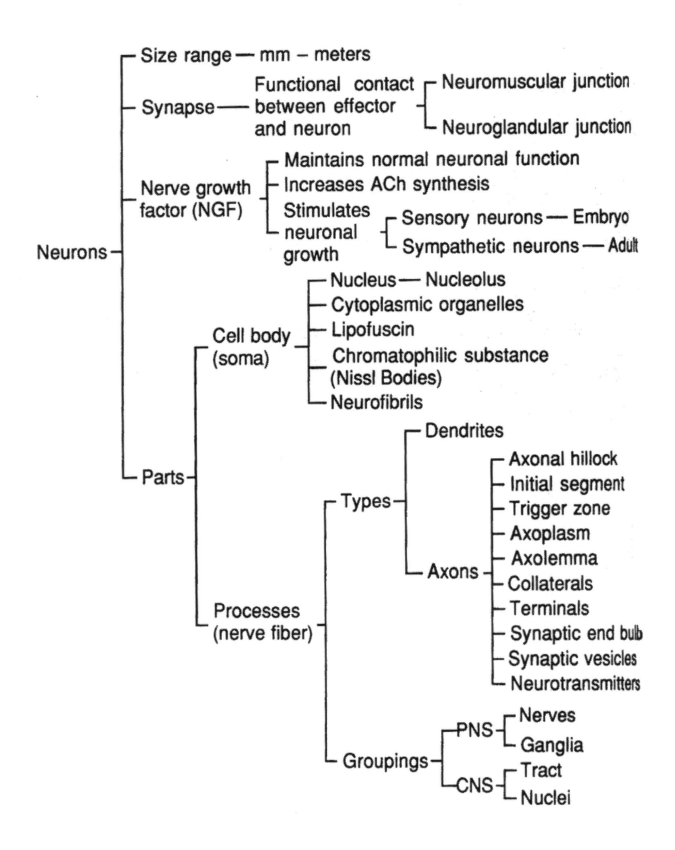

Neurons
- Size range — mm – meters
- Synapse — Functional contact between effector and neuron
  - Neuromuscular junction
  - Neuroglandular junction
- Nerve growth factor (NGF)
  - Maintains normal neuronal function
  - Increases ACh synthesis
  - Stimulates neuronal growth
    - Sensory neurons — Embryo
    - Sympathetic neurons — Adult
- Parts
  - Cell body (soma)
    - Nucleus — Nucleolus
    - Cytoplasmic organelles
    - Lipofuscin
    - Chromatophilic substance (Nissl Bodies)
    - Neurofibrils
  - Processes (nerve fiber)
    - Types
      - Dendrites
      - Axons
        - Axonal hillock
        - Initial segment
        - Trigger zone
        - Axoplasm
        - Axolemma
        - Collaterals
        - Terminals
        - Synaptic end bulb
        - Synaptic vesicles
        - Neurotransmitters
    - Groupings
      - PNS
        - Nerves
        - Ganglia
      - CNS
        - Tract
        - Nuclei

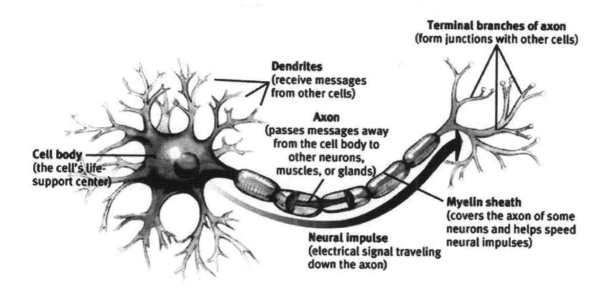

Structural Classes of Neurons

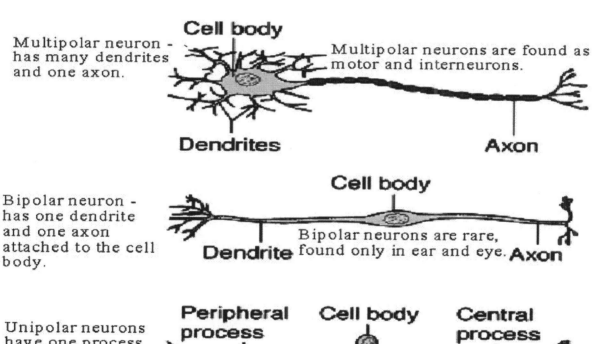

Multipolar neuron - has many dendrites and one axon.

Cell body

Multipolar neurons are found as motor and interneurons.

Dendrites   **Axon**

Bipolar neuron - has one dendrite and one axon attached to the cell body.

Cell body

Dendrite Bipolar neurons are rare, found only in ear and eye. **Axon**

Unipolar neurons have one process from the cell body, an axon. It branches to connect to receptors and the spinal cord or brain.

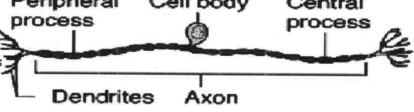

Peripheral process   **Cell body**   **Central process**

Dendrites   **Axon**

Unipolar neurons are most of the body's sensory neurons. The dendrites are found at the receptor and the axon leads to the spinal cord or brain.

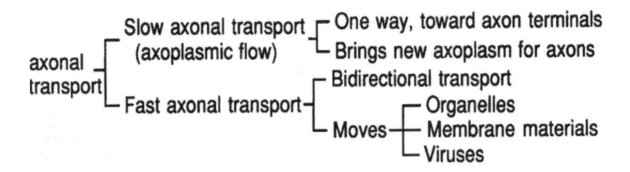

axonal transport
- Slow axonal transport (axoplasmic flow)
  - One way, toward axon terminals
  - Brings new axoplasm for axons
- Fast axonal transport
  - Bidirectional transport
  - Moves
    - Organelles
    - Membrane materials
    - Viruses

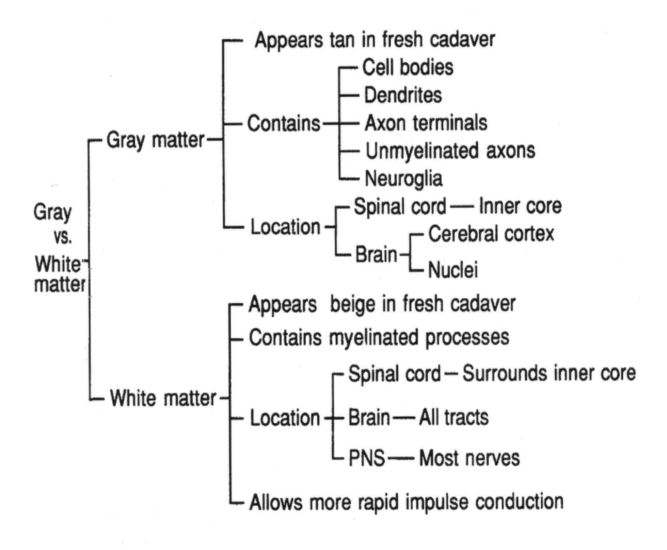

Gray vs. White matter
- Gray matter
  - Appears tan in fresh cadaver
  - Contains
    - Cell bodies
    - Dendrites
    - Axon terminals
    - Unmyelinated axons
    - Neuroglia
  - Location
    - Spinal cord — Inner core
    - Brain
      - Cerebral cortex
      - Nuclei
- White matter
  - Appears beige in fresh cadaver
  - Contains myelinated processes
  - Location
    - Spinal cord — Surrounds inner core
    - Brain — All tracts
    - PNS — Most nerves
  - Allows more rapid impulse conduction

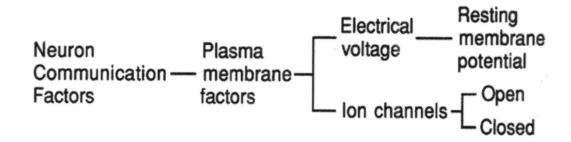

Neuron Communication Factors ─── Plasma membrane factors ┬─ Electrical voltage ─── Resting membrane potential
                                                          └─ Ion channels ┬─ Open
                                                                          └─ Closed

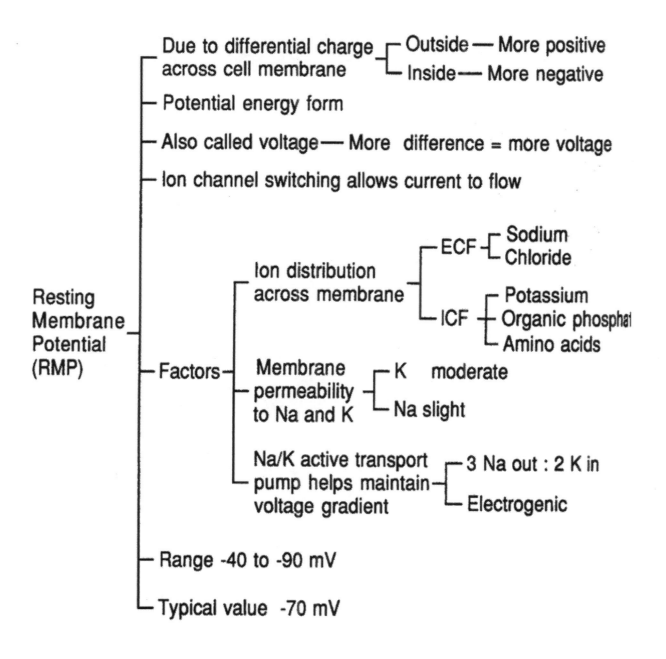

Resting Membrane Potential (RMP) ─┬─ Due to differential charge across cell membrane ┬─ Outside ─ More positive
                                  │   └─ Inside ─ More negative
                                  ├─ Potential energy form
                                  ├─ Also called voltage ─ More difference = more voltage
                                  ├─ Ion channel switching allows current to flow
                                  ├─ Factors ─┬─ Ion distribution across membrane ─┬─ ECF ─┬─ Sodium
                                  │   │   │   └─ Chloride
                                  │   │   └─ ICF ─┬─ Potassium
                                  │   │   ├─ Organic phosphat
                                  │   │   └─ Amino acids
                                  │   ├─ Membrane permeability to Na and K ─┬─ K moderate
                                  │   │   └─ Na slight
                                  │   └─ Na/K active transport pump helps maintain voltage gradient ─┬─ 3 Na out : 2 K in
                                  │   └─ Electrogenic
                                  ├─ Range -40 to -90 mV
                                  └─ Typical value -70 mV

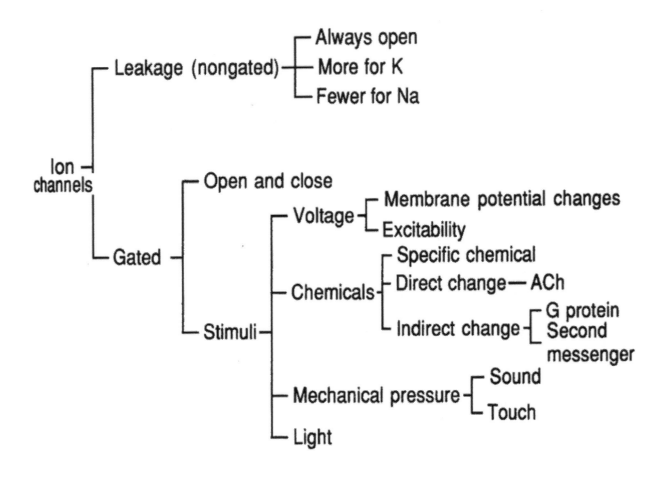

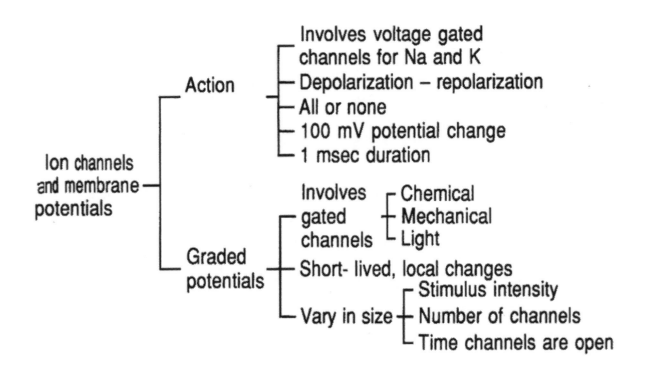

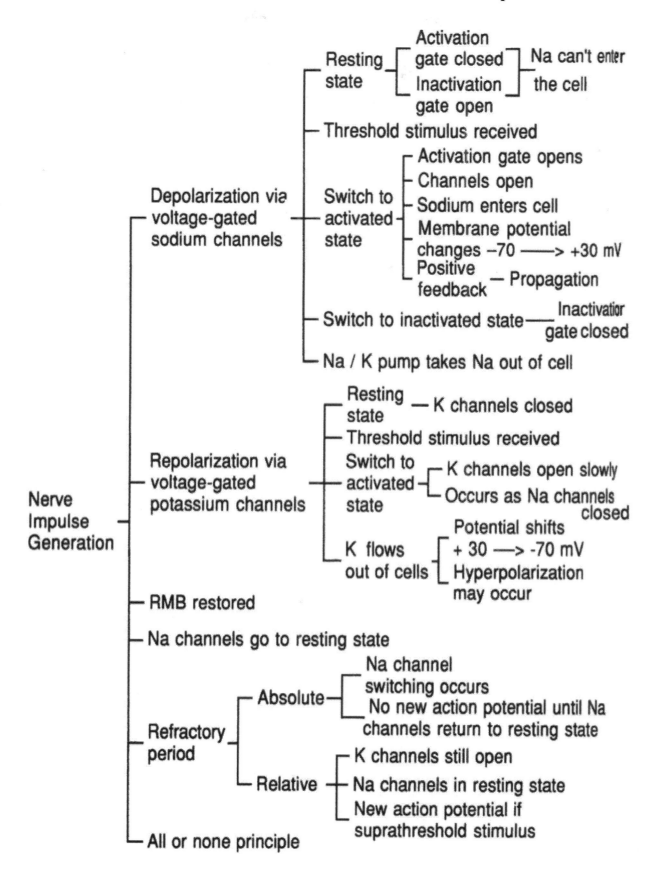

Nerve Impulse Generation
- Depolarization via voltage-gated sodium channels
  - Resting state
    - Activation gate closed
    - Inactivation gate open
    - Na can't enter the cell
  - Threshold stimulus received
  - Switch to activated state
    - Activation gate opens
    - Channels open
    - Sodium enters cell
    - Membrane potential changes −70 ——> +30 mV
    - Positive feedback — Propagation
  - Switch to inactivated state — Inactivation gate closed
  - Na / K pump takes Na out of cell
- Repolarization via voltage-gated potassium channels
  - Resting state — K channels closed
  - Threshold stimulus received
  - Switch to activated state
    - K channels open slowly
    - Occurs as Na channels closed
  - K flows out of cells
    - Potential shifts + 30 ——> -70 mV
    - Hyperpolarization may occur
- RMB restored
- Na channels go to resting state
- Refractory period
  - Absolute
    - Na channel switching occurs
    - No new action potential until Na channels return to resting state
  - Relative
    - K channels still open
    - Na channels in resting state
    - New action potential if suprathreshold stimulus
- All or none principle

(a) Resting state (cytosolic face negative)

Action Potential

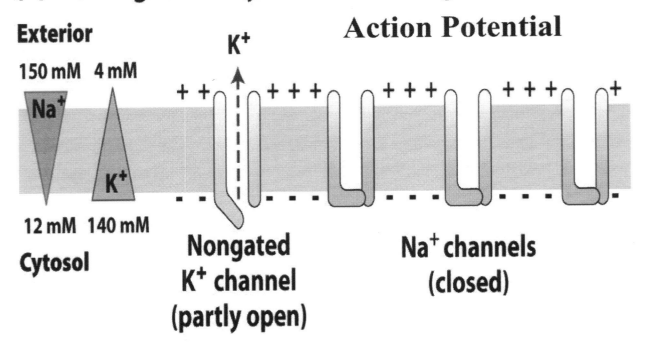

(b) Depolarized state (cytosolic face positive)

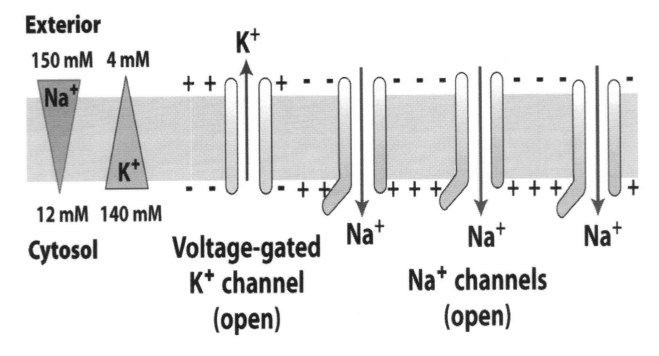

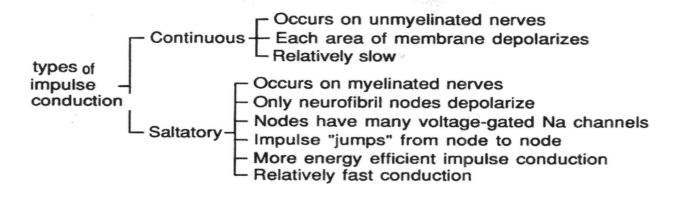

types of impulse conduction

- Continuous
  - Occurs on unmyelinated nerves
  - Each area of membrane depolarizes
  - Relatively slow
- Saltatory
  - Occurs on myelinated nerves
  - Only neurofibril nodes depolarize
  - Nodes have many voltage-gated Na channels
  - Impulse "jumps" from node to node
  - More energy efficient impulse conduction
  - Relatively fast conduction

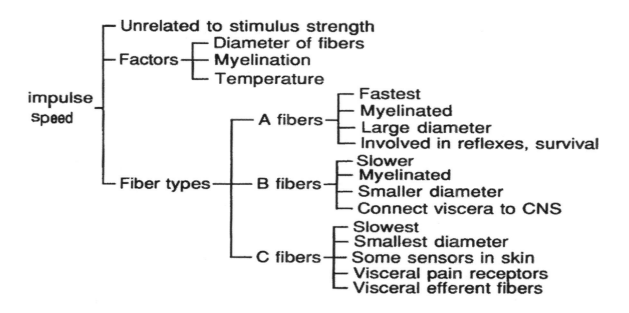

impulse speed

- Unrelated to stimulus strength
- Factors
  - Diameter of fibers
  - Myelination
  - Temperature
- Fiber types
  - A fibers
    - Fastest
    - Myelinated
    - Large diameter
    - Involved in reflexes, survival
  - B fibers
    - Slower
    - Myelinated
    - Smaller diameter
    - Connect viscera to CNS
  - C fibers
    - Slowest
    - Smallest diameter
    - Some sensors in skin
    - Visceral pain receptors
    - Visceral efferent fibers

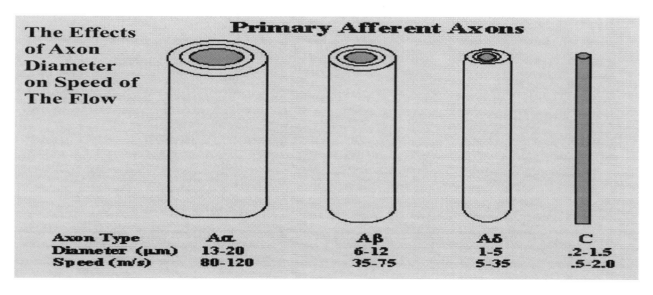

The Effects of Axon Diameter on Speed of The Flow

Primary Afferent Axons

Axon Type	Aα	Aβ	Aδ	C
Diameter (μm)	13-20	6-12	1-5	.2-1.5
Speed (m/s)	80-120	35-75	5-35	.5-2.0

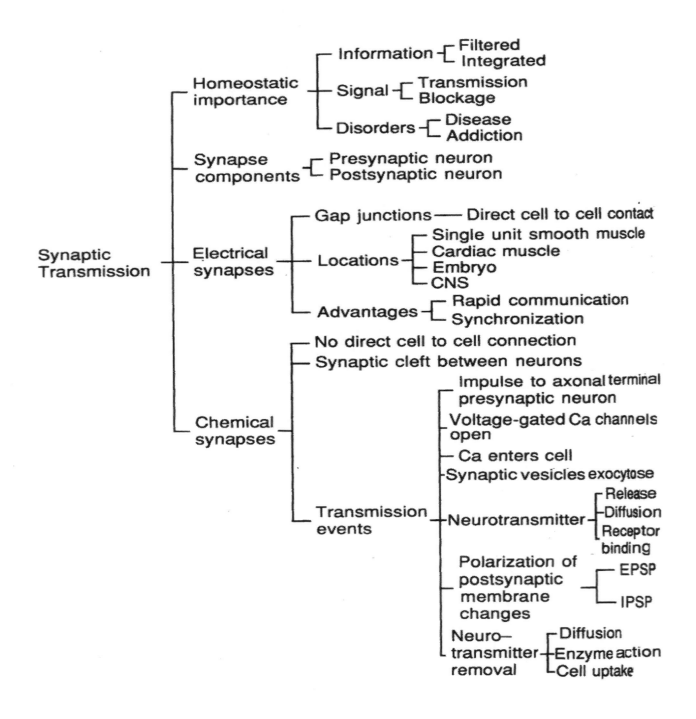

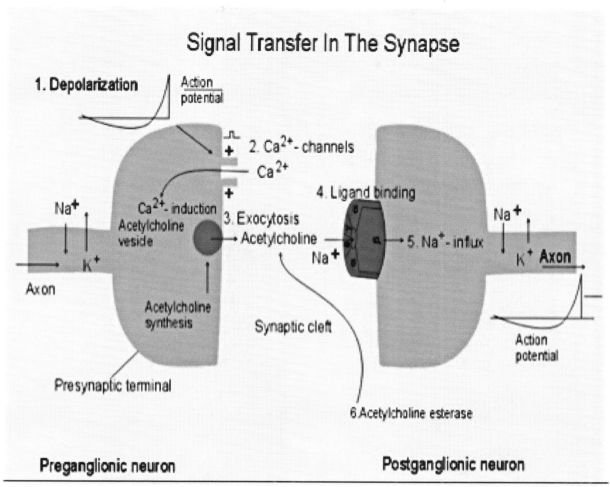

Signal Transfer In The Synapse

1. Depolarization

Action potential

2. Ca²⁺- channels

Ca²⁺

4. Ligand binding

Na⁺

Ca²⁺- induction
Acetylcholine veside

3. Exocytosis
Acetylcholine

Na⁺

5. Na⁺- influx

Na⁺

K⁺ **Axon**

Axon

Acetylcholine synthesis

Synaptic cleft

Action potential

Presynaptic terminal

6. Acetylcholine esterase

Preganglionic neuron   Postganglionic neuron

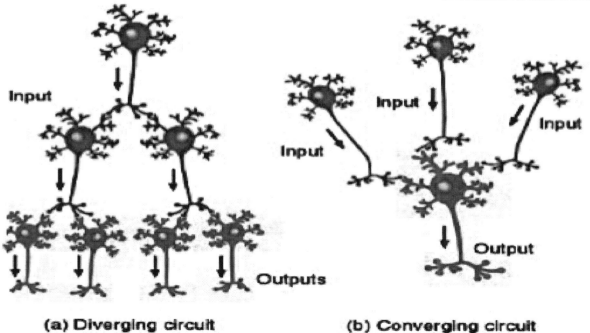

Input

Output

Input

Input

Input

Input

Outputs

Output

(a) Diverging circuit   (b) Converging circuit

Synaptic Transmission

(A) Electrical synaptic transmission with ions flowing through gap junction channels (B) Chemical synaptic transmission with synaptic cleft and ions flowing through postsynaptic channels

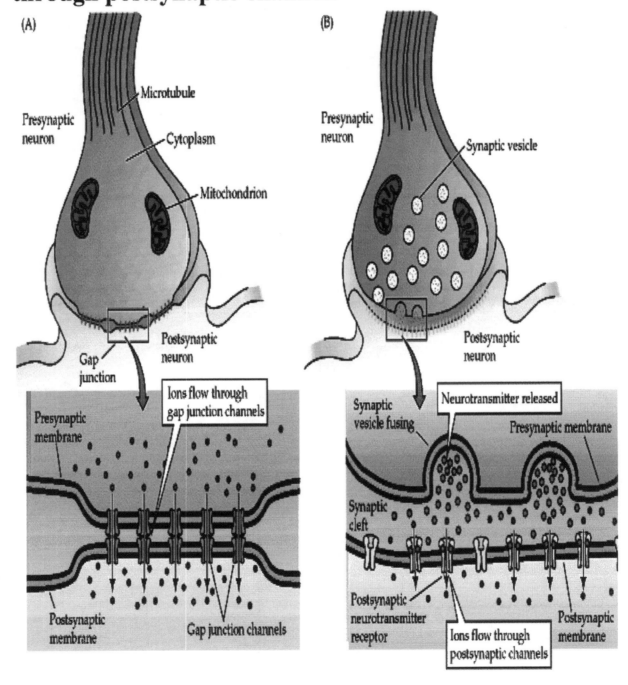

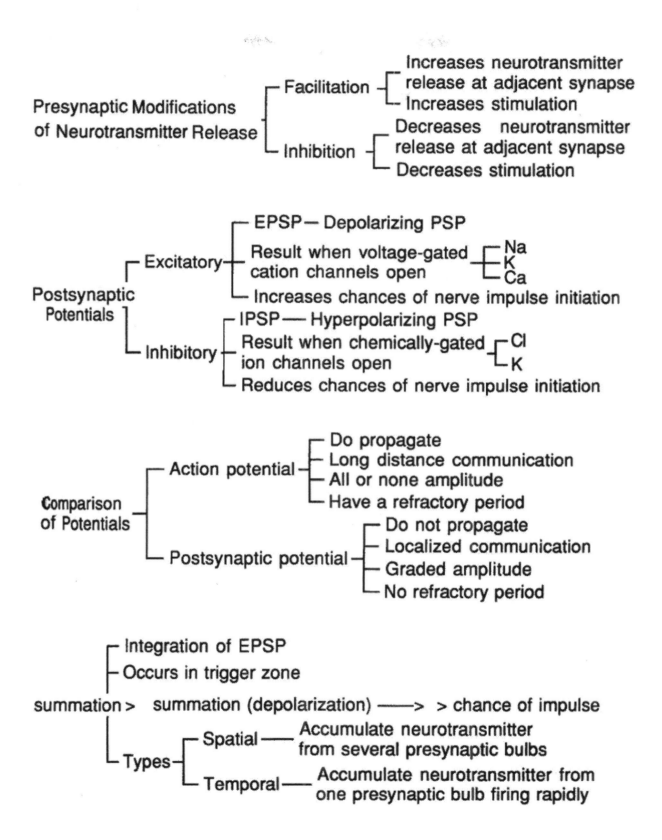

Presynaptic Modifications of Neurotransmitter Release
- Facilitation
  - Increases neurotransmitter release at adjacent synapse
  - Increases stimulation
- Inhibition
  - Decreases neurotransmitter release at adjacent synapse
  - Decreases stimulation

Postsynaptic Potentials
- Excitatory
  - EPSP — Depolarizing PSP
  - Result when voltage-gated cation channels open
    - Na
    - K
    - Ca
  - Increases chances of nerve impulse initiation
- Inhibitory
  - IPSP — Hyperpolarizing PSP
  - Result when chemically-gated ion channels open
    - Cl
    - K
  - Reduces chances of nerve impulse initiation

Comparison of Potentials
- Action potential
  - Do propagate
  - Long distance communication
  - All or none amplitude
  - Have a refractory period
- Postsynaptic potential
  - Do not propagate
  - Localized communication
  - Graded amplitude
  - No refractory period

summation
- Integration of EPSP
- Occurs in trigger zone
- summation (depolarization) ——> > chance of impulse
- Types
  - Spatial — Accumulate neurotransmitter from several presynaptic bulbs
  - Temporal — Accumulate neurotransmitter from one presynaptic bulb firing rapidly

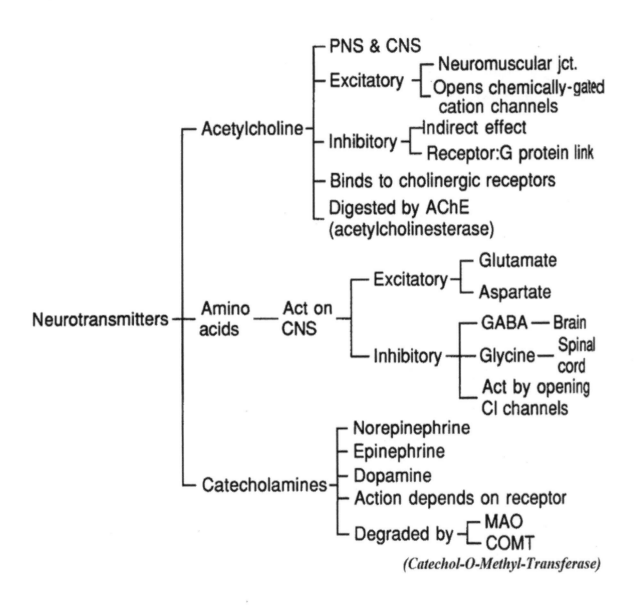

Neurotransmitters
- Acetylcholine
  - PNS & CNS
  - Excitatory
    - Neuromuscular jct.
    - Opens chemically-gated cation channels
  - Inhibitory
    - Indirect effect
    - Receptor:G protein link
  - Binds to cholinergic receptors
  - Digested by AChE (acetylcholinesterase)
- Amino acids — Act on CNS
  - Excitatory
    - Glutamate
    - Aspartate
  - Inhibitory
    - GABA — Brain
    - Glycine — Spinal cord
    - Act by opening Cl channels
- Catecholamines
  - Norepinephrine
  - Epinephrine
  - Dopamine
  - Action depends on receptor
  - Degraded by
    - MAO
    - COMT
  (Catechol-O-Methyl-Transferase)

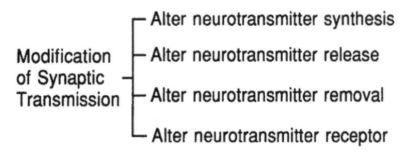

Modification of Synaptic Transmission
- Alter neurotransmitter synthesis
- Alter neurotransmitter release
- Alter neurotransmitter removal
- Alter neurotransmitter receptor

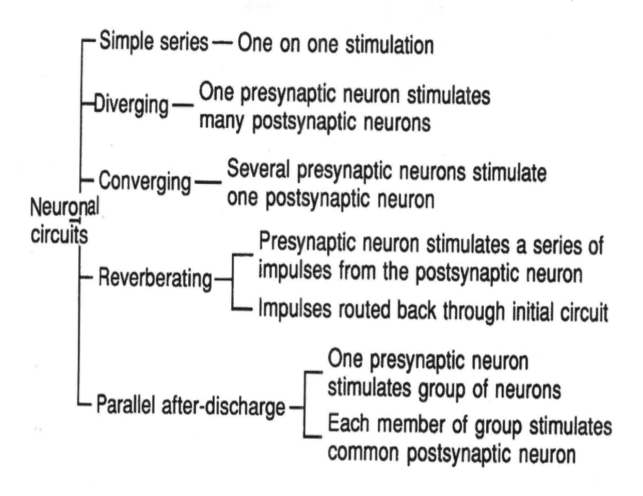

Neuronal circuits
- Simple series — One on one stimulation
- Diverging — One presynaptic neuron stimulates many postsynaptic neurons
- Converging — Several presynaptic neurons stimulate one postsynaptic neuron
- Reverberating
  - Presynaptic neuron stimulates a series of impulses from the postsynaptic neuron
  - Impulses routed back through initial circuit
- Parallel after-discharge
  - One presynaptic neuron stimulates group of neurons
  - Each member of group stimulates common postsynaptic neuron

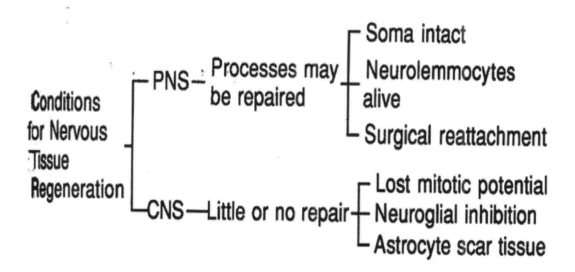

Conditions for Nervous Tissue Regeneration
- PNS — Processes may be repaired
  - Soma intact
  - Neurolemmocytes alive
  - Surgical reattachment
- CNS — Little or no repair
  - Lost mitotic potential
  - Neuroglial inhibition
  - Astrocyte scar tissue

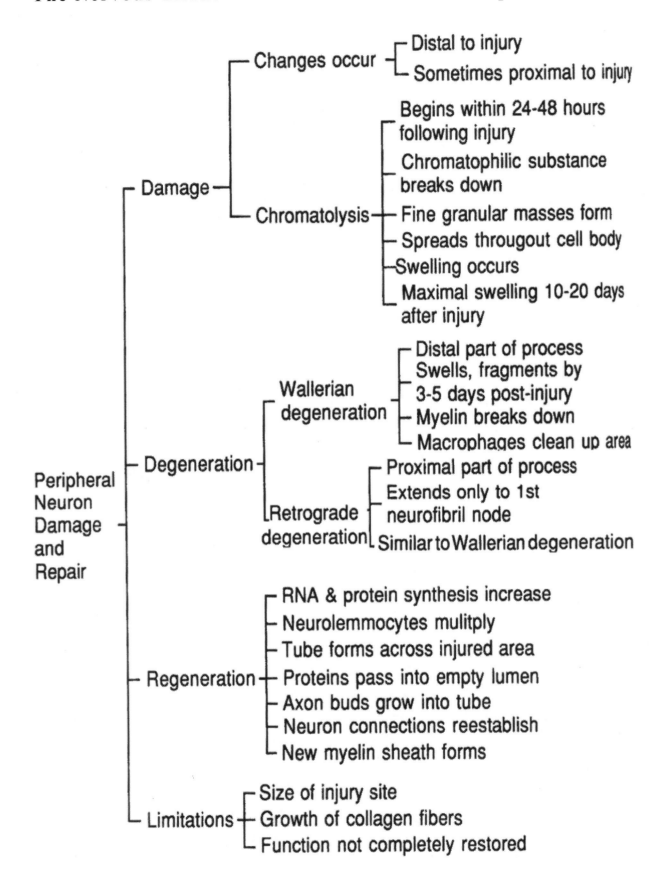

Peripheral Neuron Damage and Repair
- Damage
  - Changes occur
    - Distal to injury
    - Sometimes proximal to injury
  - Chromatolysis
    - Begins within 24-48 hours following injury
    - Chromatophilic substance breaks down
    - Fine granular masses form
    - Spreads througout cell body
    - Swelling occurs
    - Maximal swelling 10-20 days after injury
- Degeneration
  - Wallerian degeneration
    - Distal part of process Swells, fragments by 3-5 days post-injury
    - Myelin breaks down
    - Macrophages clean up area
  - Retrograde degeneration
    - Proximal part of process
    - Extends only to 1st neurofibril node
    - Similar to Wallerian degeneration
- Regeneration
  - RNA & protein synthesis increase
  - Neurolemmocytes mulitply
  - Tube forms across injured area
  - Proteins pass into empty lumen
  - Axon buds grow into tube
  - Neuron connections reestablish
  - New myelin sheath forms
- Limitations
  - Size of injury site
  - Growth of collagen fibers
  - Function not completely restored

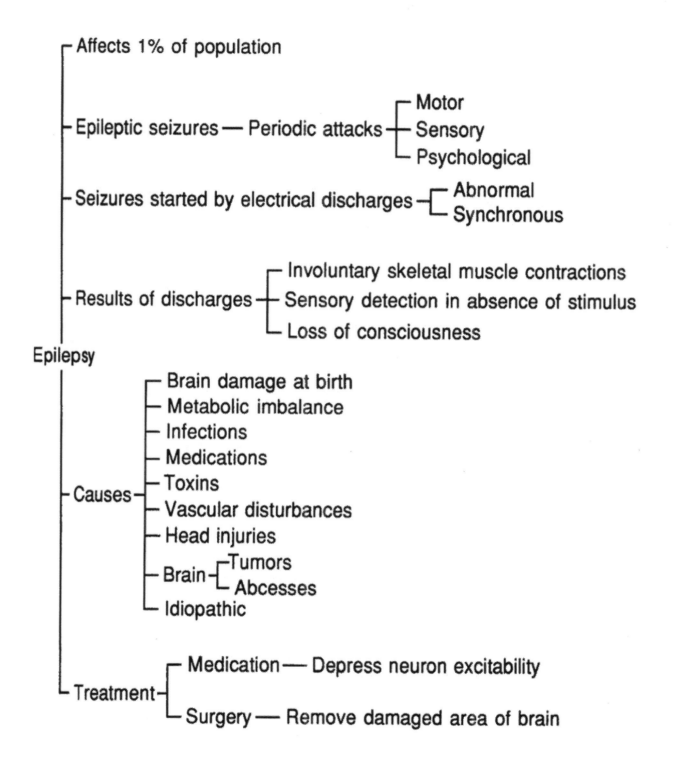

Epilepsy
- Affects 1% of population
- Epileptic seizures — Periodic attacks
  - Motor
  - Sensory
  - Psychological
- Seizures started by electrical discharges
  - Abnormal
  - Synchronous
- Results of discharges
  - Involuntary skeletal muscle contractions
  - Sensory detection in absence of stimulus
  - Loss of consciousness
- Causes
  - Brain damage at birth
  - Metabolic imbalance
  - Infections
  - Medications
  - Toxins
  - Vascular disturbances
  - Head injuries
  - Brain
    - Tumors
    - Abcesses
  - Idiopathic
- Treatment
  - Medication — Depress neuron excitability
  - Surgery — Remove damaged area of brain

CHAPTER THIRTEEN

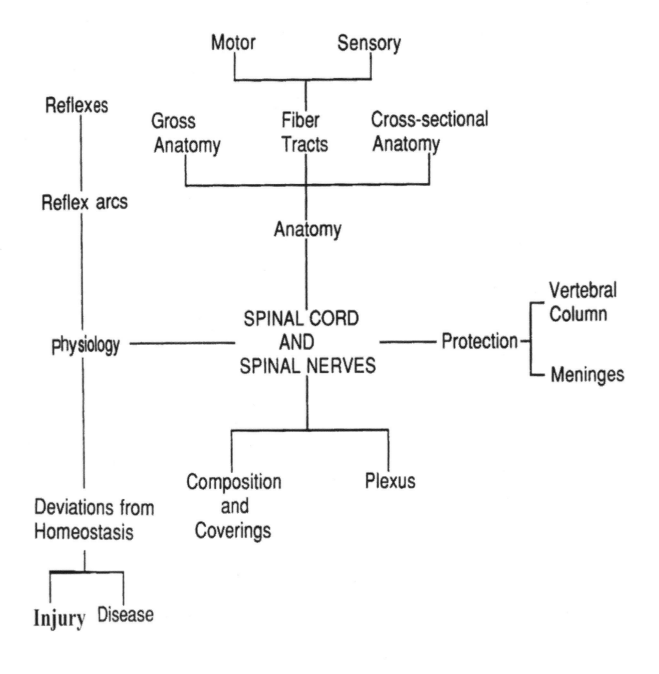

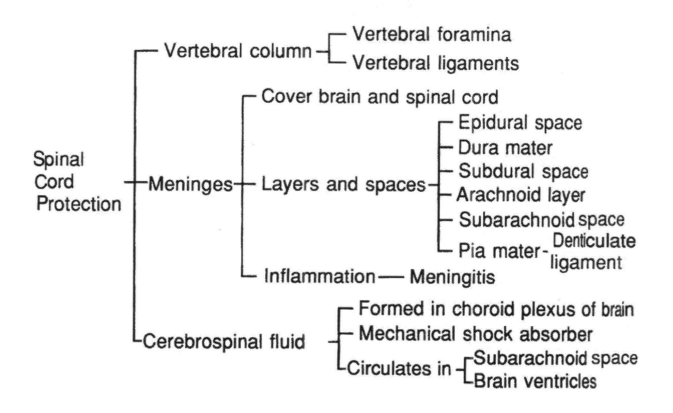

Spinal Cord Protection
- Vertebral column
  - Vertebral foramina
  - Vertebral ligaments
- Meninges
  - Cover brain and spinal cord
  - Layers and spaces
    - Epidural space
    - Dura mater
    - Subdural space
    - Arachnoid layer
    - Subarachnoid space
    - Pia mater — Denticulate ligament
  - Inflammation — Meningitis
- Cerebrospinal fluid
  - Formed in choroid plexus of brain
  - Mechanical shock absorber
  - Circulates in
    - Subarachnoid space
    - Brain ventricles

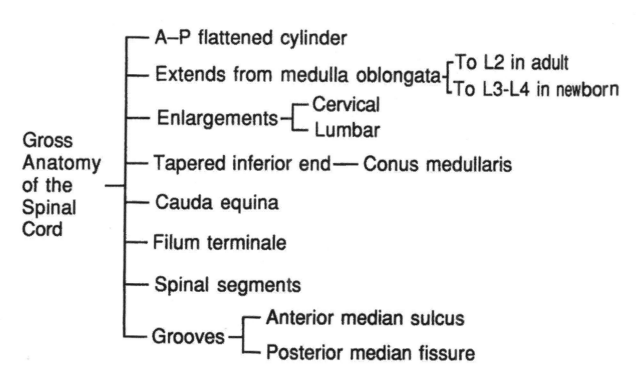

Gross Anatomy of the Spinal Cord
- A–P flattened cylinder
- Extends from medulla oblongata
  - To L2 in adult
  - To L3-L4 in newborn
- Enlargements
  - Cervical
  - Lumbar
- Tapered inferior end — Conus medullaris
- Cauda equina
- Filum terminale
- Spinal segments
- Grooves
  - Anterior median sulcus
  - Posterior median fissure

The Spinal Cord and Spinal nerves with the five groups of vertebrae- Cervical (C), Thoracic (T), Lumbar (L), Sacral (S) and Coccygeal (Co)

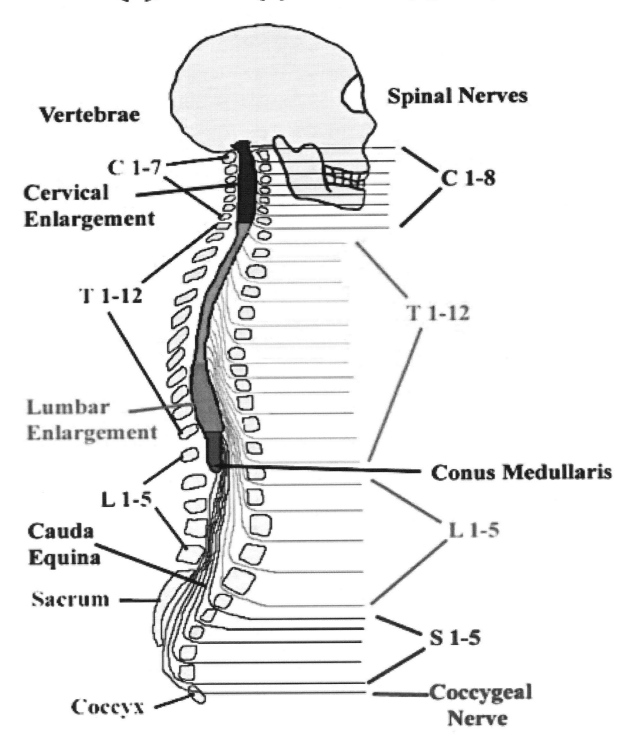

Vertebrae

Spinal Nerves

C 1-7

Cervical Enlargement

C 1-8

T 1-12

T 1-12

Lumbar Enlargement

Conus Medullaris

L 1-5

L 1-5

Cauda Equina

Sacrum

S 1-5

Coccyx

Coccygeal Nerve

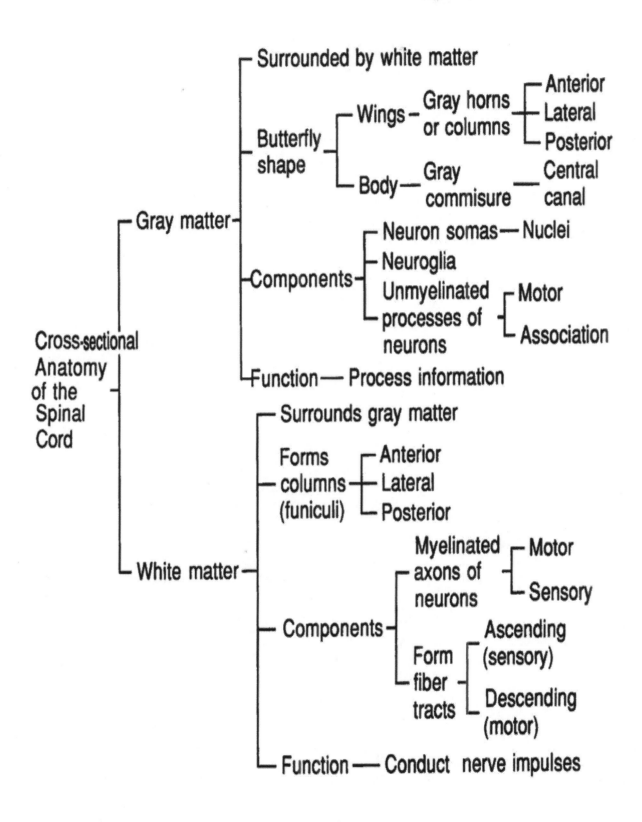

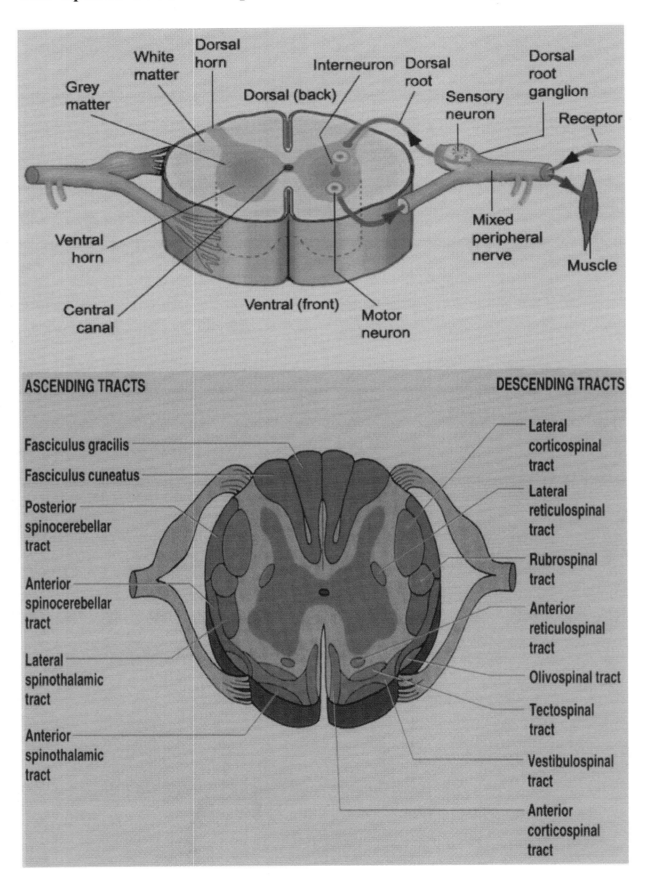

ASCENDING TRACTS

Grey matter
White matter
Dorsal horn
Dorsal (back)
Interneuron
Dorsal root
Sensory neuron
Dorsal root ganglion
Receptor
Ventral horn
Central canal
Ventral (front)
Motor neuron
Mixed peripheral nerve
Muscle

DESCENDING TRACTS

Fasciculus gracilis
Fasciculus cuneatus
Posterior spinocerebellar tract
Anterior spinocerebellar tract
Lateral spinothalamic tract
Anterior spinothalamic tract

Lateral corticospinal tract
Lateral reticulospinal tract
Rubrospinal tract
Anterior reticulospinal tract
Olivospinal tract
Tectospinal tract
Vestibulospinal tract
Anterior corticospinal tract

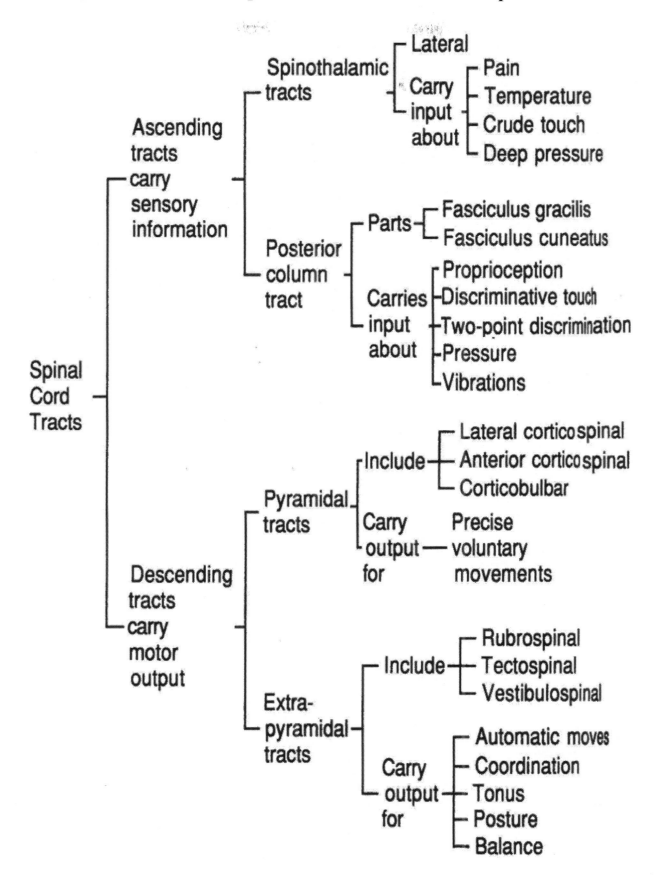

Selected descending motor pathway of the Corticospinal tract, lateral corticospinal tract (LCST) and anterior corticospinal tract (ACST)

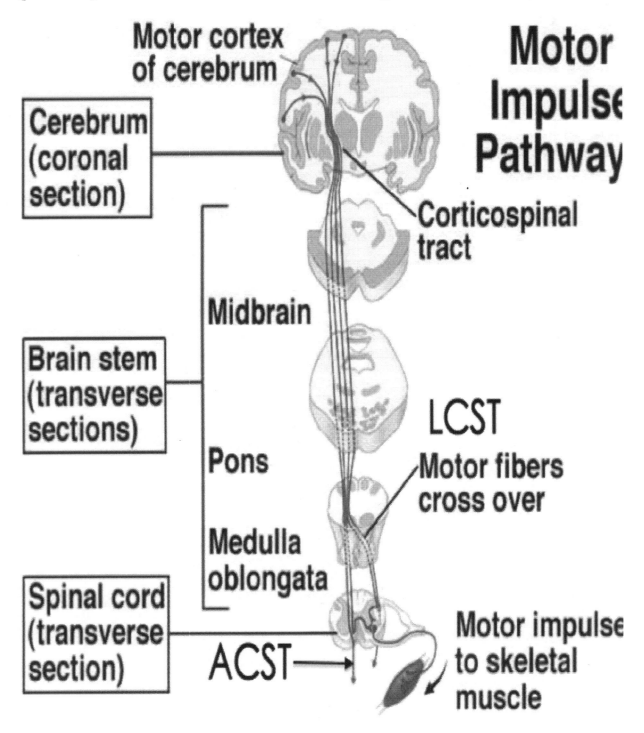

Motor cortex of cerebrum

Cerebrum (coronal section)

Motor Impulse Pathway

Corticospinal tract

Midbrain

Brain stem (transverse sections)

Pons

LCST

Motor fibers cross over

Medulla oblongata

Spinal cord (transverse section)

ACST

Motor impulse to skeletal muscle

The pathways of Pain and temperature go through the Lateral spinothalmic tract (LSTT), and pathway of the mechanosensory like touch and pressure go through anterior spinothalamic tract (ASTT)

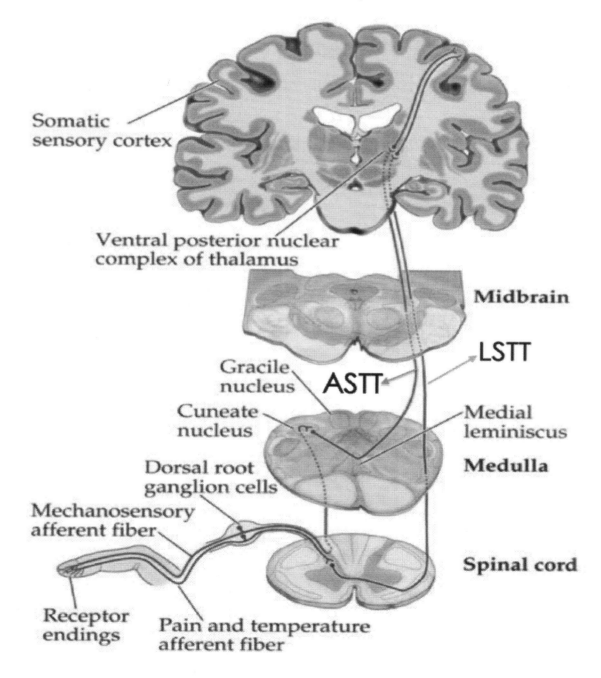

Somatic sensory cortex

Ventral posterior nuclear complex of thalamus

Midbrain

LSTT

Gracile nucleus   **ASTT**

Cuneate nucleus

Medial leminiscus

Dorsal root ganglion cells

Medulla

Mechanosensory afferent fiber

Spinal cord

Receptor endings

Pain and temperature afferent fiber

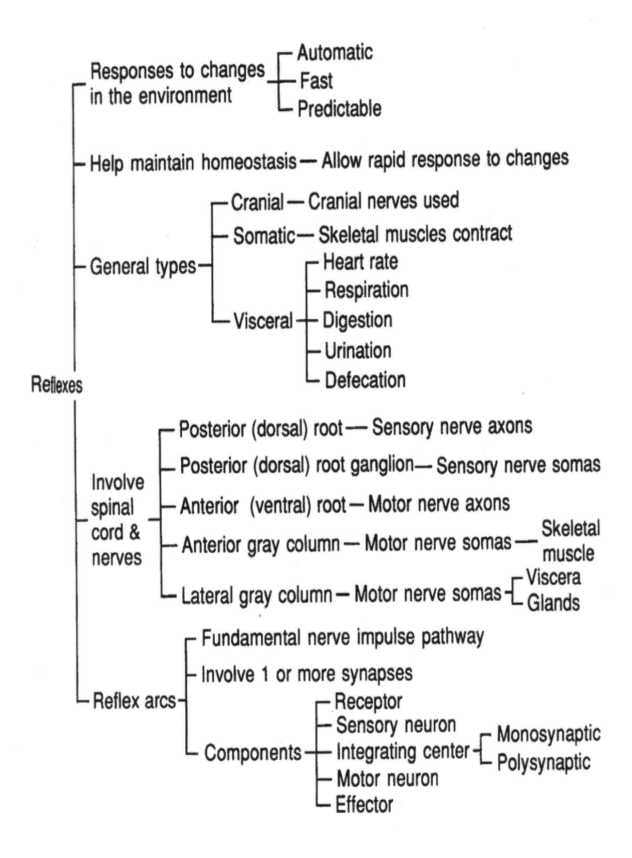

Somatic Reflex Arc

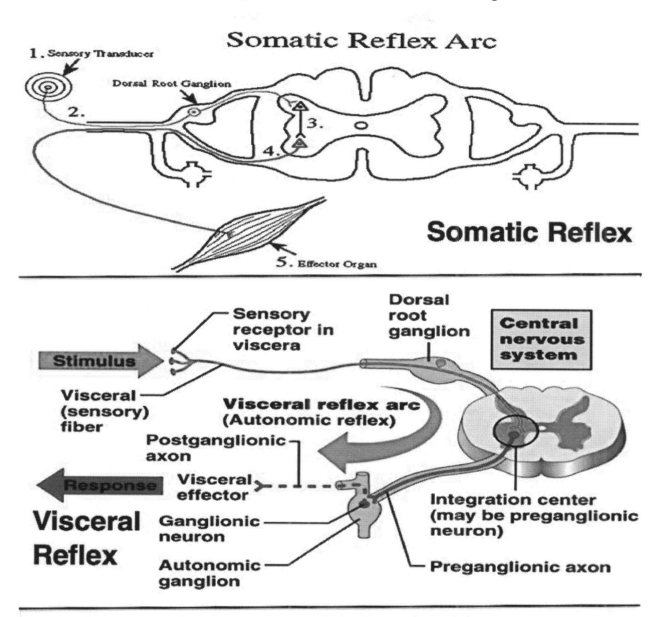

1. Sensory Transducer

Dorsal Root Ganglion

2.

3.

4.

5. Effector Organ

Somatic Reflex

Sensory receptor in viscera

Dorsal root ganglion

Central nervous system

Stimulus

Visceral reflex arc (Autonomic reflex)

Visceral (sensory) fiber

Postganglionic axon

Response

Visceral effector

Visceral Reflex

Ganglionic neuron

Autonomic ganglion

Integration center (may be preganglionic neuron)

Preganglionic axon

Pupillary Light Reflex – constriction in response to light

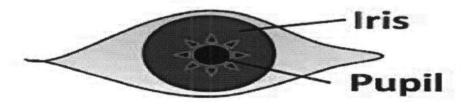

Iris

Pupil

Autonomic Cranial Reflex

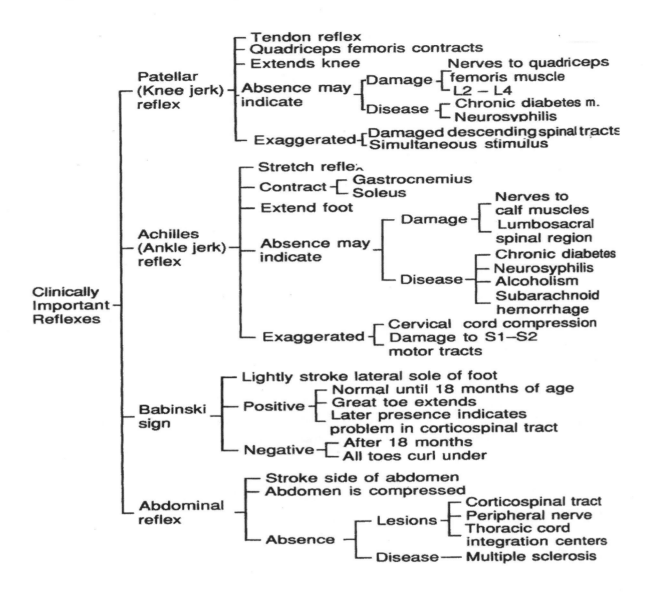

Clinically Important Reflexes

- Patellar (Knee jerk) reflex
  - Tendon reflex
  - Quadriceps femoris contracts
  - Extends knee
  - Absence may indicate
    - Damage — Nerves to quadriceps femoris muscle L2 – L4
    - Disease — Chronic diabetes m. / Neurosyphilis
  - Exaggerated — Damaged descending spinal tracts / Simultaneous stimulus

- Achilles (Ankle jerk) reflex
  - Stretch reflex
  - Contract — Gastrocnemius / Soleus
  - Extend foot
  - Absence may indicate
    - Damage — Nerves to calf muscles / Lumbosacral spinal region
    - Disease — Chronic diabetes / Neurosyphilis / Alcoholism / Subarachnoid hemorrhage
  - Exaggerated — Cervical cord compression / Damage to S1–S2 motor tracts

- Babinski sign
  - Lightly stroke lateral sole of foot
  - Positive — Normal until 18 months of age / Great toe extends / Later presence indicates problem in corticospinal tract
  - Negative — After 18 months / All toes curl under

- Abdominal reflex
  - Stroke side of abdomen
  - Abdomen is compressed
  - Absence
    - Lesions — Corticospinal tract / Peripheral nerve / Thoracic cord integration centers
    - Disease — Multiple sclerosis

DIAGRAM OF KNEE JERK STRETCH REFLEX

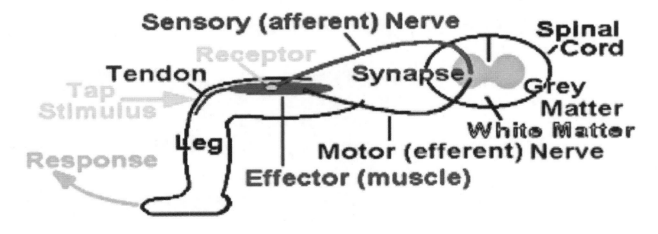

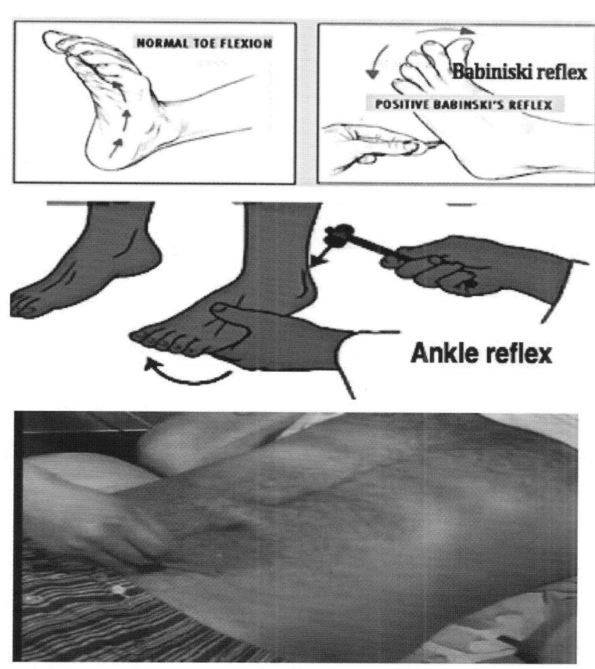

Abdominal Reflex Is a superficial neurological stimulated by stroking of the abdomen around umbilicus. It can be helpful in determining the of lesion in a neurology case. Being a superficial reflex, it is polysynaptic

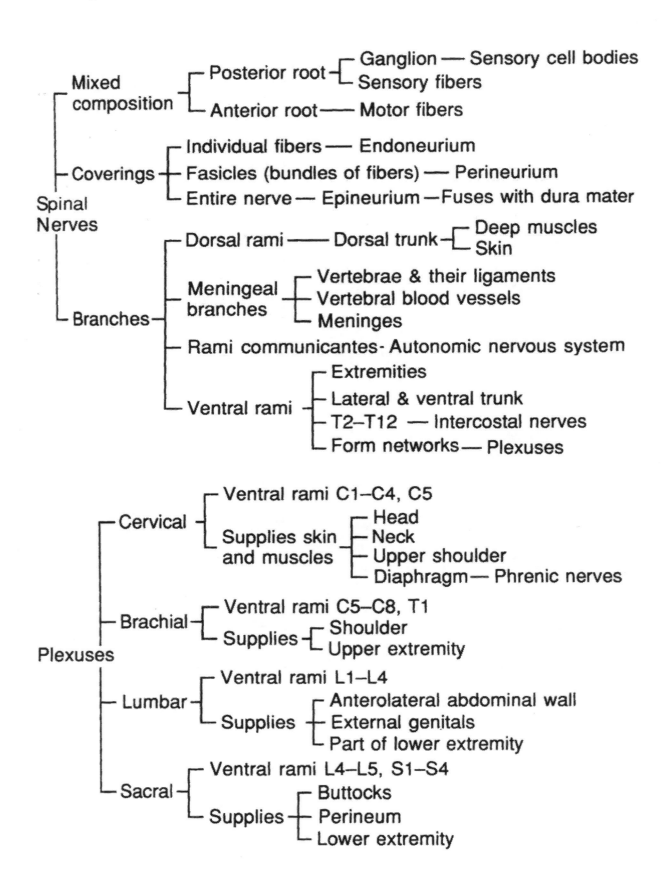

Spinal Nerves
- Mixed composition
  - Posterior root
    - Ganglion — Sensory cell bodies
    - Sensory fibers
  - Anterior root —— Motor fibers
- Coverings
  - Individual fibers — Endoneurium
  - Fasicles (bundles of fibers) — Perineurium
  - Entire nerve — Epineurium — Fuses with dura mater
- Branches
  - Dorsal rami —— Dorsal trunk
    - Deep muscles
    - Skin
  - Meningeal branches
    - Vertebrae & their ligaments
    - Vertebral blood vessels
    - Meninges
  - Rami communicantes - Autonomic nervous system
  - Ventral rami
    - Extremities
    - Lateral & ventral trunk
    - T2–T12 — Intercostal nerves
    - Form networks — Plexuses

Plexuses
- Cervical
  - Ventral rami C1–C4, C5
  - Supplies skin and muscles
    - Head
    - Neck
    - Upper shoulder
    - Diaphragm — Phrenic nerves
- Brachial
  - Ventral rami C5–C8, T1
  - Supplies
    - Shoulder
    - Upper extremity
- Lumbar
  - Ventral rami L1–L4
  - Supplies
    - Anterolateral abdominal wall
    - External genitals
    - Part of lower extremity
- Sacral
  - Ventral rami L4–L5, S1–S4
  - Supplies
    - Buttocks
    - Perineum
    - Lower extremity

(A) Nervous Plexus

(B) Spinal Map

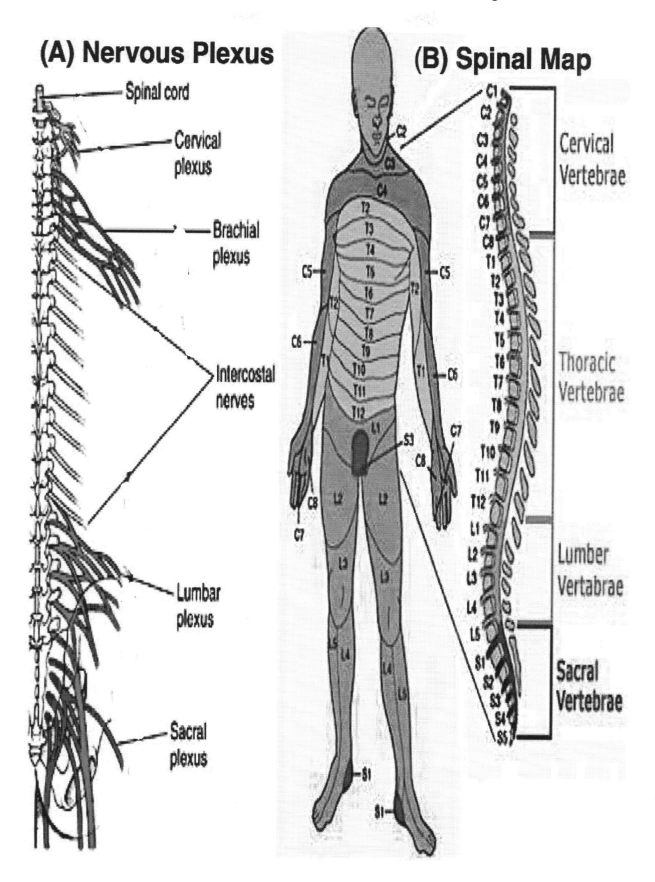

Spinal cord

Cervical plexus

Brachial plexus

Intercostal nerves

Lumbar plexus

Sacral plexus

Cervical Vertebrae

Thoracic Vertebrae

Lumber Vertabrae

Sacral Vertebrae

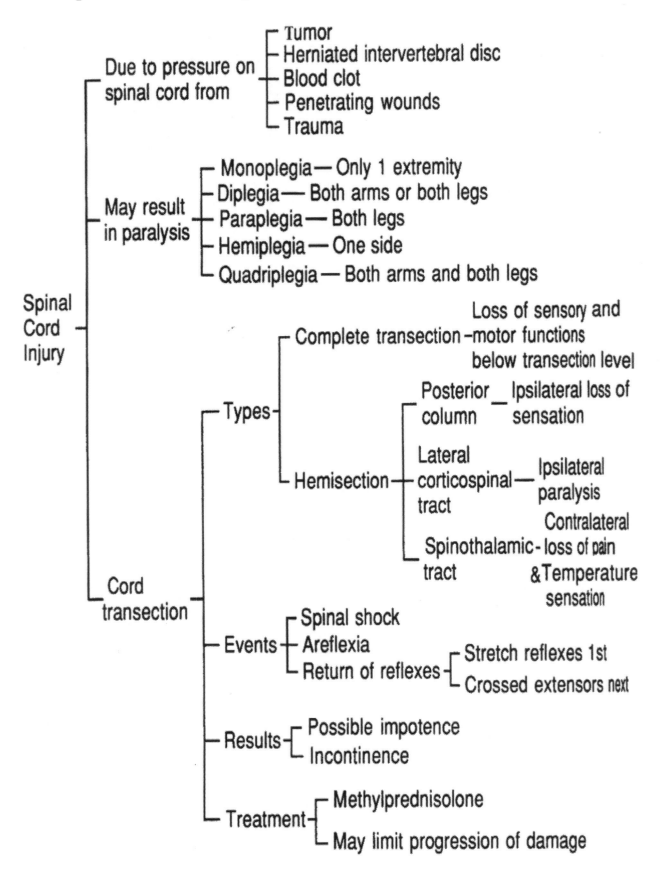

Spinal Cord Injury

Due to pressure on spinal cord from
- Tumor
- Herniated intervertebral disc
- Blood clot
- Penetrating wounds
- Trauma

May result in paralysis
- Monoplegia — Only 1 extremity
- Diplegia — Both arms or both legs
- Paraplegia — Both legs
- Hemiplegia — One side
- Quadriplegia — Both arms and both legs

Cord transection

Types
- Complete transection — Loss of sensory and motor functions below transection level
- Hemisection
  - Posterior column — Ipsilateral loss of sensation
  - Lateral corticospinal tract — Ipsilateral paralysis
  - Spinothalamic tract — Contralateral loss of pain & Temperature sensation

Events
- Spinal shock
- Areflexia
- Return of reflexes
  - Stretch reflexes 1st
  - Crossed extensors next

Results
- Possible impotence
- Incontinence

Treatment
- Methylprednisolone
- May limit progression of damage

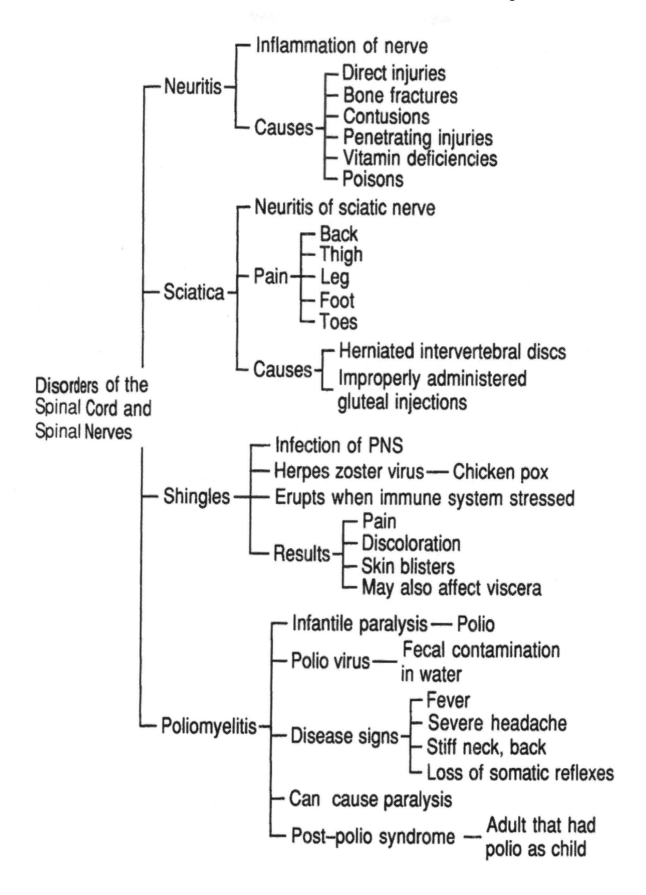

Disorders of the Spinal Cord and Spinal Nerves

- Neuritis
  - Inflammation of nerve
  - Causes
    - Direct injuries
    - Bone fractures
    - Contusions
    - Penetrating injuries
    - Vitamin deficiencies
    - Poisons
- Sciatica
  - Neuritis of sciatic nerve
  - Pain
    - Back
    - Thigh
    - Leg
    - Foot
    - Toes
  - Causes
    - Herniated intervertebral discs
    - Improperly administered gluteal injections
- Shingles
  - Infection of PNS
  - Herpes zoster virus — Chicken pox
  - Erupts when immune system stressed
  - Results
    - Pain
    - Discoloration
    - Skin blisters
    - May also affect viscera
- Poliomyelitis
  - Infantile paralysis — Polio
  - Polio virus — Fecal contamination in water
  - Disease signs
    - Fever
    - Severe headache
    - Stiff neck, back
    - Loss of somatic reflexes
  - Can cause paralysis
  - Post-polio syndrome — Adult that had polio as child

CHAPTER FOURTEEN

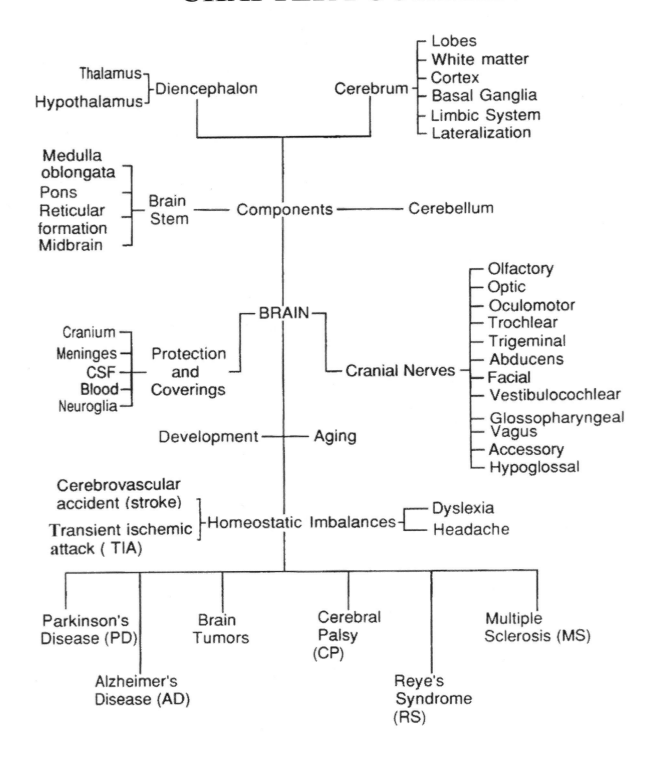

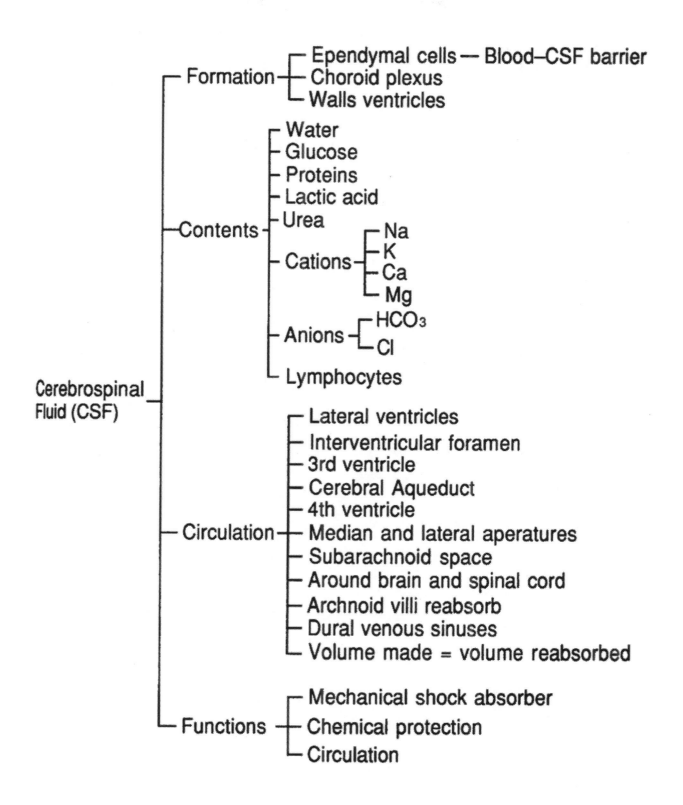

The flow of cerebrospinal fluid from the time of its formation from blood in the choroid plexuses until its reabsorbs by archanoid villi and return to the blood in the superior sagittal sinus

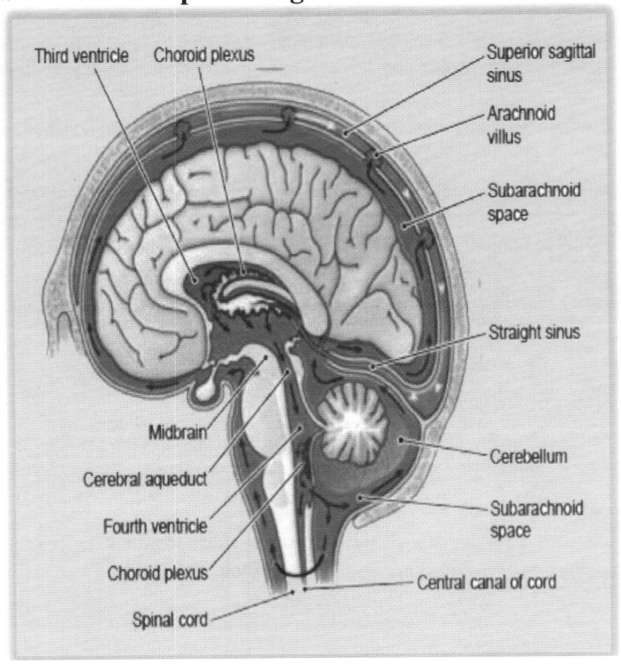

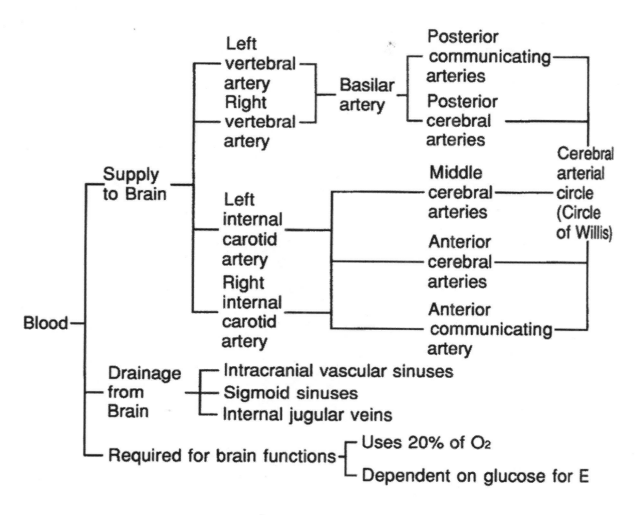

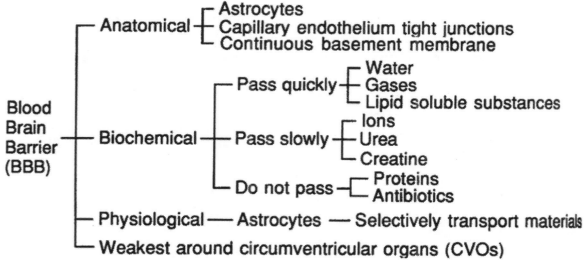

Blood Vessels of the Brain

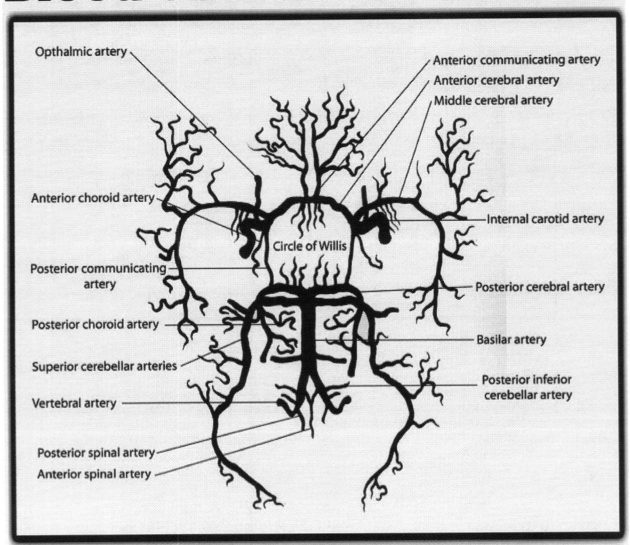

Normal protein, glucose, red blood cells and white blood cells of CSF and blood

Component	CSF	Blood
Protein	35 mg/dl	700 mg/dl
Glucose	60 mg/dl	90 mg/dl
Red blood cells	0/mm3	5 million red blood cells per micro-liter of blood
White blood cells	< 5/mm3	7000 white blood cells per micro-liter of blood

Blood-Brain Barrier

Schematic diagram of interfaces between blood, brain and cerebrospinal fluid (CSF); Arrows indicate formation of CSF at the choroid plexus, and interstitial fluid at the brain capillary. The cerebrospinal fluid is absorbed to blood at the arachnoids villi, SAS; subarachnoid space

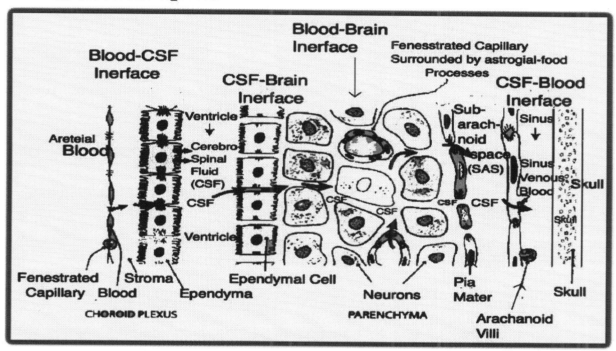

Cellular constituents of the blood–brain barrier

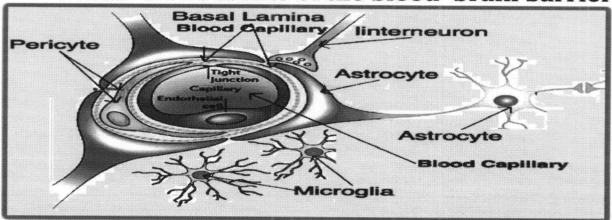

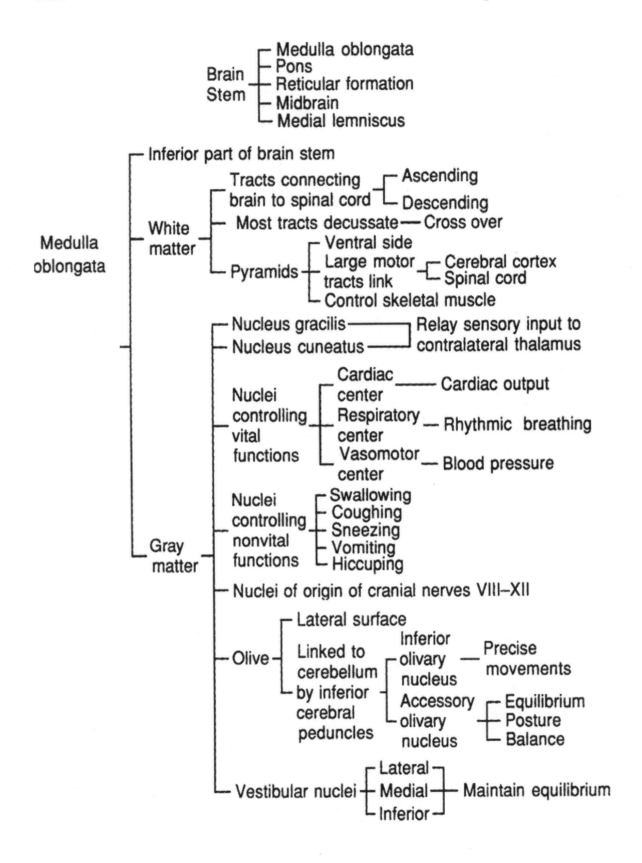

Brain Stem
— Medulla oblongata
— Pons
— Reticular formation
— Midbrain
— Medial lemniscus

Medulla oblongata
— Inferior part of brain stem
— White matter
  — Tracts connecting brain to spinal cord
    — Ascending
    — Descending
  — Most tracts decussate — Cross over
  — Pyramids
    — Ventral side
    — Large motor tracts link
      — Cerebral cortex
      — Spinal cord
    — Control skeletal muscle
— Gray matter
  — Nucleus gracilis
  — Nucleus cuneatus
    — Relay sensory input to contralateral thalamus
  — Nuclei controlling vital functions
    — Cardiac center — Cardiac output
    — Respiratory center — Rhythmic breathing
    — Vasomotor center — Blood pressure
  — Nuclei controlling nonvital functions
    — Swallowing
    — Coughing
    — Sneezing
    — Vomiting
    — Hiccuping
  — Nuclei of origin of cranial nerves VIII–XII
  — Olive
    — Lateral surface
    — Linked to cerebellum by inferior cerebral peduncles
      — Inferior olivary nucleus — Precise movements
      — Accessory olivary nucleus
        — Equilibrium
        — Posture
        — Balance
  — Vestibular nuclei
    — Lateral
    — Medial
    — Inferior
      — Maintain equilibrium

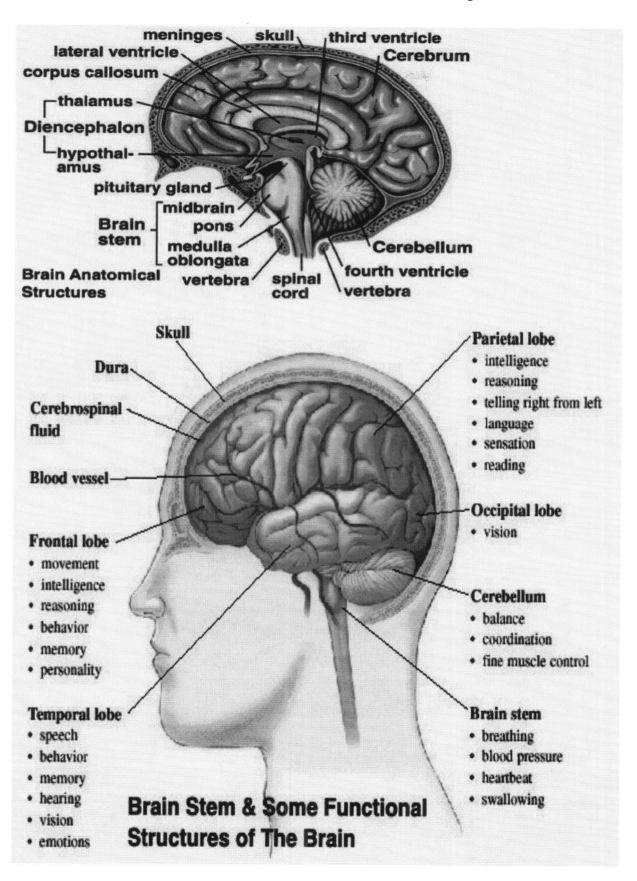

meninges   skull   third ventricle
lateral ventricle   Cerebrum
corpus callosum
thalamus
Diencephalon
hypothal-
amus
pituitary gland
Brain [midbrain
stem [pons
medulla
oblongata   spinal   fourth ventricle
Brain Anatomical   vertebra   cord   vertebra
Structures   Cerebellum

Skull

Dura

Cerebrospinal
fluid

Blood vessel

Frontal lobe
* movement
* intelligence
* reasoning
* behavior
* memory
* personality

Temporal lobe
* speech
* behavior
* memory
* hearing
* vision
* emotions

Parietal lobe
* intelligence
* reasoning
* telling right from left
* language
* sensation
* reading

Occipital lobe
* vision

Cerebellum
* balance
* coordination
* fine muscle control

Brain stem
* breathing
* blood pressure
* heartbeat
* swallowing

**Brain Stem & Some Functional
Structures of The Brain**

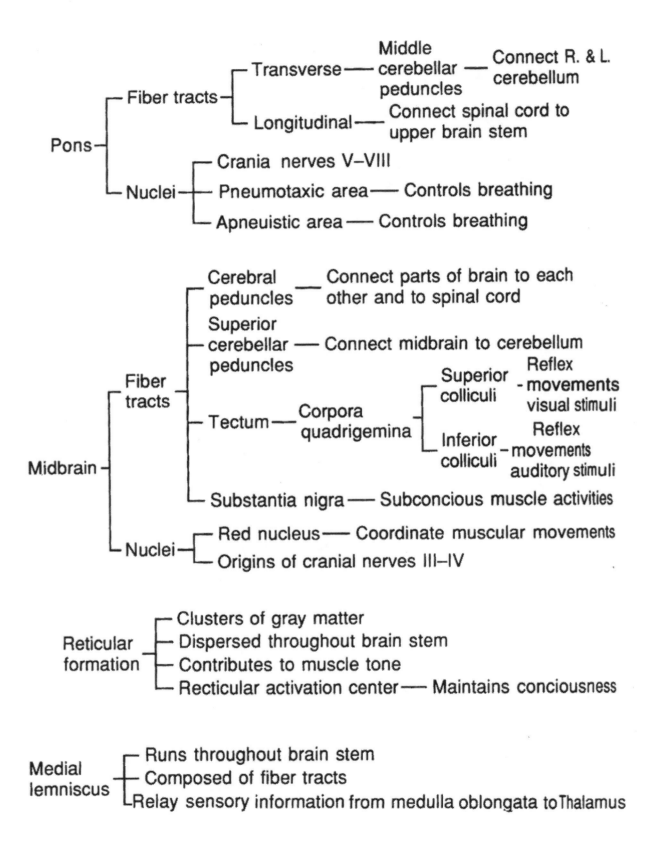

Pons
- Fiber tracts
  - Transverse — Middle cerebellar peduncles — Connect R. & L. cerebellum
  - Longitudinal — Connect spinal cord to upper brain stem
- Nuclei
  - Crania nerves V–VIII
  - Pneumotaxic area — Controls breathing
  - Apneuistic area — Controls breathing

Midbrain
- Fiber tracts
  - Cerebral peduncles — Connect parts of brain to each other and to spinal cord
  - Superior cerebellar peduncles — Connect midbrain to cerebellum
  - Tectum — Corpora quadrigemina
    - Superior colliculi — Reflex movements visual stimuli
    - Inferior colliculi — Reflex movements auditory stimuli
  - Substantia nigra — Subconcious muscle activities
- Nuclei
  - Red nucleus — Coordinate muscular movements
  - Origins of cranial nerves III–IV

Reticular formation
- Clusters of gray matter
- Dispersed throughout brain stem
- Contributes to muscle tone
- Recticular activation center — Maintains conciousness

Medial lemniscus
- Runs throughout brain stem
- Composed of fiber tracts
- Relay sensory information from medulla oblongata to Thalamus

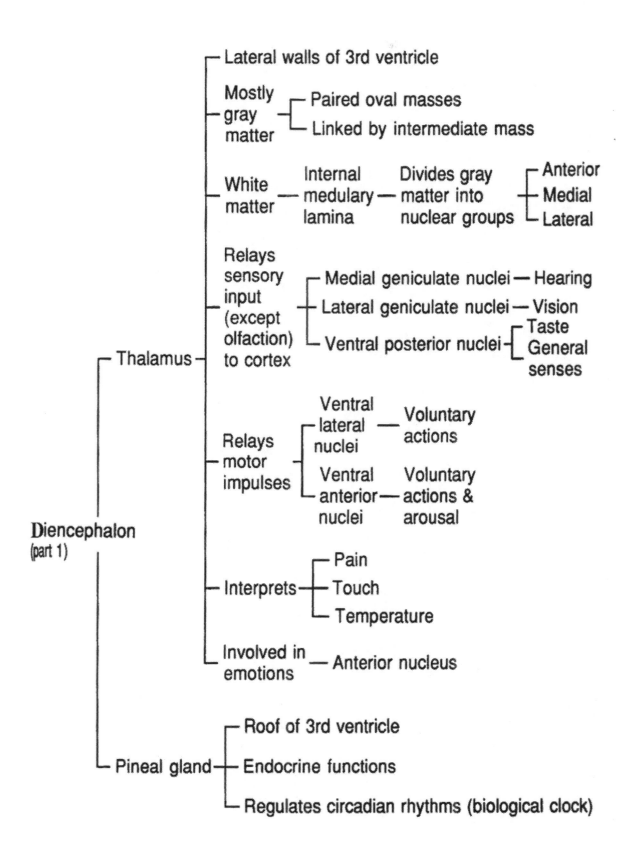

Diencephalon
(part 1)

Thalamus
- Lateral walls of 3rd ventricle
- Mostly gray matter
  - Paired oval masses
  - Linked by intermediate mass
- White matter — Internal medulary lamina — Divides gray matter into nuclear groups
  - Anterior
  - Medial
  - Lateral
- Relays sensory input (except olfaction) to cortex
  - Medial geniculate nuclei — Hearing
  - Lateral geniculate nuclei — Vision
  - Ventral posterior nuclei — Taste / General senses
- Relays motor impulses
  - Ventral lateral nuclei — Voluntary actions
  - Ventral anterior nuclei — Voluntary actions & arousal
- Interprets
  - Pain
  - Touch
  - Temperature
- Involved in emotions — Anterior nucleus

Pineal gland
- Roof of 3rd ventricle
- Endocrine functions
- Regulates circadian rhythms (biological clock)

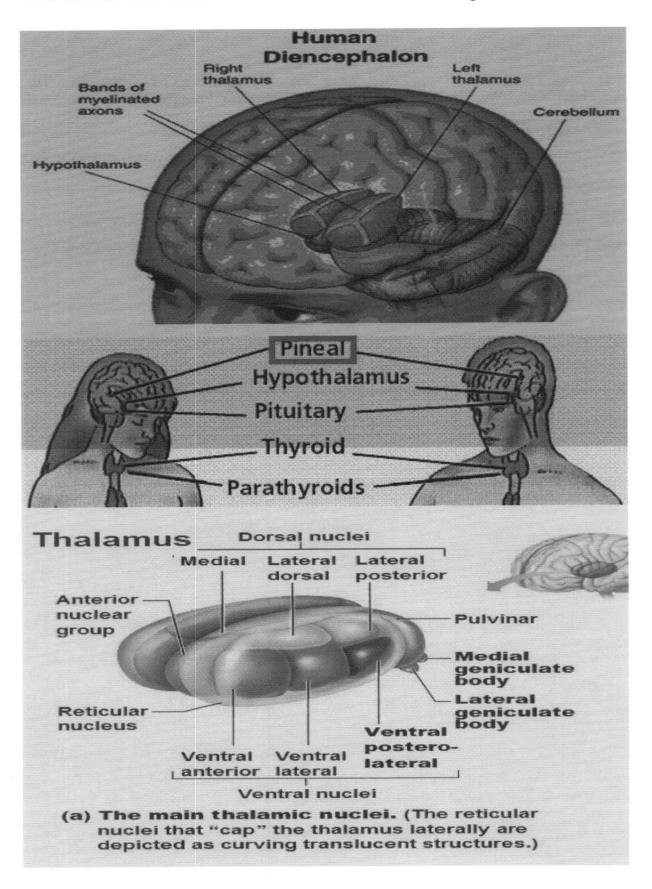

Human Diencephalon

Bands of myelinated axons

Hypothalamus

Right thalamus

Left thalamus

Cerebellum

Pineal
Hypothalamus
Pituitary
Thyroid
Parathyroids

Thalamus

Dorsal nuclei

Medial   Lateral dorsal   Lateral posterior

Anterior nuclear group

Pulvinar

Medial geniculate body

Lateral geniculate body

Reticular nucleus

Ventral anterior   Ventral lateral   Ventral postero-lateral

Ventral nuclei

(a) The main thalamic nuclei. (The reticular nuclei that "cap" the thalamus laterally are depicted as curving translucent structures.)

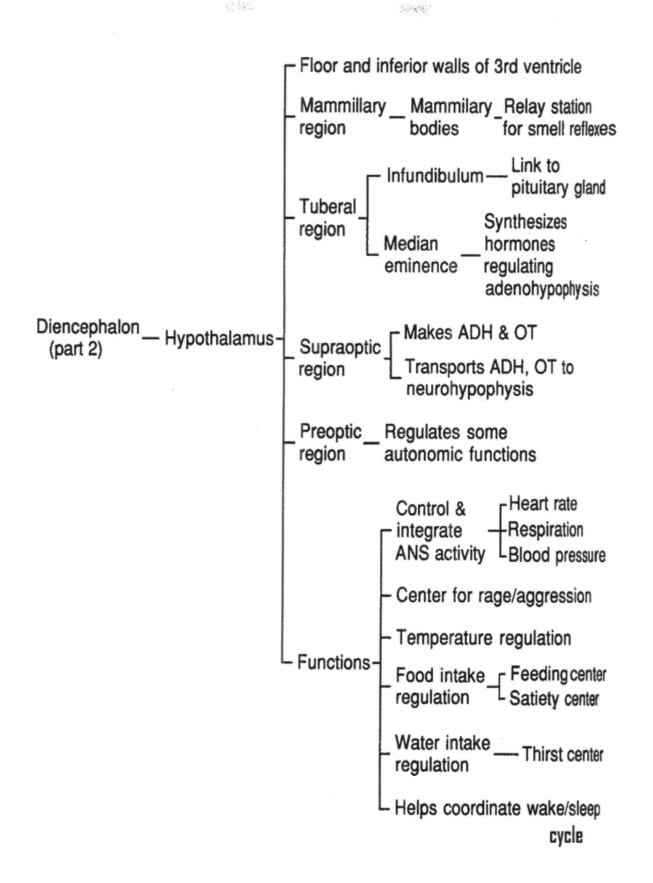

Diencephalon (part 2) — Hypothalamus

- Floor and inferior walls of 3rd ventricle
- Mammillary region — Mammilary bodies — Relay station for smell reflexes
- Tuberal region
  - Infundibulum — Link to pituitary gland
  - Median eminence — Synthesizes hormones regulating adenohypophysis
- Supraoptic region
  - Makes ADH & OT
  - Transports ADH, OT to neurohypophysis
- Preoptic region — Regulates some autonomic functions
- Functions
  - Control & integrate ANS activity
    - Heart rate
    - Respiration
    - Blood pressure
  - Center for rage/aggression
  - Temperature regulation
  - Food intake regulation
    - Feeding center
    - Satiety center
  - Water intake regulation — Thirst center
  - Helps coordinate wake/sleep cycle

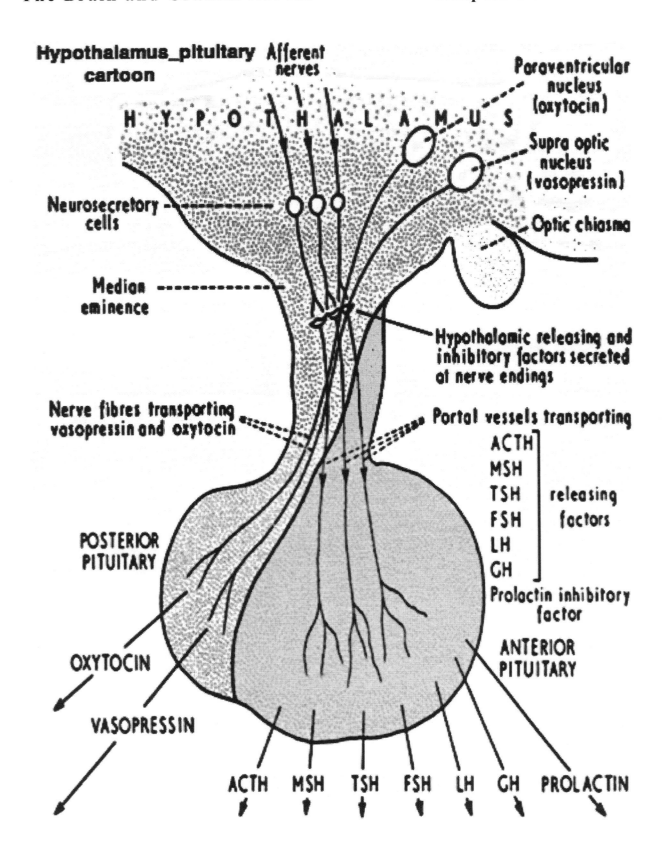

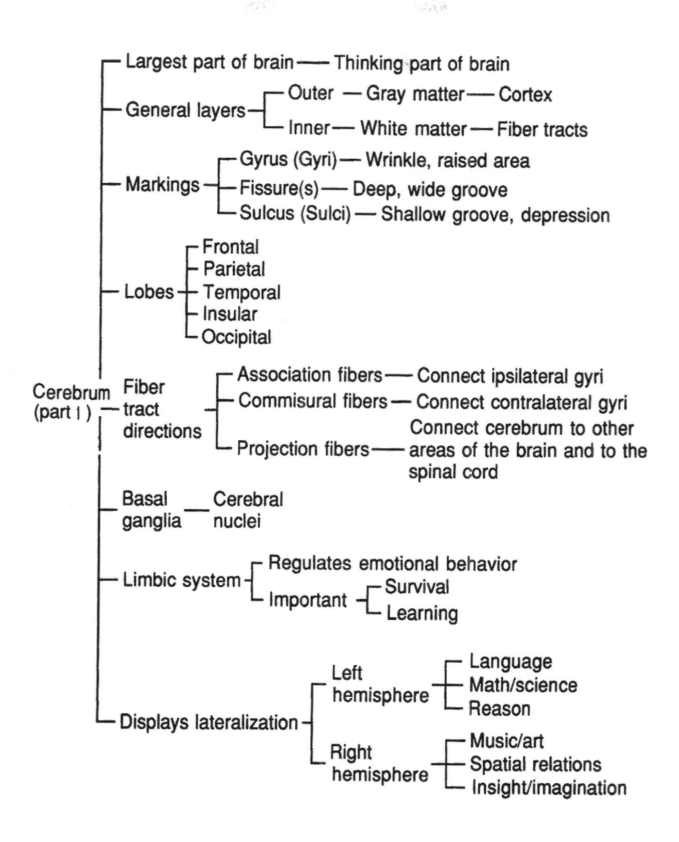

Cerebrum (part I)

- Largest part of brain —— Thinking part of brain
- General layers
  - Outer — Gray matter — Cortex
  - Inner — White matter — Fiber tracts
- Markings
  - Gyrus (Gyri) — Wrinkle, raised area
  - Fissure(s) —— Deep, wide groove
  - Sulcus (Sulci) — Shallow groove, depression
- Lobes
  - Frontal
  - Parietal
  - Temporal
  - Insular
  - Occipital
- Fiber tract directions
  - Association fibers —— Connect ipsilateral gyri
  - Commisural fibers — Connect contralateral gyri
  - Projection fibers —— Connect cerebrum to other areas of the brain and to the spinal cord
- Basal ganglia —— Cerebral nuclei
- Limbic system
  - Regulates emotional behavior
  - Important
    - Survival
    - Learning
- Displays lateralization
  - Left hemisphere
    - Language
    - Math/science
    - Reason
  - Right hemisphere
    - Music/art
    - Spatial relations
    - Insight/imagination

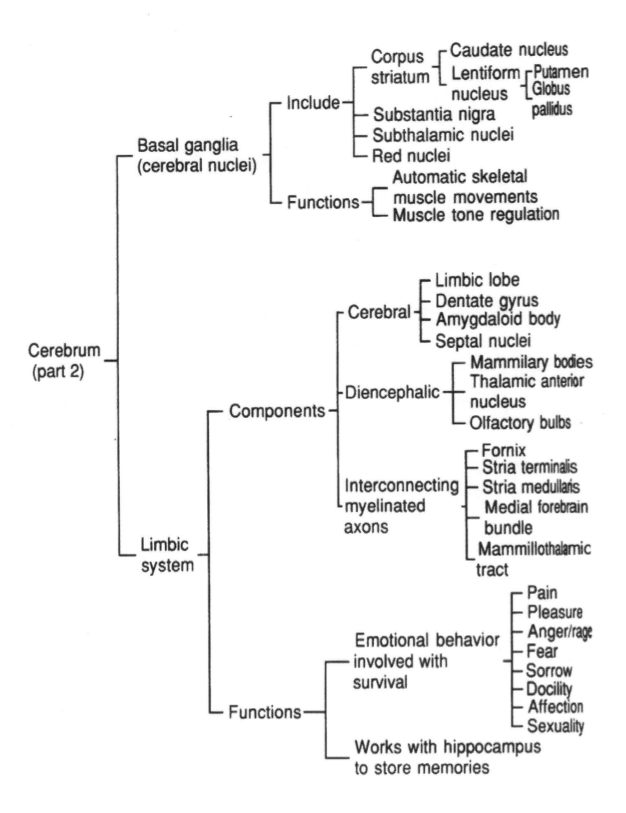

Vital Functional areas in the Brain

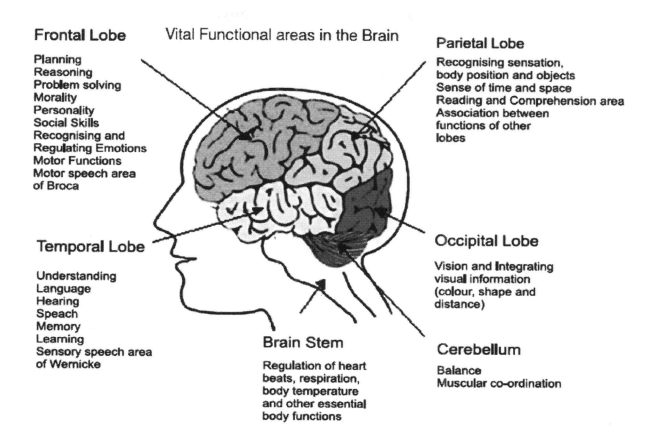

Frontal Lobe

Planning
Reasoning
Problem solving
Morality
Personality
Social Skills
Recognising and
Regulating Emotions
Motor Functions
Motor speech area
of Broca

Temporal Lobe

Understanding
Language
Hearing
Speach
Memory
Learning
Sensory speech area
of Wernicke

Brain Stem

Regulation of heart
beats, respiration,
body temperature
and other essential
body functions

Parietal Lobe

Recognising sensation,
body position and objects
Sense of time and space
Reading and Comprehension area
Association between
functions of other
lobes

Occipital Lobe

Vision and Integrating
visual information
(colour, shape and
distance)

Cerebellum

Balance
Muscular co-ordination

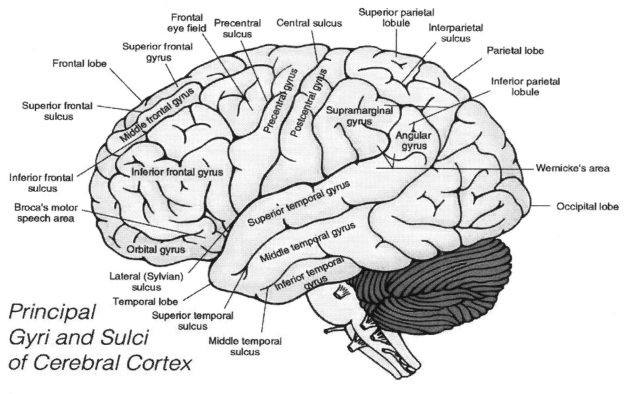

Principal Gyri and Sulci of Cerebral Cortex

Labels: Frontal eye field, Precentral sulcus, Central sulcus, Superior parietal lobule, Interparietal sulcus, Superior frontal gyrus, Parietal lobe, Frontal lobe, Precentral gyrus, Postcentral gyrus, Inferior parietal lobule, Superior frontal sulcus, Middle frontal gyrus, Supramarginal gyrus, Inferior frontal sulcus, Inferior frontal gyrus, Angular gyrus, Wernicke's area, Broca's motor speech area, Superior temporal gyrus, Occipital lobe, Orbital gyrus, Middle temporal gyrus, Lateral (Sylvian) sulcus, Inferior temporal gyrus, Temporal lobe, Superior temporal sulcus, Middle temporal sulcus

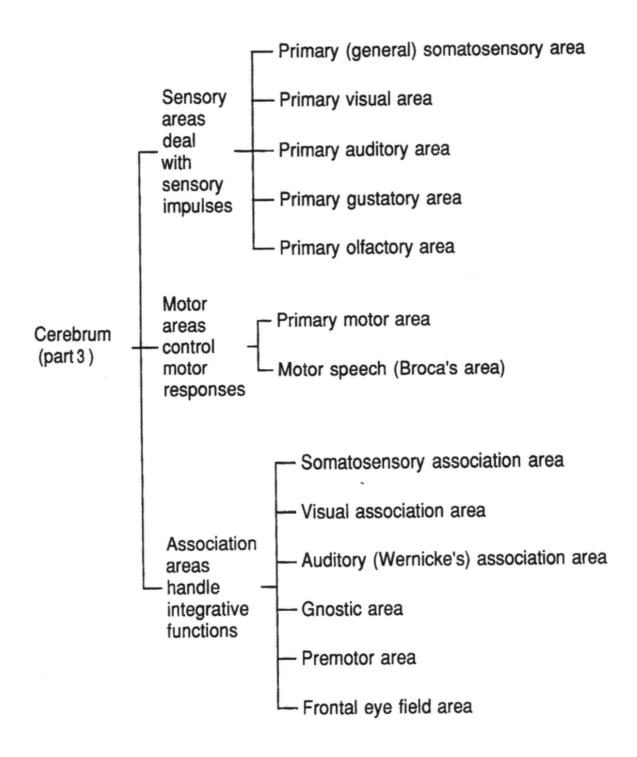

Cerebrum (part 3)

- Sensory areas deal with sensory impulses
  - Primary (general) somatosensory area
  - Primary visual area
  - Primary auditory area
  - Primary gustatory area
  - Primary olfactory area
- Motor areas control motor responses
  - Primary motor area
  - Motor speech (Broca's area)
- Association areas handle integrative functions
  - Somatosensory association area
  - Visual association area
  - Auditory (Wernicke's) association area
  - Gnostic area
  - Premotor area
  - Frontal eye field area

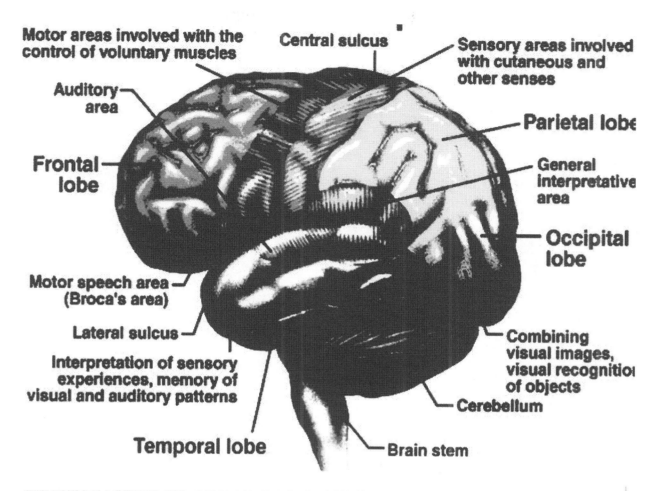

Motor areas involved with the control of voluntary muscles

Central sulcus

Sensory areas involved with cutaneous and other senses

Auditory area

Parietal lobe

Frontal lobe

General interpretative area

Motor speech area (Broca's area)

Occipital lobe

Lateral sulcus

Interpretation of sensory experiences, memory of visual and auditory patterns

Combining visual images, visual recognition of objects

Cerebellum

Temporal lobe

Brain stem

BRODMANN'S CLASSIFICATION SYSTEM

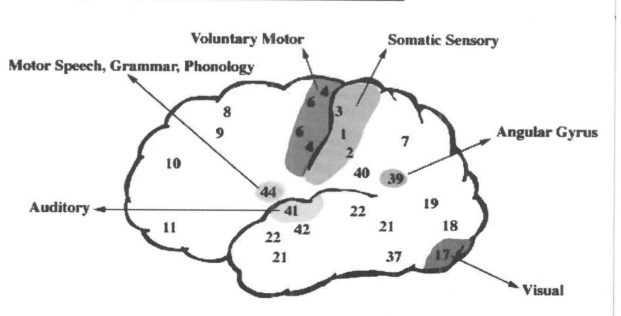

Voluntary Motor

Somatic Sensory

Motor Speech, Grammar, Phonology

Angular Gyrus

Auditory

Visual

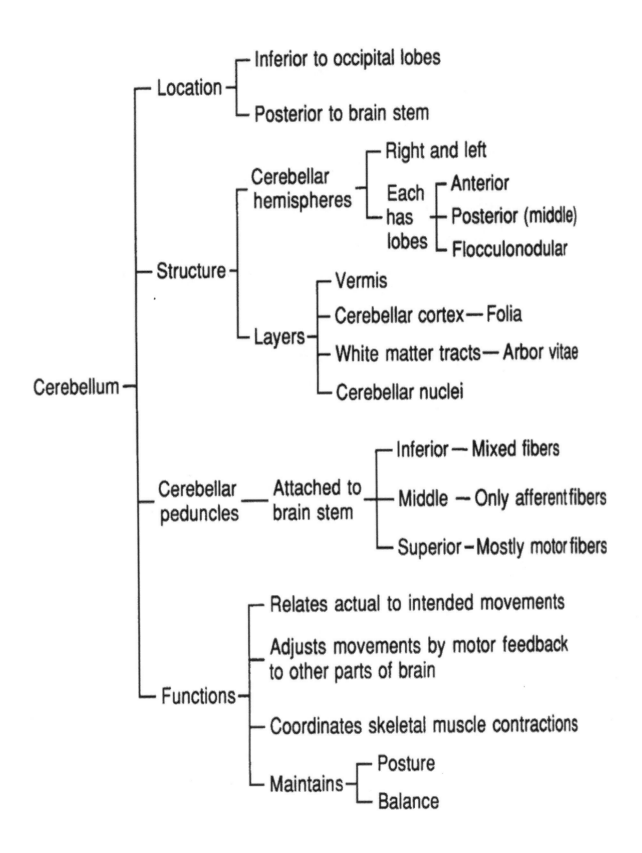

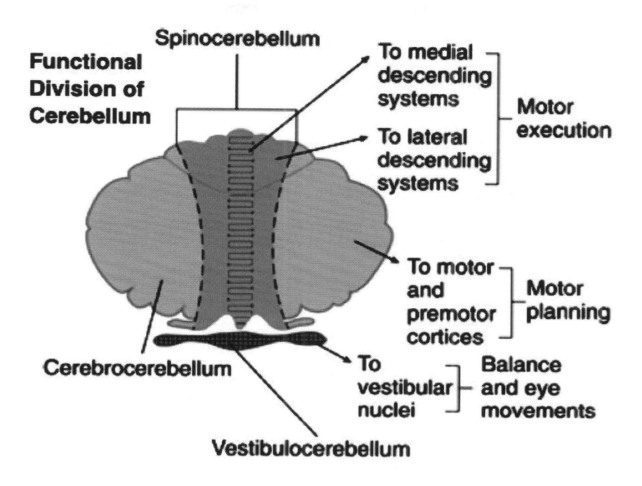

Functional Division of Cerebellum

Spinocerebellum

To medial descending systems

To lateral descending systems

Motor execution

To motor and premotor cortices

Motor planning

Cerebrocerebellum

To vestibular nuclei

Balance and eye movements

Vestibulocerebellum

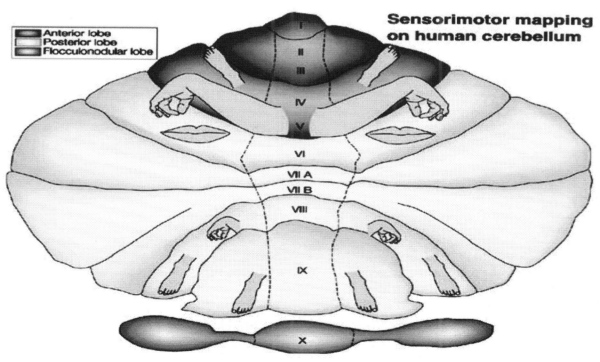

Anterior lobe
Posterior lobe
Flocculonodular lobe

Sensorimotor mapping on human cerebellum

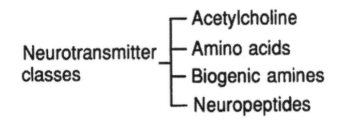

Neurotransmitter classes
- Acetylcholine
- Amino acids
- Biogenic amines
- Neuropeptides

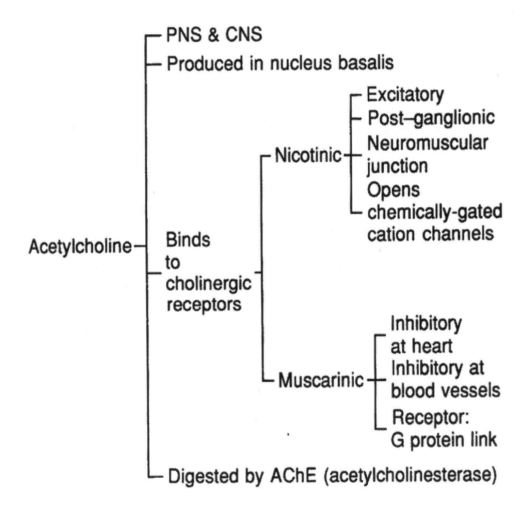

Acetylcholine
- PNS & CNS
- Produced in nucleus basalis
- Binds to cholinergic receptors
  - Nicotinic
    - Excitatory
    - Post–ganglionic
    - Neuromuscular junction
    - Opens chemically-gated cation channels
  - Muscarinic
    - Inhibitory at heart
    - Inhibitory at blood vessels
    - Receptor: G protein link
- Digested by AChE (acetylcholinesterase)

Amino acids
- Excitatory — Brain
  - Glutamate
  - Aspartate
- Inhibitory
  - Brain — Gamma aminobutyric acid — GABA
  - Spinal cord — Glycine

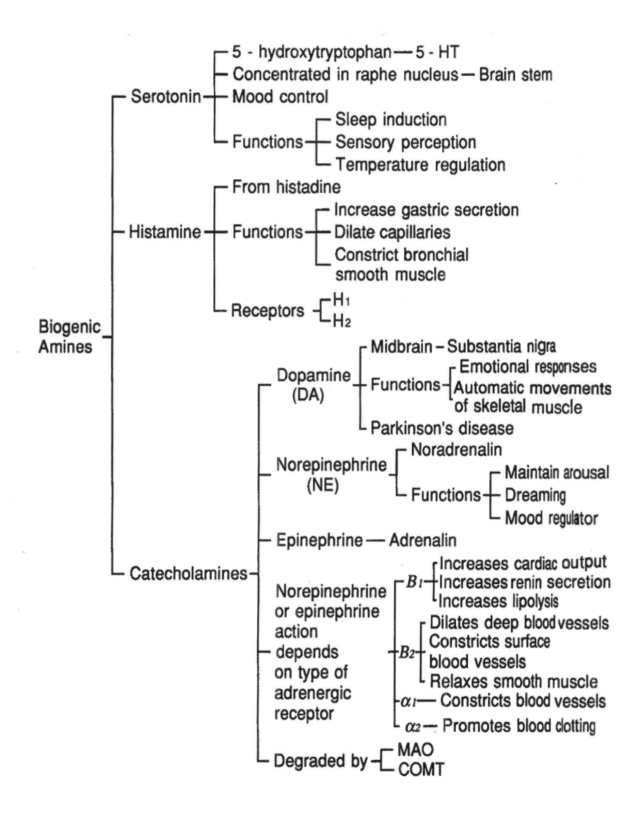

Biogenic Amines

- Serotonin
  - 5 - hydroxytryptophan — 5 - HT
  - Concentrated in raphe nucleus — Brain stem
  - Mood control
  - Functions
    - Sleep induction
    - Sensory perception
    - Temperature regulation
- Histamine
  - From histadine
  - Functions
    - Increase gastric secretion
    - Dilate capillaries
    - Constrict bronchial smooth muscle
  - Receptors
    - H_1
    - H_2
- Catecholamines
  - Dopamine (DA)
    - Midbrain — Substantia nigra
    - Functions
      - Emotional responses
      - Automatic movements of skeletal muscle
    - Parkinson's disease
  - Norepinephrine (NE)
    - Noradrenalin
    - Functions
      - Maintain arousal
      - Dreaming
      - Mood regulator
  - Epinephrine — Adrenalin
  - Norepinephrine or epinephrine action depends on type of adrenergic receptor
    - B_1
      - Increases cardiac output
      - Increases renin secretion
      - Increases lipolysis
    - B_2
      - Dilates deep blood vessels
      - Constricts surface blood vessels
      - Relaxes smooth muscle
    - α_1 — Constricts blood vessels
    - α_2 — Promotes blood clotting
  - Degraded by
    - MAO
    - COMT

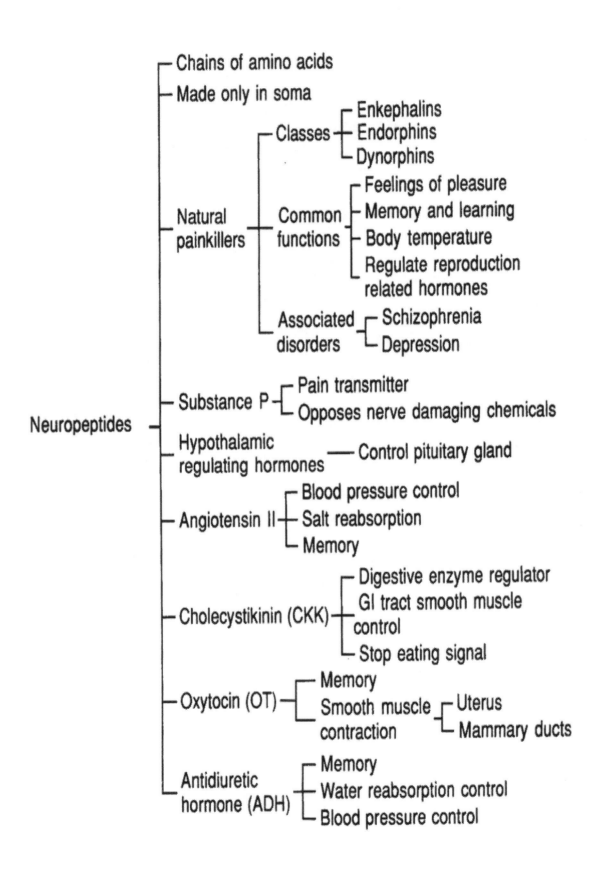

Neuropeptides
- Chains of amino acids
- Made only in soma
- Natural painkillers
  - Classes
    - Enkephalins
    - Endorphins
    - Dynorphins
  - Common functions
    - Feelings of pleasure
    - Memory and learning
    - Body temperature
    - Regulate reproduction related hormones
  - Associated disorders
    - Schizophrenia
    - Depression
- Substance P
  - Pain transmitter
  - Opposes nerve damaging chemicals
- Hypothalamic regulating hormones
  - Control pituitary gland
- Angiotensin II
  - Blood pressure control
  - Salt reabsorption
  - Memory
- Cholecystikinin (CKK)
  - Digestive enzyme regulator
  - GI tract smooth muscle control
  - Stop eating signal
- Oxytocin (OT)
  - Memory
  - Smooth muscle contraction
    - Uterus
    - Mammary ducts
- Antidiuretic hormone (ADH)
  - Memory
  - Water reabsorption control
  - Blood pressure control

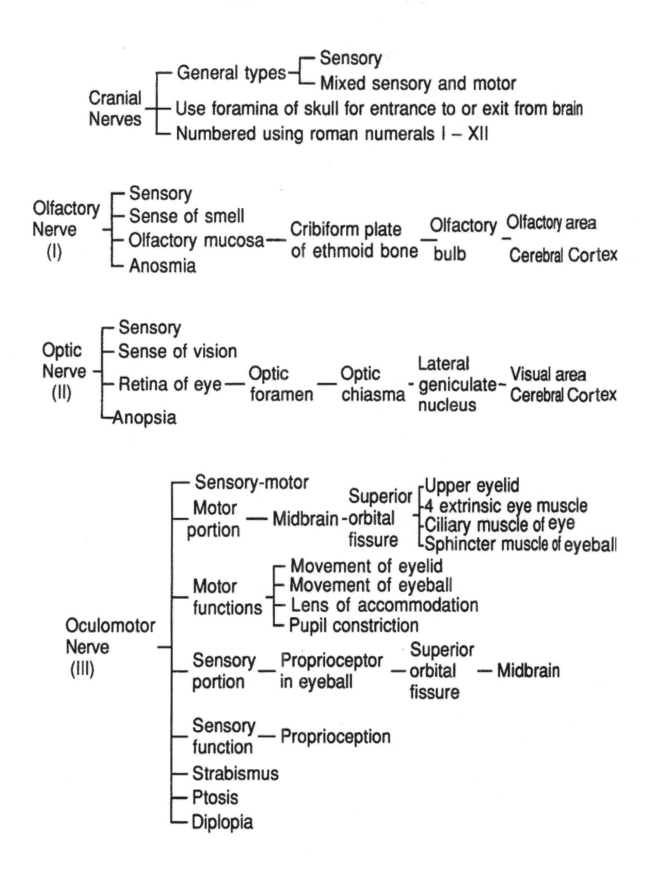

Cranial Nerves
- General types
  - Sensory
  - Mixed sensory and motor
- Use foramina of skull for entrance to or exit from brain
- Numbered using roman numerals I – XII

Olfactory Nerve (I)
- Sensory
- Sense of smell
- Olfactory mucosa — Cribiform plate of ethmoid bone — Olfactory bulb — Olfactory area — Cerebral Cortex
- Anosmia

Optic Nerve (II)
- Sensory
- Sense of vision
- Retina of eye — Optic foramen — Optic chiasma — Lateral geniculate nucleus — Visual area Cerebral Cortex
- Anopsia

Oculomotor Nerve (III)
- Sensory-motor
- Motor portion — Midbrain — Superior orbital fissure
  - Upper eyelid
  - 4 extrinsic eye muscle
  - Ciliary muscle of eye
  - Sphincter muscle of eyeball
- Motor functions
  - Movement of eyelid
  - Movement of eyeball
  - Lens of accommodation
  - Pupil constriction
- Sensory portion — Proprioceptor in eyeball — Superior orbital fissure — Midbrain
- Sensory function — Proprioception
- Strabismus
- Ptosis
- Diplopia

Cranial Nerve		General Function	Cranial Exit Opening
I	Olfactory	Sense of Smell	Cribriform Plate of the Ethmoid
II	Optic	Sight	Optic Foramen
III	Oculomotor	Eye Movement	Superior Orbital Fissure
IV	Trochlear	Eye Movement	Superior Orbital Fissure
V	Trigeminal	Face: sensory, motor	Superior Orbital Fissure
VI	Abducens	Eye Movement	Superior Orbital Fissure
VII	Facial	Face: expression, and sensory	Stylomastoid Foramen
VIII	Vestibulocochlear	Hearing and Balance	Internal Acoustic Meatus
IX	Glossopharyngeal	Tongue and Throat - motor and sensory	Jugular Foramen
X	Vagus	Parasympathetic	Jugular Foramen
XI	Accessory	Head, neck, shoulder - movement & swallowing	Jugular Foramen
XII	Hypoglossal	Speech, Chewing and Swallowing	Hypoglossal Canal

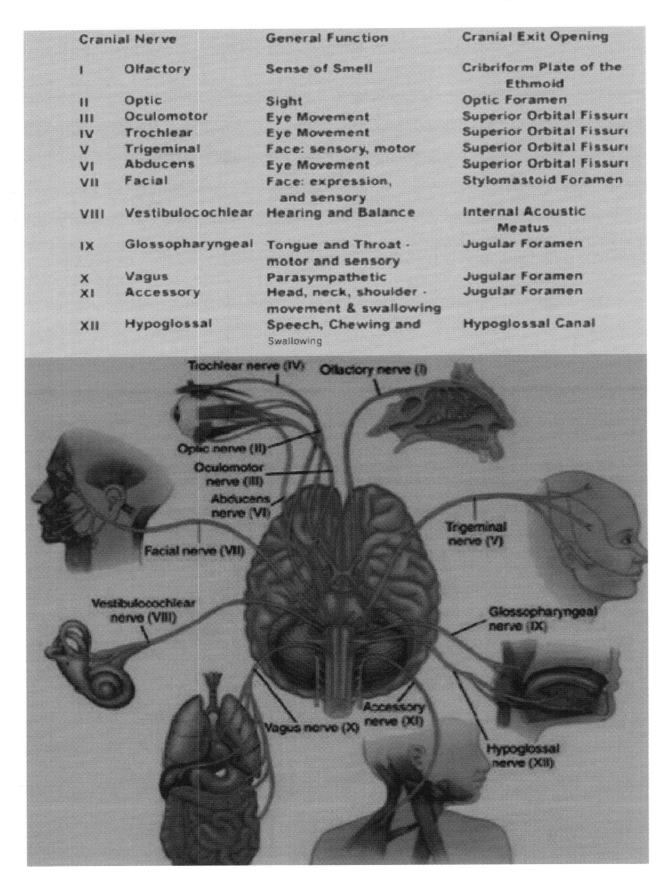

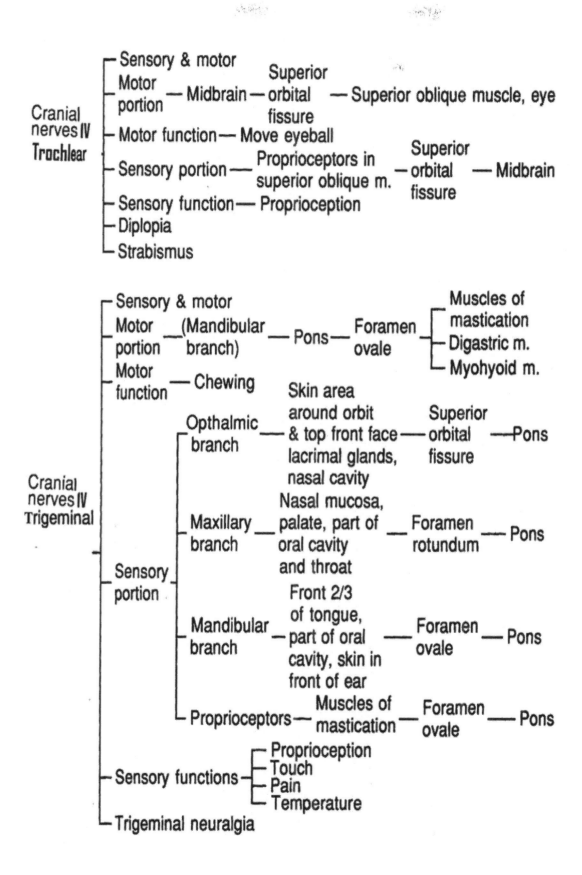

Cranial nerves IV Trochlear
- Sensory & motor
- Motor portion — Midbrain — Superior orbital fissure — Superior oblique muscle, eye
- Motor function — Move eyeball
- Sensory portion — Proprioceptors in superior oblique m. — Superior orbital fissure — Midbrain
- Sensory function — Proprioception
- Diplopia
- Strabismus

Cranial nerves IV Trigeminal
- Sensory & motor
- Motor portion — (Mandibular branch) — Pons — Foramen ovale — Muscles of mastication / Digastric m. / Myohyoid m.
- Motor function — Chewing
- Sensory portion
  - Opthalmic branch — Skin area around orbit & top front face lacrimal glands, nasal cavity — Superior orbital fissure — Pons
  - Maxillary branch — Nasal mucosa, palate, part of oral cavity and throat — Foramen rotundum — Pons
  - Mandibular branch — Front 2/3 of tongue, part of oral cavity, skin in front of ear — Foramen ovale — Pons
  - Proprioceptors — Muscles of mastication — Foramen ovale — Pons
- Sensory functions — Proprioception / Touch / Pain / Temperature
- Trigeminal neuralgia

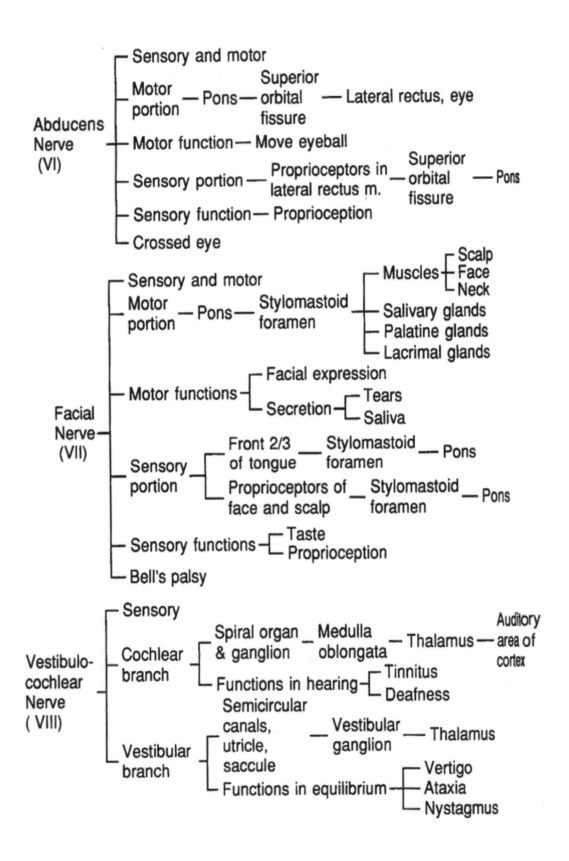

Abducens Nerve (VI)
- Sensory and motor
- Motor portion — Pons — Superior orbital fissure — Lateral rectus, eye
- Motor function — Move eyeball
- Sensory portion — Proprioceptors in lateral rectus m. — Superior orbital fissure — Pons
- Sensory function — Proprioception
- Crossed eye

Facial Nerve (VII)
- Sensory and motor
- Motor portion — Pons — Stylomastoid foramen — Muscles — Scalp / Face / Neck; Salivary glands; Palatine glands; Lacrimal glands
- Motor functions — Facial expression; Secretion — Tears / Saliva
- Sensory portion — Front 2/3 of tongue — Stylomastoid foramen — Pons; Proprioceptors of face and scalp — Stylomastoid foramen — Pons
- Sensory functions — Taste / Proprioception
- Bell's palsy

Vestibulo-cochlear Nerve (VIII)
- Sensory
- Cochlear branch — Spiral organ & ganglion — Medulla oblongata — Thalamus — Auditory area of cortex; Functions in hearing — Tinnitus / Deafness
- Vestibular branch — Semicircular canals, utricle, saccule — Vestibular ganglion — Thalamus; Functions in equilibrium — Vertigo / Ataxia / Nystagmus

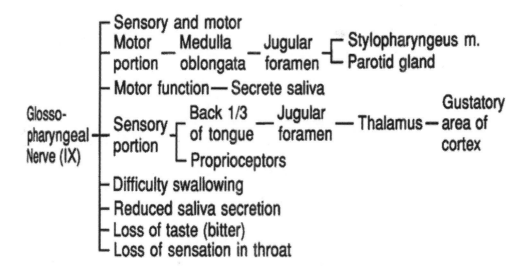

Glosso-pharyngeal Nerve (IX)
- Sensory and motor
  - Motor portion — Medulla oblongata — Jugular foramen
    - Stylopharyngeus m.
    - Parotid gland
- Motor function — Secrete saliva
- Sensory portion
  - Back 1/3 of tongue — Jugular foramen — Thalamus — Gustatory area of cortex
  - Proprioceptors
- Difficulty swallowing
- Reduced saliva secretion
- Loss of taste (bitter)
- Loss of sensation in throat

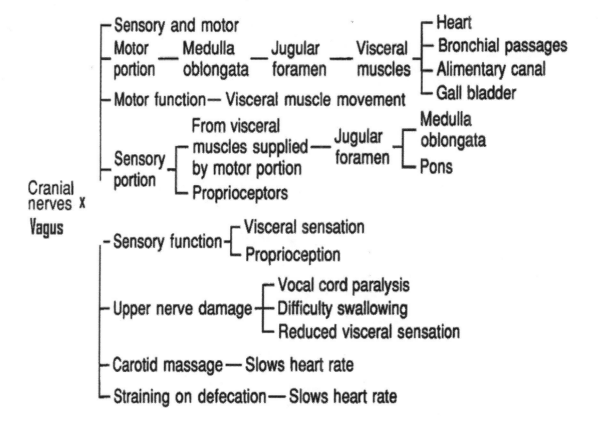

Cranial nerves X Vagus
- Sensory and motor
  - Motor portion — Medulla oblongata — Jugular foramen — Visceral muscles
    - Heart
    - Bronchial passages
    - Alimentary canal
    - Gall bladder
- Motor function — Visceral muscle movement
- Sensory portion
  - From visceral muscles supplied by motor portion — Jugular foramen
    - Medulla oblongata
    - Pons
  - Proprioceptors
- Sensory function
  - Visceral sensation
  - Proprioception
- Upper nerve damage
  - Vocal cord paralysis
  - Difficulty swallowing
  - Reduced visceral sensation
- Carotid massage — Slows heart rate
- Straining on defecation — Slows heart rate

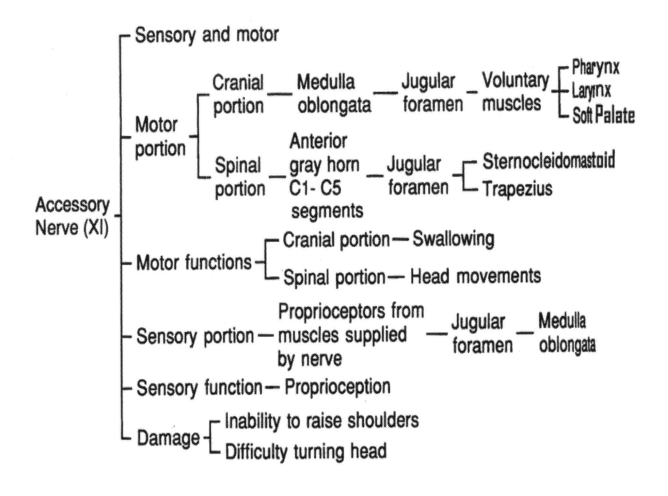

Accessory Nerve (XI)
- Sensory and motor
- Motor portion
  - Cranial portion — Medulla oblongata — Jugular foramen — Voluntary muscles
    - Pharynx
    - Larynx
    - Soft Palate
  - Spinal portion — Anterior gray horn C1- C5 segments — Jugular foramen
    - Sternocleidomastoid
    - Trapezius
- Motor functions
  - Cranial portion — Swallowing
  - Spinal portion — Head movements
- Sensory portion — Proprioceptors from muscles supplied by nerve — Jugular foramen — Medulla oblongata
- Sensory function — Proprioception
- Damage
  - Inability to raise shoulders
  - Difficulty turning head

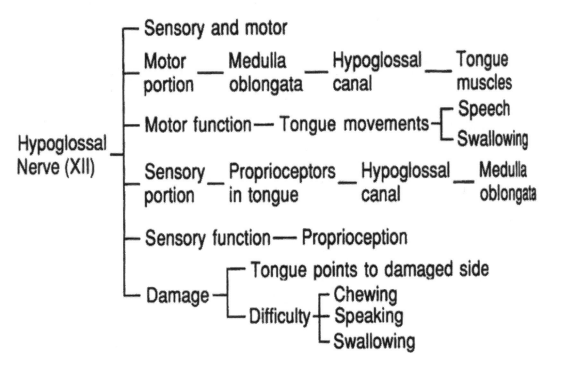

Hypoglossal Nerve (XII)
- Sensory and motor
- Motor portion — Medulla oblongata — Hypoglossal canal — Tongue muscles
- Motor function — Tongue movements
  - Speech
  - Swallowing
- Sensory portion — Proprioceptors in tongue — Hypoglossal canal — Medulla oblongata
- Sensory function — Proprioception
- Damage
  - Tongue points to damaged side
  - Difficulty
    - Chewing
    - Speaking
    - Swallowing

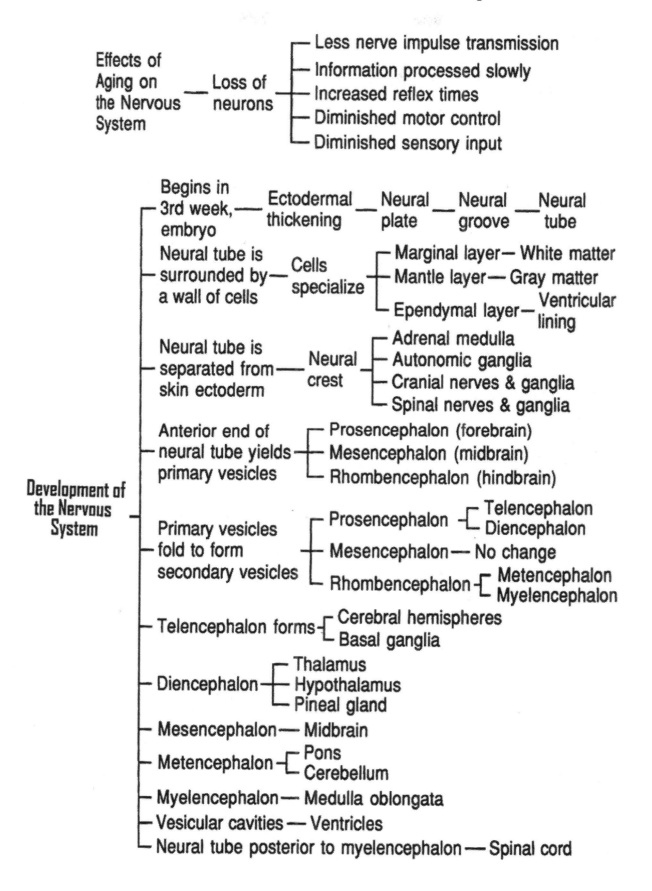

Effects of Aging on the Nervous System — Loss of neurons
— Less nerve impulse transmission
— Information processed slowly
— Increased reflex times
— Diminished motor control
— Diminished sensory input

Development of the Nervous System

Begins in 3rd week, embryo — Ectodermal thickening — Neural plate — Neural groove — Neural tube

Neural tube is surrounded by a wall of cells — Cells specialize
— Marginal layer — White matter
— Mantle layer — Gray matter
— Ependymal layer — Ventricular lining

Neural tube is separated from skin ectoderm — Neural crest
— Adrenal medulla
— Autonomic ganglia
— Cranial nerves & ganglia
— Spinal nerves & ganglia

Anterior end of neural tube yields primary vesicles
— Prosencephalon (forebrain)
— Mesencephalon (midbrain)
— Rhombencephalon (hindbrain)

Primary vesicles fold to form secondary vesicles
— Prosencephalon — Telencephalon / Diencephalon
— Mesencephalon — No change
— Rhombencephalon — Metencephalon / Myelencephalon

Telencephalon forms — Cerebral hemispheres / Basal ganglia

Diencephalon — Thalamus / Hypothalamus / Pineal gland

Mesencephalon — Midbrain

Metencephalon — Pons / Cerebellum

Myelencephalon — Medulla oblongata

Vesicular cavities — Ventricles

Neural tube posterior to myelencephalon — Spinal cord

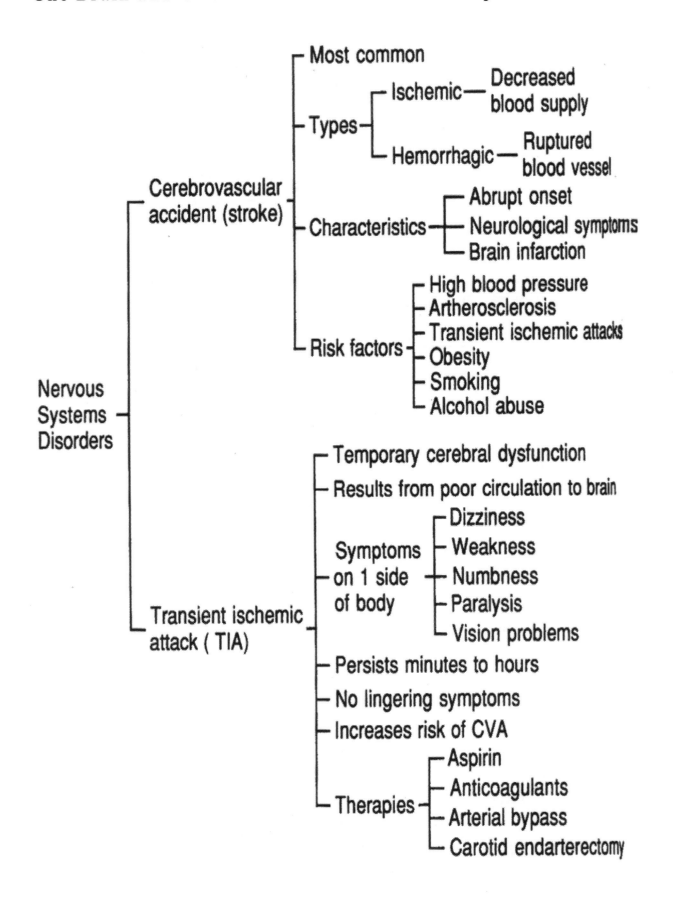

Nervous Systems Disorders

- Cerebrovascular accident (stroke)
  - Most common
  - Types
    - Ischemic — Decreased blood supply
    - Hemorrhagic — Ruptured blood vessel
  - Characteristics
    - Abrupt onset
    - Neurological symptoms
    - Brain infarction
  - Risk factors
    - High blood pressure
    - Artherosclerosis
    - Transient ischemic attacks
    - Obesity
    - Smoking
    - Alcohol abuse
- Transient ischemic attack (TIA)
  - Temporary cerebral dysfunction
  - Results from poor circulation to brain
  - Symptoms on 1 side of body
    - Dizziness
    - Weakness
    - Numbness
    - Paralysis
    - Vision problems
  - Persists minutes to hours
  - No lingering symptoms
  - Increases risk of CVA
  - Therapies
    - Aspirin
    - Anticoagulants
    - Arterial bypass
    - Carotid endarterectomy

Transient-ischemic-attack-pictur

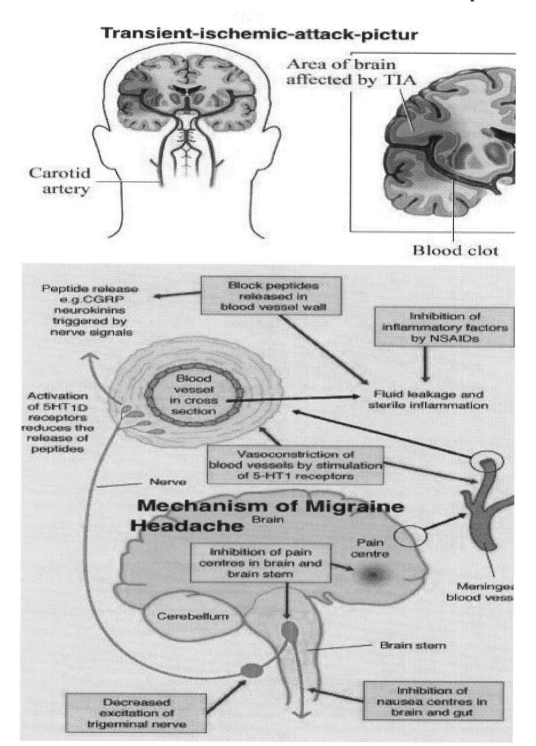

Area of brain affected by TIA

Carotid artery

Blood clot

Peptide release e.g.CGRP neurokinins triggered by nerve signals

Block peptides released in blood vessel wall

Inhibition of inflammatory factors by NSAIDs

Activation of 5HT1D receptors reduces the release of peptides

Blood vessel in cross section

Fluid leakage and sterile inflammation

Nerve

Vasoconstriction of blood vessels by stimulation of 5-HT1 receptors

Mechanism of Migraine Headache   Brain

Pain centre

Inhibition of pain centres in brain and brain stem

Meningeal blood vess

Cerebellum

Brain stem

Decreased excitation of trigeminal nerve

Inhibition of nausea centres in brain and gut

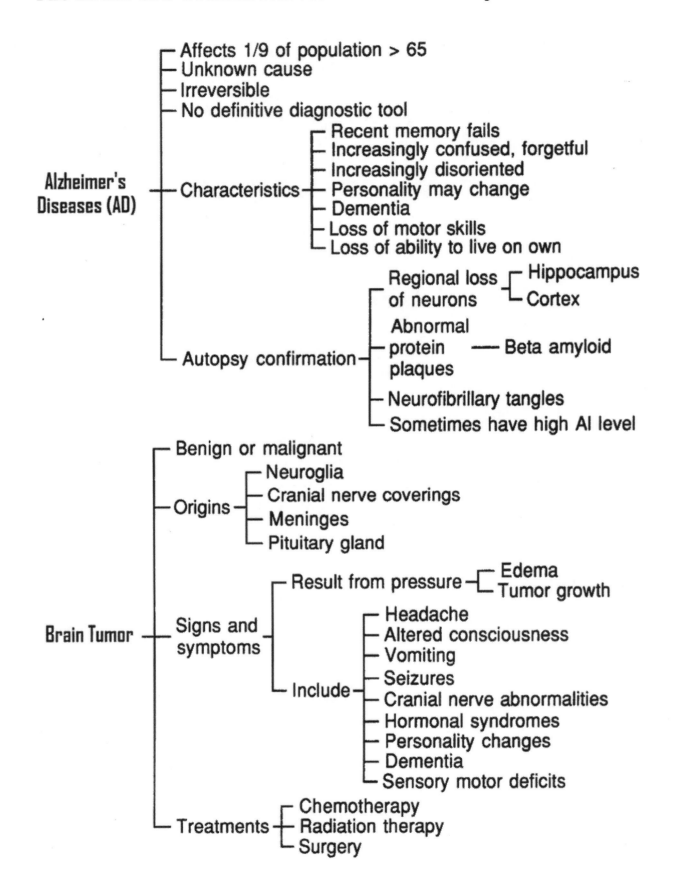

Alzheimer's Diseases (AD)
- Affects 1/9 of population > 65
- Unknown cause
- Irreversible
- No definitive diagnostic tool
- Characteristics
  - Recent memory fails
  - Increasingly confused, forgetful
  - Increasingly disoriented
  - Personality may change
  - Dementia
  - Loss of motor skills
  - Loss of ability to live on own
- Autopsy confirmation
  - Regional loss of neurons
    - Hippocampus
    - Cortex
  - Abnormal protein plaques — Beta amyloid
  - Neurofibrillary tangles
  - Sometimes have high Al level

Brain Tumor
- Benign or malignant
- Origins
  - Neuroglia
  - Cranial nerve coverings
  - Meninges
  - Pituitary gland
- Signs and symptoms
  - Result from pressure
    - Edema
    - Tumor growth
  - Include
    - Headache
    - Altered consciousness
    - Vomiting
    - Seizures
    - Cranial nerve abnormalities
    - Hormonal syndromes
    - Personality changes
    - Dementia
    - Sensory motor deficits
- Treatments
  - Chemotherapy
  - Radiation therapy
  - Surgery

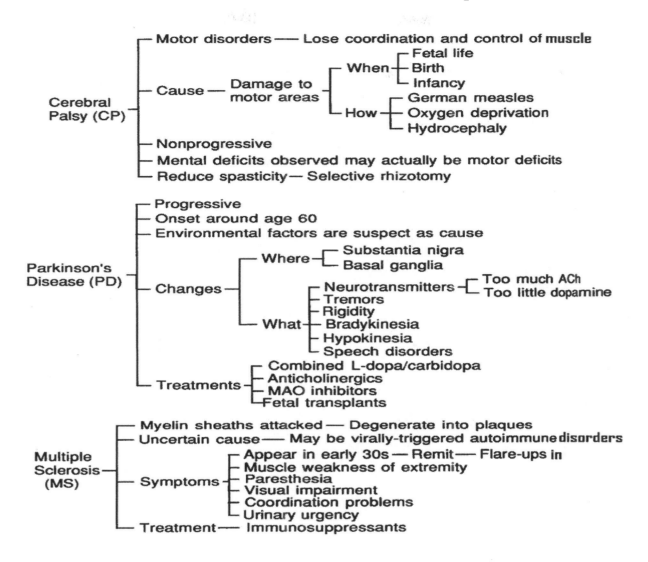

Cerebral Palsy (CP)
- Motor disorders —— Lose coordination and control of muscle
- Cause —— Damage to motor areas
  - When
    - Fetal life
    - Birth
    - Infancy
  - How
    - German measles
    - Oxygen deprivation
    - Hydrocephaly
- Nonprogressive
- Mental deficits observed may actually be motor deficits
- Reduce spasticity — Selective rhizotomy

Parkinson's Disease (PD)
- Progressive
- Onset around age 60
- Environmental factors are suspect as cause
- Changes
  - Where
    - Substantia nigra
    - Basal ganglia
  - What
    - Neurotransmitters
      - Too much ACh
      - Too little dopamine
    - Tremors
    - Rigidity
    - Bradykinesia
    - Hypokinesia
    - Speech disorders
- Treatments
  - Combined L-dopa/carbidopa
  - Anticholinergics
  - MAO inhibitors
  - Fetal transplants

Multiple Sclerosis (MS)
- Myelin sheaths attacked — Degenerate into plaques
- Uncertain cause —— May be virally-triggered autoimmune disorders
- Symptoms
  - Appear in early 30s — Remit —— Flare-ups in
  - Muscle weakness of extremity
  - Paresthesia
  - Visual impairment
  - Coordination problems
  - Urinary urgency
- Treatment — Immunosuppressants

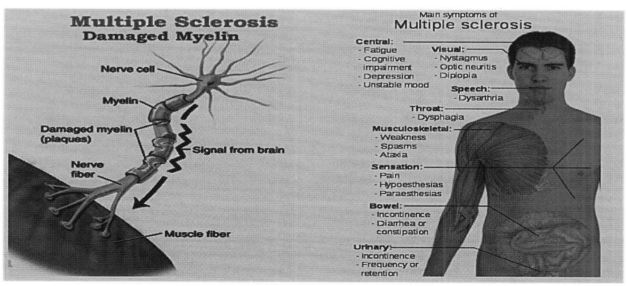

Multiple Sclerosis
Damaged Myelin
- Nerve cell
- Myelin
- Damaged myelin (plaques)
- Nerve fiber
- Signal from brain
- Muscle fiber

Main symptoms of
Multiple sclerosis

Central:
- Fatigue
- Cognitive impairment
- Depression
- Unstable mood

Visual:
- Nystagmus
- Optic neuritis
- Diplopia

Speech:
- Dysarthria

Throat:
- Dysphagia

Musculoskeletal:
- Weakness
- Spasms
- Ataxia

Sensation:
- Pain
- Hypoesthesias
- Paraesthesias

Bowel:
- Incontinence
- Diarrhea or constipation

Urinary:
- Incontinence
- Frequency or retention

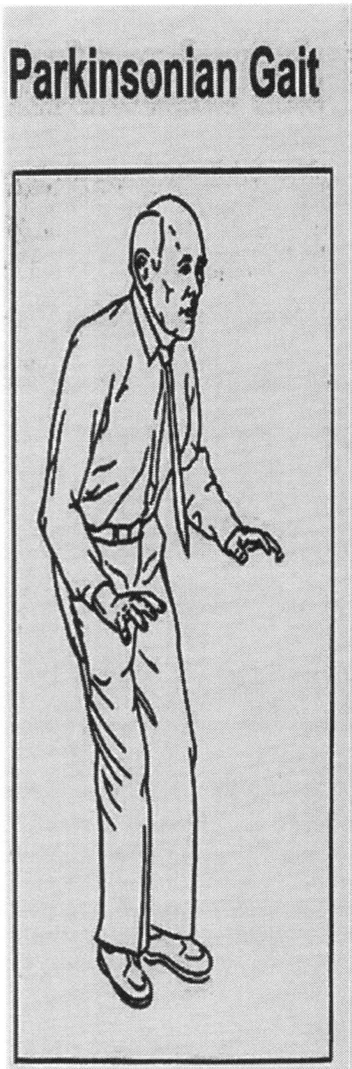

Parkinsonian Gait

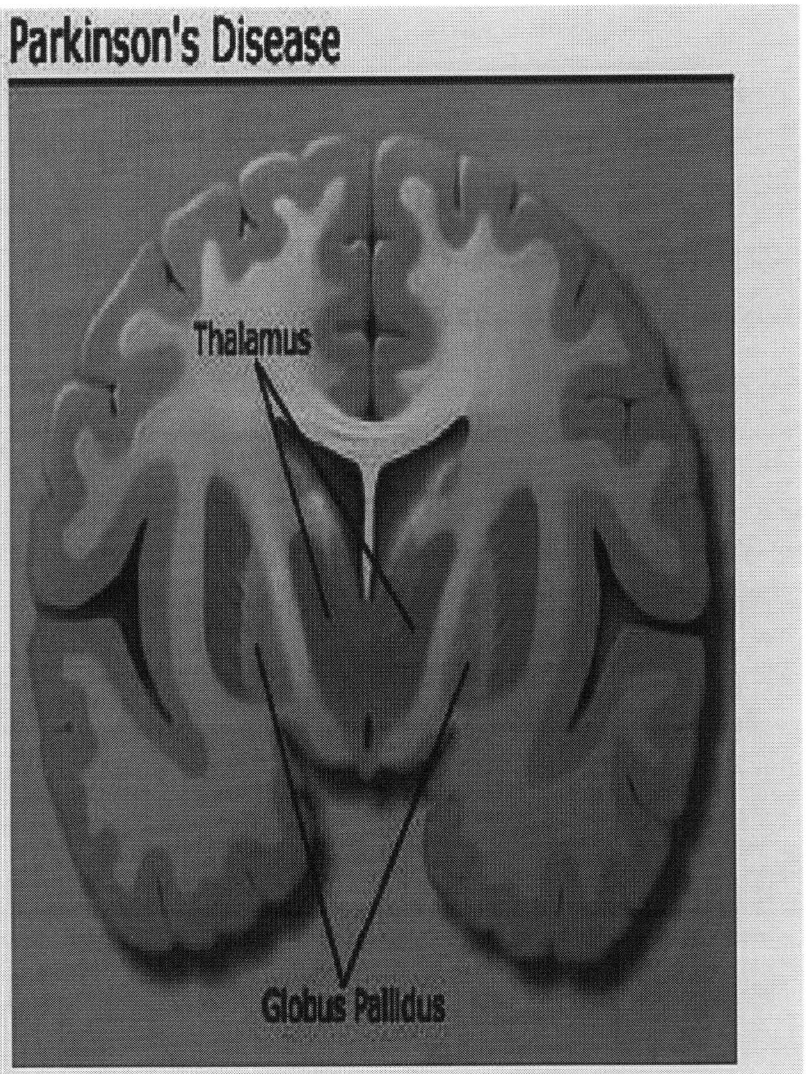

Parkinson's Disease

Thalamus

Globus Pallidus

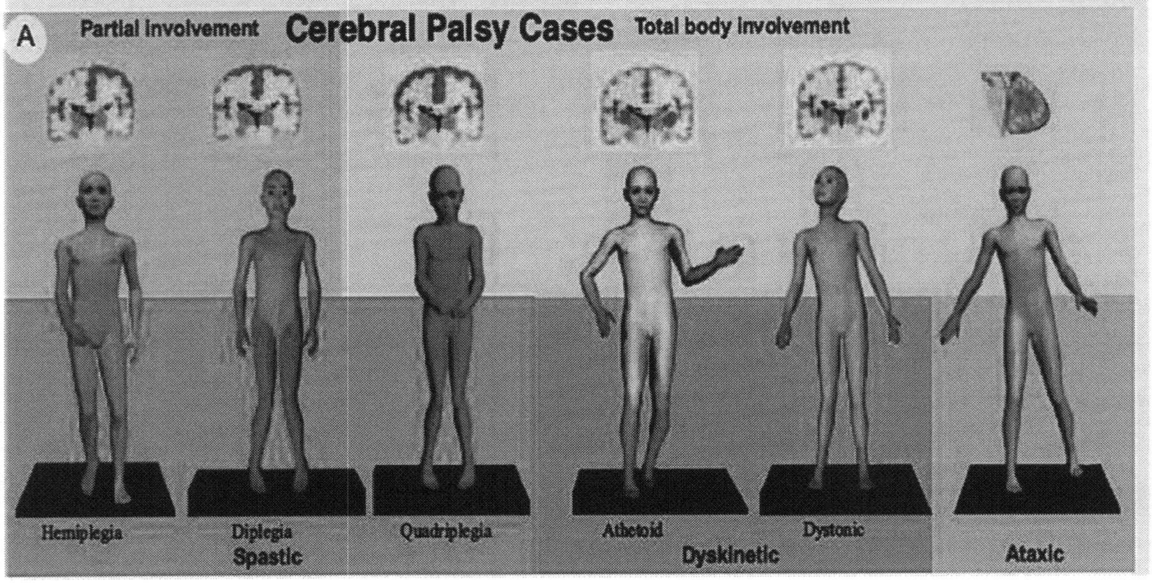

Cerebral Palsy Cases

A   Partial involvement   Total body involvement

Hemiplegia   Diplegia   Quadriplegia   Athetoid   Dystonic   Ataxic

Spastic   **Dyskinetic**

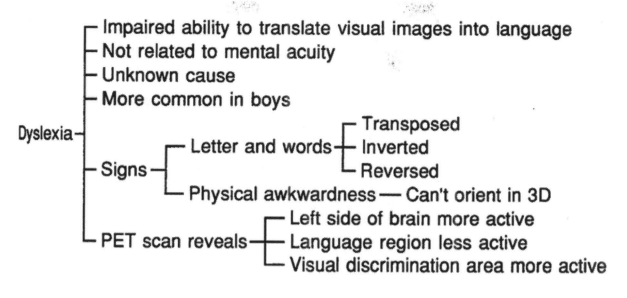

Dyslexia
- Impaired ability to translate visual images into language
- Not related to mental acuity
- Unknown cause
- More common in boys
- Signs
  - Letter and words
    - Transposed
    - Inverted
    - Reversed
  - Physical awkwardness — Can't orient in 3D
- PET scan reveals
  - Left side of brain more active
  - Language region less active
  - Visual discrimination area more active

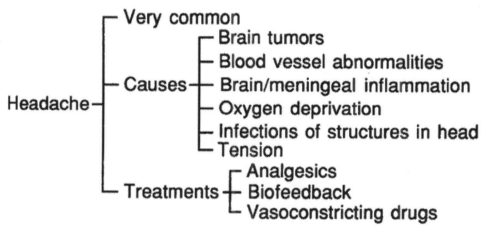

Headache
- Very common
- Causes
  - Brain tumors
  - Blood vessel abnormalities
  - Brain/meningeal inflammation
  - Oxygen deprivation
  - Infections of structures in head
  - Tension
- Treatments
  - Analgesics
  - Biofeedback
  - Vasoconstricting drugs

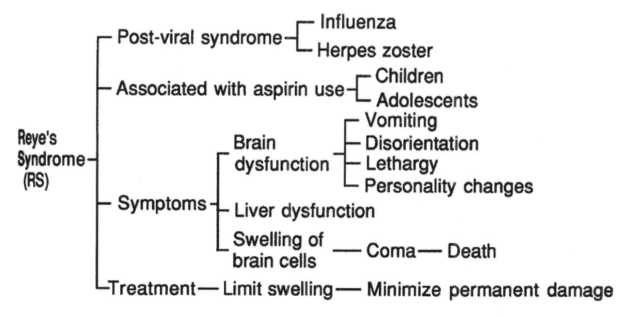

Reye's Syndrome (RS)
- Post-viral syndrome
  - Influenza
  - Herpes zoster
- Associated with aspirin use
  - Children
  - Adolescents
- Symptoms
  - Brain dysfunction
    - Vomiting
    - Disorientation
    - Lethargy
    - Personality changes
  - Liver dysfunction
  - Swelling of brain cells — Coma — Death
- Treatment — Limit swelling — Minimize permanent damage

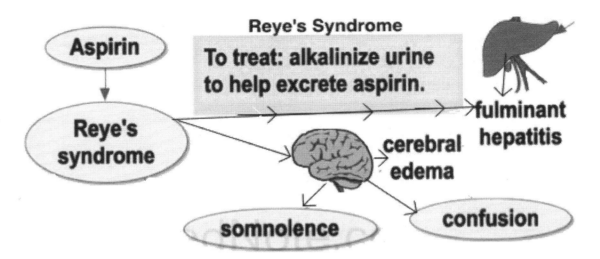

Reye's Syndrome

Aspirin

To treat: alkalinize urine to help excrete aspirin.

Reye's syndrome → cerebral edema → fulminant hepatitis

somnolence

confusion

Aspirin is contraindicated in children. Reye's syndrome can be fatal. Choose acetaminophen instead.

Healthy | Alzheimer's

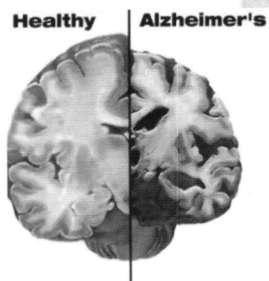

Brain Tumor

Meningioma

Glioblastoma

Deep tumor

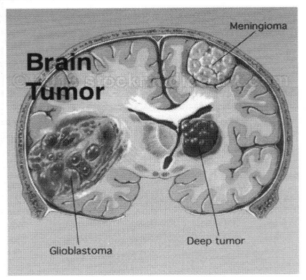

dysl∈xia

Peas hep rong wef

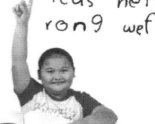

- **Reading gives me headaches**
- **The words are always moving**
- **I get so tired**
- **I hate to read**

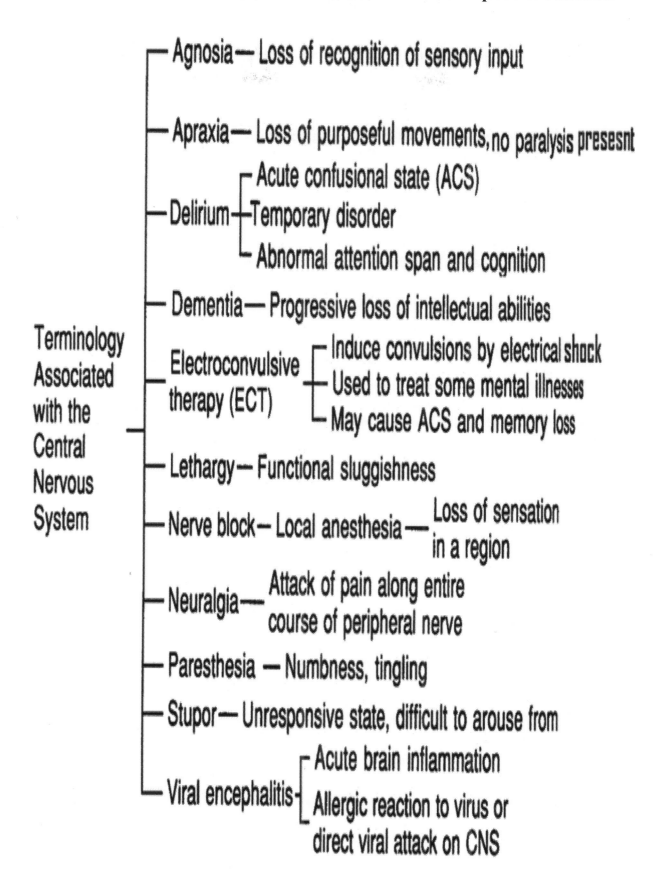

Terminology Associated with the Central Nervous System

- Agnosia — Loss of recognition of sensory input
- Apraxia — Loss of purposeful movements, no paralysis presesnt
- Delirium
  - Acute confusional state (ACS)
  - Temporary disorder
  - Abnormal attention span and cognition
- Dementia — Progressive loss of intellectual abilities
- Electroconvulsive therapy (ECT)
  - Induce convulsions by electrical shock
  - Used to treat some mental illnesses
  - May cause ACS and memory loss
- Lethargy — Functional sluggishness
- Nerve block — Local anesthesia — Loss of sensation in a region
- Neuralgia — Attack of pain along entire course of peripheral nerve
- Paresthesia — Numbness, tingling
- Stupor — Unresponsive state, difficult to arouse from
- Viral encephalitis
  - Acute brain inflammation
  - Allergic reaction to virus or direct viral attack on CNS

CHAPTER FIFTEEN

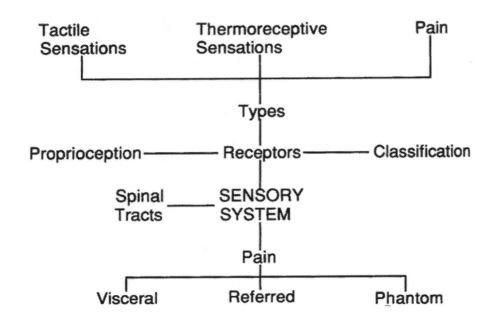

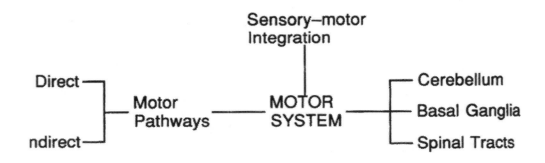

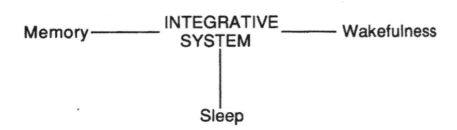

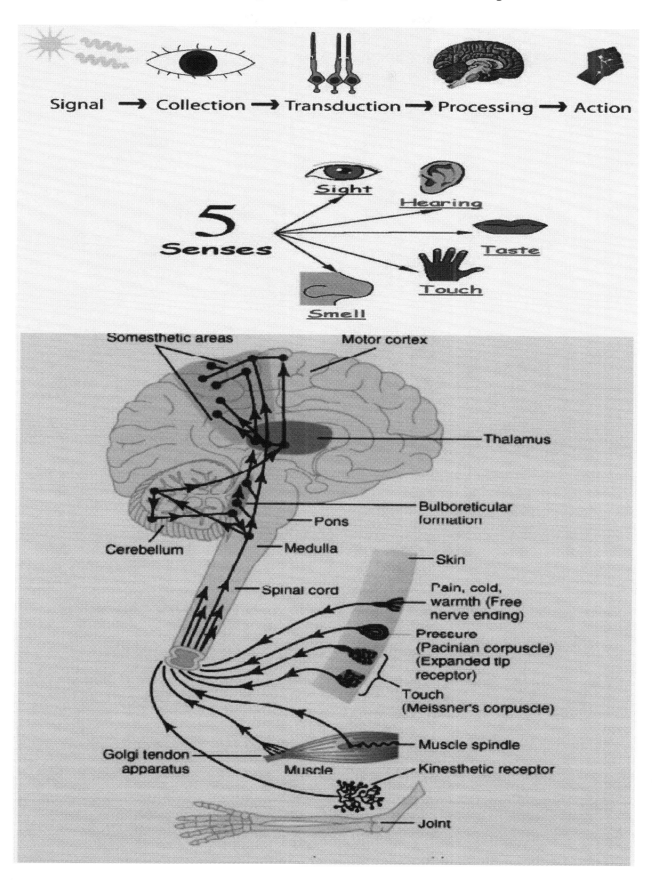

Signal → Collection → Transduction → Processing → Action

5 Senses

Sight
Hearing
Taste
Touch
Smell

Somesthetic areas
Motor cortex
Thalamus
Bulboreticular formation
Pons
Cerebellum
Medulla
Skin
Spinal cord
Pain, cold, warmth (Free nerve ending)
Pressure (Pacinian corpuscle) (Expanded tip receptor)
Touch (Meissner's corpuscle)
Golgi tendon apparatus
Muscle
Muscle spindle
Kinesthetic receptor
Joint

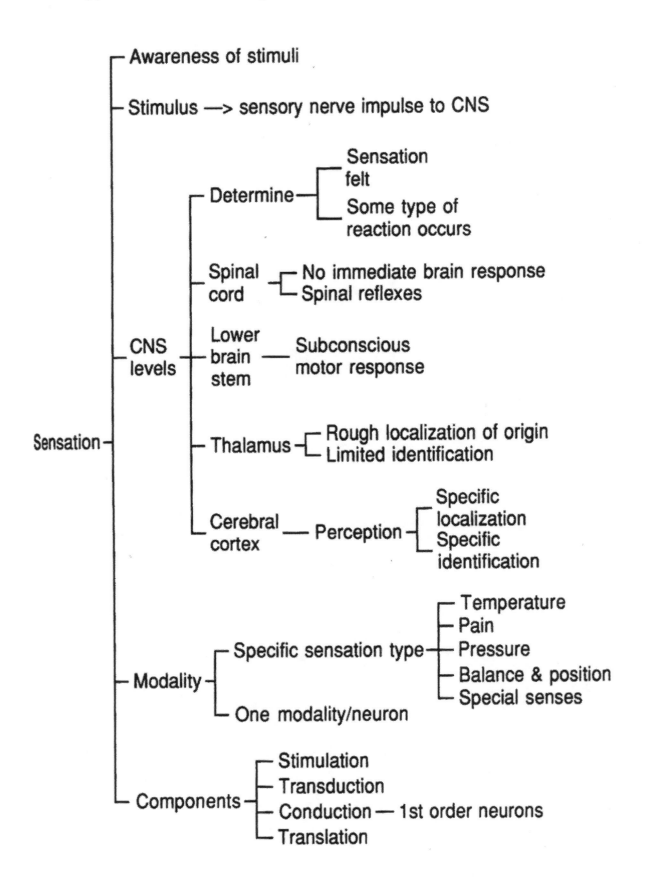

Sensation
- Awareness of stimuli
- Stimulus —> sensory nerve impulse to CNS
- CNS levels
  - Determine
    - Sensation felt
    - Some type of reaction occurs
  - Spinal cord
    - No immediate brain response
    - Spinal reflexes
  - Lower brain stem — Subconscious motor response
  - Thalamus
    - Rough localization of origin
    - Limited identification
  - Cerebral cortex — Perception
    - Specific localization
    - Specific identification
- Modality
  - Specific sensation type
    - Temperature
    - Pain
    - Pressure
    - Balance & position
    - Special senses
  - One modality/neuron
- Components
  - Stimulation
  - Transduction
  - Conduction — 1st order neurons
  - Translation

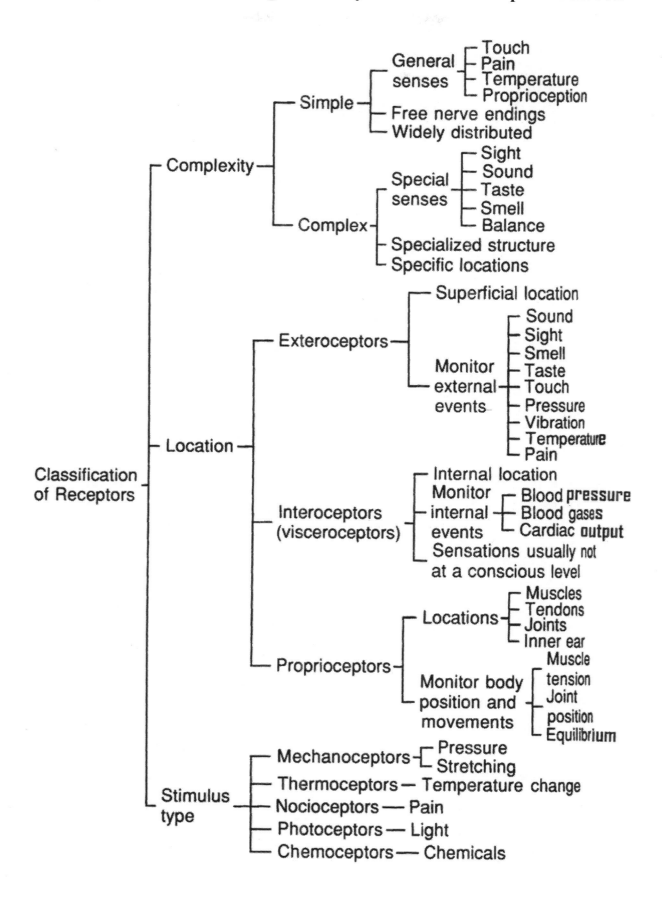

Classification of Receptors

- Complexity
  - Simple
    - General senses
      - Touch
      - Pain
      - Temperature
      - Proprioception
    - Free nerve endings
    - Widely distributed
  - Complex
    - Special senses
      - Sight
      - Sound
      - Taste
      - Smell
      - Balance
    - Specialized structure
    - Specific locations
- Location
  - Exteroceptors
    - Superficial location
    - Monitor external events
      - Sound
      - Sight
      - Smell
      - Taste
      - Touch
      - Pressure
      - Vibration
      - Temperature
      - Pain
  - Interoceptors (visceroceptors)
    - Internal location
    - Monitor internal events
      - Blood pressure
      - Blood gases
      - Cardiac output
    - Sensations usually not at a conscious level
  - Proprioceptors
    - Locations
      - Muscles
      - Tendons
      - Joints
      - Inner ear
    - Monitor body position and movements
      - Muscle tension
      - Joint position
      - Equilibrium
- Stimulus type
  - Mechanoceptors
    - Pressure
    - Stretching
  - Thermoceptors — Temperature change
  - Nocioceptors — Pain
  - Photoceptors — Light
  - Chemoceptors — Chemicals

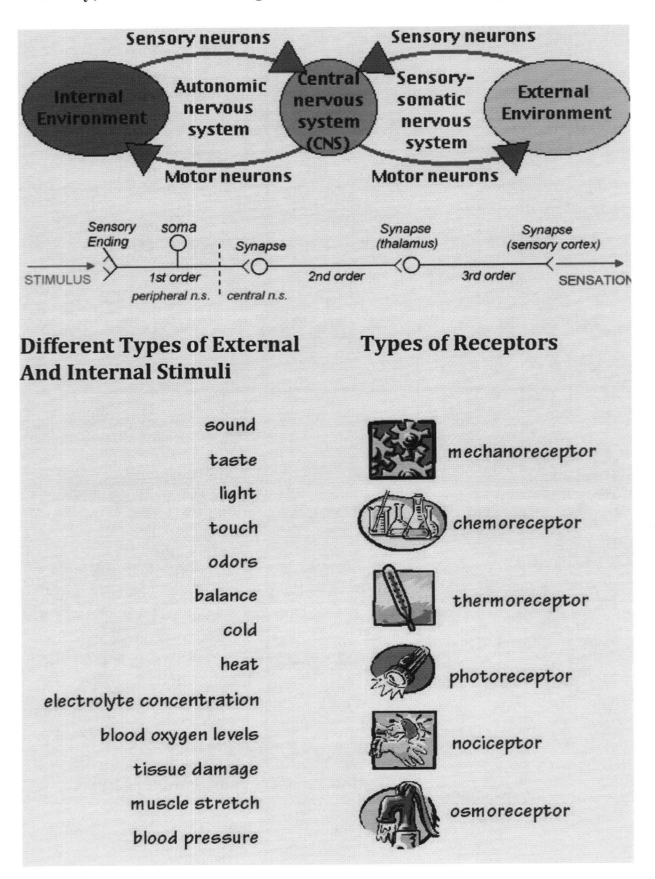

Different Types of External And Internal Stimuli

sound

taste

light

touch

odors

balance

cold

heat

electrolyte concentration

blood oxygen levels

tissue damage

muscle stretch

blood pressure

Types of Receptors

mechanoreceptor

chemoreceptor

thermoreceptor

photoreceptor

nociceptor

osmoreceptor

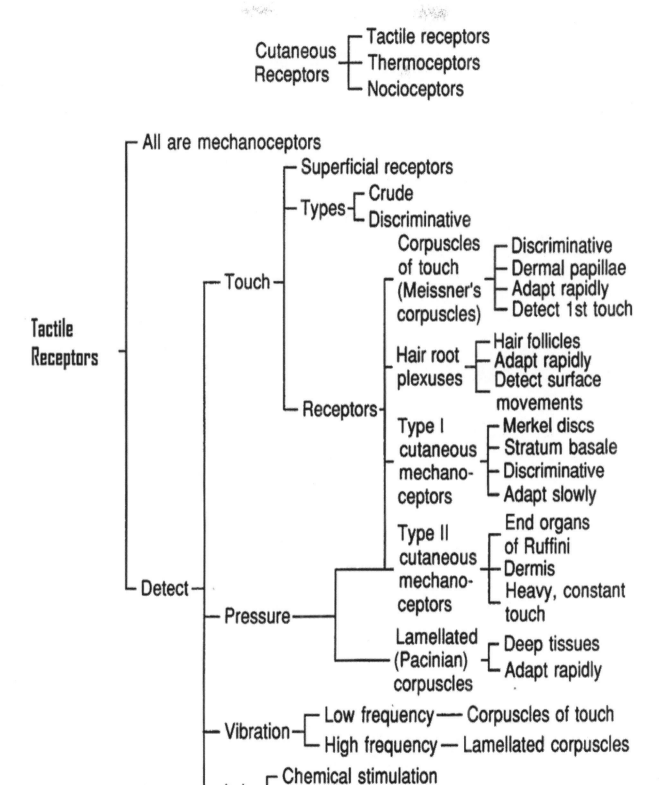

Thermoceptors ── Free nerve endings ── Detect ┬ Hot
                                              └ Cold

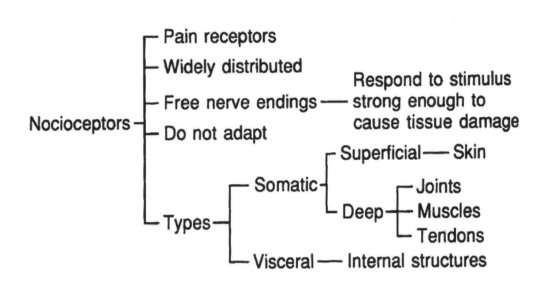

Nocioceptors ┬ Pain receptors
             ├ Widely distributed
             ├ Free nerve endings ── Respond to stimulus strong enough to cause tissue damage
             ├ Do not adapt
             └ Types ┬ Somatic ┬ Superficial ── Skin
                     │   └ Deep ┬ Joints
                     │   ├ Muscles
                     │   └ Tendons
                     └ Visceral ── Internal structures

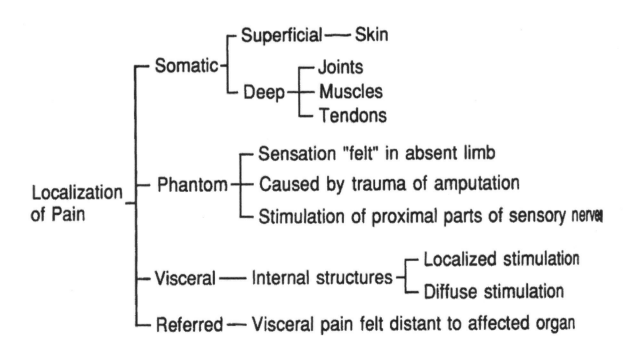

Localization of Pain ┬ Somatic ┬ Superficial ── Skin
                     │   └ Deep ┬ Joints
                     │   ├ Muscles
                     │   └ Tendons
                     ├ Phantom ┬ Sensation "felt" in absent limb
                     │   ├ Caused by trauma of amputation
                     │   └ Stimulation of proximal parts of sensory nerve
                     ├ Visceral ── Internal structures ┬ Localized stimulation
                     │   └ Diffuse stimulation
                     └ Referred ── Visceral pain felt distant to affected organ

Common sites of referred pain from different visceral organs

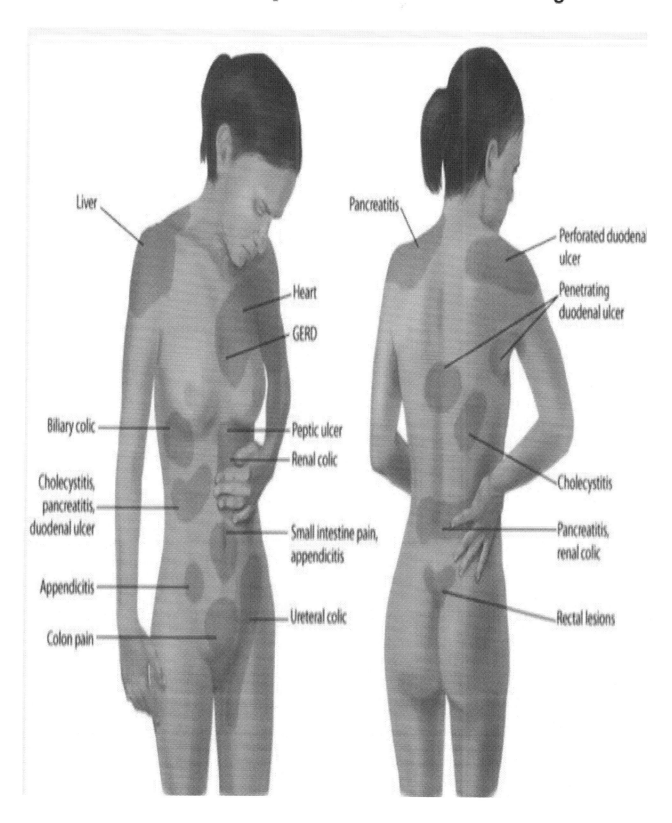

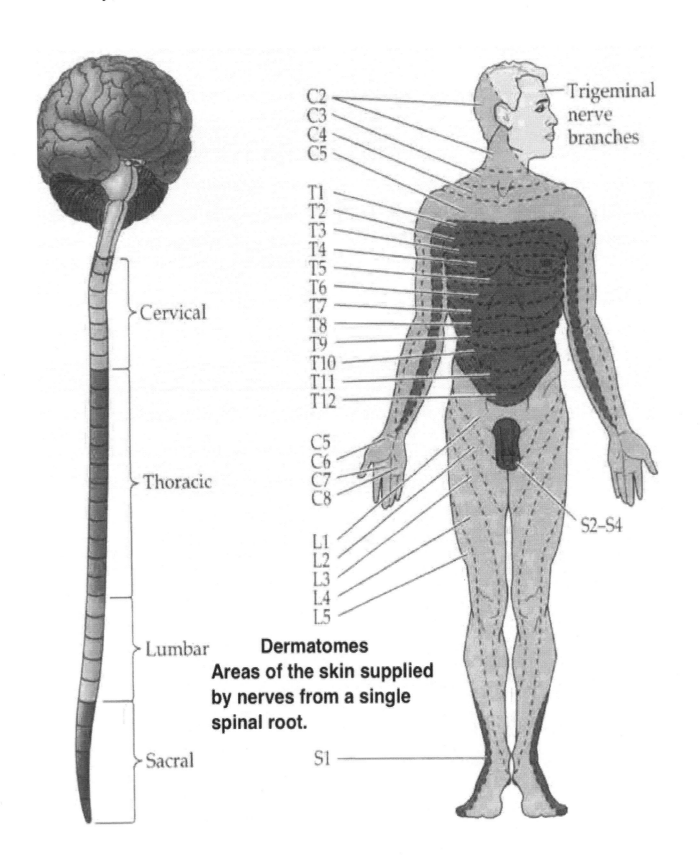

C2
C3
C4
C5

T1
T2
T3
T4
T5
T6
T7
T8
T9
T10
T11
T12

C5
C6
C7
C8

L1
L2
L3
L4
L5

S1

Trigeminal nerve branches

S2–S4

Cervical

Thoracic

Lumbar

Sacral

Dermatomes
Areas of the skin supplied
by nerves from a single
spinal root.

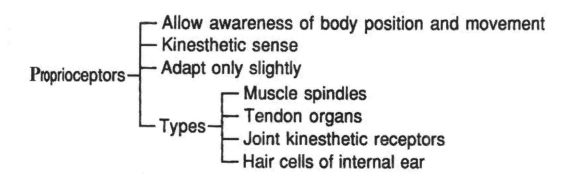

Proprioceptors
- Allow awareness of body position and movement
- Kinesthetic sense
- Adapt only slightly
- Types
  - Muscle spindles
  - Tendon organs
  - Joint kinesthetic receptors
  - Hair cells of internal ear

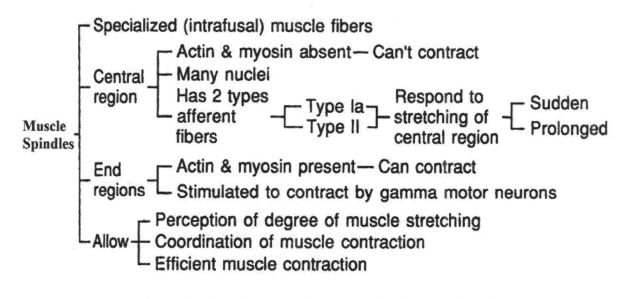

Muscle Spindles
- Specialized (intrafusal) muscle fibers
- Central region
  - Actin & myosin absent — Can't contract
  - Many nuclei
  - Has 2 types afferent fibers
    - Type Ia
    - Type II
    - Respond to stretching of central region
      - Sudden
      - Prolonged
- End regions
  - Actin & myosin present — Can contract
  - Stimulated to contract by gamma motor neurons
- Allow
  - Perception of degree of muscle stretching
  - Coordination of muscle contraction
  - Efficient muscle contraction

Tendon organs
- Located at junction between tendon and muscle
- Protect tendon/muscle from excess tension
- Monitor contraction force
- Type Ib fibers carry nerve impulses to CNS

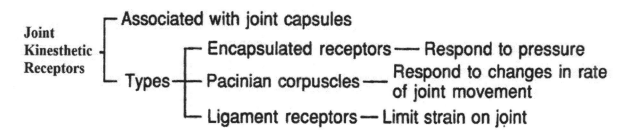

Joint Kinesthetic Receptors
- Associated with joint capsules
- Types
  - Encapsulated receptors — Respond to pressure
  - Pacinian corpuscles — Respond to changes in rate of joint movement
  - Ligament receptors — Limit strain on joint

Sense organs in different parts of the body

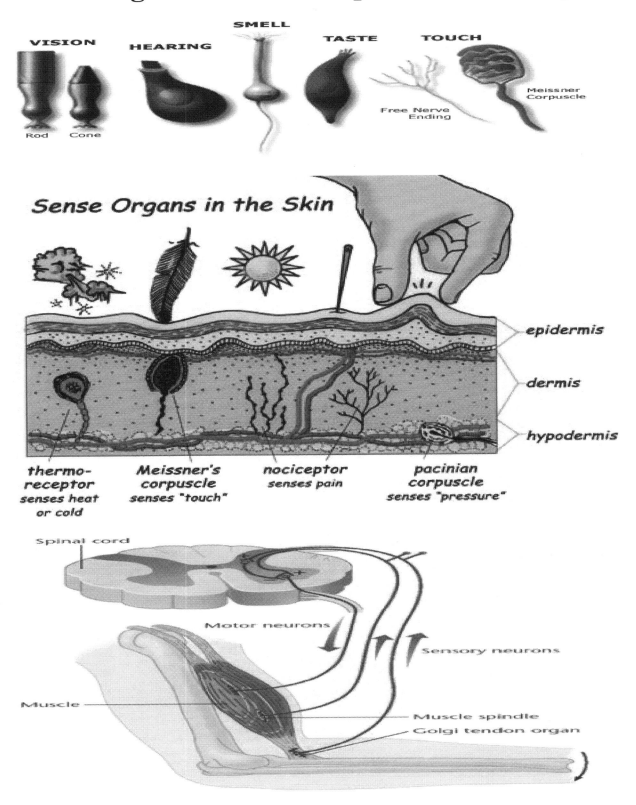

VISION

Rod   Cone

HEARING

SMELL

TASTE

TOUCH

Free Nerve Ending

Meissner Corpuscle

Sense Organs in the Skin

epidermis

dermis

hypodermis

thermo-receptor
senses heat or cold

Meissner's corpuscle
senses "touch"

nociceptor
senses pain

pacinian corpuscle
senses "pressure"

Spinal cord

Motor neurons

Sensory neurons

Muscle

Muscle spindle

Golgi tendon organ

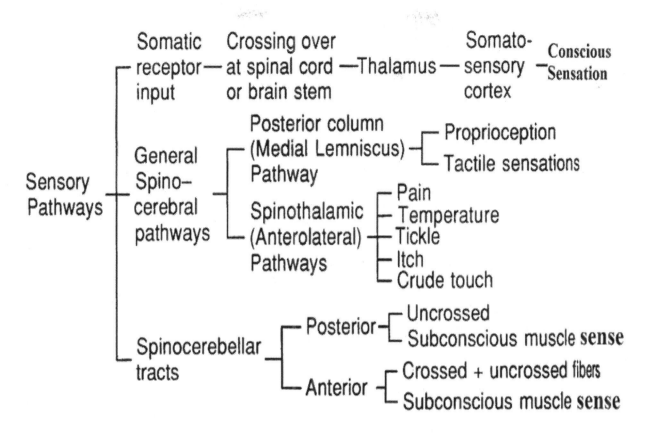

Sensory Pathways
- Somatic receptor input — Crossing over at spinal cord or brain stem — Thalamus — Somato-sensory cortex — Conscious Sensation
- General Spino-cerebral pathways
  - Posterior column (Medial Lemniscus) Pathway
    - Proprioception
    - Tactile sensations
  - Spinothalamic (Anterolateral) Pathways
    - Pain
    - Temperature
    - Tickle
    - Itch
    - Crude touch
- Spinocerebellar tracts
  - Posterior
    - Uncrossed
    - Subconscious muscle sense
  - Anterior
    - Crossed + uncrossed fibers
    - Subconscious muscle sense

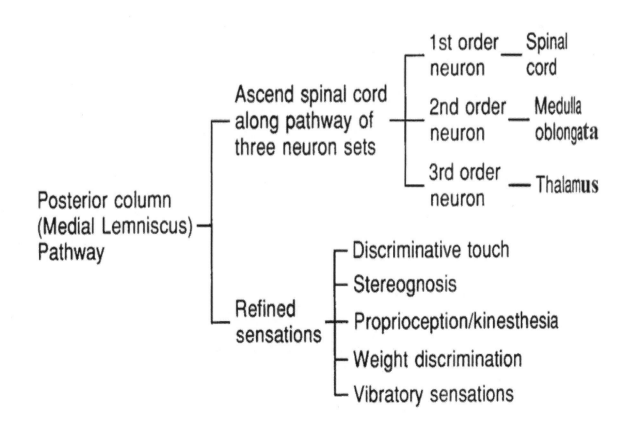

Posterior column (Medial Lemniscus) Pathway
- Ascend spinal cord along pathway of three neuron sets
  - 1st order neuron — Spinal cord
  - 2nd order neuron — Medulla oblongata
  - 3rd order neuron — Thalamus
- Refined sensations
  - Discriminative touch
  - Stereognosis
  - Proprioception/kinesthesia
  - Weight discrimination
  - Vibratory sensations

Posterior column-medial lemniscus pathways (PCML)

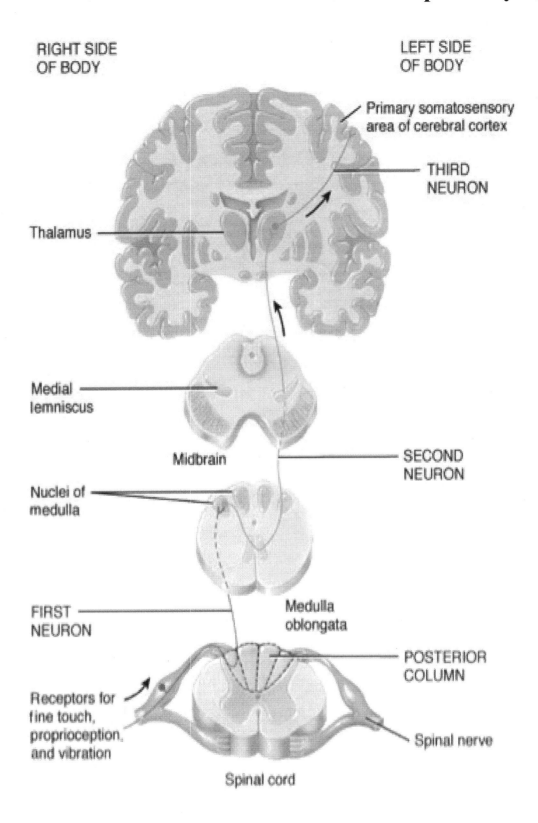

RIGHT SIDE
OF BODY

LEFT SIDE
OF BODY

Primary somatosensory
area of cerebral cortex

THIRD
NEURON

Thalamus

Medial
lemniscus

Midbrain

SECOND
NEURON

Nuclei of
medulla

FIRST
NEURON

Medulla
oblongata

POSTERIOR
COLUMN

Receptors for
fine touch,
proprioception,
and vibration

Spinal nerve

Spinal cord

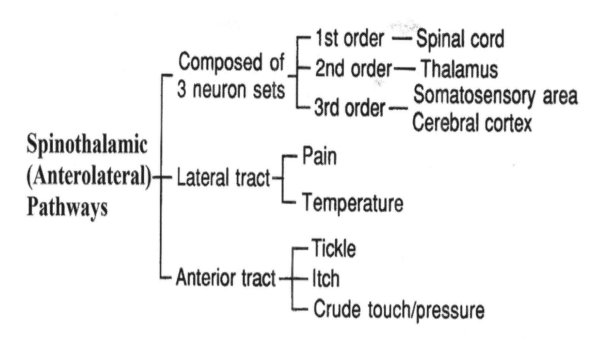

Spinothalamic (Anterolateral) Pathways
- Composed of 3 neuron sets
  - 1st order — Spinal cord
  - 2nd order — Thalamus
  - 3rd order — Somatosensory area Cerebral cortex
- Lateral tract
  - Pain
  - Temperature
- Anterior tract
  - Tickle
  - Itch
  - Crude touch/pressure

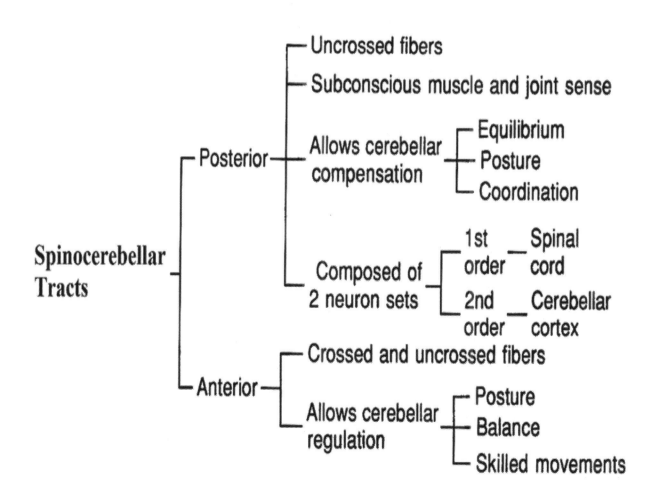

Spinocerebellar Tracts
- Posterior
  - Uncrossed fibers
  - Subconscious muscle and joint sense
  - Allows cerebellar compensation
    - Equilibrium
    - Posture
    - Coordination
  - Composed of 2 neuron sets
    - 1st order — Spinal cord
    - 2nd order — Cerebellar cortex
- Anterior
  - Crossed and uncrossed fibers
  - Allows cerebellar regulation
    - Posture
    - Balance
    - Skilled movements

Anterior Spinothalamic tracts

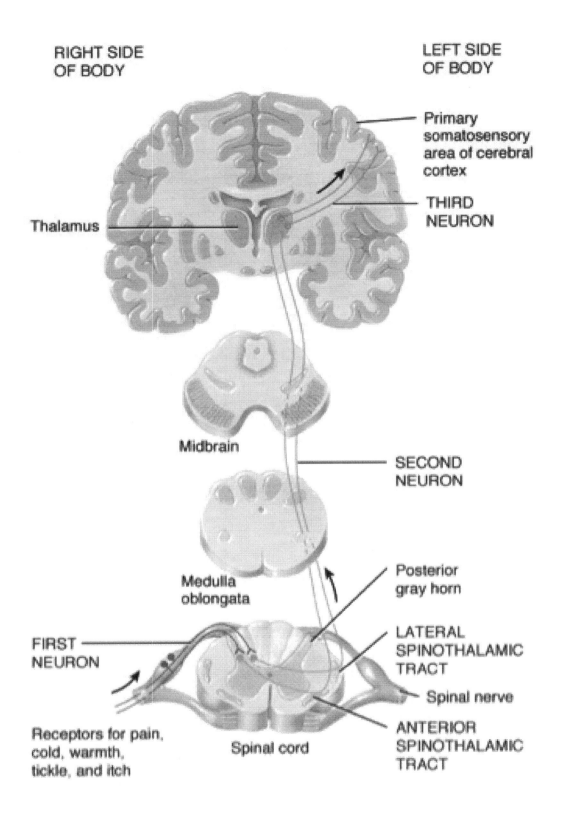

RIGHT SIDE
OF BODY

LEFT SIDE
OF BODY

Primary
somatosensory
area of cerebral
cortex

THIRD
NEURON

Thalamus

Midbrain

SECOND
NEURON

Medulla
oblongata

Posterior
gray horn

FIRST
NEURON

LATERAL
SPINOTHALAMIC
TRACT

Spinal nerve

Receptors for pain,
cold, warmth,
tickle, and itch

Spinal cord

ANTERIOR
SPINOTHALAMIC
TRACT

Posterior spinocerebellar and anterior spinocerebellar tracts

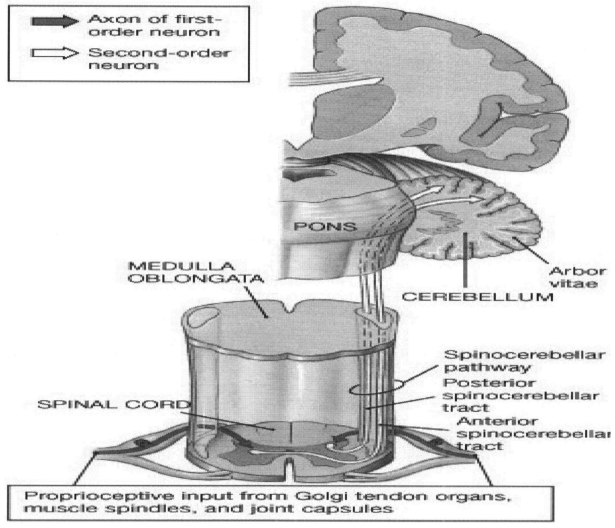

Axon of first-order neuron

Second-order neuron

PONS

MEDULLA OBLONGATA

Arbor vitae

CEREBELLUM

SPINAL CORD

Spinocerebellar pathway

Posterior spinocerebellar tract

Anterior spinocerebellar tract

Proprioceptive input from Golgi tendon organs, muscle spindles, and joint capsules

The final common pathway transmits all central nervous system commands to the skeletal muscles. This path is influenced by sensory input from the muscle spindles and tendon organs (dashed lines) and descending signals from the cerebral cortex and brain stem. The cerebellum and basal ganglia influence the motor function indirectly, using brain stem and cortical pathways.

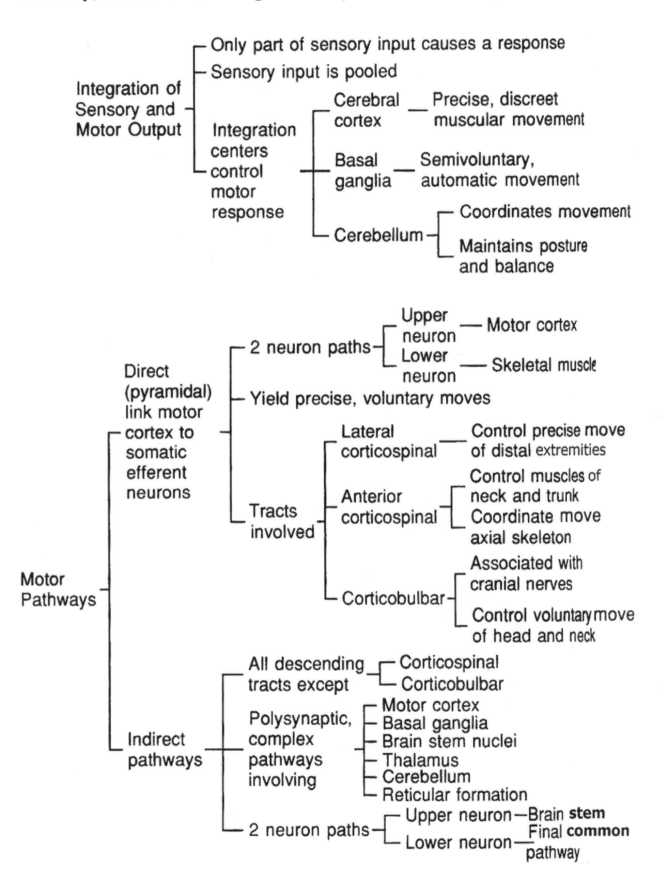

Integration of Sensory and Motor Output
- Only part of sensory input causes a response
- Sensory input is pooled
- Integration centers control motor response
  - Cerebral cortex — Precise, discreet muscular movement
  - Basal ganglia — Semivoluntary, automatic movement
  - Cerebellum
    - Coordinates movement
    - Maintains posture and balance

Motor Pathways
- Direct (pyramidal) link motor cortex to somatic efferent neurons
  - 2 neuron paths
    - Upper neuron — Motor cortex
    - Lower neuron — Skeletal muscle
  - Yield precise, voluntary moves
  - Tracts involved
    - Lateral corticospinal — Control precise move of distal extremities
    - Anterior corticospinal
      - Control muscles of neck and trunk
      - Coordinate move axial skeleton
    - Corticobulbar
      - Associated with cranial nerves
      - Control voluntary move of head and neck
- Indirect pathways
  - All descending tracts except
    - Corticospinal
    - Corticobulbar
  - Polysynaptic, complex pathways involving
    - Motor cortex
    - Basal ganglia
    - Brain stem nuclei
    - Thalamus
    - Cerebellum
    - Reticular formation
  - 2 neuron paths
    - Upper neuron — Brain **stem**
    - Lower neuron — Final **common** pathway

Motor pathways: Pyramidal (Corticospinal) tracts
Degree of representation of the different muscles of the body in the motor cortex

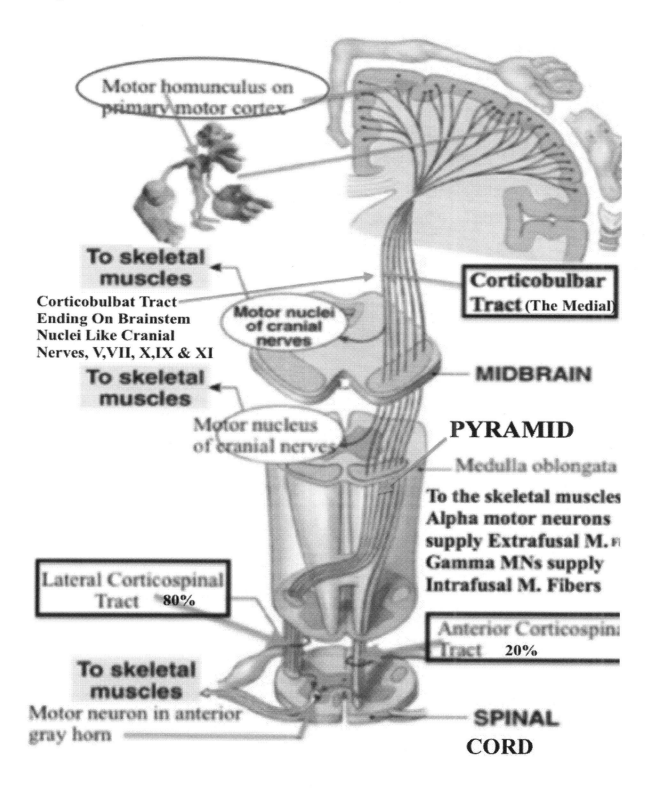

Motor homunculus on primary motor cortex

To skeletal muscles

Corticobulbat Tract Ending On Brainstem Nuclei Like Cranial Nerves, V,VII, X,IX & XI

Motor nuclei of cranial nerves

Corticobulbar Tract (The Medial)

To skeletal muscles

Motor nucleus of cranial nerves

MIDBRAIN

PYRAMID

Medulla oblongata

To the skeletal muscles Alpha motor neurons supply Extrafusal M. F Gamma MNs supply Intrafusal M. Fibers

Lateral Corticospinal Tract   80%

Anterior Corticospinal Tract   20%

To skeletal muscles

Motor neuron in anterior gray horn

SPINAL CORD

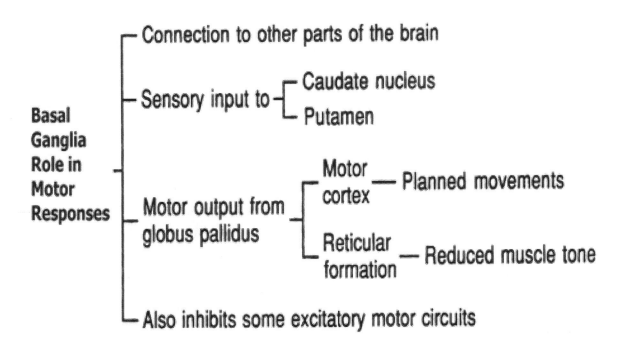

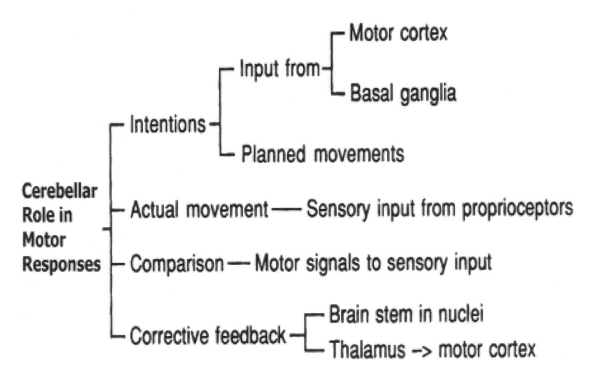

Connectivity diagram showing excitatory glutamatergic pathways as red, inhibitory GABAergic pathways as blue, and modulatory dopaminergic pathways as magenta

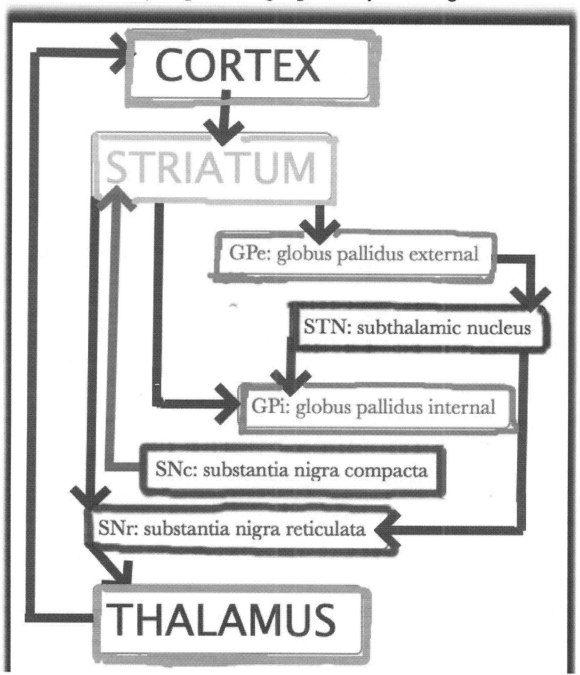

The left side of this figure shows the basic neuronal circuit of the cerebellum, with excitatory neurons shown in red and the Purkinje cell (an inhibitory neuron) shown in black. To the right is shown the physical relationship of the deep cerebellar nuclei to the cerebellar cortex with its three layers.

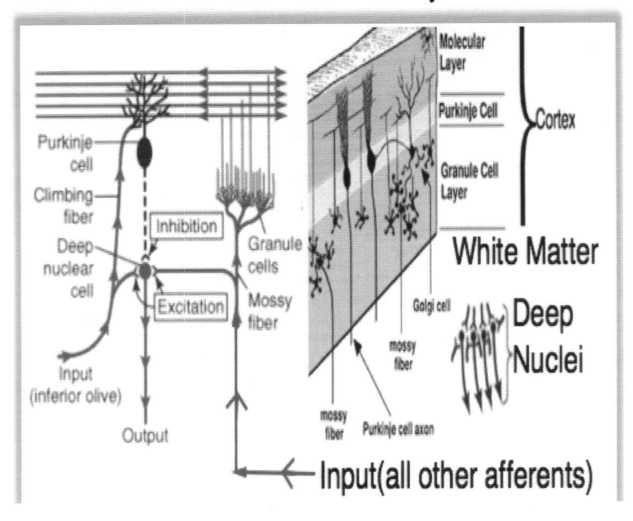

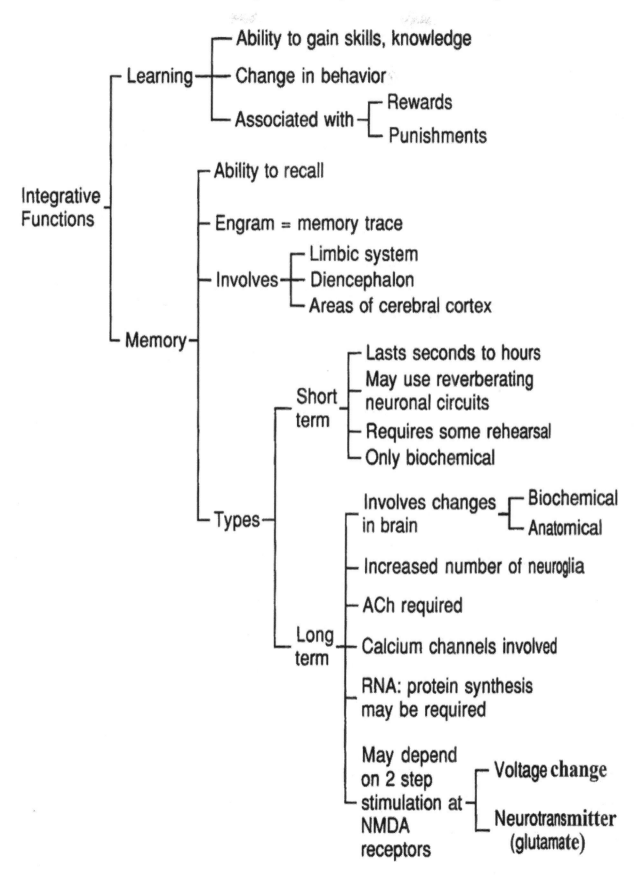

Integrative Functions

Learning
- Ability to gain skills, knowledge
- Change in behavior
- Associated with
  - Rewards
  - Punishments

Memory
- Ability to recall
- Engram = memory trace
- Involves
  - Limbic system
  - Diencephalon
  - Areas of cerebral cortex
- Types
  - Short term
    - Lasts seconds to hours
    - May use reverberating neuronal circuits
    - Requires some rehearsal
    - Only biochemical
  - Long term
    - Involves changes in brain
      - Biochemical
      - Anatomical
    - Increased number of neuroglia
    - ACh required
    - Calcium channels involved
    - RNA: protein synthesis may be required
    - May depend on 2 step stimulation at NMDA receptors
      - Voltage change
      - Neurotransmitter (glutamate)

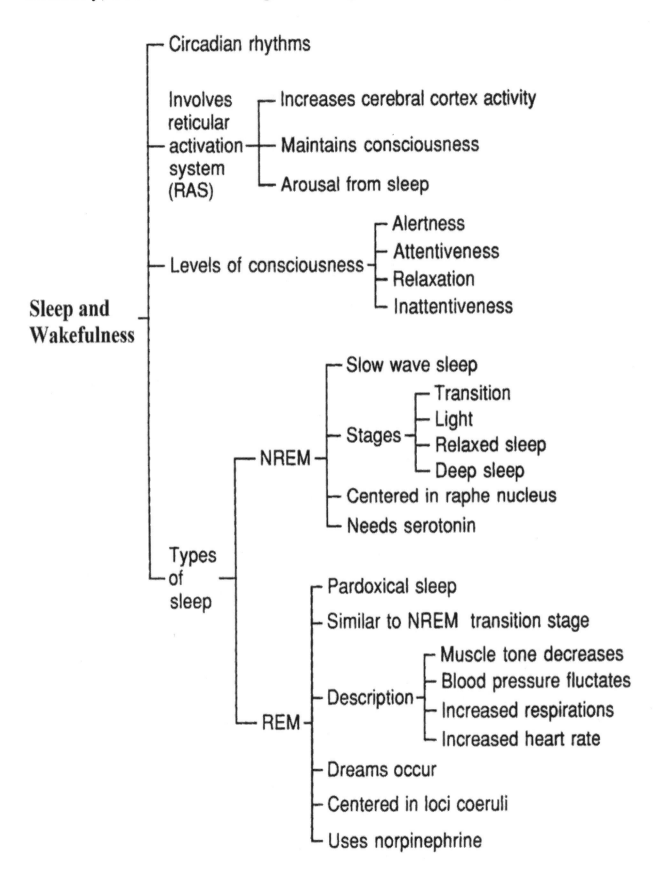

Sleep and Wakefulness

- Circadian rhythms
- Involves reticular activation system (RAS)
  - Increases cerebral cortex activity
  - Maintains consciousness
  - Arousal from sleep
- Levels of consciousness
  - Alertness
  - Attentiveness
  - Relaxation
  - Inattentiveness
- Types of sleep
  - NREM
    - Slow wave sleep
    - Stages
      - Transition
      - Light
      - Relaxed sleep
      - Deep sleep
    - Centered in raphe nucleus
    - Needs serotonin
  - REM
    - Pardoxical sleep
    - Similar to NREM transition stage
    - Description
      - Muscle tone decreases
      - Blood pressure fluctates
      - Increased respirations
      - Increased heart rate
    - Dreams occur
    - Centered in loci coeruli
    - Uses norpinephrine

CHAPTER SIXTEEN

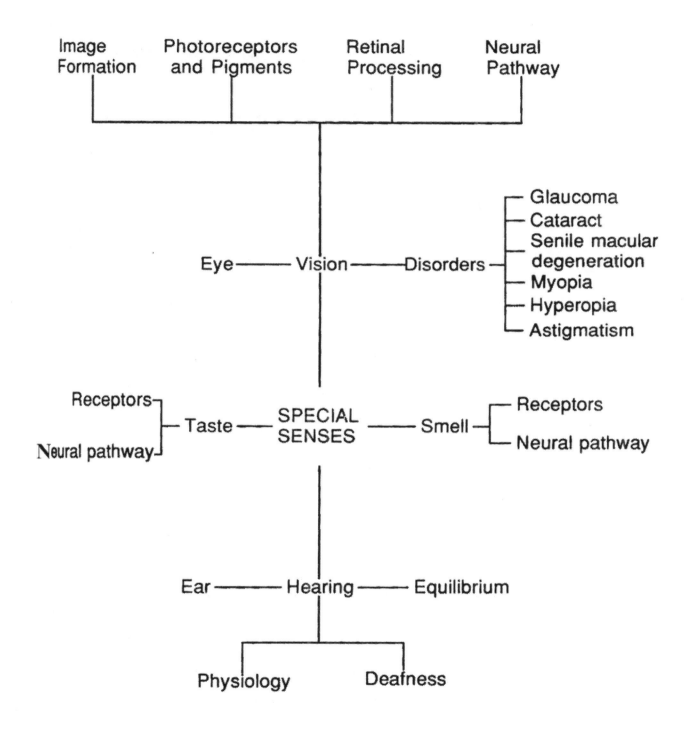

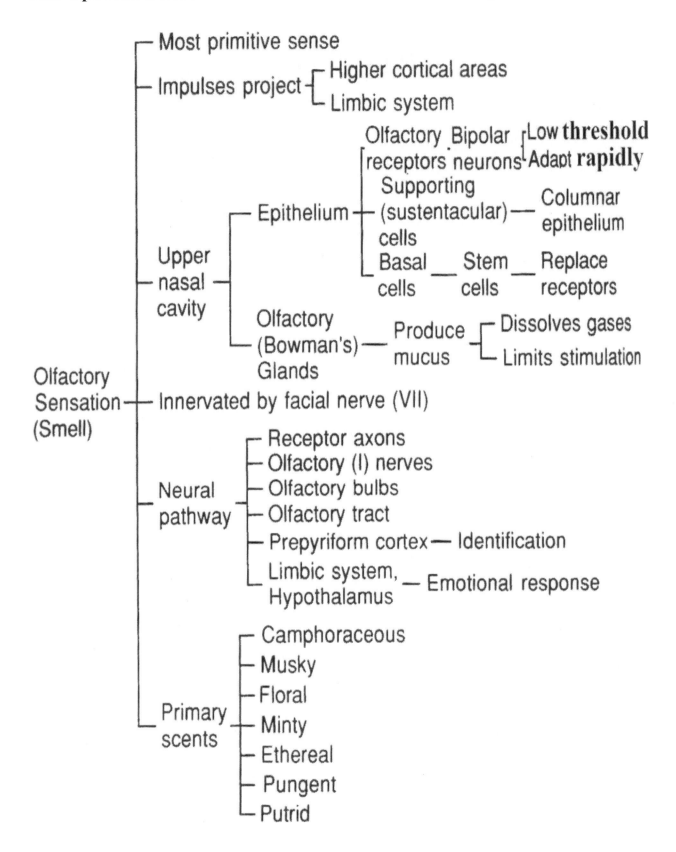

Olfactory Sensation (Smell)
- Most primitive sense
- Impulses project
  - Higher cortical areas
  - Limbic system
- Upper nasal cavity
  - Epithelium
    - Olfactory receptors Bipolar neurons
      - Low **threshold**
      - Adapt **rapidly**
    - Supporting (sustentacular) cells — Columnar epithelium
    - Basal cells — Stem cells — Replace receptors
  - Olfactory (Bowman's) Glands — Produce mucus
    - Dissolves gases
    - Limits stimulation
- Innervated by facial nerve (VII)
- Neural pathway
  - Receptor axons
  - Olfactory (I) nerves
  - Olfactory bulbs
  - Olfactory tract
  - Prepyriform cortex — Identification
  - Limbic system, Hypothalamus — Emotional response
- Primary scents
  - Camphoraceous
  - Musky
  - Floral
  - Minty
  - Ethereal
  - Pungent
  - Putrid

(A) Anatomy of Smell, (B) Organization of the olfactory membrane, olfactory bulb, and connections to the olfactory tract

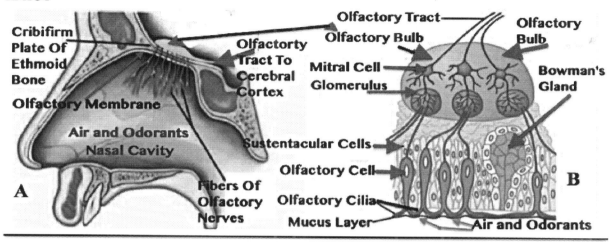

Olfactory bulb functional anatomy: Abbreviations: M - Mitral cells; T - tufted cells; Gr - Granulle cells; PG - Periglomerular cells; OSN - Olfactory sensory neurons.

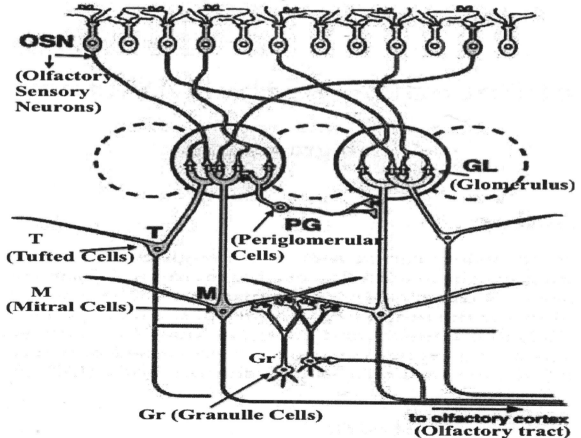

Main Characteristics Of Gustation (Sense of Taste)

The Gustation receptors cells for taste are located in taste buds on the surface of the tongue, roof of mouth, throat, and epiglottis.

Substances to be tasted must be in solution in saliva.

The five primary tastes are SALT, SWEET, BITTER, SOUR, and UMAMI.

The senses of smell and taste are closely associated. If one's ability to smell is impaired, the ability to taste will be greatly diminished.

Adaptation to taste occurs quickly and the threshold for taste varies for each of the primary tastes.

Gustatory cells convey their impulses to the facial (VII), glossopharyngeal (IX), vagus (X) cranial nerves, medulla, thalamus, cerebral cortex, limbic system and hypothalamus.

Main Characteristics Of Olfaction (Sense of Smell)

The Olfaction receptors are located in the nasal epithelium in the superior portion of the nasal cavity and consist of three types of cells: olfactory receptor cells, supporting cells, and basal cells.

In order to be smelled, substances must be volatile, water-soluble, and lipid-soluble.

The chemical theory assumes that there are different receptor molecules in the membranes of the olfactory hairs, each capable of reacting with a particular stimulus. The interaction of the olfactory receptor cells and the odorant molecules produce **a transduction**. This is followed by the initiation of a nerve impulse.

Adaptation to odors occurs quickly, and the threshold of smell is low.

Olfactory cells convey nerve impulses to the olfactory nerves (cranial nerve I), olfactory bulbs, olfactory tracts, cerebral cortex, limbic system and hypothalamus.

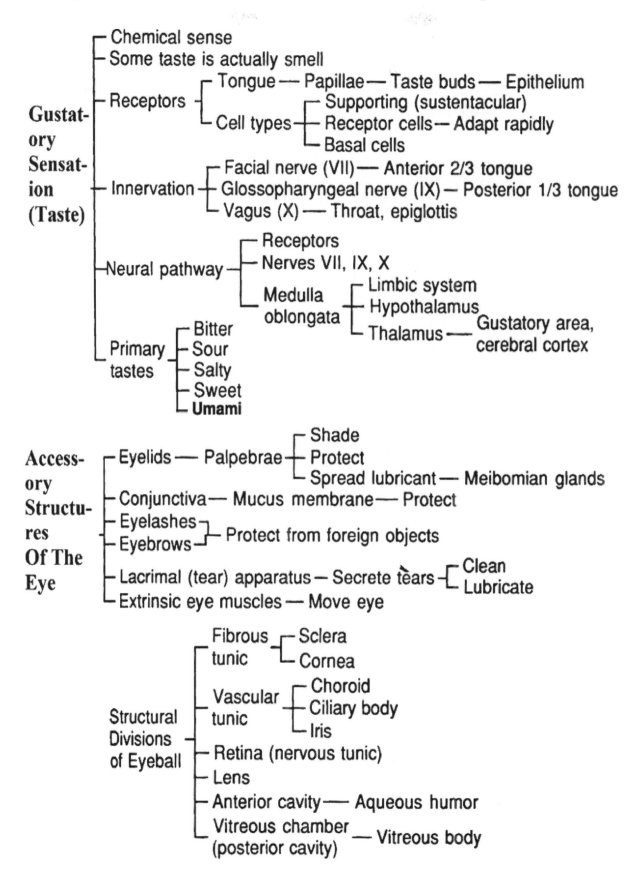

Gustatory Sensation (Taste)
- Chemical sense
- Some taste is actually smell
- Receptors
  - Tongue — Papillae — Taste buds — Epithelium
  - Cell types
    - Supporting (sustentacular)
    - Receptor cells — Adapt rapidly
    - Basal cells
- Innervation
  - Facial nerve (VII) — Anterior 2/3 tongue
  - Glossopharyngeal nerve (IX) — Posterior 1/3 tongue
  - Vagus (X) — Throat, epiglottis
- Neural pathway
  - Receptors
  - Nerves VII, IX, X
  - Medulla oblongata
    - Limbic system
    - Hypothalamus
    - Thalamus — Gustatory area, cerebral cortex
- Primary tastes
  - Bitter
  - Sour
  - Salty
  - Sweet
  - **Umami**

Accessory Structures Of The Eye
- Eyelids — Palpebrae
  - Shade
  - Protect
  - Spread lubricant — Meibomian glands
- Conjunctiva — Mucus membrane — Protect
- Eyelashes
- Eyebrows
  - Protect from foreign objects
- Lacrimal (tear) apparatus — Secrete tears
  - Clean
  - Lubricate
- Extrinsic eye muscles — Move eye

Structural Divisions of Eyeball
- Fibrous tunic
  - Sclera
  - Cornea
- Vascular tunic
  - Choroid
  - Ciliary body
  - Iris
- Retina (nervous tunic)
- Lens
- Anterior cavity — Aqueous humor
- Vitreous chamber (posterior cavity) — Vitreous body

(A) Tongue contains taste buds- (the Foliate, Filiform, Fungiform and Circumvallated papillae) Papillae are sensitive to sweet, sour, salty, bitter tastes and Umami. (B) Taste buds contain taste cells that end in taste pores and gustatory hairs, which bear receptors proteins

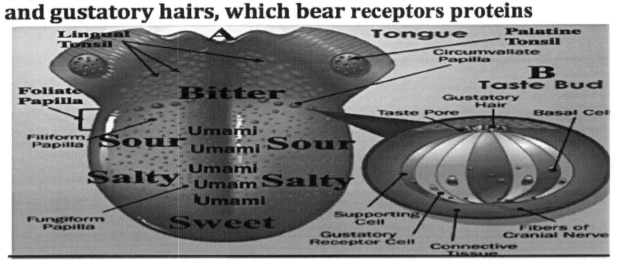

(A) Smell and taste center (B) Olfactory receptor and (C) Taste receptor

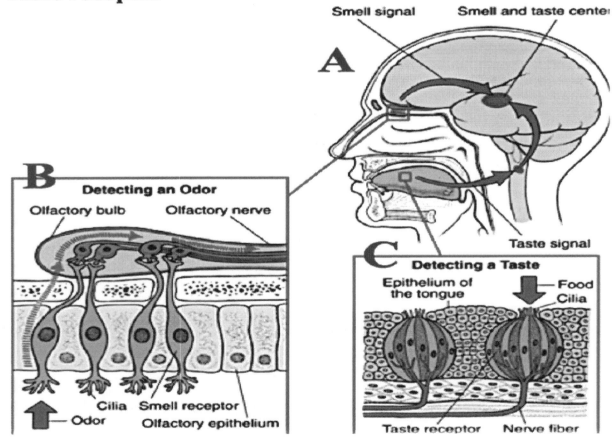

Transverse section of the eyeball and its appendage

1. Aqueous chamber
2. Choroid
3. Ciliary muscle
4. Ciliary processes
5. Cornea
6. Crystalline lens
7. Frontal bone
8. Frontal sinus
9. Inferior oblique muscle
10. Inferior ophthalmic vein
11. Inferior rectus muscle
12. Inferior tarsus
13. Iris
14. Lateral rectus muscle
15. Maxillary sinus
16. Optic nerve
17. Ora serrata
18. Pupil of the iris
19. Retina
20. Retinal artery and vein
21. Sclera
22. Sphenoid sinus
23. Pterygopalatine ganglion
24. Superior oblique muscle
25. Superior rectus muscle
26. Superior tarsus
27. Suspensory ligament
28. Vitreous chamber

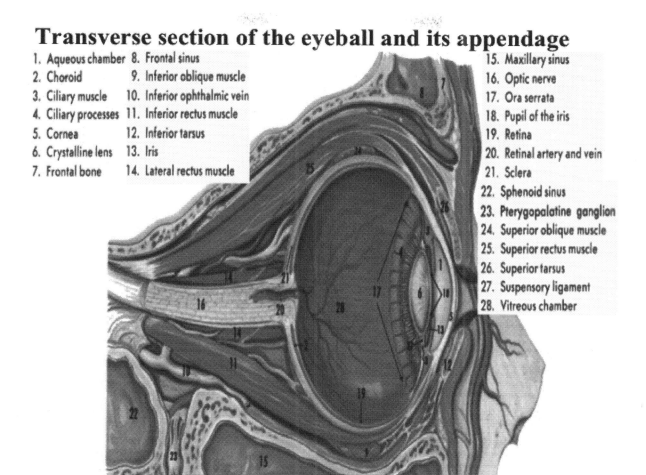

Parts the Eye And Their Functions

Parts the Eye	Functions of the parts of the eye
Sclera	Protect and supports eyeball
Cornea	Reflects light rays
Pupil	Admits light
Choroid	Absorbs stray light
Ciliary body	Hold the lens in place, Accommodation
Iris	Regulates light entrance
Retina	Contains sensory receptors for light
Rods	Make black and white vision possible
Cones	Make color vision possible
Fovea centralis	Make acute vision possible
Lens	Refracts and focuses light rays
Humors	Transmit light rays and support eyeball
Optic nerve	Transmits impulse to the brain

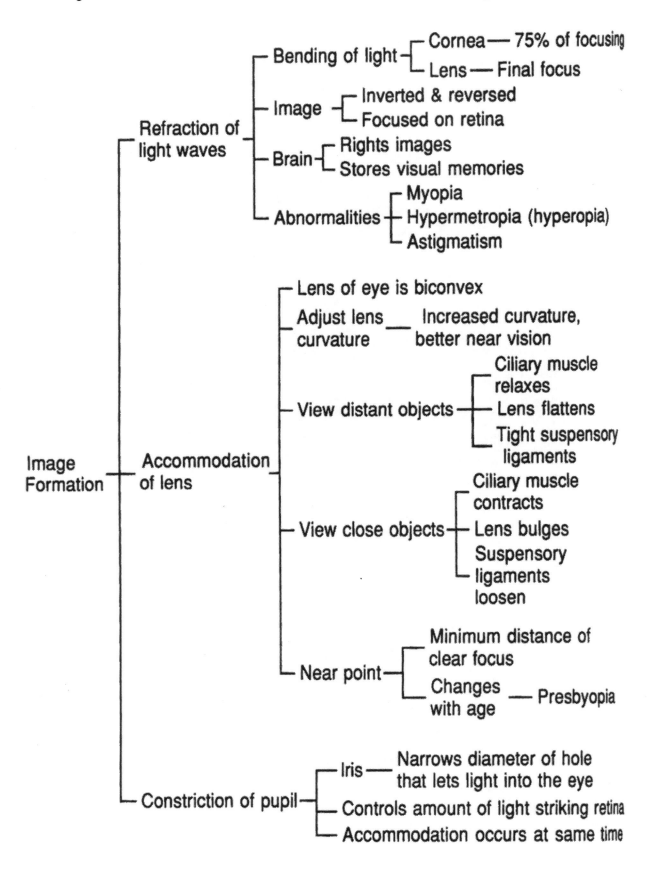

Image Formation

Refraction of light waves
- Bending of light
  - Cornea — 75% of focusing
  - Lens — Final focus
- Image
  - Inverted & reversed
  - Focused on retina
- Brain
  - Rights images
  - Stores visual memories
- Abnormalities
  - Myopia
  - Hypermetropia (hyperopia)
  - Astigmatism

Accommodation of lens
- Lens of eye is biconvex
- Adjust lens curvature — Increased curvature, better near vision
- View distant objects
  - Ciliary muscle relaxes
  - Lens flattens
  - Tight suspensory ligaments
- View close objects
  - Ciliary muscle contracts
  - Lens bulges
  - Suspensory ligaments loosen
- Near point
  - Minimum distance of clear focus
  - Changes with age — Presbyopia

Constriction of pupil
- Iris — Narrows diameter of hole that lets light into the eye
- Controls amount of light striking retina
- Accommodation occurs at same time

Reflection of light in the eye

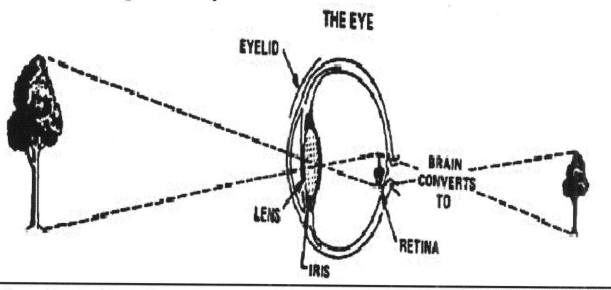

Eye focusing (accommodation); Normal, Nearsighted (Myopia) and Farsighted (Hyperopia) Vision

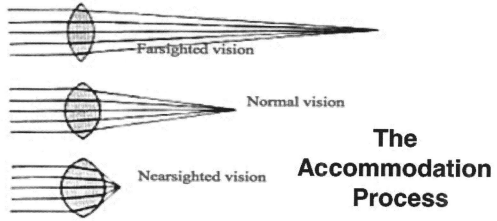

Farsighted vision

Normal vision

Nearsighted vision

The Accommodation Process

The shapes of the lens determines the focusing

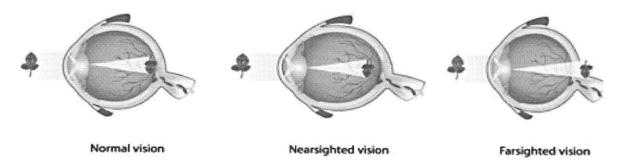

Normal vision   Nearsighted vision   Farsighted vision

Autonomic innervations of the eye: showing also the reflex arc of the light reflex. The sympathetic fibers innervate the dilator iridis muscles, which are responsible for dilating the iris. The sphincter pupillae muscle is innervated by the parasympathetic system. When the sympathetic innervations are interrupted, the parasympathetic system is unopposed and the pupil dilates.

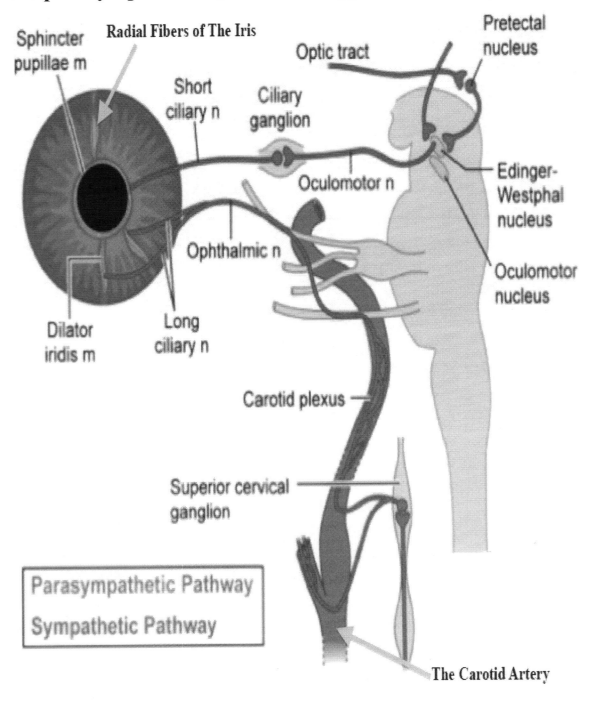

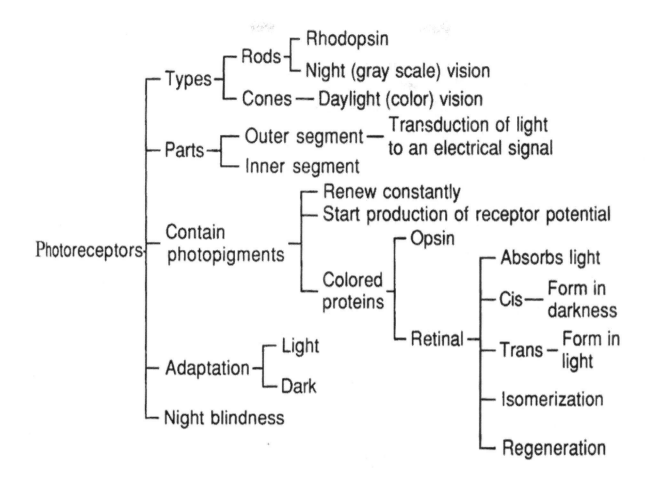

Photoreceptors
- Types
  - Rods
    - Rhodopsin
    - Night (gray scale) vision
  - Cones — Daylight (color) vision
- Parts
  - Outer segment — Transduction of light to an electrical signal
  - Inner segment
- Contain photopigments
  - Renew constantly
  - Start production of receptor potential
  - Colored proteins
    - Opsin
    - Retinal
      - Absorbs light
      - Cis — Form in darkness
      - Trans — Form in light
      - Isomerization
      - Regeneration
- Adaptation
  - Light
  - Dark
- Night blindness

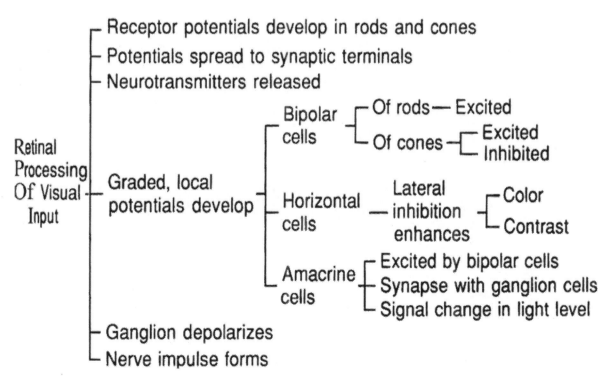

Retinal Processing Of Visual Input
- Receptor potentials develop in rods and cones
- Potentials spread to synaptic terminals
- Neurotransmitters released
- Graded, local potentials develop
  - Bipolar cells
    - Of rods — Excited
    - Of cones
      - Excited
      - Inhibited
  - Horizontal cells — Lateral inhibition enhances
    - Color
    - Contrast
  - Amacrine cells
    - Excited by bipolar cells
    - Synapse with ganglion cells
    - Signal change in light level
- Ganglion depolarizes
- Nerve impulse forms

Organization of the Human Retina:

Photoreceptor layer (Rods and Cones), Nuclear layer (Nuclei of Rods and Cones), Outer Plexiform layer (junction of rods, cones, horizontal and bipolar cells), Inner nuclear layer (nuclei of horizontal, amacrine and bipolar cells), Inner Plexiform layer (junction of ganglion, amacrine and bipolar cells), Ganglion layer (nuclei of ganglion cells), Nerve fiber layer (fibers of the optic nerve going to the brain cortex)

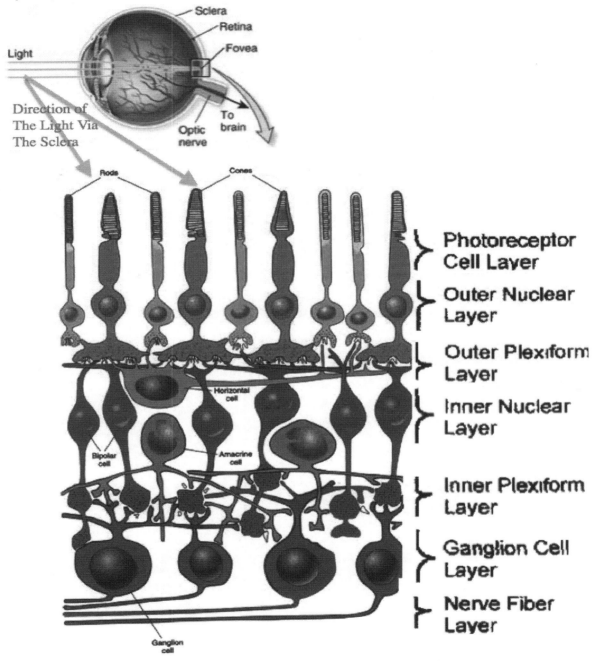

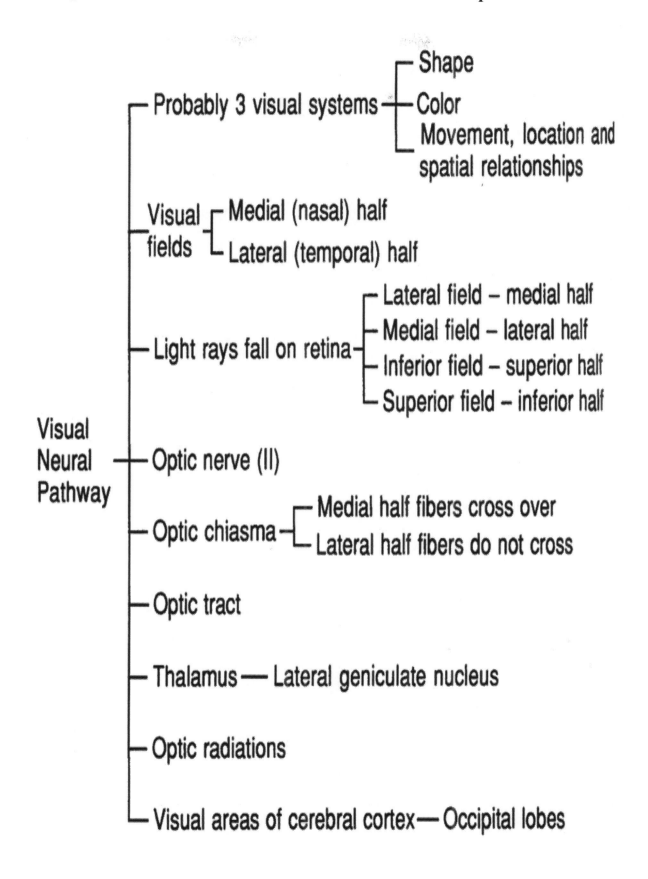

Visual Neural Pathway

- Probably 3 visual systems
  - Shape
  - Color
  - Movement, location and spatial relationships
- Visual fields
  - Medial (nasal) half
  - Lateral (temporal) half
- Light rays fall on retina
  - Lateral field – medial half
  - Medial field – lateral half
  - Inferior field – superior half
  - Superior field – inferior half
- Optic nerve (II)
- Optic chiasma
  - Medial half fibers cross over
  - Lateral half fibers do not cross
- Optic tract
- Thalamus — Lateral geniculate nucleus
- Optic radiations
- Visual areas of cerebral cortex — Occipital lobes

There are Four Photoreceptor types in human retina; Short-Wavelength Cones (Blue), Medium-Wavelength Cones (Green), Long-Wavelength (Red) and The Rods

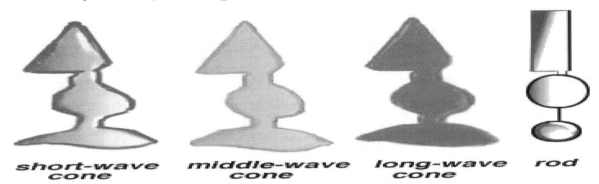

short-wave cone   middle-wave cone   long-wave cone   rod

Visual Pathway

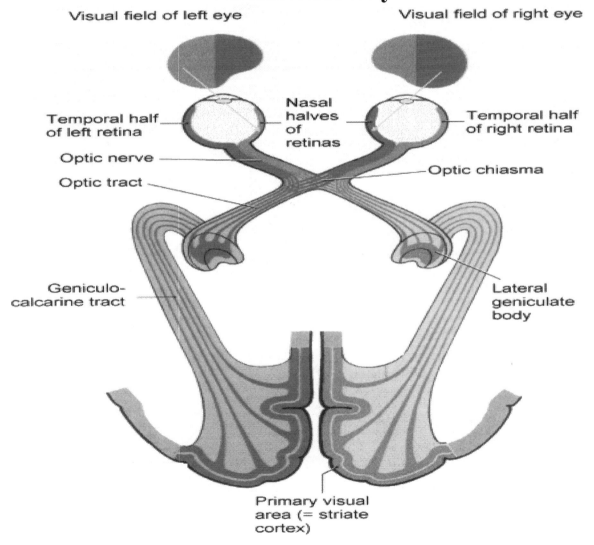

Visual field of left eye   Visual field of right eye

Temporal half of left retina

Nasal halves of retinas

Temporal half of right retina

Optic nerve

Optic tract

Optic chiasma

Geniculo-calcarine tract

Lateral geniculate body

Primary visual area (= striate cortex)

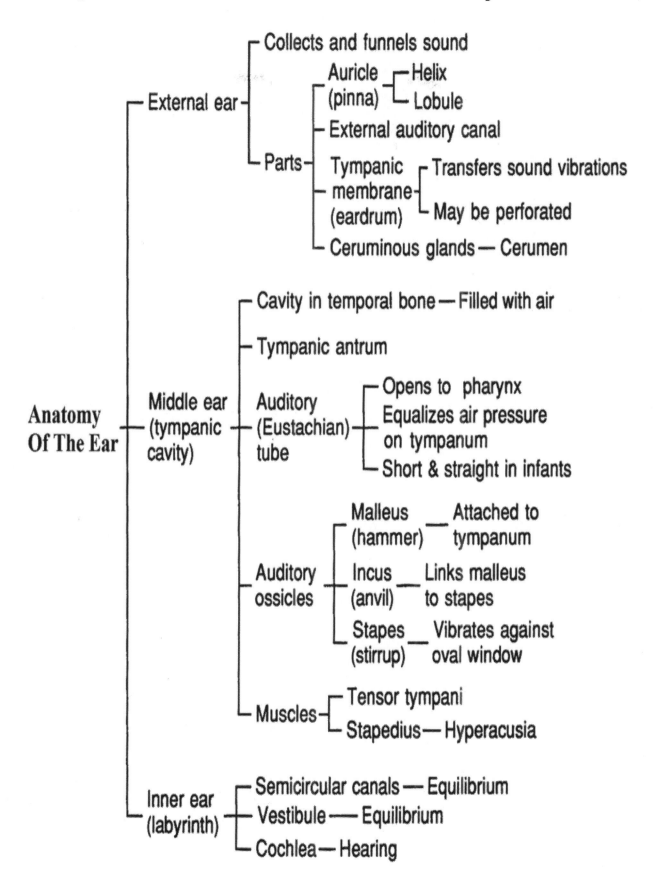

Anatomy Of The Ear

- External ear
  - Collects and funnels sound
  - Parts
    - Auricle (pinna)
      - Helix
      - Lobule
    - External auditory canal
    - Tympanic membrane (eardrum)
      - Transfers sound vibrations
      - May be perforated
    - Ceruminous glands — Cerumen

- Middle ear (tympanic cavity)
  - Cavity in temporal bone — Filled with air
  - Tympanic antrum
  - Auditory (Eustachian) tube
    - Opens to pharynx
    - Equalizes air pressure on tympanum
    - Short & straight in infants
  - Auditory ossicles
    - Malleus (hammer) — Attached to tympanum
    - Incus (anvil) — Links malleus to stapes
    - Stapes (stirrup) — Vibrates against oval window
  - Muscles
    - Tensor tympani
    - Stapedius — Hyperacusia

- Inner ear (labyrinth)
  - Semicircular canals — Equilibrium
  - Vestibule — Equilibrium
  - Cochlea — Hearing

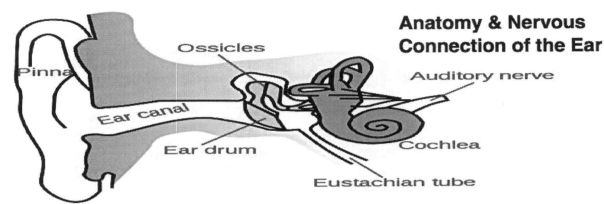

Anatomy & Nervous Connection of the Ear

The principle central connections of the hearing, solid colored lines show the ascending pathways to the primary auditory cortex while the broken lines are the descending connections

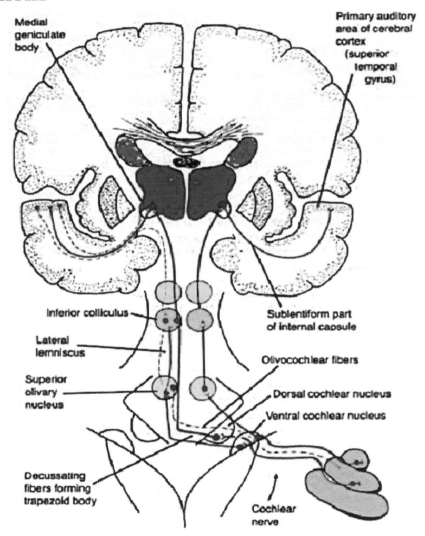

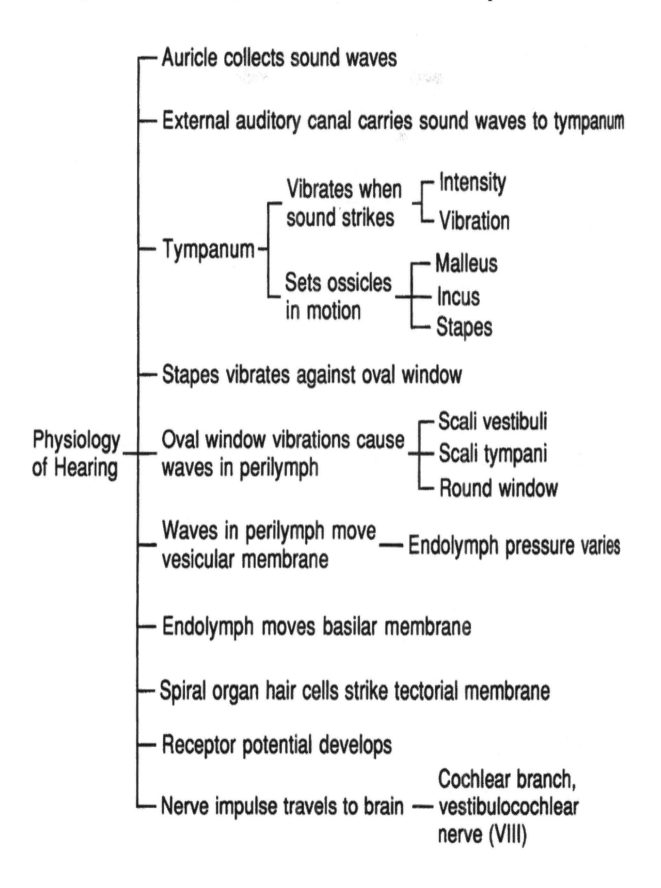

Physiology of Hearing

- Auricle collects sound waves
- External auditory canal carries sound waves to tympanum
- Tympanum
  - Vibrates when sound strikes
    - Intensity
    - Vibration
  - Sets ossicles in motion
    - Malleus
    - Incus
    - Stapes
- Stapes vibrates against oval window
- Oval window vibrations cause waves in perilymph
  - Scali vestibuli
  - Scali tympani
  - Round window
- Waves in perilymph move vesicular membrane — Endolymph pressure varies
- Endolymph moves basilar membrane
- Spiral organ hair cells strike tectorial membrane
- Receptor potential develops
- Nerve impulse travels to brain — Cochlear branch, vestibulocochlear nerve (VIII)

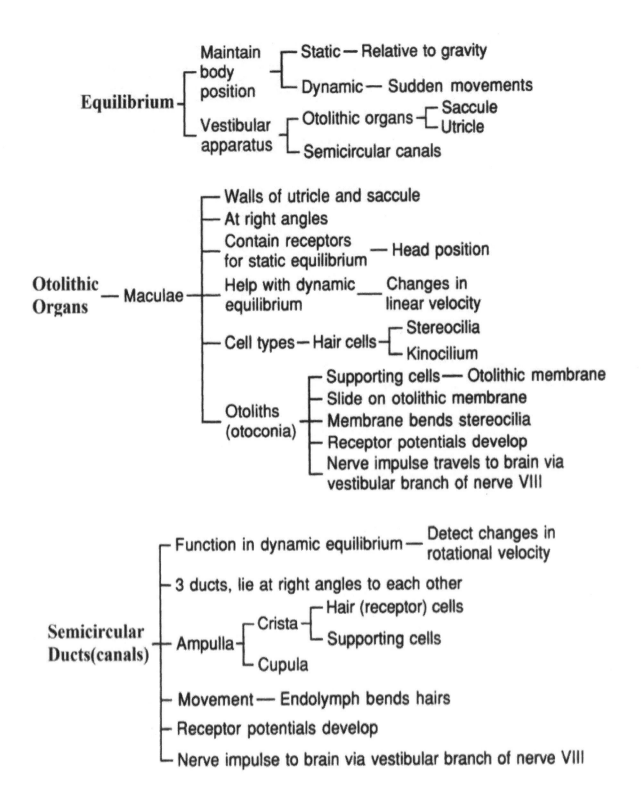

Role of the vestibular system in control of posture, eye movements and perception of orientation

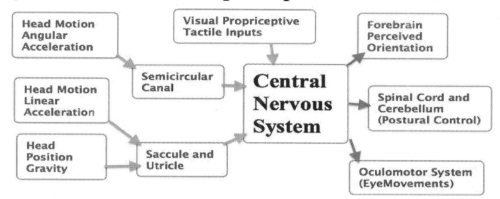

Schematic representations of Vestibulo-spinal and Vestibulo-Ocular pathways

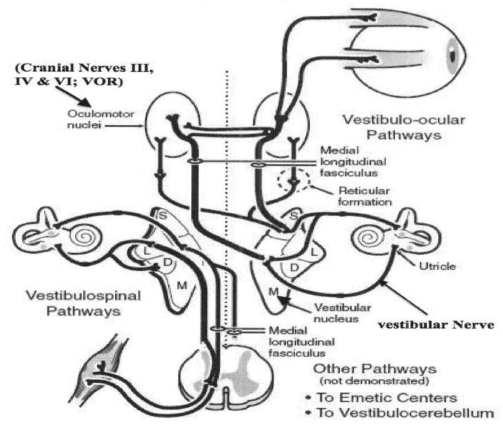

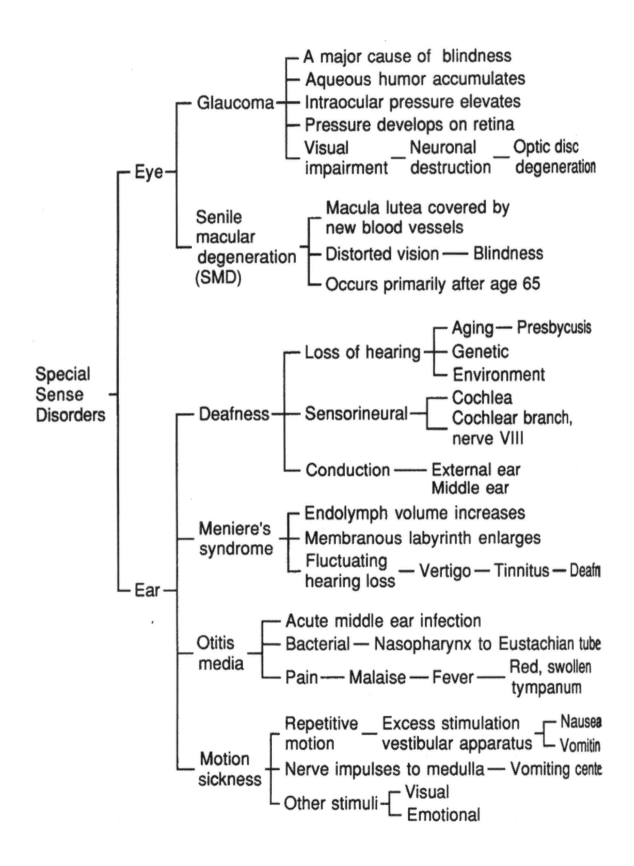

Special Sense Disorders

- Eye
  - Glaucoma
    - A major cause of blindness
    - Aqueous humor accumulates
    - Intraocular pressure elevates
    - Pressure develops on retina
    - Visual impairment — Neuronal destruction — Optic disc degeneration
  - Senile macular degeneration (SMD)
    - Macula lutea covered by new blood vessels
    - Distorted vision — Blindness
    - Occurs primarily after age 65
- Ear
  - Deafness
    - Loss of hearing
      - Aging — Presbycusis
      - Genetic
      - Environment
    - Sensorineural
      - Cochlea
      - Cochlear branch, nerve VIII
    - Conduction — External ear / Middle ear
  - Meniere's syndrome
    - Endolymph volume increases
    - Membranous labyrinth enlarges
    - Fluctuating hearing loss — Vertigo — Tinnitus — Deafn
  - Otitis media
    - Acute middle ear infection
    - Bacterial — Nasopharynx to Eustachian tube
    - Pain — Malaise — Fever — Red, swollen tympanum
  - Motion sickness
    - Repetitive motion — Excess stimulation vestibular apparatus — Nausea / Vomitin
    - Nerve impulses to medulla — Vomiting cente
    - Other stimuli — Visual / Emotional

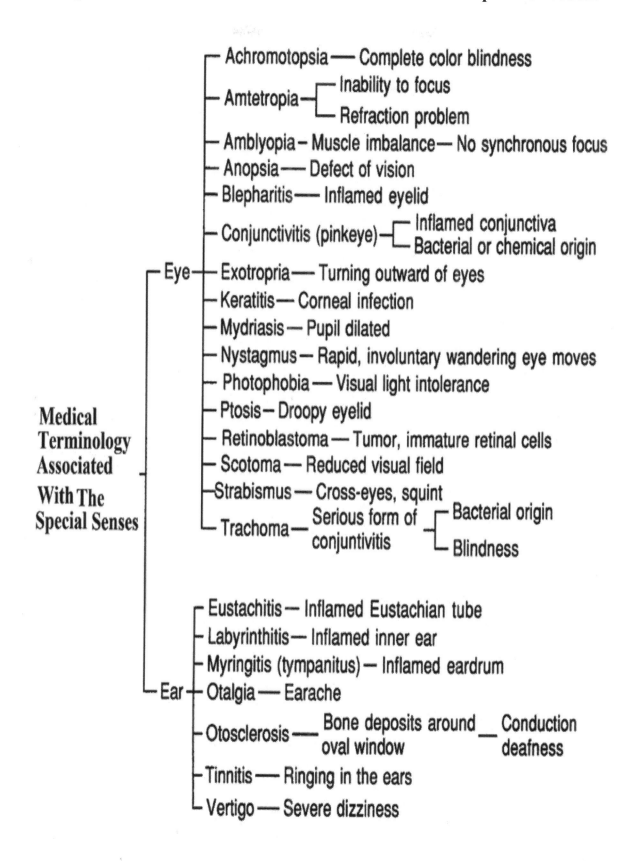

Medical Terminology Associated With The Special Senses

Eye
- Achromotopsia — Complete color blindness
- Amtetropia
  - Inability to focus
  - Refraction problem
- Amblyopia – Muscle imbalance — No synchronous focus
- Anopsia — Defect of vision
- Blepharitis — Inflamed eyelid
- Conjunctivitis (pinkeye)
  - Inflamed conjunctiva
  - Bacterial or chemical origin
- Exotropria — Turning outward of eyes
- Keratitis — Corneal infection
- Mydriasis — Pupil dilated
- Nystagmus — Rapid, involuntary wandering eye moves
- Photophobia — Visual light intolerance
- Ptosis – Droopy eyelid
- Retinoblastoma — Tumor, immature retinal cells
- Scotoma — Reduced visual field
- Strabismus — Cross-eyes, squint
- Trachoma — Serious form of conjuntivitis
  - Bacterial origin
  - Blindness

Ear
- Eustachitis — Inflamed Eustachian tube
- Labyrinthitis — Inflamed inner ear
- Myringitis (tympanitus) — Inflamed eardrum
- Otalgia — Earache
- Otosclerosis — Bone deposits around oval window — Conduction deafness
- Tinnitis — Ringing in the ears
- Vertigo — Severe dizziness

CHAPTER SEVENTEEN

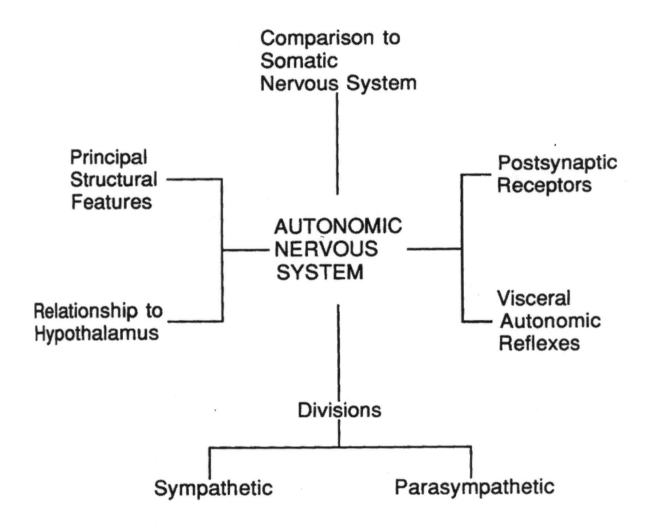

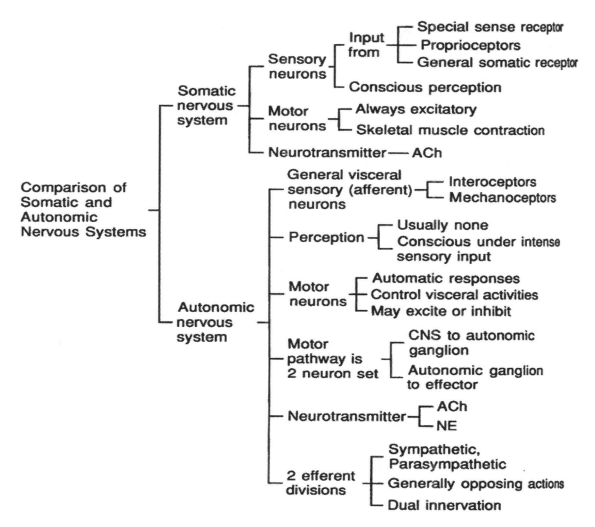

Comparison of Autonomic and Somatic Nervous Systems

Somatic	Autonomic
Conscious or voluntary regulation	Functions without conscious awareness (involuntary)
Fibers do not synapse after they leave the CNS (single neuron from CNS to effector organ).	Fibers synapse once at a ganglion after they leave the CNS (two-neuron chain). Motor control.
Innervates skeletal muscle fibers, always stimulatory	Innervates smooth muscle, cardiac muscle, and glands; either stimulates or inhibits

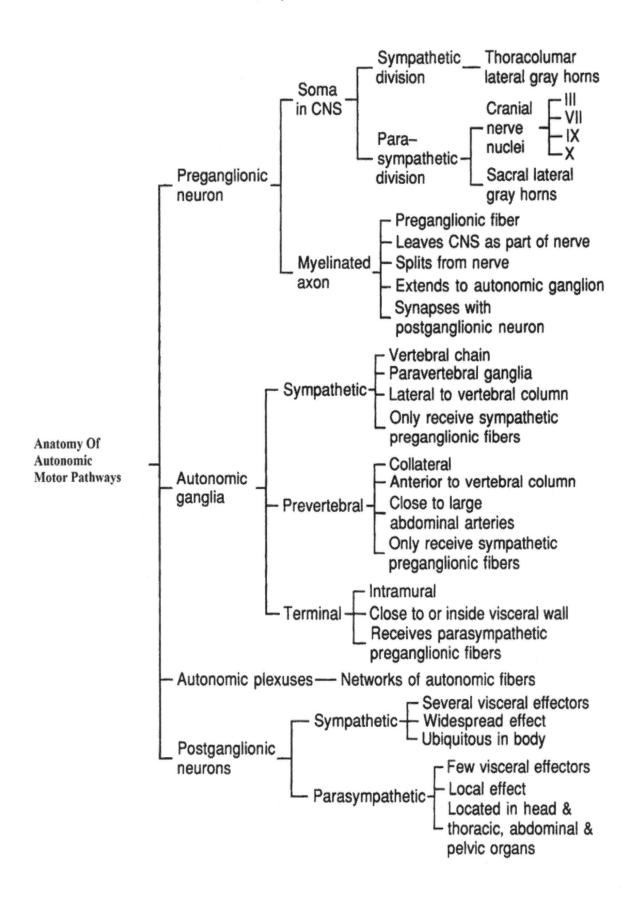

Autonomic Motor Pathways

	Sympathetic	Parasympathetic
Type of control	Involuntary	Involuntary
Number of neurons per message	Two (preganglionic shorter than postganglionic)	Two (preganglionic longer than postganglionic)
Location of motor fiber	Thoracolumbar spinal nerves	Cranial (e.g., vagus) and sacral spinal nerves
Neurotransmitter	Norepinephrine	Acetylcholine
Effectors	Smooth and cardiac muscle, glands	Smooth and cardiac muscle, glands

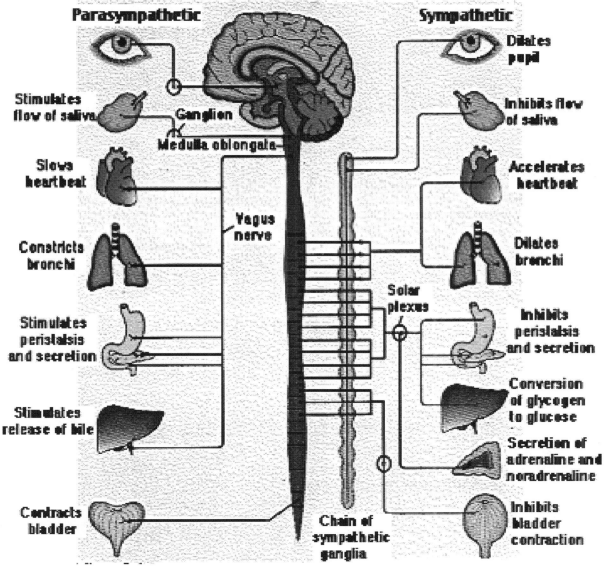

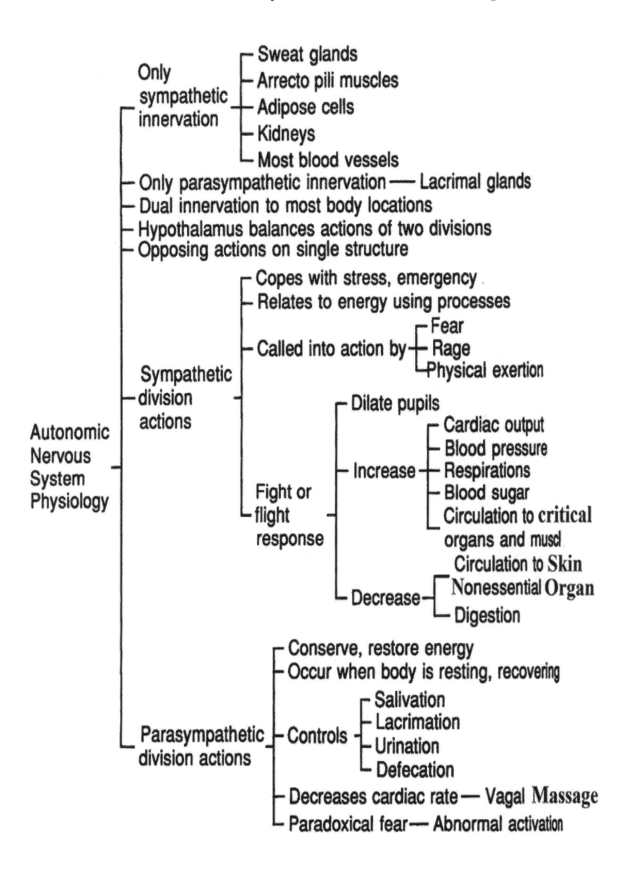

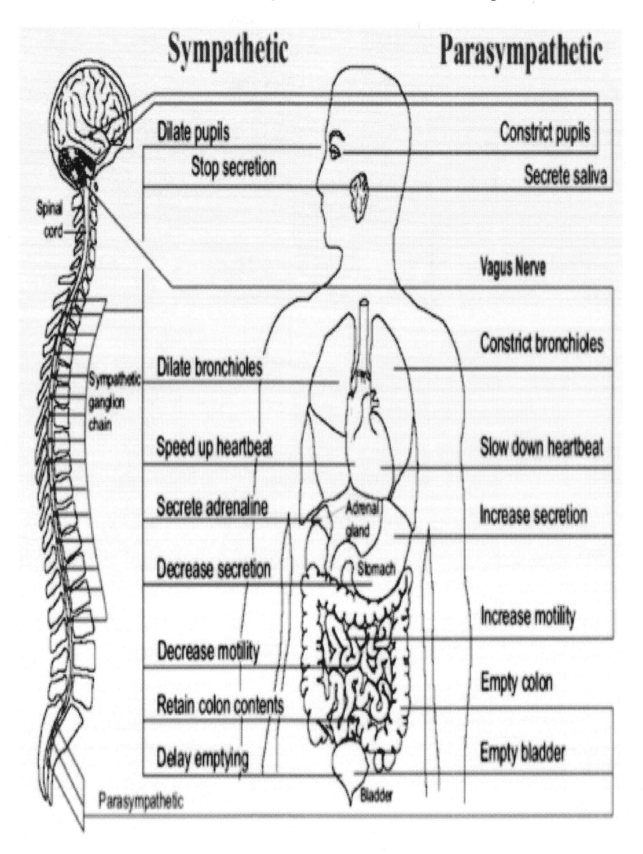

Sympathetic

Parasympathetic

Dilate pupils — Constrict pupils

Stop secretion — Secrete saliva

Vagus Nerve

Dilate bronchioles — Constrict bronchioles

Speed up heartbeat — Slow down heartbeat

Secrete adrenaline — Increase secretion

Decrease secretion — Increase motility

Decrease motility — Empty colon

Retain colon contents — Empty bladder

Delay emptying

Spinal cord

Sympathetic ganglion chain

Parasympathetic

Adrenal gland

Stomach

Bladder

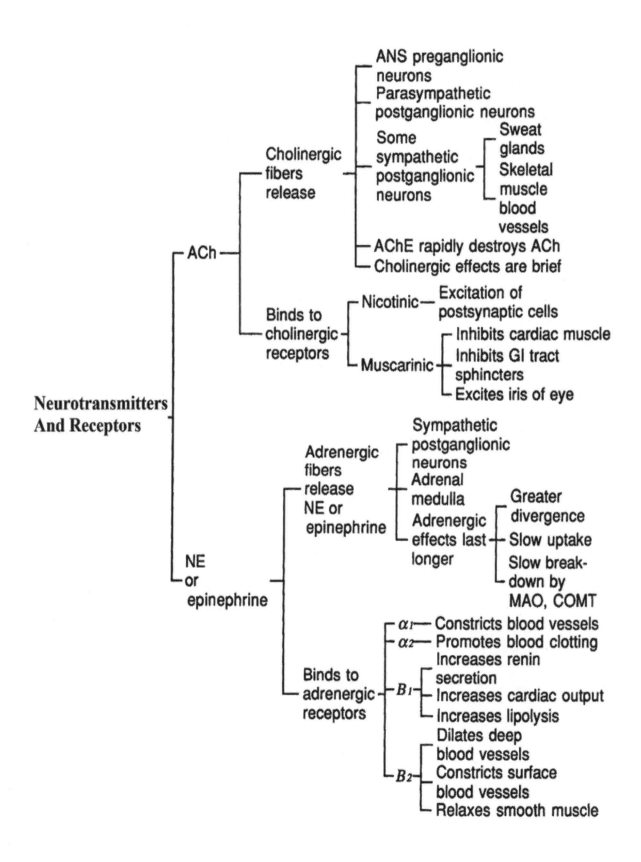

Neurotransmitters And Receptors

- ACh
  - Cholinergic fibers release
    - ANS preganglionic neurons
    - Parasympathetic postganglionic neurons
    - Some sympathetic postganglionic neurons
      - Sweat glands
      - Skeletal muscle blood vessels
    - AChE rapidly destroys ACh
    - Cholinergic effects are brief
  - Binds to cholinergic receptors
    - Nicotinic — Excitation of postsynaptic cells
    - Muscarinic
      - Inhibits cardiac muscle
      - Inhibits GI tract sphincters
      - Excites iris of eye
- NE or epinephrine
  - Adrenergic fibers release NE or epinephrine
    - Sympathetic postganglionic neurons
    - Adrenal medulla
    - Adrenergic effects last longer
      - Greater divergence
      - Slow uptake
      - Slow breakdown by MAO, COMT
  - Binds to adrenergic receptors
    - α_1 — Constricts blood vessels
    - α_2 — Promotes blood clotting
    - B_1
      - Increases renin secretion
      - Increases cardiac output
      - Increases lipolysis
    - B_2
      - Dilates deep blood vessels
      - Constricts surface blood vessels
      - Relaxes smooth muscle

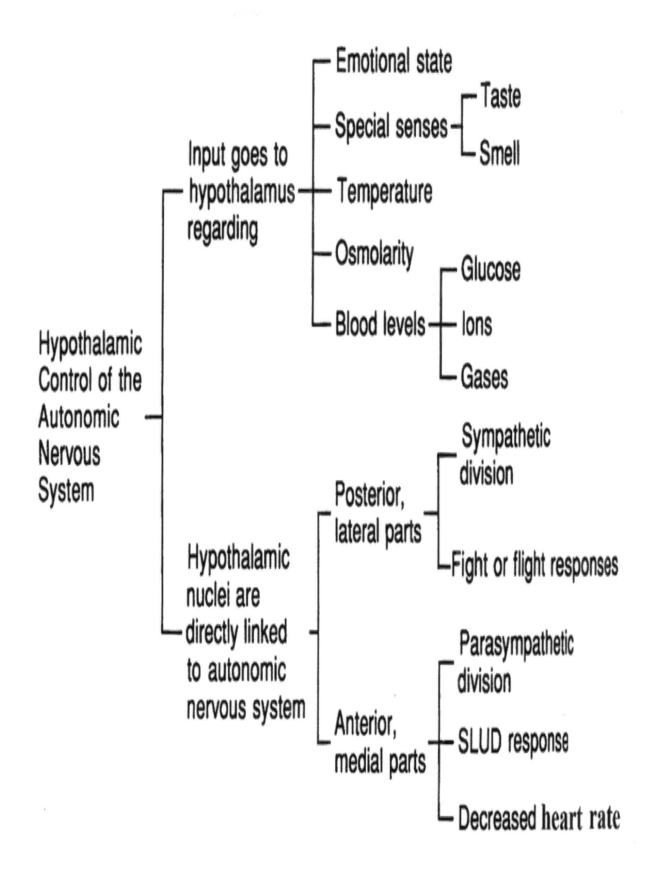

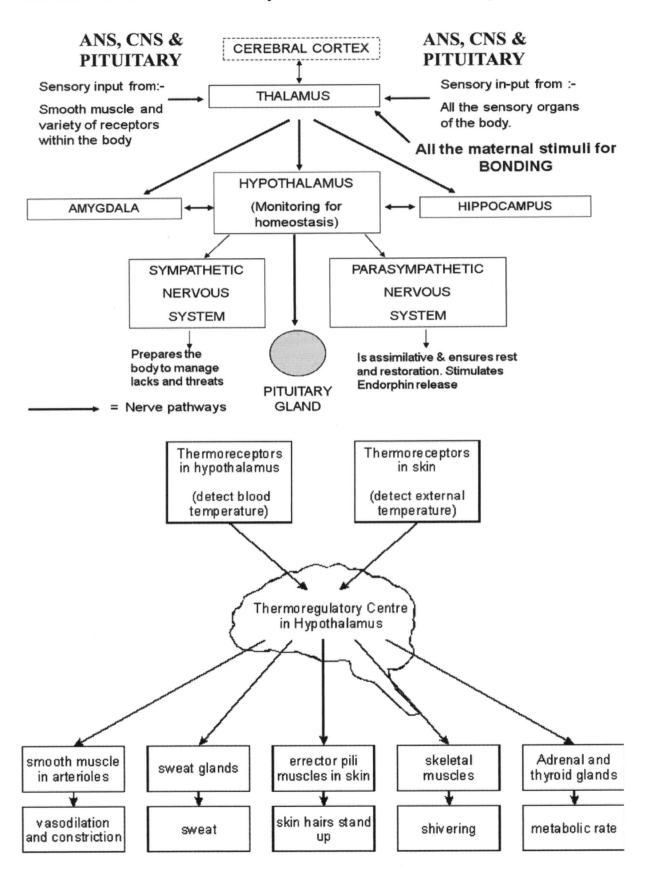

ANS, CNS & PITUITARY

Sensory input from:-

Smooth muscle and variety of receptors within the body

CEREBRAL CORTEX

THALAMUS

ANS, CNS & PITUITARY

Sensory in-put from :-

All the sensory organs of the body.

All the maternal stimuli for BONDING

HYPOTHALAMUS (Monitoring for homeostasis)

AMYGDALA

HIPPOCAMPUS

SYMPATHETIC NERVOUS SYSTEM

PARASYMPATHETIC NERVOUS SYSTEM

Prepares the body to manage lacks and threats

PITUITARY GLAND

Is assimilative & ensures rest and restoration. Stimulates Endorphin release

⟶ = Nerve pathways

Thermoreceptors in hypothalamus (detect blood temperature)

Thermoreceptors in skin (detect external temperature)

Thermoregulatory Centre in Hypothalamus

smooth muscle in arterioles → vasodilation and constriction

sweat glands → sweat

errector pili muscles in skin → skin hairs stand up

skeletal muscles → shivering

Adrenal and thyroid glands → metabolic rate

CHAPTER EIGHTEEN

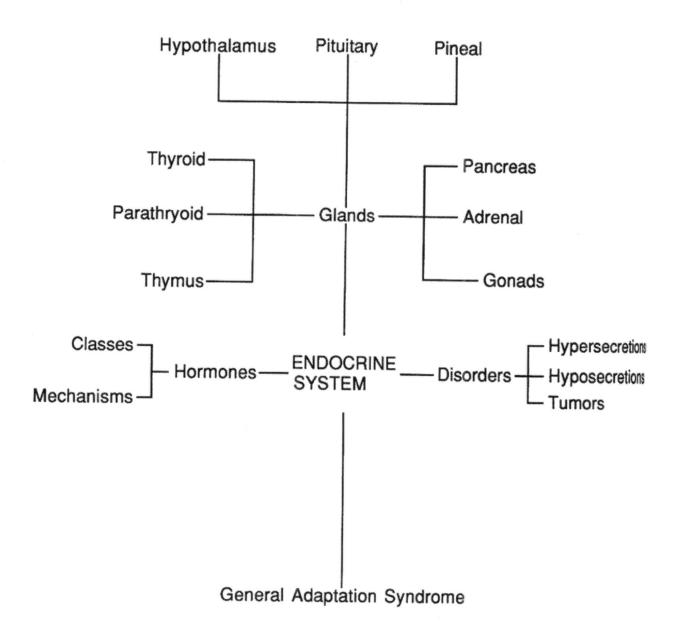

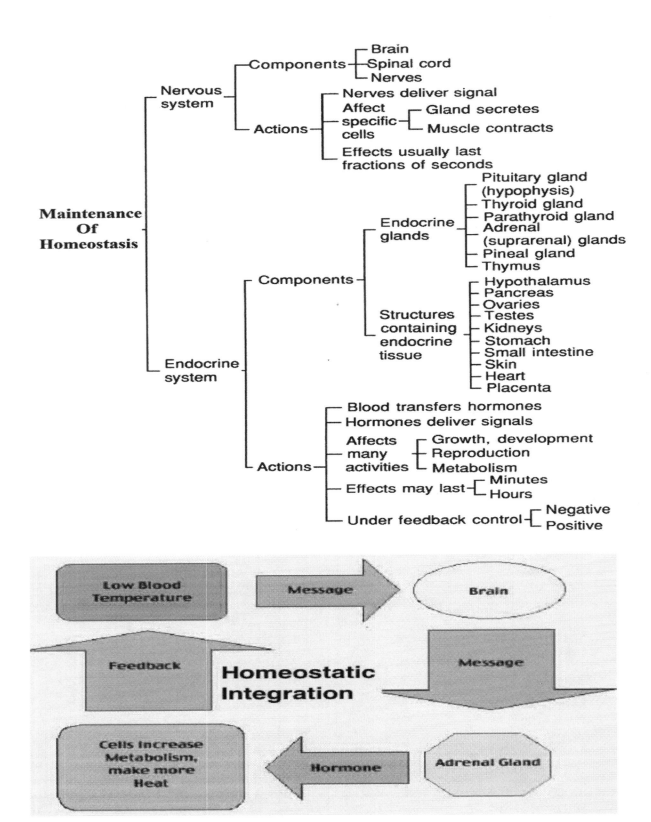

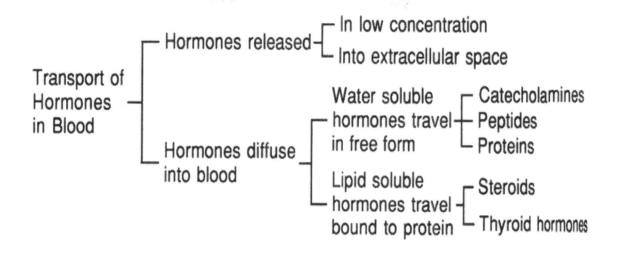

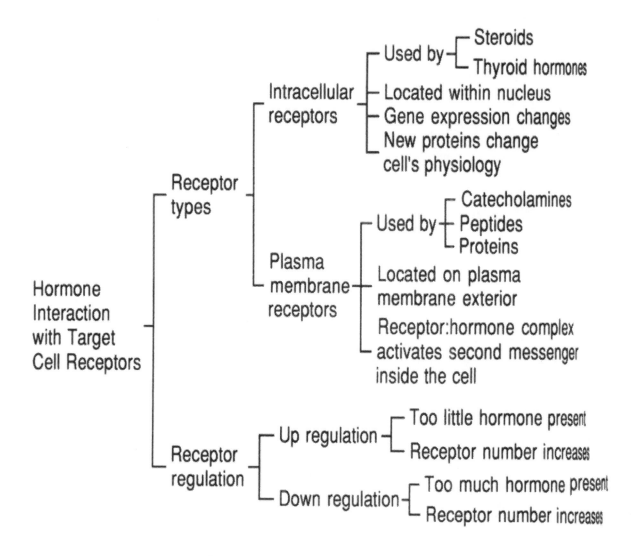

Mechanisms of hormone action

More than fifty human hormones have been identified; all act by binding to receptor molecules. The binding hormone changes the shape of the receptor causing the response to the hormone. There are two mechanisms of hormone action on all target cells. These are (A) Peptide hormone receptors e.g. thyroid-stimulating hormone, follicle-stimulating hormone, luteinizing hormone and insulin (B) Steroid hormone receptors (intracellular receptors) e. g. glucocorticoids, estrogens, androgens, thyroid hormone (T3), calcitriol (the active form of vitamin D), and the retinoids (vitamin A)

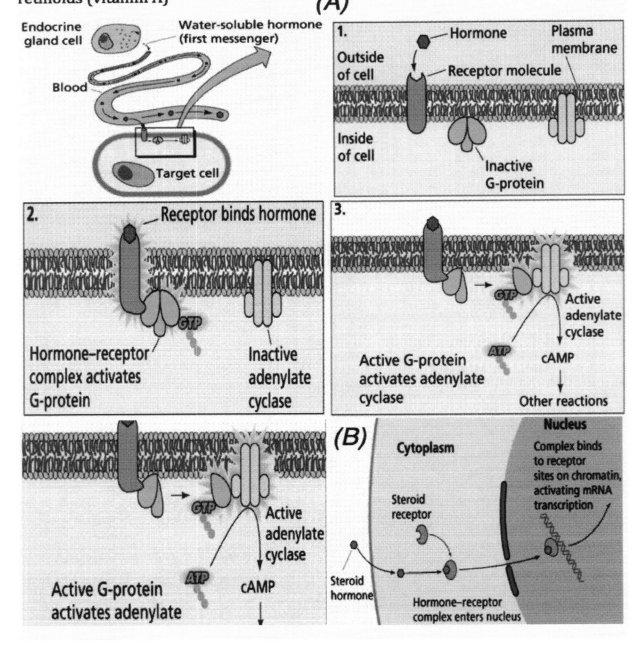

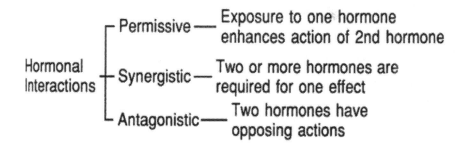

Hormonal Interactions
- Permissive — Exposure to one hormone enhances action of 2nd hormone
- Synergistic — Two or more hormones are required for one effect
- Antagonistic — Two hormones have opposing actions

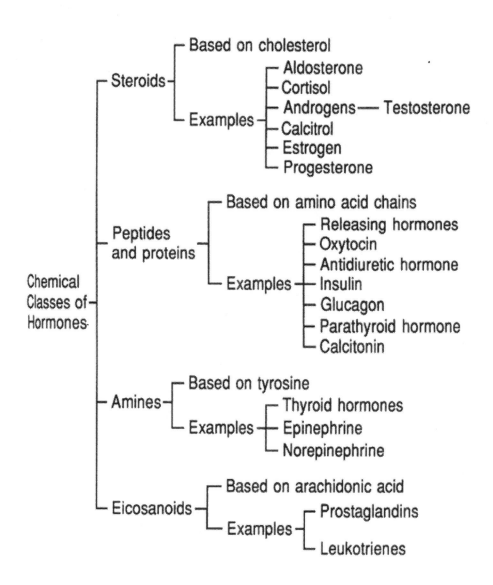

Chemical Classes of Hormones
- Steroids
  - Based on cholesterol
  - Examples
    - Aldosterone
    - Cortisol
    - Androgens — Testosterone
    - Calcitrol
    - Estrogen
    - Progesterone
- Peptides and proteins
  - Based on amino acid chains
  - Examples
    - Releasing hormones
    - Oxytocin
    - Antidiuretic hormone
    - Insulin
    - Glucagon
    - Parathyroid hormone
    - Calcitonin
- Amines
  - Based on tyrosine
  - Examples
    - Thyroid hormones
    - Epinephrine
    - Norepinephrine
- Eicosanoids
  - Based on arachidonic acid
  - Examples
    - Prostaglandins
    - Leukotrienes

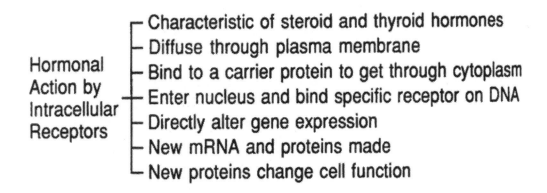

Hormonal Action by Intracellular Receptors
- Characteristic of steroid and thyroid hormones
- Diffuse through plasma membrane
- Bind to a carrier protein to get through cytoplasm
- Enter nucleus and bind specific receptor on DNA
- Directly alter gene expression
- New mRNA and proteins made
- New proteins change cell function

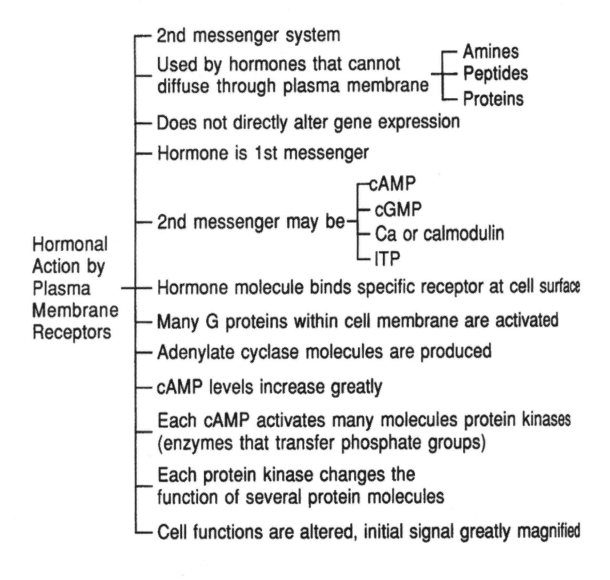

Hormonal Action by Plasma Membrane Receptors
- 2nd messenger system
- Used by hormones that cannot diffuse through plasma membrane
  - Amines
  - Peptides
  - Proteins
- Does not directly alter gene expression
- Hormone is 1st messenger
- 2nd messenger may be
  - cAMP
  - cGMP
  - Ca or calmodulin
  - ITP
- Hormone molecule binds specific receptor at cell surface
- Many G proteins within cell membrane are activated
- Adenylate cyclase molecules are produced
- cAMP levels increase greatly
- Each cAMP activates many molecules protein kinases (enzymes that transfer phosphate groups)
- Each protein kinase changes the function of several protein molecules
- Cell functions are altered, initial signal greatly magnified

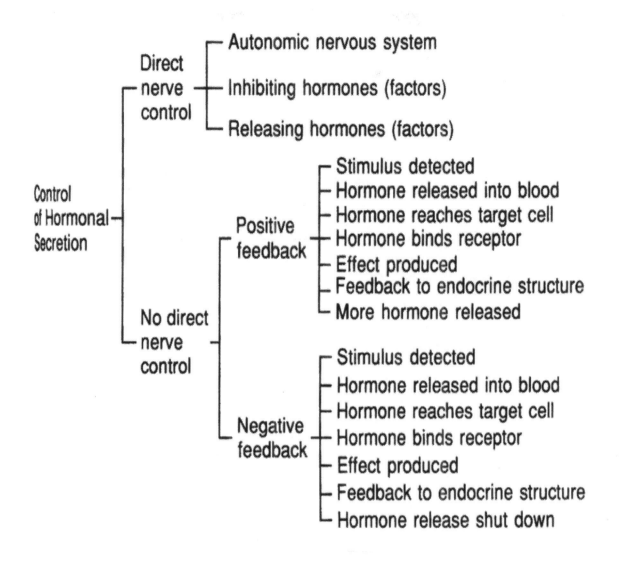

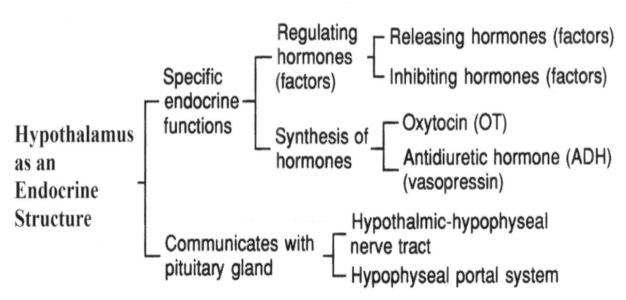

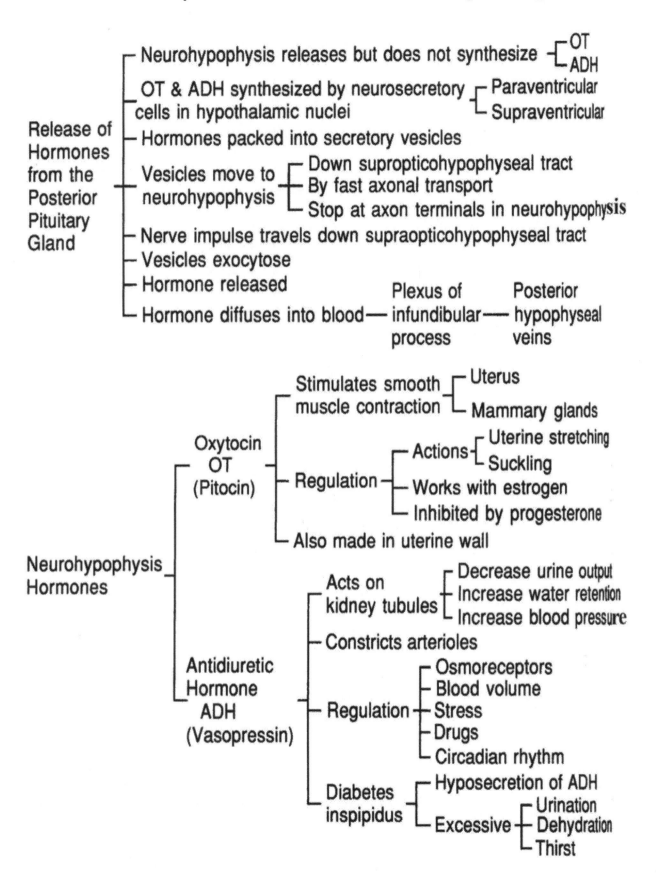

Release of Hormones from the Posterior Pituitary Gland
- Neurohypophysis releases but does not synthesize
  - OT
  - ADH
- OT & ADH synthesized by neurosecretory cells in hypothalamic nuclei
  - Paraventricular
  - Supraventricular
- Hormones packed into secretory vesicles
- Vesicles move to neurohypophysis
  - Down supropticohypophyseal tract
  - By fast axonal transport
  - Stop at axon terminals in neurohypophysis
- Nerve impulse travels down supraopticohypophyseal tract
- Vesicles exocytose
- Hormone released
- Hormone diffuses into blood — Plexus of infundibular process — Posterior hypophyseal veins

Neurohypophysis Hormones
- Oxytocin OT (Pitocin)
  - Stimulates smooth muscle contraction
    - Uterus
    - Mammary glands
  - Regulation
    - Actions
      - Uterine stretching
      - Suckling
    - Works with estrogen
    - Inhibited by progesterone
  - Also made in uterine wall
- Antidiuretic Hormone ADH (Vasopressin)
  - Acts on kidney tubules
    - Decrease urine output
    - Increase water retention
    - Increase blood pressure
  - Constricts arterioles
  - Regulation
    - Osmoreceptors
    - Blood volume
    - Stress
    - Drugs
    - Circadian rhythm
  - Diabetes inspipidus
    - Hyposecretion of ADH
    - Excessive
      - Urination
      - Dehydration
      - Thirst

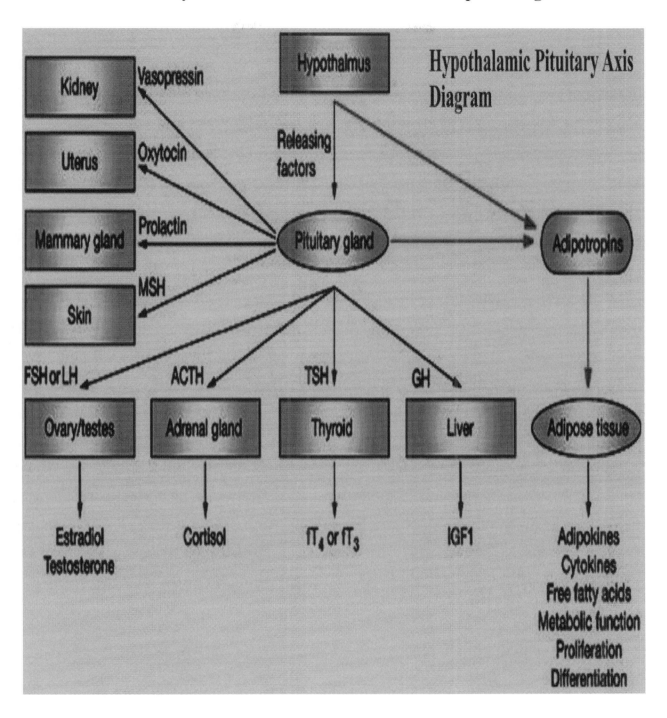

Hypothalamic Pituitary Axis Diagram

(A): Endocrine Glands, Hormones, and Their Functions and Structure

Gland/Tissue	Hormones	Major Functions
Hypothalamus	1-Thyrotropin-releasing hormone (TRH)	Stimulates secretion of TSH and prolactin
	2-Corticotropin-releasing hormone (CRH)	Causes release of ACTH
	3- Growth hormone-releasing hormone (GHRH) Growth hormone inhibitory hormone (GHIH) (somatostatin)	Causes release of growth hormone Inhibits release of growth hormone
	4-Gonadotropin-releasing hormone (GnRH)	Causes release of LH and FSH
	5- Dopamine or prolactin-inhibiting factor (PIF)	nhibits release of prolactin
Anterior pituitary	1-Growth hormone	Stimulates protein synthesis and overall growthof most cells and tissues
	2-Thyroid-stimulating hormone (TSH)	Stimulates synthesis and secretion of thyroid
	3-Adrenocorticotropic hormone (ACTH)	Stimulates synthesis and secretion of adrenocortical hormones (cortisol, androgens, and aldosterone)
	4-Prolactin	Promotes development of the female breasts and secretion of milk
	5-Follicle-stimulating hormone (FSH)	Causes growth of follicles in the ovaries and sperm maturation in Sertoli cells of testes
	6- Luteinizing hormone (LH)	Stimulates testosterone synthesis in Leydig cells of testes; stimulates ovulation, formation of corpus luteum, and estrogen and progesterone synthesis in ovaries
Posterior pituitary	1-Antidiuretic hormone (ADH) (also called vasopressin)	Increases water reabsorption by the kidneys and causes vasoconstriction and increased blood pressure
	2-Oxytocin	Stimulates milk ejection from breasts and uterine contractions
Thyroid	1-Thyroxine (T4) and triiodothyronine (T3)	Increases the rates of chemical reactions in most cells, thus increasing body metabolic rate
	2-Calcitonin	Promotes deposition of calcium in the bones and decreases extracellular fluid calcium ion concentration

(B): Endocrine Glands, Hormones, and Their Functions and Structure

Gland/Tissue	Hormones	Major Functions	Chemical Structure
Adrenal cortex	1-Cortisol	Has multiple metabolic functions for controlling metabolism of proteins, carbohydrates, and fats; also has anti-inflammatory effects	Steroid
	2-Aldosterone 3-Androgen	Increases renal sodium reabsorption, potassium secretion, and hydrogen ion secretion' Androgen(testostrone)	Steroid
Adrenal medulla	1-Norepinephrine, epinephrine	Same effects as sympathetic stimulation	Amine
Pancreas	1-Insulin (b cells)	Promotes glucose entry in many cells, and in this way controls carbohydrate metabolism	Peptide
	2-Glucagon (a cells)	Increases synthesis and release of glucose from the liver into the body fluids	Peptide
Parathyroid	1-Parathyroid hormone (PTH)	Controls serum calcium ion concentration by increasing calcium absorption by the gut and kidneys and releasing calcium from bones	Peptide
Testes	1-Testosterone	Promotes development of male reproductive system and male secondary sexual characteristics	Steroid
Ovaries	1-Estrogens	Promotes growth and development of female reproductive system, female breasts, and female secondary sexual characteristics	Steroid
	2-Progesterone	Stimulates secretion of "uterine milk" by the uterine endometrial glands and promotes development of secretory apparatus of breasts	Steroid
Placenta	1-Human chorionic gonadotropin (HCG)	Promotes growth of corpus luteum and secretion of estrogens and progesterone by corpus luteum	Peptide
	2-Human somatomammotropin	Probably helps promote development of some fetal tissues as well as the mother's breasts	Peptide
	3-Estrogens	See actions of estrogens from ovaries	Steroid
	4-Progesterone	See actions of progesterone from ovaries	Steroid
Kidney	1-Renin	Catalyzes conversion of angiotensinogen to angiotensin I (acts as an enzyme)	Peptide
	2- 1,25-2-Dihydroxycholecalciferol	Increases intestinal absorption of calcium and bone mineralization	Steroid
	3- Erythropoietin	Increases erythrocyte production	Peptide
Heart	1- Atrial natriuretic peptide (ANP)	Increases sodium excretion by kidneys, reduces blood pressure	Peptide
Stomach	1-Gastrin	Stimulates HCl secretion by parietal cells	Peptide
Small intestine	1-Secretin	Stimulates pancreatic acinar cells to release bicarbonate and water	Peptide
	2-Cholecystokinin (CCK)	Stimulates gallbladder contraction and release of pancreatic enzymes	Peptide
Adipocytes	1-Leptin	Inhibits appetite, stimulates thermogenesis	Peptide

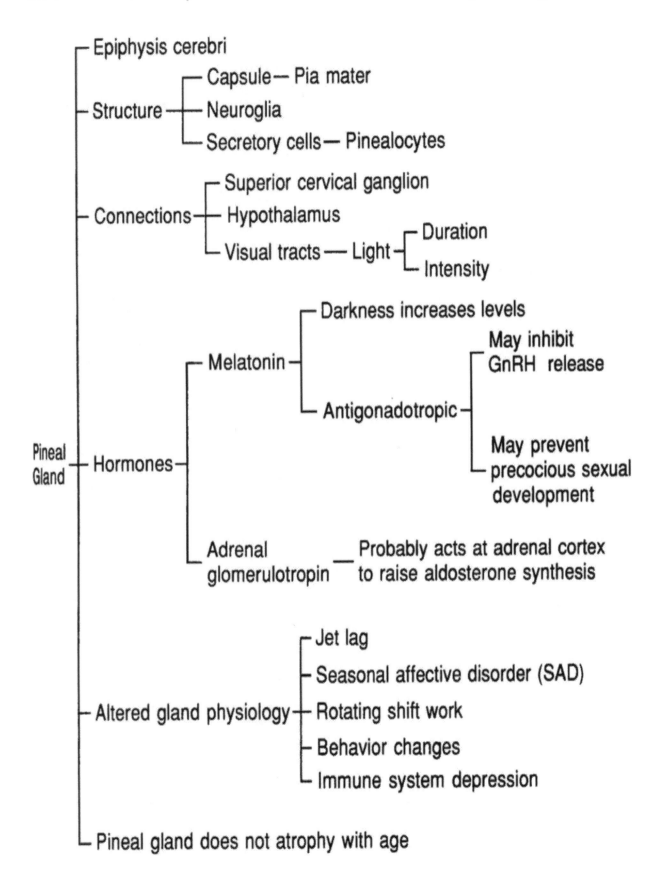

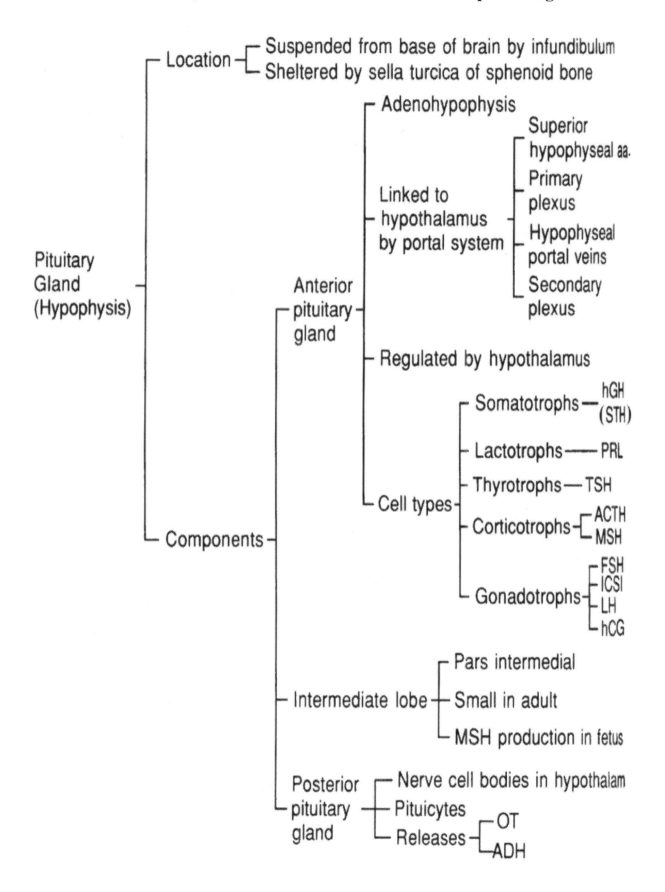

Pituitary Gland (Hypophysis)

- Location
  - Suspended from base of brain by infundibulum
  - Sheltered by sella turcica of sphenoid bone

- Components
  - Anterior pituitary gland
    - Adenohypophysis
    - Linked to hypothalamus by portal system
      - Superior hypophyseal aa.
      - Primary plexus
      - Hypophyseal portal veins
      - Secondary plexus
    - Regulated by hypothalamus
    - Cell types
      - Somatotrophs — hGH (STH)
      - Lactotrophs — PRL
      - Thyrotrophs — TSH
      - Corticotrophs
        - ACTH
        - MSH
      - Gonadotrophs
        - FSH
        - ICSI
        - LH
        - hCG
  - Intermediate lobe
    - Pars intermedial
    - Small in adult
    - MSH production in fetus
  - Posterior pituitary gland
    - Nerve cell bodies in hypothalam
    - Pituicytes
    - Releases
      - OT
      - ADH

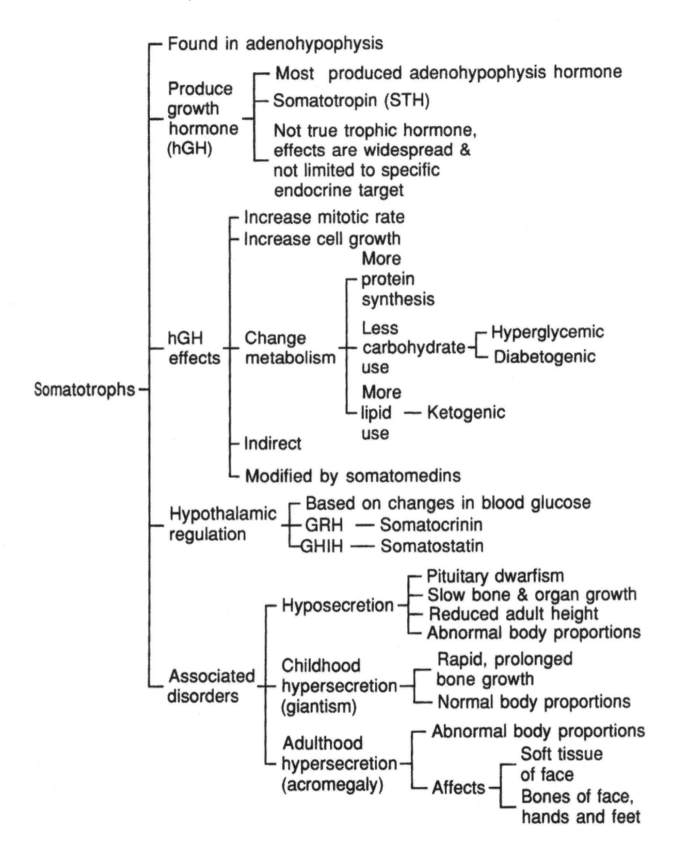

Somatotrophs
- Found in adenohypophysis
- Produce growth hormone (hGH)
  - Most produced adenohypophysis hormone
  - Somatotropin (STH)
  - Not true trophic hormone, effects are widespread & not limited to specific endocrine target
- hGH effects
  - Increase mitotic rate
  - Increase cell growth
  - Change metabolism
    - More protein synthesis
    - Less carbohydrate use
      - Hyperglycemic
      - Diabetogenic
    - More lipid use — Ketogenic
  - Indirect
  - Modified by somatomedins
- Hypothalamic regulation
  - Based on changes in blood glucose
  - GRH — Somatocrinin
  - GHIH — Somatostatin
- Associated disorders
  - Hyposecretion
    - Pituitary dwarfism
    - Slow bone & organ growth
    - Reduced adult height
    - Abnormal body proportions
  - Childhood hypersecretion (giantism)
    - Rapid, prolonged bone growth
    - Normal body proportions
  - Adulthood hypersecretion (acromegaly)
    - Abnormal body proportions
    - Affects
      - Soft tissue of face
      - Bones of face, hands and feet

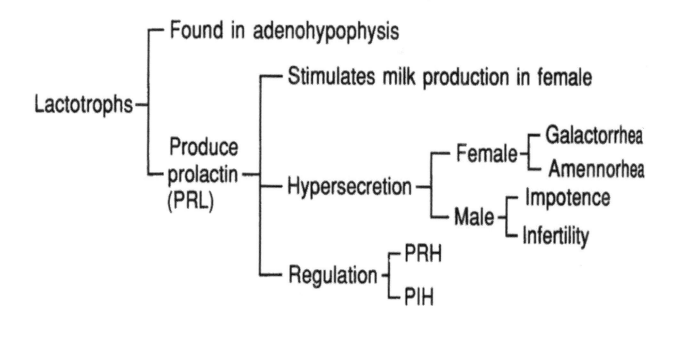

Lactotrophs
- Found in adenohypophysis
- Produce prolactin (PRL)
  - Stimulates milk production in female
  - Hypersecretion
    - Female
      - Galactorrhea
      - Amennorhea
    - Male
      - Impotence
      - Infertility
  - Regulation
    - PRH
    - PIH

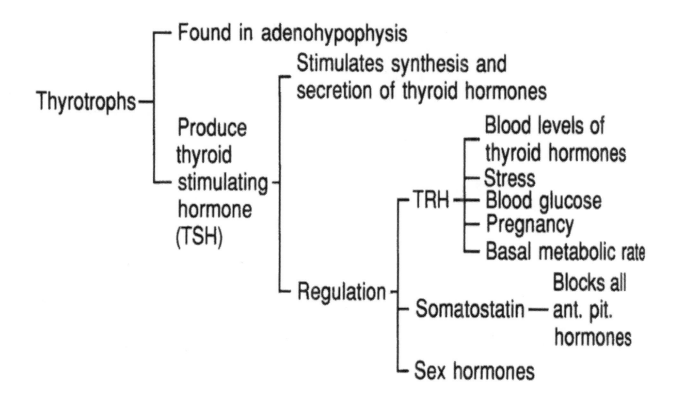

Thyrotrophs
- Found in adenohypophysis
- Produce thyroid stimulating hormone (TSH)
  - Stimulates synthesis and secretion of thyroid hormones
  - Regulation
    - TRH
      - Blood levels of thyroid hormones
      - Stress
      - Blood glucose
      - Pregnancy
      - Basal metabolic rate
    - Somatostatin — Blocks all ant. pit. hormones
    - Sex hormones

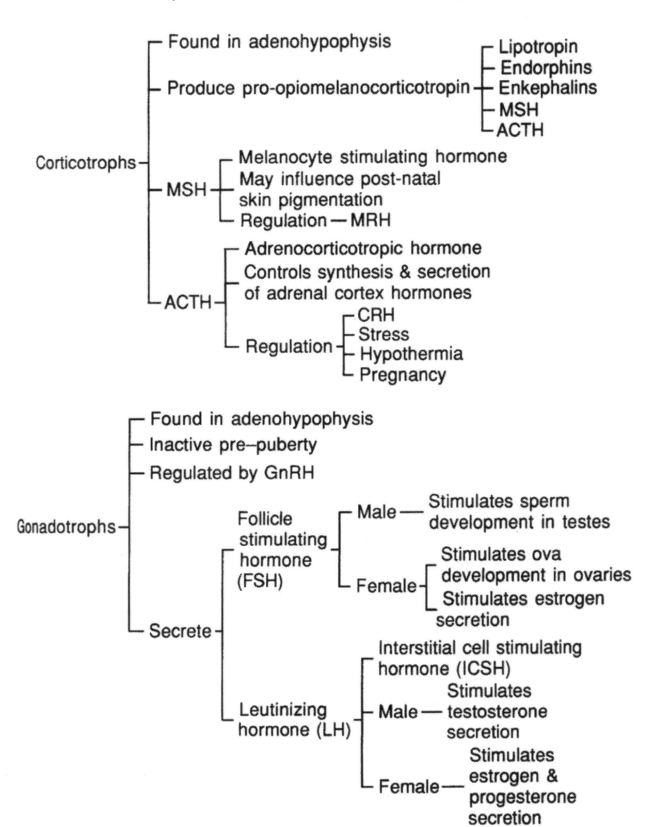

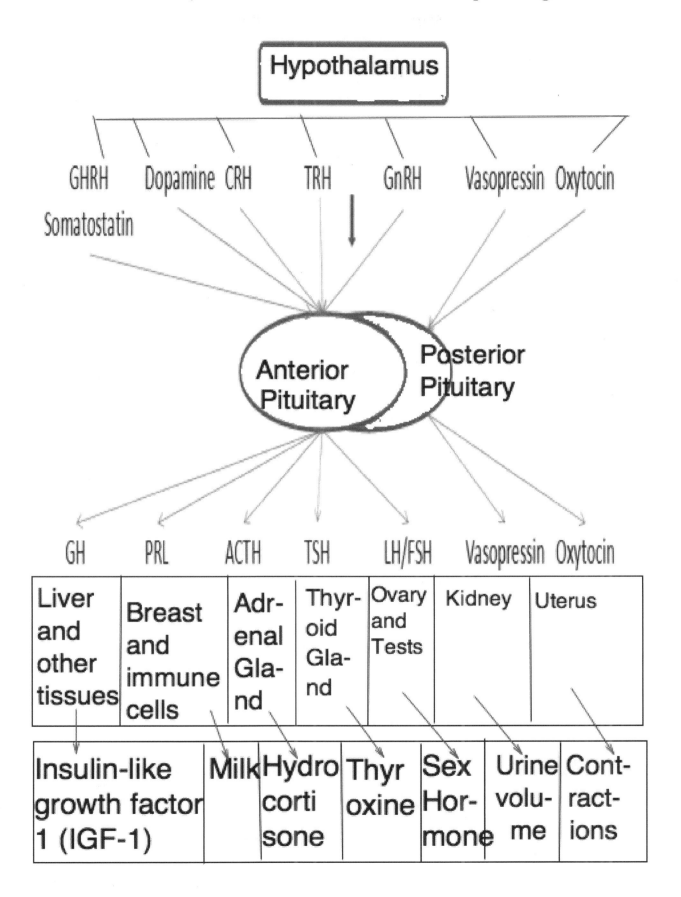

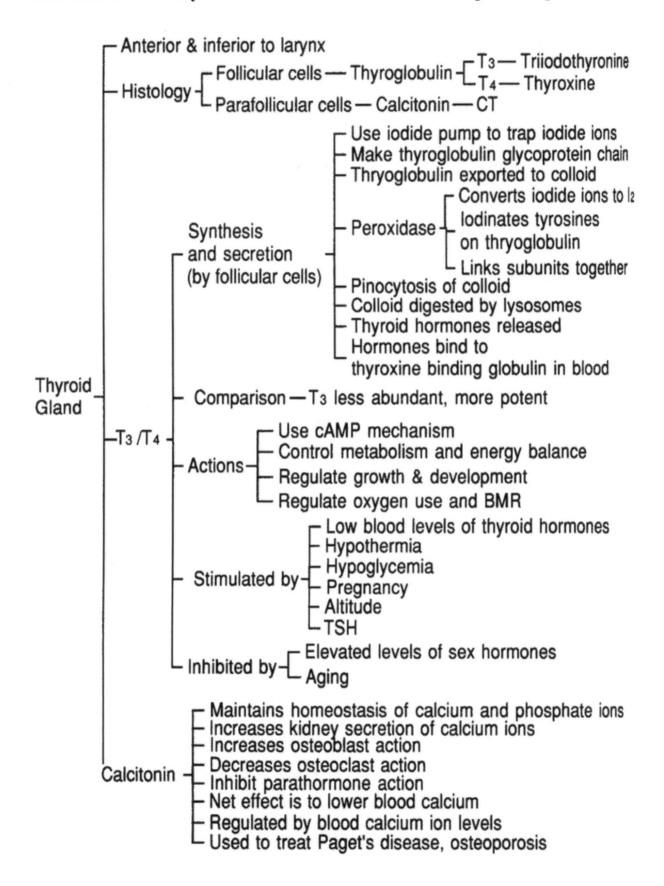

Thyroid Gland
- Anterior & inferior to larynx
- Histology
  - Follicular cells — Thyroglobulin
    - T3 — Triiodothyronine
    - T4 — Thyroxine
  - Parafollicular cells — Calcitonin — CT
- T3 /T4
  - Synthesis and secretion (by follicular cells)
    - Use iodide pump to trap iodide ions
    - Make thyroglobulin glycoprotein chain
    - Thryoglobulin exported to colloid
    - Peroxidase
      - Converts iodide ions to I2
      - Iodinates tyrosines on thryoglobulin
      - Links subunits together
    - Pinocytosis of colloid
    - Colloid digested by lysosomes
    - Thyroid hormones released
    - Hormones bind to thyroxine binding globulin in blood
  - Comparison — T3 less abundant, more potent
  - Actions
    - Use cAMP mechanism
    - Control metabolism and energy balance
    - Regulate growth & development
    - Regulate oxygen use and BMR
  - Stimulated by
    - Low blood levels of thyroid hormones
    - Hypothermia
    - Hypoglycemia
    - Pregnancy
    - Altitude
    - TSH
  - Inhibited by
    - Elevated levels of sex hormones
    - Aging
- Calcitonin
  - Maintains homeostasis of calcium and phosphate ions
  - Increases kidney secretion of calcium ions
  - Increases osteoblast action
  - Decreases osteoclast action
  - Inhibit parathormone action
  - Net effect is to lower blood calcium
  - Regulated by blood calcium ion levels
  - Used to treat Paget's disease, osteoporosis

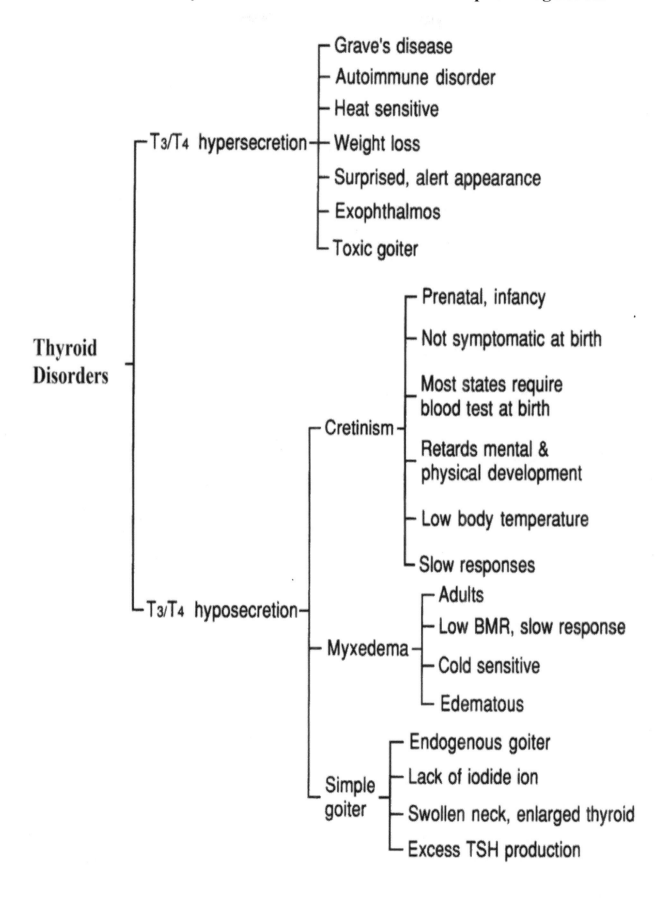

Thyroid Disorders

T3/T4 hypersecretion
- Grave's disease
- Autoimmune disorder
- Heat sensitive
- Weight loss
- Surprised, alert appearance
- Exophthalmos
- Toxic goiter

T3/T4 hyposecretion

Cretinism
- Prenatal, infancy
- Not symptomatic at birth
- Most states require blood test at birth
- Retards mental & physical development
- Low body temperature
- Slow responses

Myxedema
- Adults
- Low BMR, slow response
- Cold sensitive
- Edematous

Simple goiter
- Endogenous goiter
- Lack of iodide ion
- Swollen neck, enlarged thyroid
- Excess TSH production

A. Thyroid gland Anterior View B. Thyroid histology, follicular cells (stored thyroid hormone), parafollicular cells, which secrete Calcitonin

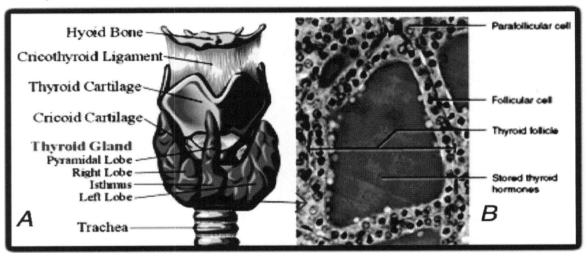

Manifestations of Hypothyroid and Hyperthyroid States

Effects on:	Hypothyroidism	Hyperthyroidism
Basal metabolic rate	Decreased	Increased
Sensitivity to catecholamines	Decreased	Increased
General features	Myxedematous features Deep voice Impaired growth (child)	Exophthalmos (in Graves disease) Lid lag Decreased blinking
Blood cholesterol levels	Increased	Decreased
General behavior	Mental retardation (infant) Mental and physical sluggishness Somnolence	Restlessness, irritability, anxiety Hyperkinesis Wakefulness
Cardiovascular function	Decreased cardiac output Bradycardia	Increased cardiac output Tachycardia and palpitations
Gastrointestinal function	Constipation Decreased appetite	Diarrhea Increased appetite
Respiratory function	Hypoventilation	Dyspnea
Muscle tone and reflexes	Decreased	Increased, with tremor and fibrillatory twitching
Temperature tolerance	Cold intolerance	Heat intolerance
Skin and hair	Decreased sweating Coarse and dry skin and hair	Increased sweating Thin and silky skin and hair
Weight	Gain	Loss

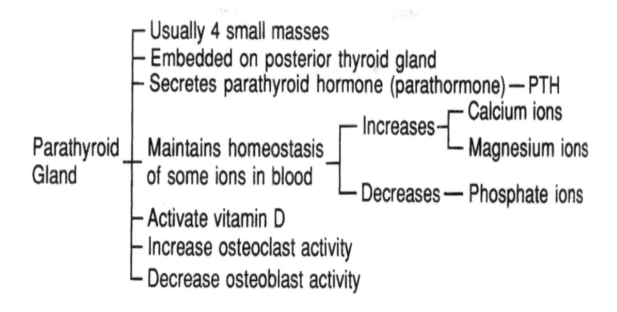

Parathyroid Gland
- Usually 4 small masses
- Embedded on posterior thyroid gland
- Secretes parathyroid hormone (parathormone) — PTH
- Maintains homeostasis of some ions in blood
  - Increases
    - Calcium ions
    - Magnesium ions
  - Decreases — Phosphate ions
- Activate vitamin D
- Increase osteoclast activity
- Decrease osteoblast activity

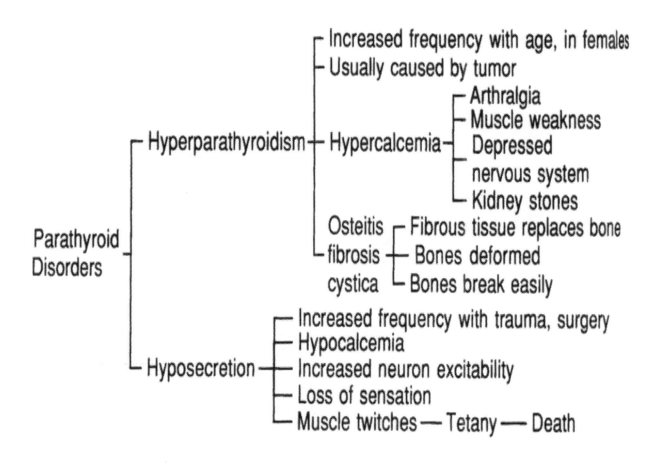

Parathyroid Disorders
- Hyperparathyroidism
  - Increased frequency with age, in females
  - Usually caused by tumor
  - Hypercalcemia
    - Arthralgia
    - Muscle weakness
    - Depressed nervous system
    - Kidney stones
  - Osteitis fibrosis cystica
    - Fibrous tissue replaces bone
    - Bones deformed
    - Bones break easily
- Hyposecretion
  - Increased frequency with trauma, surgery
  - Hypocalcemia
  - Increased neuron excitability
  - Loss of sensation
  - Muscle twitches — Tetany — Death

The parathyroid glands, parathyroid hormone (PTH) blood, bone, kidney and gastrointestinal

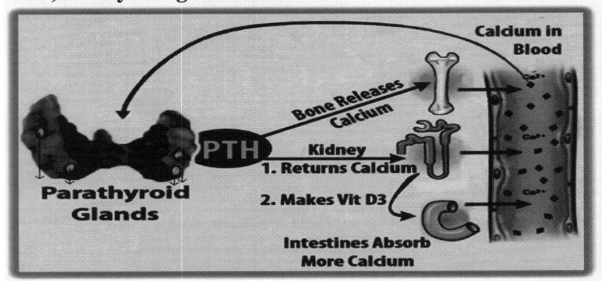

Regulation of serum calcium concentration by parathyroid hormone; Calcitriol (also called 1,25-dihydroxycholecalciferol or 1,25-dihydroxyvitamin D3), Calcitonin CT, (also known as thyrocalcitonin)

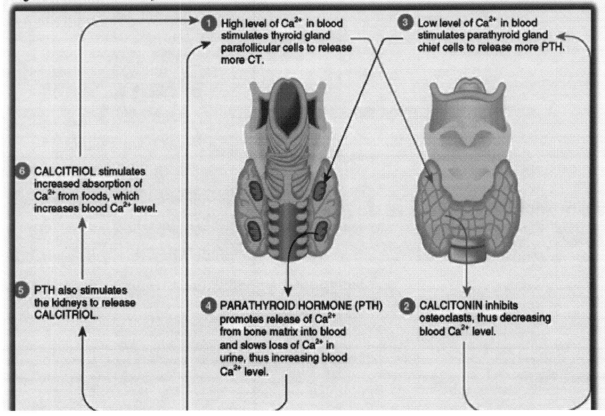

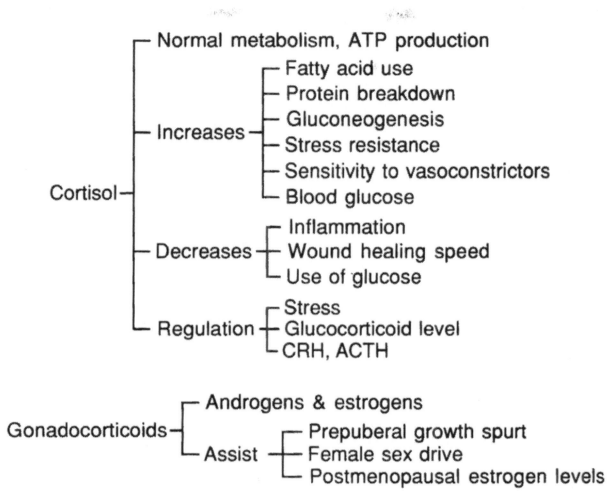

Cortisol
- Normal metabolism, ATP production
- Increases
  - Fatty acid use
  - Protein breakdown
  - Gluconeogenesis
  - Stress resistance
  - Sensitivity to vasoconstrictors
  - Blood glucose
- Decreases
  - Inflammation
  - Wound healing speed
  - Use of glucose
- Regulation
  - Stress
  - Glucocorticoid level
  - CRH, ACTH

Gonadocorticoids
- Androgens & estrogens
- Assist
  - Prepuberal growth spurt
  - Female sex drive
  - Postmenopausal estrogen levels

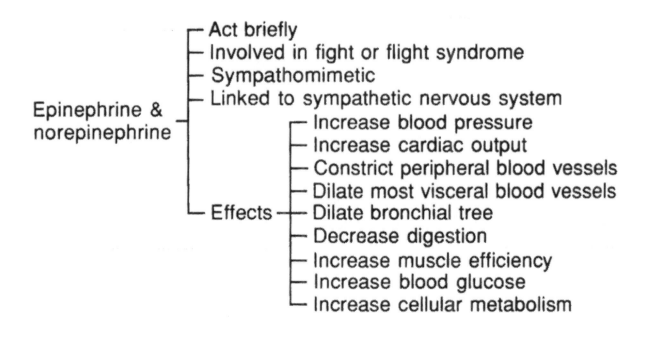

Epinephrine & norepinephrine
- Act briefly
- Involved in fight or flight syndrome
- Sympathomimetic
- Linked to sympathetic nervous system
- Effects
  - Increase blood pressure
  - Increase cardiac output
  - Constrict peripheral blood vessels
  - Dilate most visceral blood vessels
  - Dilate bronchial tree
  - Decrease digestion
  - Increase muscle efficiency
  - Increase blood glucose
  - Increase cellular metabolism

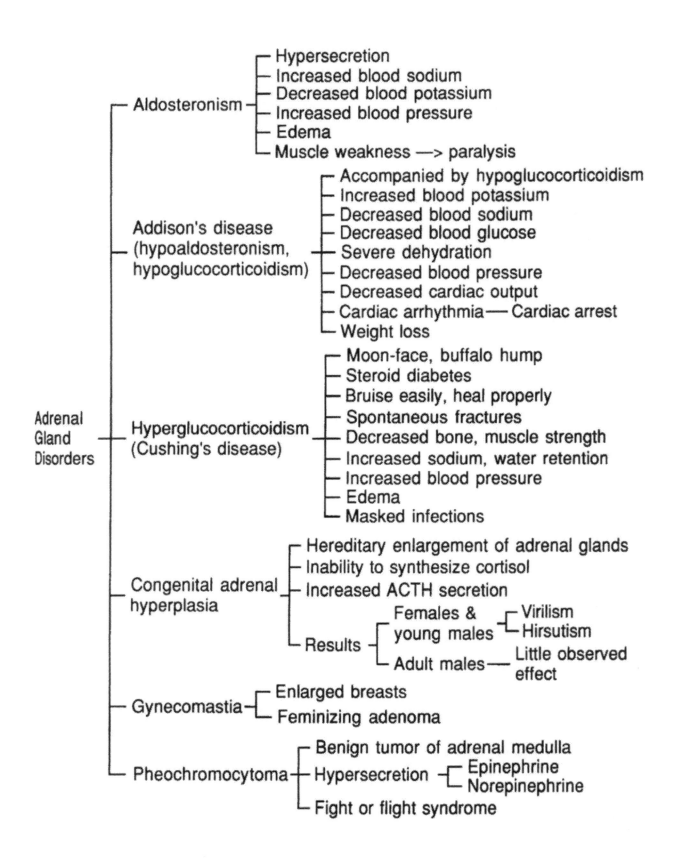

- Adrenal Gland Disorders
  - Aldosteronism
    - Hypersecretion
    - Increased blood sodium
    - Decreased blood potassium
    - Increased blood pressure
    - Edema
    - Muscle weakness —> paralysis
  - Addison's disease (hypoaldosteronism, hypoglucocorticoidism)
    - Accompanied by hypoglucocorticoidism
    - Increased blood potassium
    - Decreased blood sodium
    - Decreased blood glucose
    - Severe dehydration
    - Decreased blood pressure
    - Decreased cardiac output
    - Cardiac arrhythmia — Cardiac arrest
    - Weight loss
  - Hyperglucocorticoidism (Cushing's disease)
    - Moon-face, buffalo hump
    - Steroid diabetes
    - Bruise easily, heal properly
    - Spontaneous fractures
    - Decreased bone, muscle strength
    - Increased sodium, water retention
    - Increased blood pressure
    - Edema
    - Masked infections
  - Congenital adrenal hyperplasia
    - Hereditary enlargement of adrenal glands
    - Inability to synthesize cortisol
    - Increased ACTH secretion
    - Results
      - Females & young males
        - Virilism
        - Hirsutism
      - Adult males — Little observed effect
  - Gynecomastia
    - Enlarged breasts
    - Feminizing adenoma
  - Pheochromocytoma
    - Benign tumor of adrenal medulla
    - Hypersecretion
      - Epinephrine
      - Norepinephrine
    - Fight or flight syndrome

Major actions of cortisols on metabolism

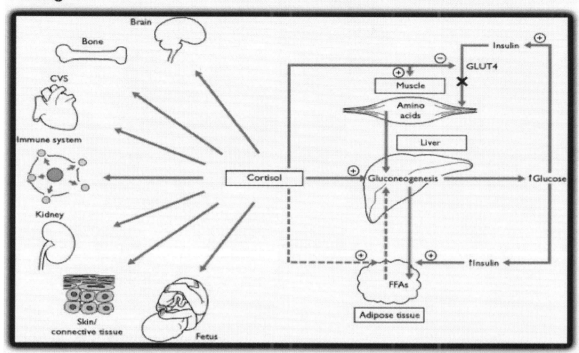

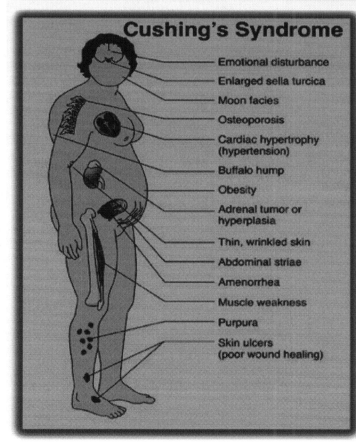

Cushing's Syndrome

- Emotional disturbance
- Enlarged sella turcica
- Moon facies
- Osteoporosis
- Cardiac hypertrophy (hypertension)
- Buffalo hump
- Obesity
- Adrenal tumor or hyperplasia
- Thin, wrinkled skin
- Abdominal striae
- Amenorrhea
- Muscle weakness
- Purpura
- Skin ulcers (poor wound healing)

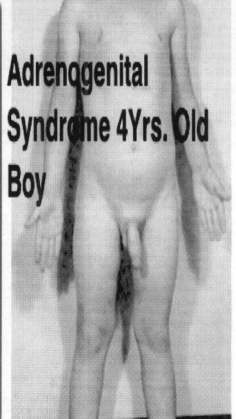

Adrenogenital Syndrome 4Yrs. Old Boy

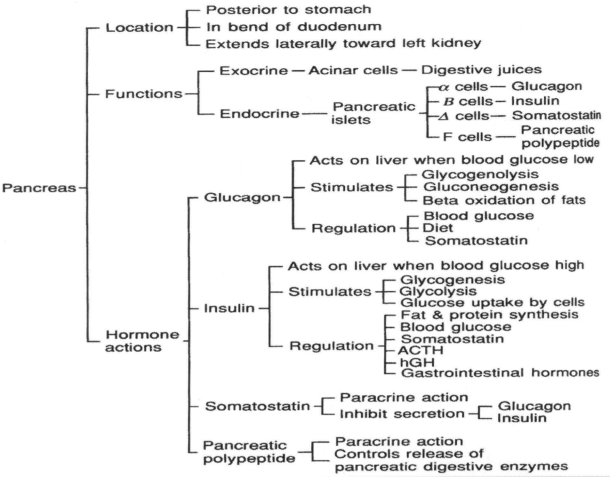

Pancreas
- Location
  - Posterior to stomach
  - In bend of duodenum
  - Extends laterally toward left kidney
- Functions
  - Exocrine — Acinar cells — Digestive juices
  - Endocrine — Pancreatic islets
    - α cells — Glucagon
    - B cells — Insulin
    - Δ cells — Somatostatin
    - F cells — Pancreatic polypeptide
- Hormone actions
  - Glucagon
    - Acts on liver when blood glucose low
    - Stimulates
      - Glycogenolysis
      - Gluconeogenesis
      - Beta oxidation of fats
    - Regulation
      - Blood glucose
      - Diet
      - Somatostatin
  - Insulin
    - Acts on liver when blood glucose high
    - Stimulates
      - Glycogenesis
      - Glycolysis
      - Glucose uptake by cells
    - Regulation
      - Fat & protein synthesis
      - Blood glucose
      - Somatostatin
      - ACTH
      - hGH
      - Gastrointestinal hormones
  - Somatostatin
    - Paracrine action
    - Inhibit secretion
      - Glucagon
      - Insulin
  - Pancreatic polypeptide
    - Paracrine action
    - Controls release of pancreatic digestive enzymes

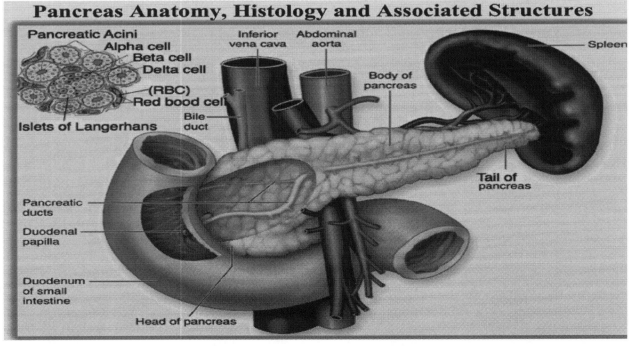

Pancreas Anatomy, Histology and Associated Structures

Pancreatic Acini
Alpha cell
Beta cell
Delta cell
(RBC)
Red bood cell
Islets of Langerhans

Inferior vena cava
Abdominal aorta
Spleen
Body of pancreas
Bile duct
Tail of pancreas
Pancreatic ducts
Duodenal papilla
Duodenum of small intestine
Head of pancreas

Insulin and Glucagon Regulation Of Glucose

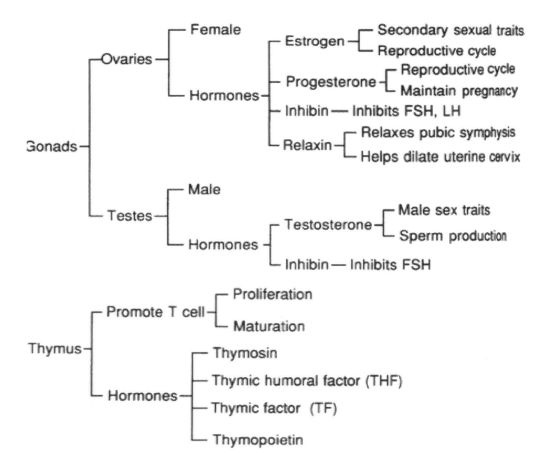

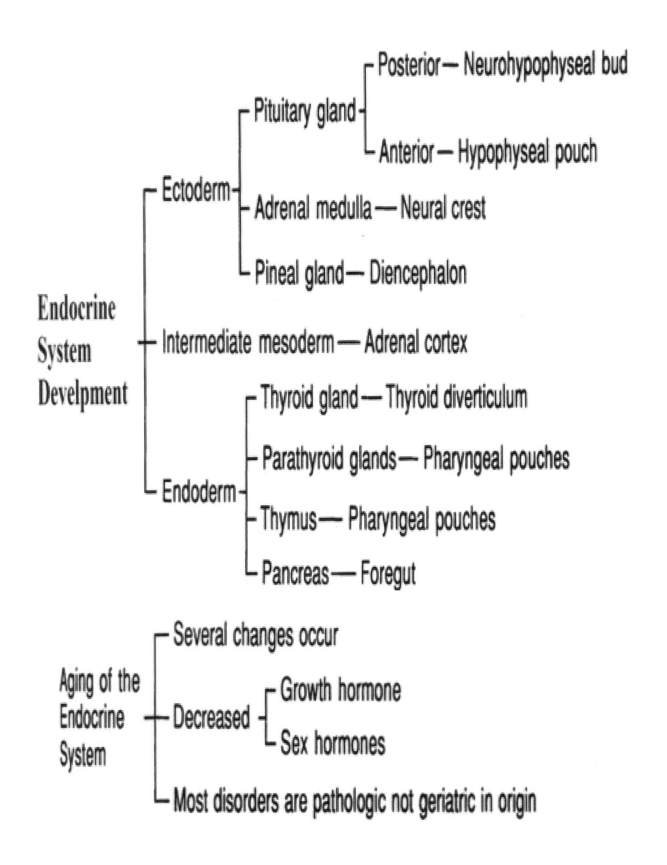

Endocrine System Develpment
- Ectoderm
  - Pituitary gland
    - Posterior — Neurohypophyseal bud
    - Anterior — Hypophyseal pouch
  - Adrenal medulla — Neural crest
  - Pineal gland — Diencephalon
- Intermediate mesoderm — Adrenal cortex
- Endoderm
  - Thyroid gland — Thyroid diverticulum
  - Parathyroid glands — Pharyngeal pouches
  - Thymus — Pharyngeal pouches
  - Pancreas — Foregut

Aging of the Endocrine System
- Several changes occur
- Decreased
  - Growth hormone
  - Sex hormones
- Most disorders are pathologic not geriatric in origin

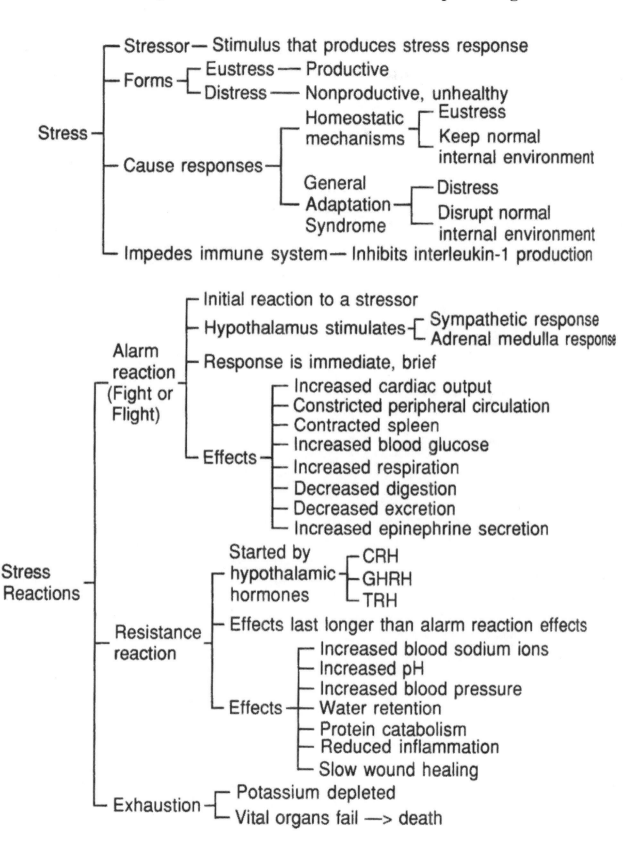

Stress Curve Phases, Good Stress And Bad Stress

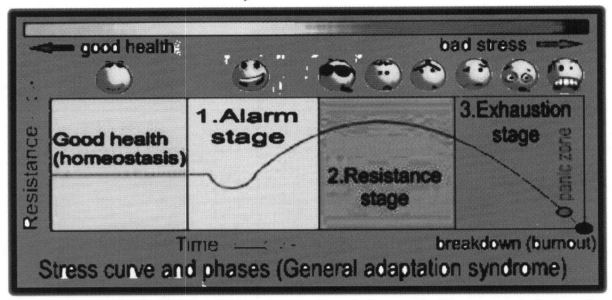

Stress curve and phases (General adaptation syndrome)

The Adrenal Gland (Suprarenal); Adrenal Cortex, Adrenal Medulla and Pheochromocytoma

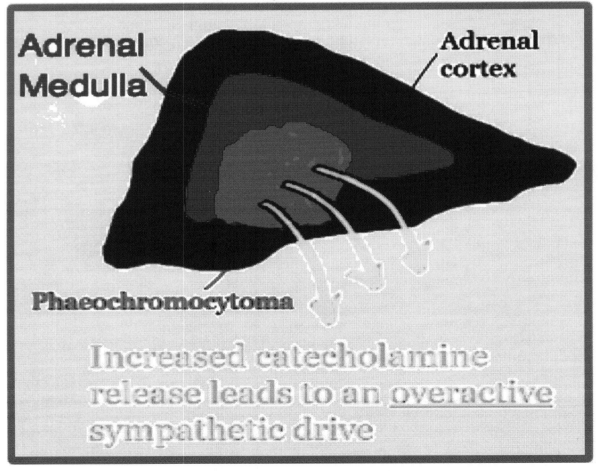

CHAPTER NINETEEN

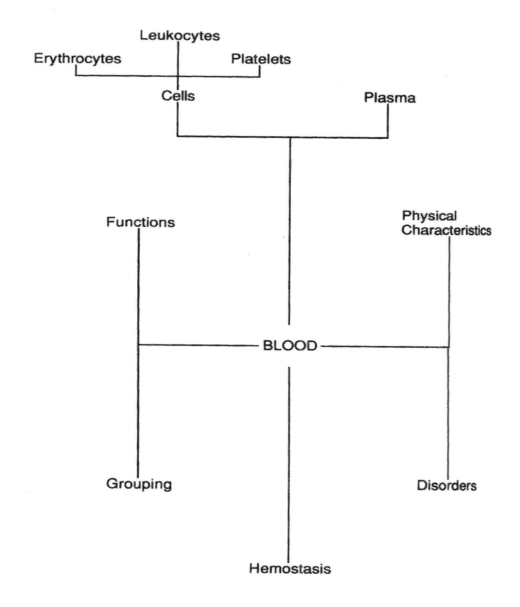

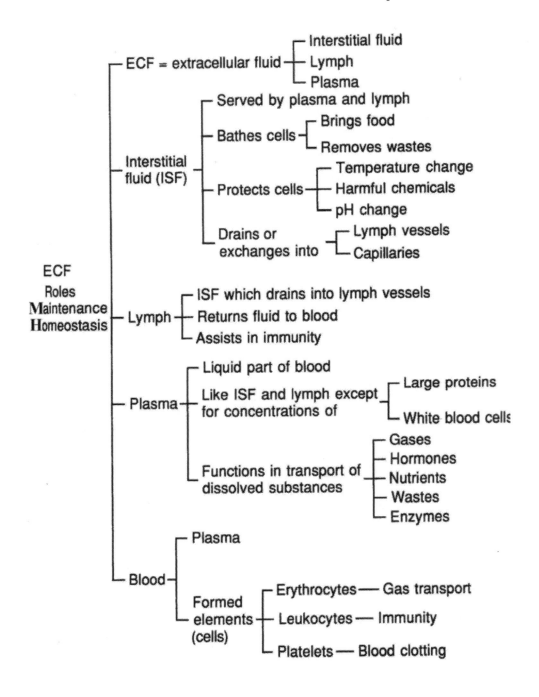

ECF
Roles
Maintenance
Homeostasis

- ECF = extracellular fluid
  - Interstitial fluid
  - Lymph
  - Plasma
- Interstitial fluid (ISF)
  - Served by plasma and lymph
  - Bathes cells
    - Brings food
    - Removes wastes
  - Protects cells
    - Temperature change
    - Harmful chemicals
    - pH change
  - Drains or exchanges into
    - Lymph vessels
    - Capillaries
- Lymph
  - ISF which drains into lymph vessels
  - Returns fluid to blood
  - Assists in immunity
- Plasma
  - Liquid part of blood
  - Like ISF and lymph except for concentrations of
    - Large proteins
    - White blood cells
  - Functions in transport of dissolved substances
    - Gases
    - Hormones
    - Nutrients
    - Wastes
    - Enzymes
- Blood
  - Plasma
  - Formed elements (cells)
    - Erythrocytes — Gas transport
    - Leukocytes — Immunity
    - Platelets — Blood clotting

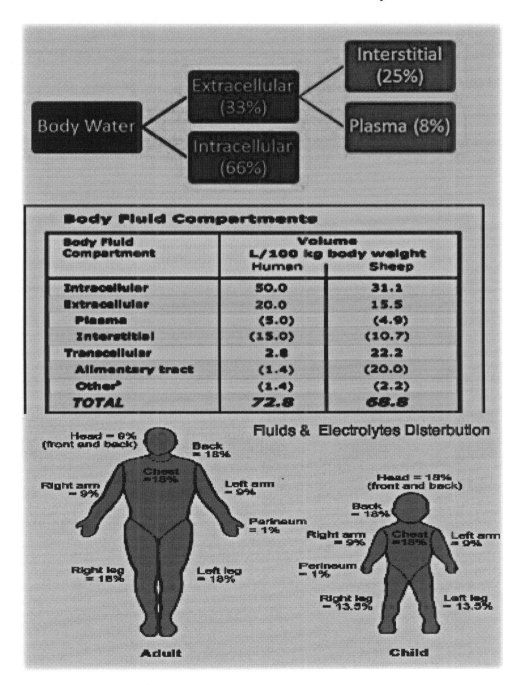

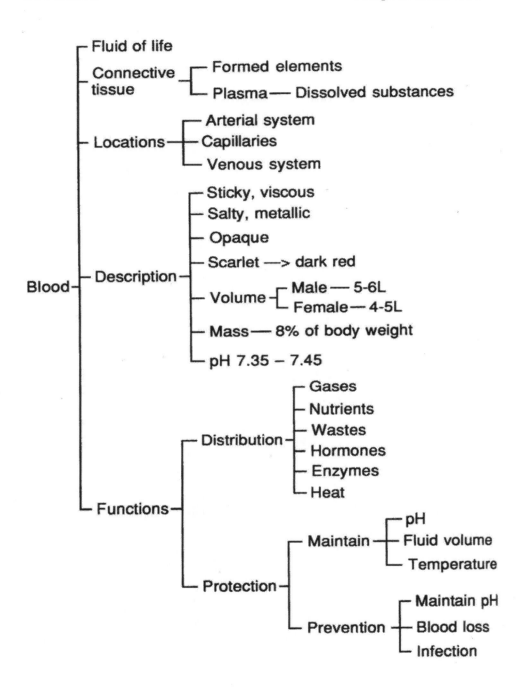

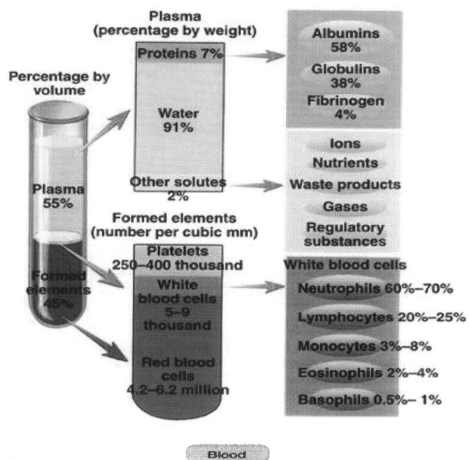

Plasma (percentage by weight)

Proteins 7%

Water 91%

Other solutes 2%

Percentage by volume

Plasma 55%

Formed elements 45%

Albumins 58%

Globulins 38%

Fibrinogen 4%

Ions
Nutrients
Waste products
Gases
Regulatory substances

Formed elements (number per cubic mm)

Platelets 250–400 thousand

White blood cells 5–9 thousand

Red blood cells 4.2–6.2 million

White blood cells
Neutrophils 60%–70%
Lymphocytes 20%–25%
Monocytes 3%–8%
Eosinophils 2%–4%
Basophils 0.5%–1%

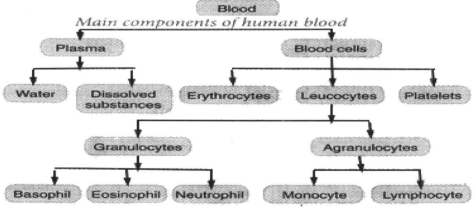

Main components of human blood

Blood

Plasma — Blood cells

Water — Dissolved substances

Erythrocytes — Leucocytes — Plateleets

Granulocytes — Agranulocytes

Basophil — Eosinophil — Neutrophil

Monocyte — Lymphocyte

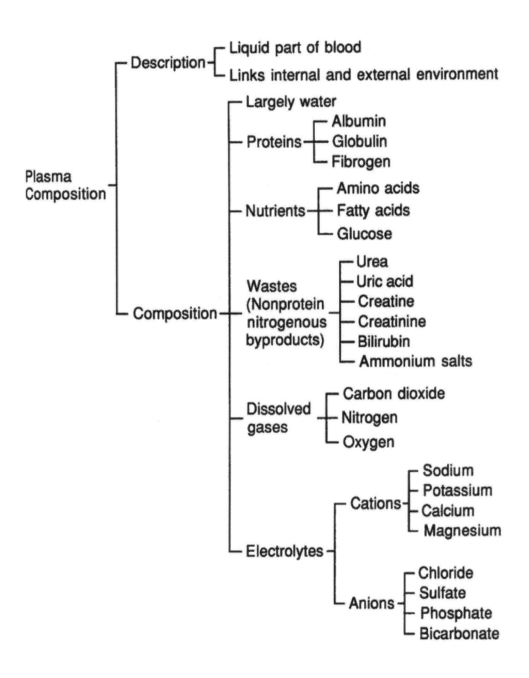

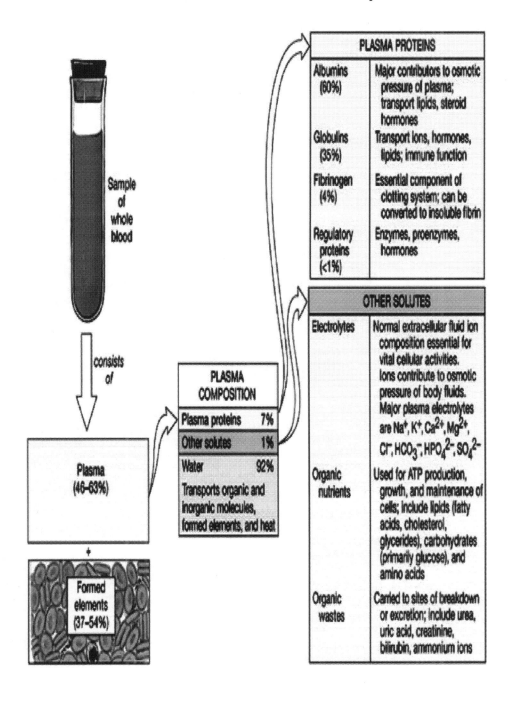

PLASMA PROTEINS	
Albumins (60%)	Major contributors to osmotic pressure of plasma; transport lipids, steroid hormones
Globulins (35%)	Transport ions, hormones, lipids; immune function
Fibrinogen (4%)	Essential component of clotting system; can be converted to insoluble fibrin
Regulatory proteins (<1%)	Enzymes, proenzymes, hormones

Sample of whole blood

consists of

PLASMA COMPOSITION	
Plasma proteins	7%
Other solutes	1%
Water	92%
Transports organic and inorganic molecules, formed elements, and heat	

Plasma (46–63%)

Formed elements (37–54%)

OTHER SOLUTES	
Electrolytes	Normal extracellular fluid ion composition essential for vital cellular activities. Ions contribute to osmotic pressure of body fluids. Major plasma electrolytes are Na^+, K^+, Ca^{2+}, Mg^{2+}, Cl^-, HCO_3^-, HPO_4^{2-}, SO_4^{2-}
Organic nutrients	Used for ATP production, growth, and maintenance of cells; include lipids (fatty acids, cholesterol, glycerides), carbohydrates (primarily glucose), and amino acids
Organic wastes	Carried to sites of breakdown or excretion; include urea, uric acid, creatinine, bilirubin, ammonium ions

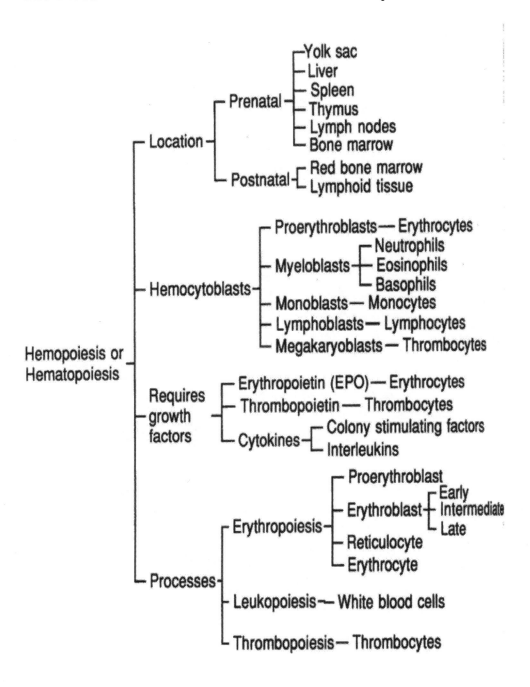

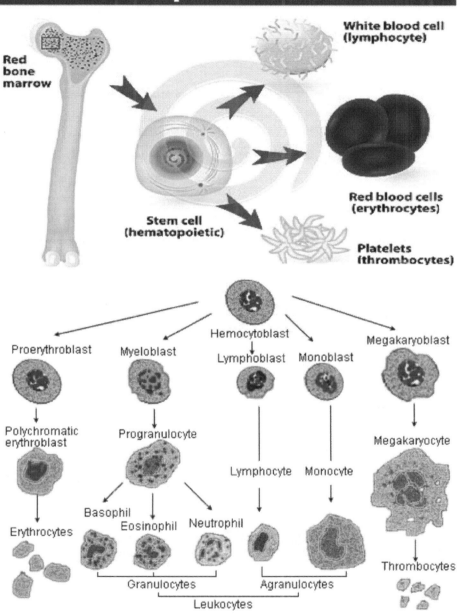

Haematopoiesis & Stem cell

Red bone marrow

Stem cell (hematopoietic)

White blood cell (lymphocyte)

Red blood cells (erythrocytes)

Platelets (thrombocytes)

Hemocytoblast

Proerythroblast   Myeloblast   Lymphoblast   Monoblast   Megakaryoblast

Polychromatic erythroblast   Progranulocyte

Lymphocyte   Monocyte   Megakaryocyte

Erythrocytes   Basophil   Eosinophil   Neutrophil

Granulocytes   Agranulocytes   Thrombocytes

Leukocytes

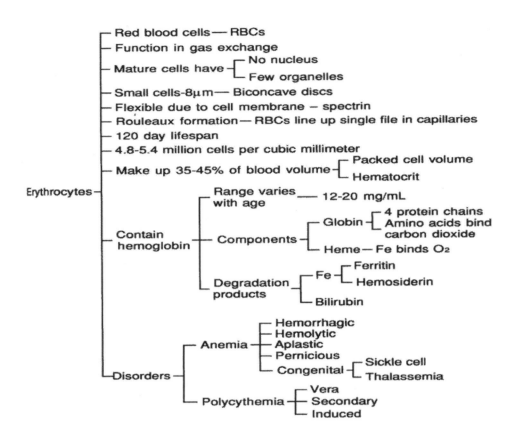

```
Erythrocytes ─┬─ Red blood cells ── RBCs
              ├─ Function in gas exchange
              ├─ Mature cells ─┬─ No nucleus
              │                └─ Few organelles
              ├─ Small cells-8μm ── Biconcave discs
              ├─ Flexible due to cell membrane ─ spectrin
              ├─ Rouleaux formation ── RBCs line up single file in capillaries
              ├─ 120 day lifespan
              ├─ 4.8-5.4 million cells per cubic millimeter
              ├─ Make up 35-45% of blood volume ─┬─ Packed cell volume
              │                                   └─ Hematocrit
              ├─ Contain ─┬─ Range varies ── 12-20 mg/mL
              │  hemoglobin│  with age
              │            ├─ Components ─┬─ Globin ─┬─ 4 protein chains
              │            │              │          └─ Amino acids bind
              │            │              │             carbon dioxide
              │            │              └─ Heme ─ Fe binds O₂
              │            └─ Degradation ─┬─ Fe ─┬─ Ferritin
              │               products     │      └─ Hemosiderin
              │                            └─ Bilirubin
              └─ Disorders ─┬─ Anemia ─┬─ Hemorrhagic
                            │          ├─ Hemolytic
                            │          ├─ Aplastic
                            │          ├─ Pernicious
                            │          └─ Congenital ─┬─ Sickle cell
                            │                         └─ Thalassemia
                            └─ Polycythemia ─┬─ Vera
                                             ├─ Secondary
                                             └─ Induced
```

Mechanisms of Erythrocyte Control of O₂ Delivery

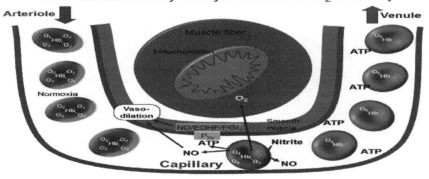

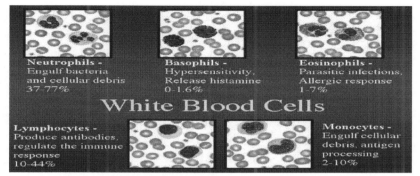

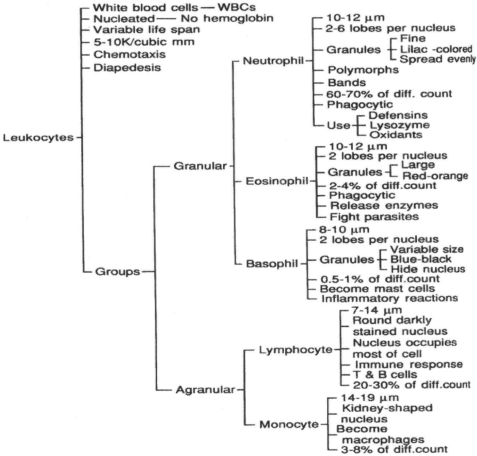

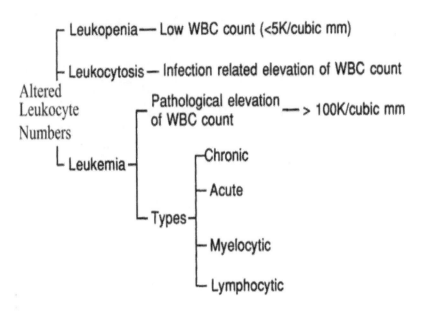

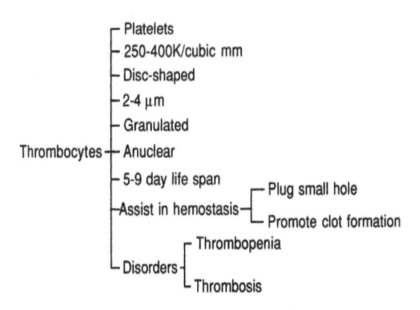

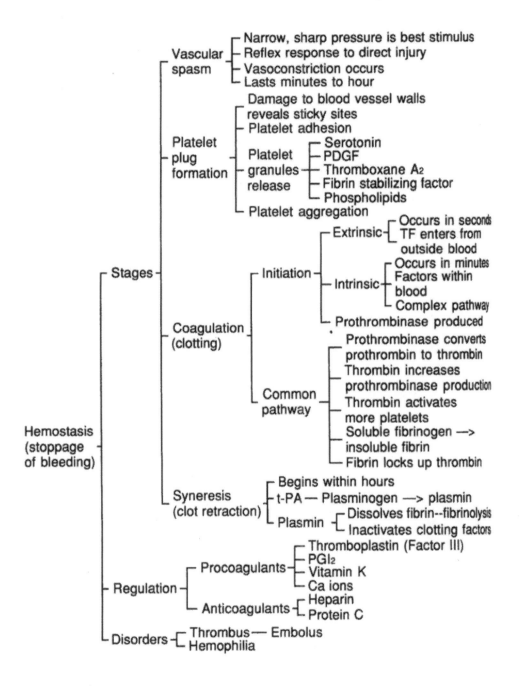

Hemostasis (stoppage of bleeding)

- Stages
  - Vascular spasm
    - Narrow, sharp pressure is best stimulus
    - Reflex response to direct injury
    - Vasoconstriction occurs
    - Lasts minutes to hour
  - Platelet plug formation
    - Damage to blood vessel walls reveals sticky sites
    - Platelet adhesion
    - Platelet granules release
      - Serotonin
      - PDGF
      - Thromboxane A₂
      - Fibrin stabilizing factor
      - Phospholipids
    - Platelet aggregation
  - Coagulation (clotting)
    - Initiation
      - Extrinsic
        - Occurs in seconds
        - TF enters from outside blood
      - Intrinsic
        - Occurs in minutes
        - Factors within blood
        - Complex pathway
      - Prothrombinase produced
    - Common pathway
      - Prothrombinase converts prothrombin to thrombin
      - Thrombin increases prothrombinase production
      - Thrombin activates more platelets
      - Soluble fibrinogen —> insoluble fibrin
      - Fibrin locks up thrombin
  - Syneresis (clot retraction)
    - Begins within hours
    - t-PA — Plasminogen —> plasmin
    - Plasmin
      - Dissolves fibrin--fibrinolysis
      - Inactivates clotting factors
- Regulation
  - Procoagulants
    - Thromboplastin (Factor III)
    - PGI₂
    - Vitamin K
    - Ca ions
  - Anticoagulants
    - Heparin
    - Protein C
- Disorders
  - Thrombus — Embolus
  - Hemophilia

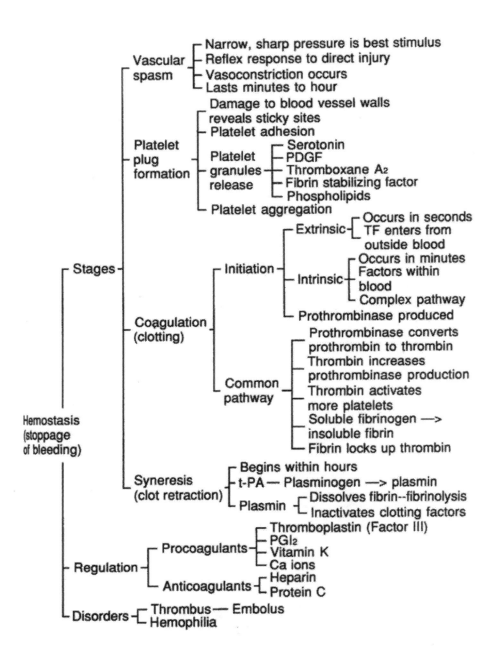

Hemostasis (stoppage of bleeding)

- Stages
  - Vascular spasm
    - Narrow, sharp pressure is best stimulus
    - Reflex response to direct injury
    - Vasoconstriction occurs
    - Lasts minutes to hour
  - Platelet plug formation
    - Damage to blood vessel walls reveals sticky sites
    - Platelet adhesion
    - Platelet granules release
      - Serotonin
      - PDGF
      - Thromboxane A_2
      - Fibrin stabilizing factor
      - Phospholipids
    - Platelet aggregation
  - Coagulation (clotting)
    - Initiation
      - Extrinsic
        - Occurs in seconds
        - TF enters from outside blood
      - Intrinsic
        - Occurs in minutes
        - Factors within blood
        - Complex pathway
      - Prothrombinase produced
    - Common pathway
      - Prothrombinase converts prothrombin to thrombin
      - Thrombin increases prothrombinase production
      - Thrombin activates more platelets
      - Soluble fibrinogen —> insoluble fibrin
      - Fibrin locks up thrombin
  - Syneresis (clot retraction)
    - Begins within hours
    - t-PA — Plasminogen —> plasmin
    - Plasmin
      - Dissolves fibrin--fibrinolysis
      - Inactivates clotting factors
- Regulation
  - Procoagulants
    - Thromboplastin (Factor III)
    - PGI_2
    - Vitamin K
    - Ca ions
  - Anticoagulants
    - Heparin
    - Protein C
- Disorders
  - Thrombus — Embolus
  - Hemophilia

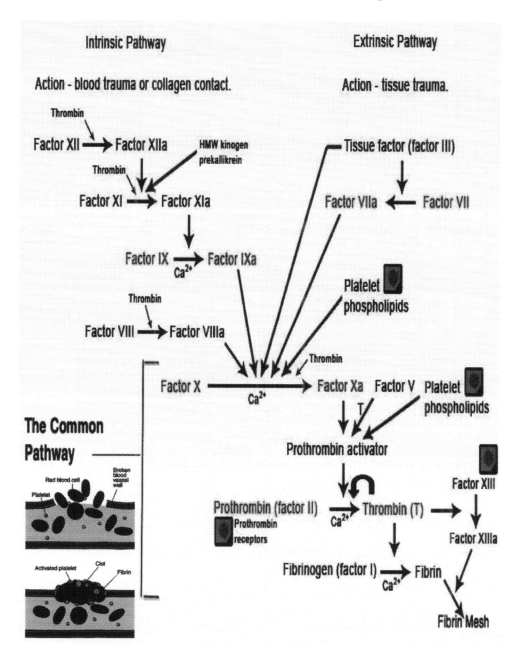

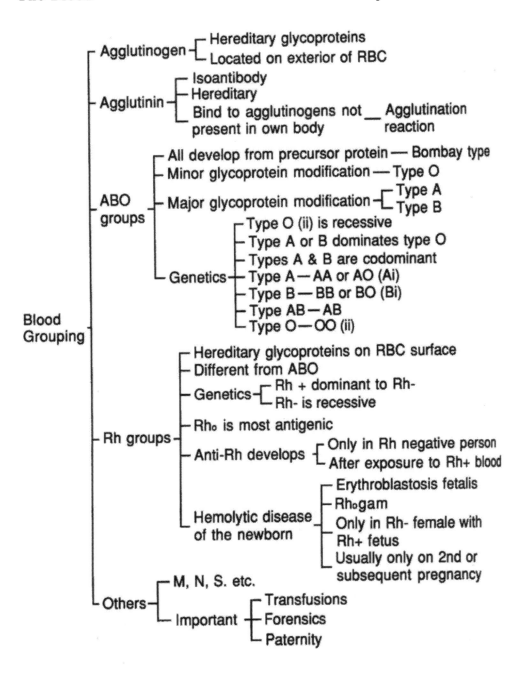

Blood Types according to Antigens-Antibodies

Red blood cells	Antigen A	Antigen B	Antigens A and B	Neither antigen A nor B

Plasma	Anti-B antibody	Anti-A antibody	Neither Anti-A nor Anti-B antibodies	Anti-A and Anti-B antibodies
				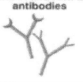

Type A
Red blood cells with type A surface antigens and plasma with anti-B antibodies

Type B
Red blood cells with type B surface antigens and plasma with anti-A antibodies

Type AB
Red blood cells with both anti-A and anti-B surface antigens, and neither anti-A nor anti-B plasma antibodies

Type O
Red blood cells with neither type A nor type B surface antigens, but both anti-A and anti-B plasma antibodies

The Agglutination Process

(a) No agglutination reaction. Type A blood donated to a type A recipient does not cause an agglutination reaction because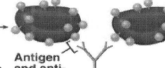

Type A blood of donor   +   Anti-B antibody in type A blood of recipient   →   Antigen and antibody do not match   No agglutination

the anti-B antibodies in the recipient do not combine with the type A antigens on the red blood cells in the donated blood.

(b) Agglutination reaction. Type A blood donated to a type B recipient causes an agglutination reaction because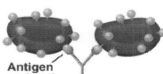

Type A blood of donor   +   Anti-A antibody in type B blood of recipient   →   Antigen and antibody match   Agglutination

the anti-A antibodies in the recipient combine with the type A antigens on the red blood cells in the donated blood.

Cross-Matching Test

Recipient's blood			Reactions with donor's red blood cells			
ABO antigens	ABO antibodies	ABO blood type	Donor type O cells	Donor type A cells	Donor type B cells	Donor type AB cells
None	Anti-A Anti-B	O				
A	Anti-B	A				
B	Anti-A	B				
A & B	None	AB				

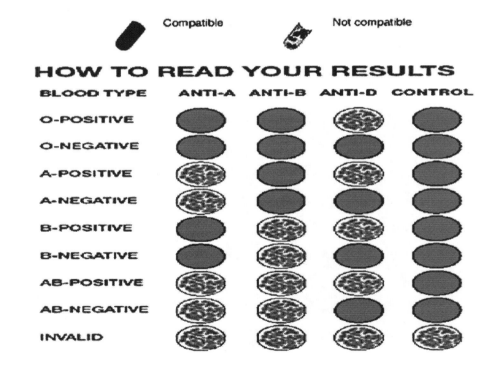

Compatible   Not compatible

HOW TO READ YOUR RESULTS

BLOOD TYPE	ANTI-A	ANTI-B	ANTI-D	CONTROL
O-POSITIVE				
O-NEGATIVE				
A-POSITIVE				
A-NEGATIVE				
B-POSITIVE				
B-NEGATIVE				
AB-POSITIVE				
AB-NEGATIVE				
INVALID				

ERYTHROBLASTOSIS FETALIS

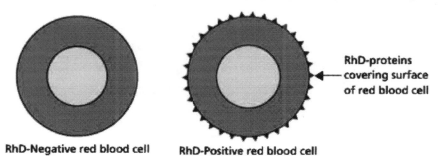

RhD-Negative red blood cell   RhD-Positive red blood cell

RhD-proteins covering surface of red blood cell

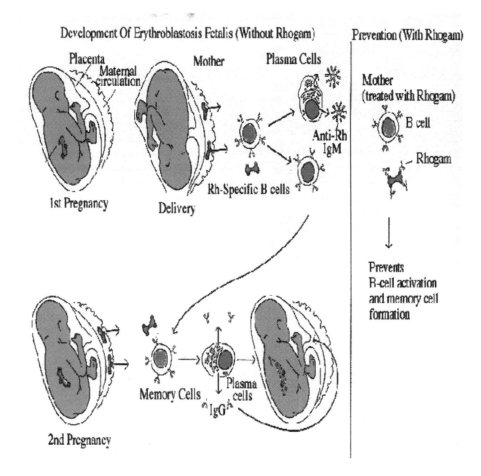

Hereditary Linkage to the Antigen

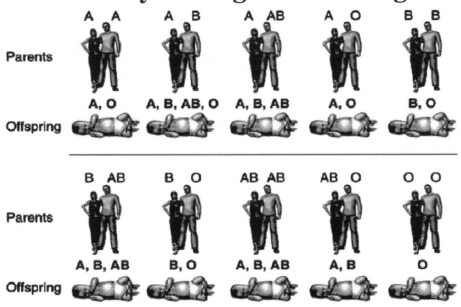

Summary of Possible Child Blood Types

Parent A Blood Type	Parent B Blood Type	Possible Child Blood Types
A	A	A, O
A	B	A, AB, B, O
A	AB	A, AB, B
AB	AB	A, AB, B
B	B	B, O
B	AB	A, AB, B
O	O	O
O	A	A, O
O	B	O, B
O	AB	A, B
Rh+	Rh-	Rh+, Rh-
Rh-	Rh-	Rh-
Rh+	Rh+	Rh+, Rh-

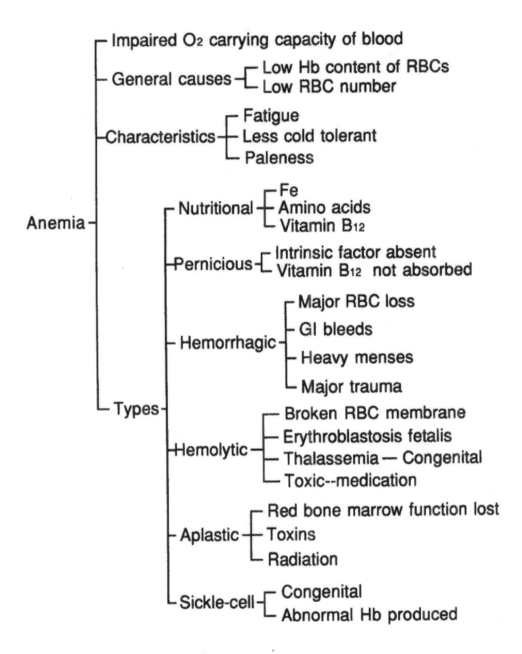

Anemia
- Impaired O_2 carrying capacity of blood
- General causes
  - Low Hb content of RBCs
  - Low RBC number
- Characteristics
  - Fatigue
  - Less cold tolerant
  - Paleness
- Types
  - Nutritional
    - Fe
    - Amino acids
    - Vitamin B_{12}
  - Pernicious
    - Intrinsic factor absent
    - Vitamin B_{12} not absorbed
  - Hemorrhagic
    - Major RBC loss
    - GI bleeds
    - Heavy menses
    - Major trauma
  - Hemolytic
    - Broken RBC membrane
    - Erythroblastosis fetalis
    - Thalassemia — Congenital
    - Toxic--medication
  - Aplastic
    - Red bone marrow function lost
    - Toxins
    - Radiation
  - Sickle-cell
    - Congenital
    - Abnormal Hb produced

Anemia Severity Classification

According to the National Cancer Institute and the National Institutes of Health, anemia can be classified into five grades.

Grade	Hb level (g/dL)	Description
1	10 - lower limit of normal	Mild
2	8 - <10	Moderate
3	6.5 - <8	Severe
4	Life threatening	Life threatening
5	Death	Death

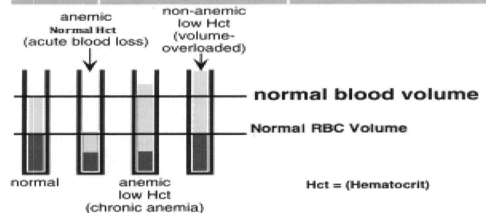

Hct = (Hematocrit)

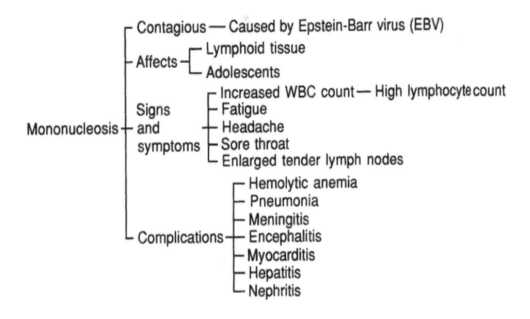

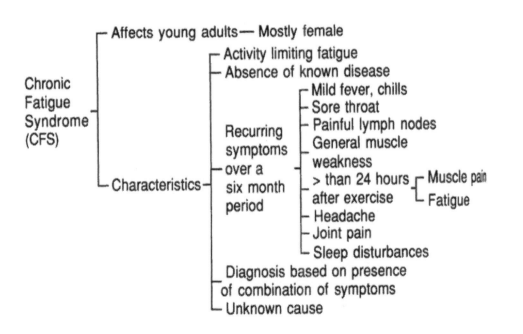

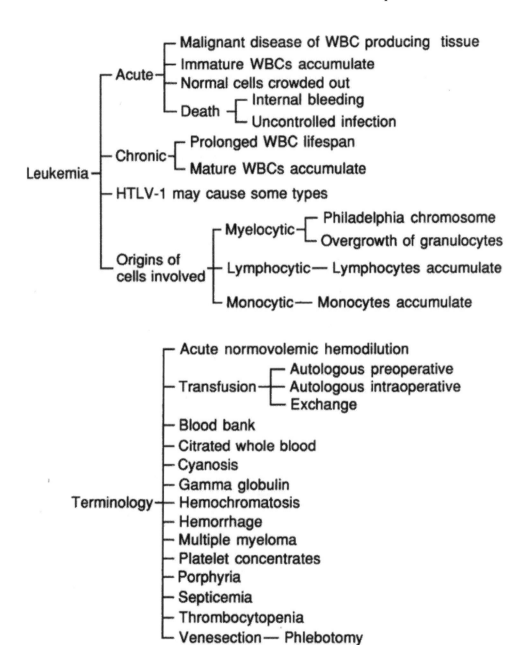

Leukemia
- Acute
  - Malignant disease of WBC producing tissue
  - Immature WBCs accumulate
  - Normal cells crowded out
  - Death
    - Internal bleeding
    - Uncontrolled infection
- Chronic
  - Prolonged WBC lifespan
  - Mature WBCs accumulate
- HTLV-1 may cause some types
- Origins of cells involved
  - Myelocytic
    - Philadelphia chromosome
    - Overgrowth of granulocytes
  - Lymphocytic — Lymphocytes accumulate
  - Monocytic — Monocytes accumulate

Terminology
- Acute normovolemic hemodilution
- Transfusion
  - Autologous preoperative
  - Autologous intraoperative
  - Exchange
- Blood bank
- Citrated whole blood
- Cyanosis
- Gamma globulin
- Hemochromatosis
- Hemorrhage
- Multiple myeloma
- Platelet concentrates
- Porphyria
- Septicemia
- Thrombocytopenia
- Venesection — Phlebotomy

CHAPTER TWENTY

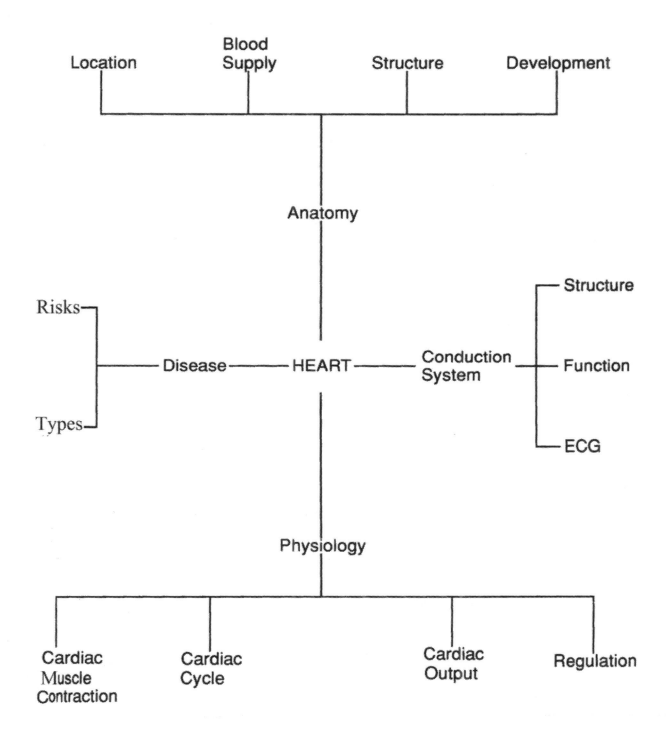

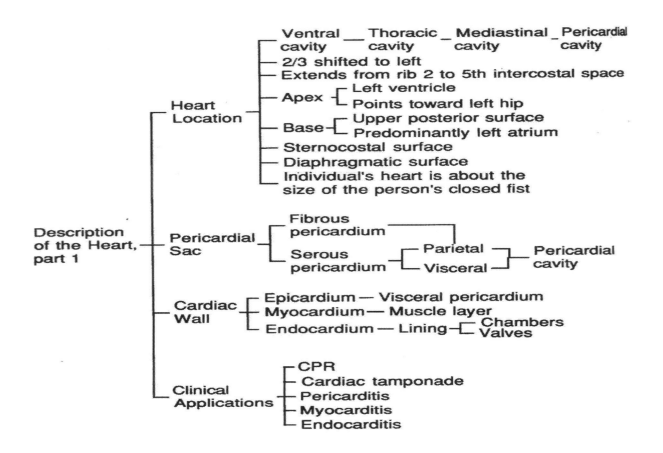

Description of the Heart, part 1

- Heart Location
  - Ventral cavity __ Thoracic cavity _ Mediastinal cavity _ Pericardial cavity
  - 2/3 shifted to left
  - Extends from rib 2 to 5th intercostal space
  - Apex
    - Left ventricle
    - Points toward left hip
  - Base
    - Upper posterior surface
    - Predominantly left atrium
  - Sternocostal surface
  - Diaphragmatic surface
  - Individual's heart is about the size of the person's closed fist

- Pericardial Sac
  - Fibrous pericardium
  - Serous pericardium
    - Parietal
    - Visceral — Pericardial cavity

- Cardiac Wall
  - Epicardium — Visceral pericardium
  - Myocardium — Muscle layer
  - Endocardium — Lining — Chambers / Valves

- Clinical Applications
  - CPR
  - Cardiac tamponade
  - Pericarditis
  - Myocarditis
  - Endocarditis

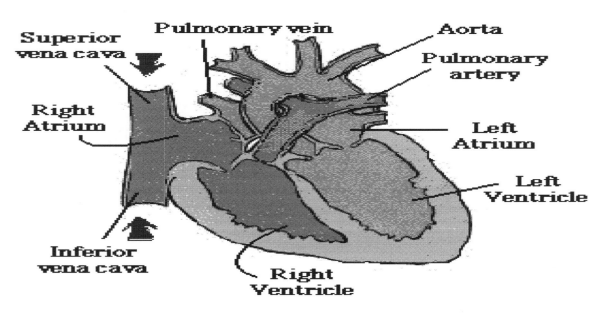

Superior vena cava
Pulmonary vein
Aorta
Pulmonary artery
Right Atrium
Left Atrium
Left Ventricle
Inferior vena cava
Right Ventricle

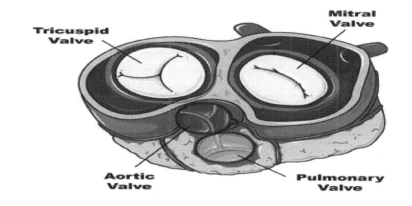

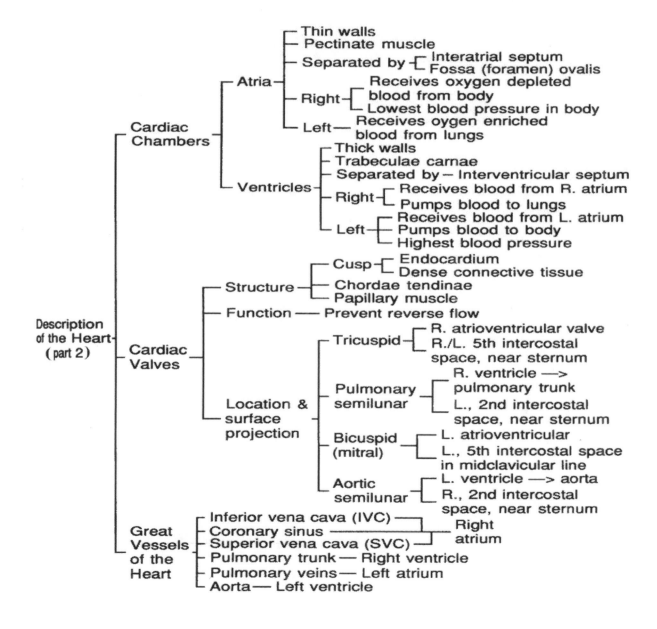

Description of the Heart (part 2)

Cardiac Chambers

- Atria
  - Thin walls
  - Pectinate muscle
  - Separated by
    - Interatrial septum
    - Fossa (foramen) ovalis
  - Right
    - Receives oxygen depleted blood from body
    - Lowest blood pressure in body
  - Left
    - Receives oxygen enriched blood from lungs
- Ventricles
  - Thick walls
  - Trabeculae carnae
  - Separated by — Interventricular septum
  - Right
    - Receives blood from R. atrium
    - Pumps blood to lungs
  - Left
    - Receives blood from L. atrium
    - Pumps blood to body
    - Highest blood pressure

Cardiac Valves

- Structure
  - Cusp
    - Endocardium
    - Dense connective tissue
  - Chordae tendinae
  - Papillary muscle
- Function — Prevent reverse flow
- Location & surface projection
  - Tricuspid
    - R. atrioventricular valve
    - R./L. 5th intercostal space, near sternum
  - Pulmonary semilunar
    - R. ventricle —> pulmonary trunk
    - L., 2nd intercostal space, near sternum
  - Bicuspid (mitral)
    - L. atrioventricular
    - L., 5th intercostal space in midclavicular line
  - Aortic semilunar
    - L. ventricle —> aorta
    - R., 2nd intercostal space, near sternum

Great Vessels of the Heart

- Inferior vena cava (IVC) — Right atrium
- Coronary sinus — Right atrium
- Superior vena cava (SVC) — Right atrium
- Pulmonary trunk — Right ventricle
- Pulmonary veins — Left atrium
- Aorta — Left ventricle

3

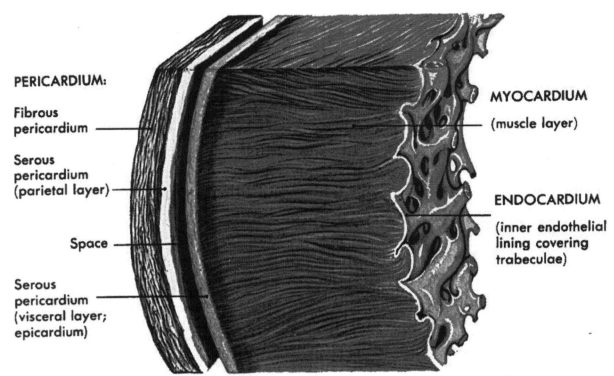

PERICARDIUM:

Fibrous
pericardium

Serous
pericardium
(parietal layer)

Space

Serous
pericardium
(visceral layer;
epicardium)

MYOCARDIUM
(muscle layer)

ENDOCARDIUM
(inner endothelial
lining covering
trabeculae)

Section of the heart wall showing the components of
the outer pericardium (heart sac), muscle layer
(myocardium), and inner lining (endocardium).

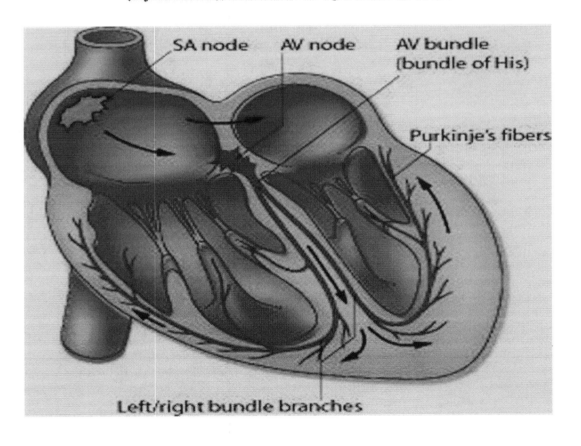

SA node   AV node   AV bundle
(bundle of His)

Purkinje's fibers

Left/right bundle branches

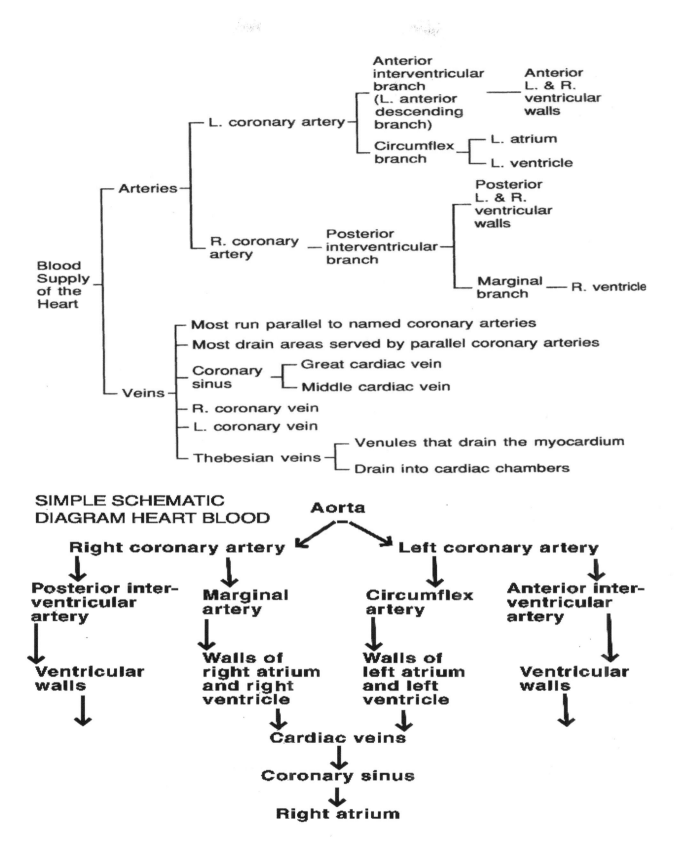

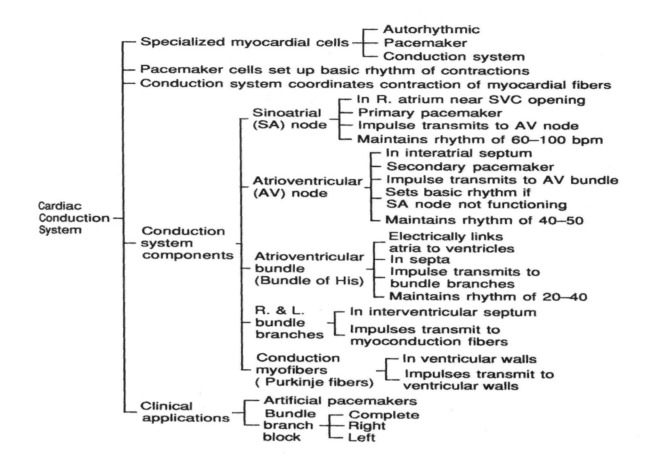

Cardiac Conduction System
- Specialized myocardial cells
  - Autorhythmic
  - Pacemaker
  - Conduction system
- Pacemaker cells set up basic rhythm of contractions
- Conduction system coordinates contraction of myocardial fibers
- Conduction system components
  - Sinoatrial (SA) node
    - In R. atrium near SVC opening
    - Primary pacemaker
    - Impulse transmits to AV node
    - Maintains rhythm of 60–100 bpm
  - Atrioventricular (AV) node
    - In interatrial septum
    - Secondary pacemaker
    - Impulse transmits to AV bundle
    - Sets basic rhythm if SA node not functioning
    - Maintains rhythm of 40–50
  - Atrioventricular bundle (Bundle of His)
    - Electrically links atria to ventricles
    - In septa
    - Impulse transmits to bundle branches
    - Maintains rhythm of 20–40
  - R. & L. bundle branches
    - In interventricular septum
    - Impulses transmit to myoconduction fibers
  - Conduction myofibers (Purkinje fibers)
    - In ventricular walls
    - Impulses transmit to ventricular walls
- Clinical applications
  - Artificial pacemakers
  - Bundle branch block
    - Complete
    - Right
    - Left

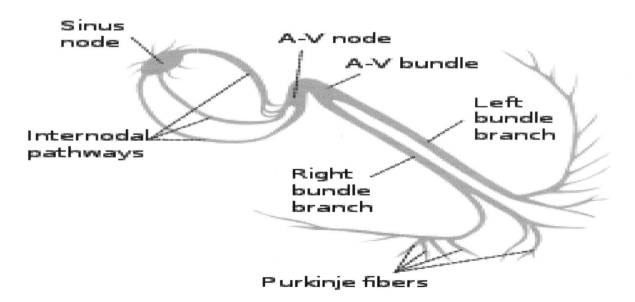

Sinus node

A-V node

A-V bundle

Left bundle branch

Internodal pathways

Right bundle branch

Purkinje fibers

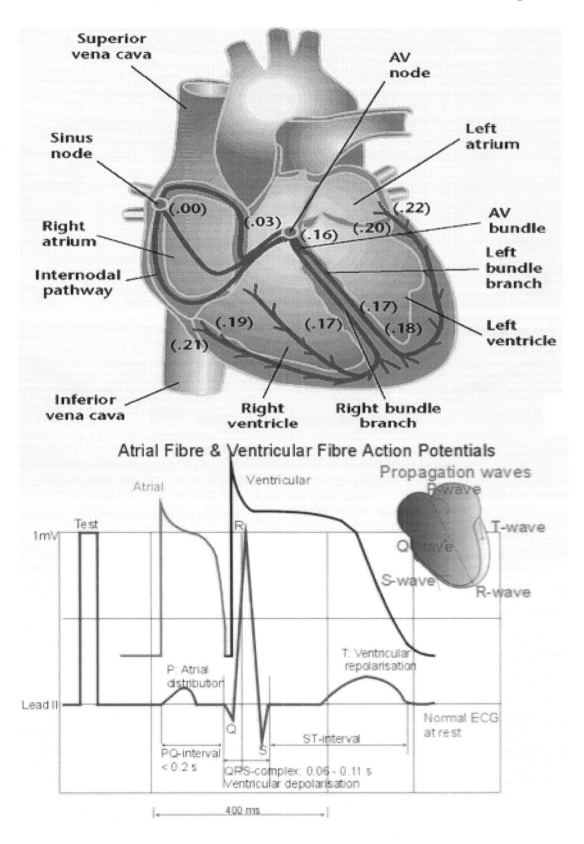

Atrial Fibre & Ventricular Fibre Action Potentials

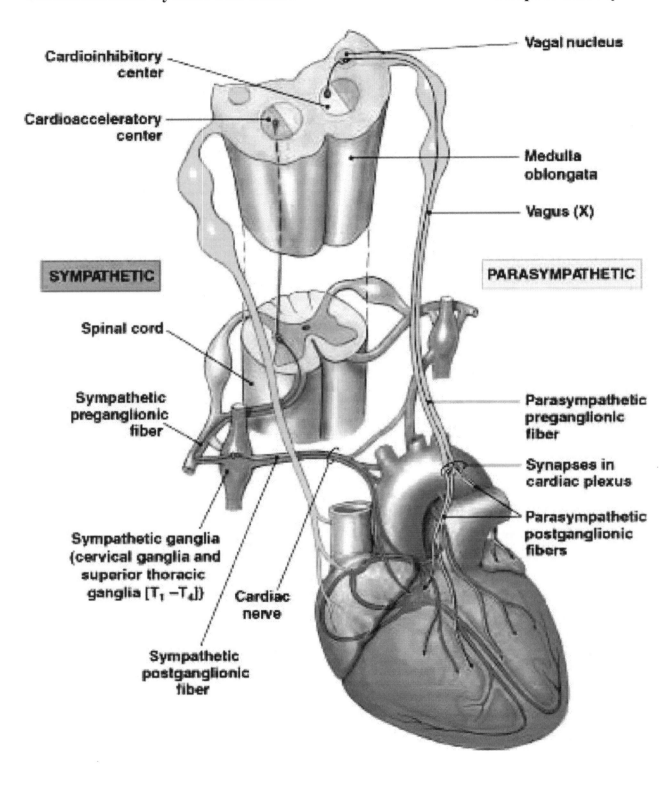

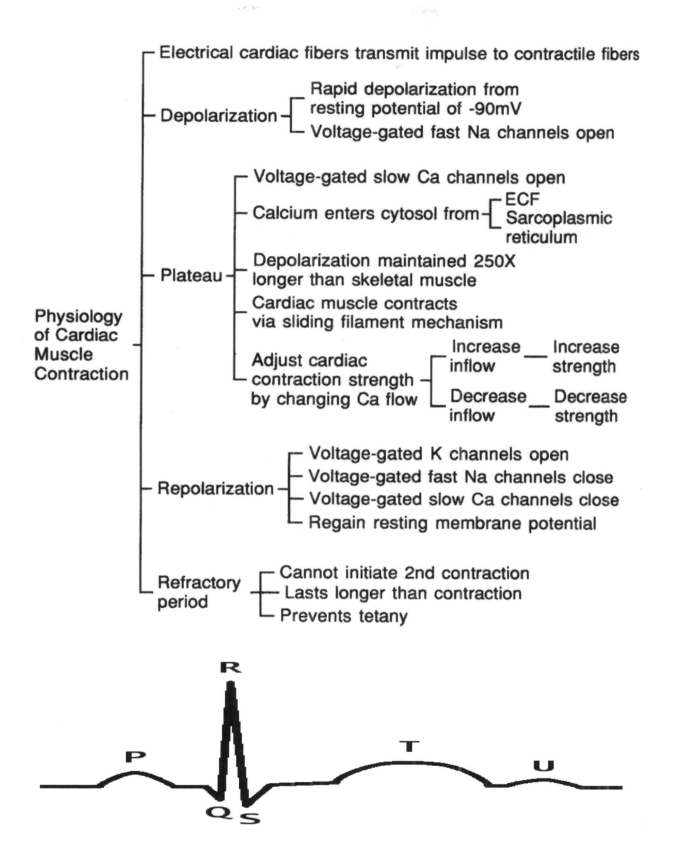

Physiology of Cardiac Muscle Contraction

- Electrical cardiac fibers transmit impulse to contractile fibers
- Depolarization
  - Rapid depolarization from resting potential of -90mV
  - Voltage-gated fast Na channels open
- Plateau
  - Voltage-gated slow Ca channels open
  - Calcium enters cytosol from
    - ECF
    - Sarcoplasmic reticulum
  - Depolarization maintained 250X longer than skeletal muscle
  - Cardiac muscle contracts via sliding filament mechanism
  - Adjust cardiac contraction strength by changing Ca flow
    - Increase inflow __ Increase strength
    - Decrease inflow __ Decrease strength
- Repolarization
  - Voltage-gated K channels open
  - Voltage-gated fast Na channels close
  - Voltage-gated slow Ca channels close
  - Regain resting membrane potential
- Refractory period
  - Cannot initiate 2nd contraction
  - Lasts longer than contraction
  - Prevents tetany

R

P   Q S   T   U

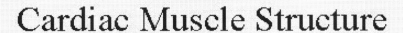

Microscopic Anatomy of Heart Muscle

Cardiac Muscle Structure

Intercalated disks are anchoring structures containing gap junctions

Cardiac muscle cells are faintly striated, branching, mononucleated cells, which connect by means of intercalated disks to form a functional network.

The action potential travels through all cells connected together forming a functional <u>syncytium</u> in which cells function as a unit.

nucleus

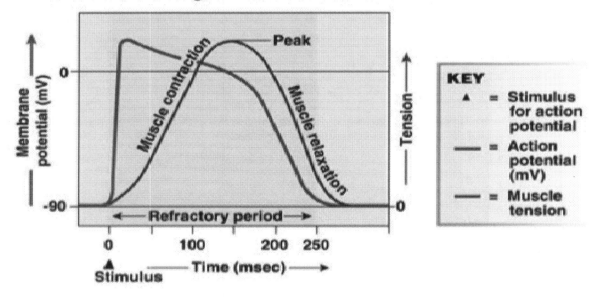

Cardiac muscle fiber: The refractory period lasts almost as long as the entire muscle twitch.

ECG (EKG)
Electrocardiagram

- Recording of electrical activity of heart
- P wave
  - Atrial depolarize 0.1 sec before atrial contraction
  - Impulse spreads from SA to AV node
  - Widened may indicate
    - Atrial enlargement
    - Mitral stenosis
- PQ or PR interval
  - Normally 0.2 sec
  - Time between beginning of atrial contraction and beginning of ventricular contraction
  - Impulse travels SA node —> AV node —> AV bundle —> bundle branches —> conduction myofibers
  - Prolonged may indicate
    - Ischemia/scarring
    - AV node damage
- Q wave — Deep and wide may indicate M.I.
- R wave — Increased size may indicate ventricular hypertrophy
- QRS complex
  - Ventricles depolarize
  - < 0.12 sec prior to contraction
  - Atria repolarize concurrently
  - > 0.12 sec may indicate bundle branch block
- QT interval — Ventricles contract
- ST interval
  - Absolute refractory period
  - Heart can't be forced to contract at this time
  - Time between end of depolarization and beginning of repolarization of ventricles
  - Plateau period
  - Elevated — May indicate M.I.
  - Depressed
    - Ischemia/scarring
    - Digitalis effect
- T wave
  - Ventricles repolarize
  - Relative refractory period
  - Contraction at this point can yield ventricular fibrillation
  - Elevated when K levels are high
  - Inverted when ischemia/scarring present
- U wave
  - Sometimes seen between T and P waves
  - May indicate myconduction fiber repolarization
  - Occurs
    - In conjunction with PVCs
    - Electrolyte imbalance
    - Medication effects

11

ECG of Normal Sinus Rhythm

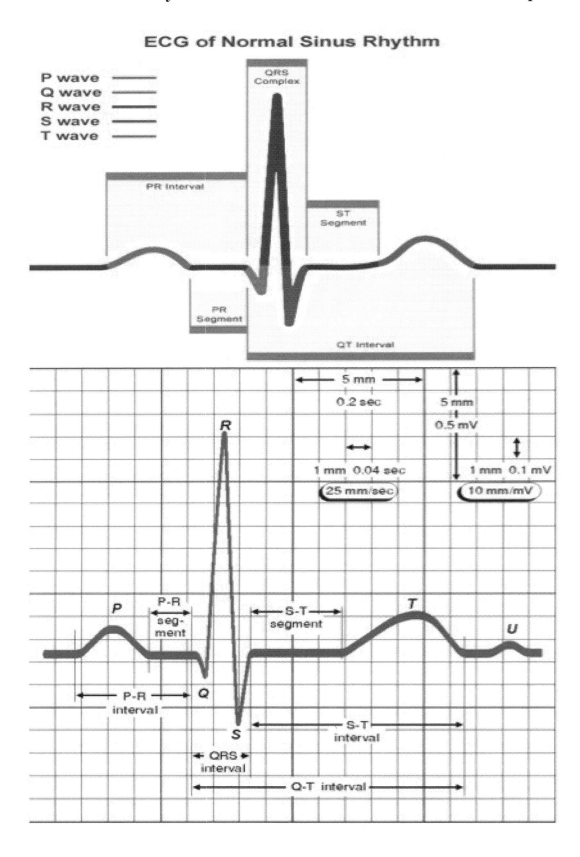

P wave ——
Q wave ——
R wave ——
S wave ——
T wave ——

QRS Complex

PR Interval

ST Segment

PR Segment

QT Interval

5 mm
0.2 sec

5 mm
0.5 mV

1 mm 0.04 sec

1 mm 0.1 mV

25 mm/sec

10 mm/mV

R

P

P-R seg-ment

S-T segment

T

U

P-R interval

Q

S

S-T interval

QRS interval

Q-T interval

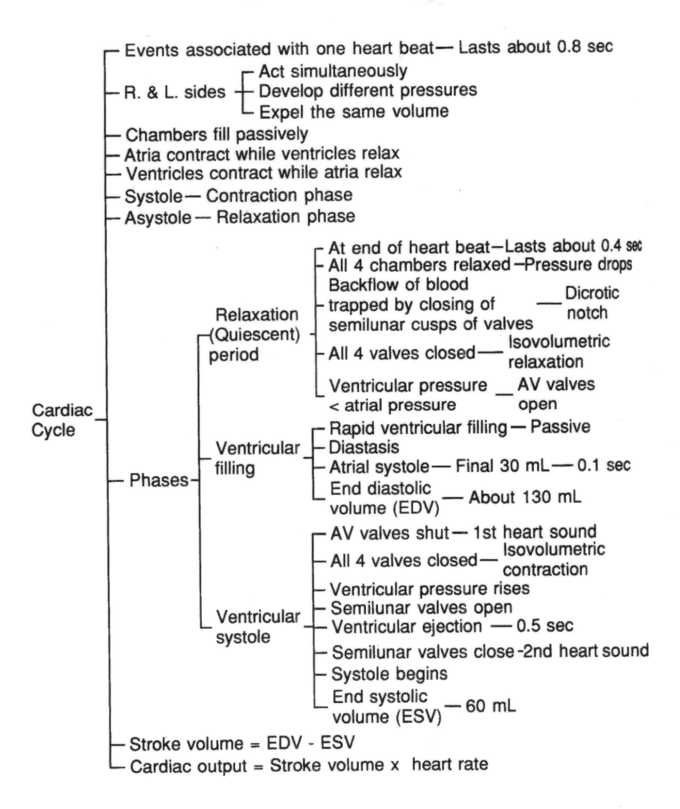

Cardiac Cycle
- Events associated with one heart beat — Lasts about 0.8 sec
- R. & L. sides
  - Act simultaneously
  - Develop different pressures
  - Expel the same volume
- Chambers fill passively
- Atria contract while ventricles relax
- Ventricles contract while atria relax
- Systole — Contraction phase
- Asystole — Relaxation phase
- Phases
  - Relaxation (Quiescent) period
    - At end of heart beat — Lasts about 0.4 sec
    - All 4 chambers relaxed — Pressure drops
    - Backflow of blood trapped by closing of semilunar cusps of valves — Dicrotic notch
    - All 4 valves closed — Isovolumetric relaxation
    - Ventricular pressure < atrial pressure — AV valves open
  - Ventricular filling
    - Rapid ventricular filling — Passive
    - Diastasis
    - Atrial systole — Final 30 mL — 0.1 sec
    - End diastolic volume (EDV) — About 130 mL
  - Ventricular systole
    - AV valves shut — 1st heart sound
    - All 4 valves closed — Isovolumetric contraction
    - Ventricular pressure rises
    - Semilunar valves open
    - Ventricular ejection — 0.5 sec
    - Semilunar valves close - 2nd heart sound
    - Systole begins
    - End systolic volume (ESV) — 60 mL
- Stroke volume = EDV - ESV
- Cardiac output = Stroke volume x heart rate

13

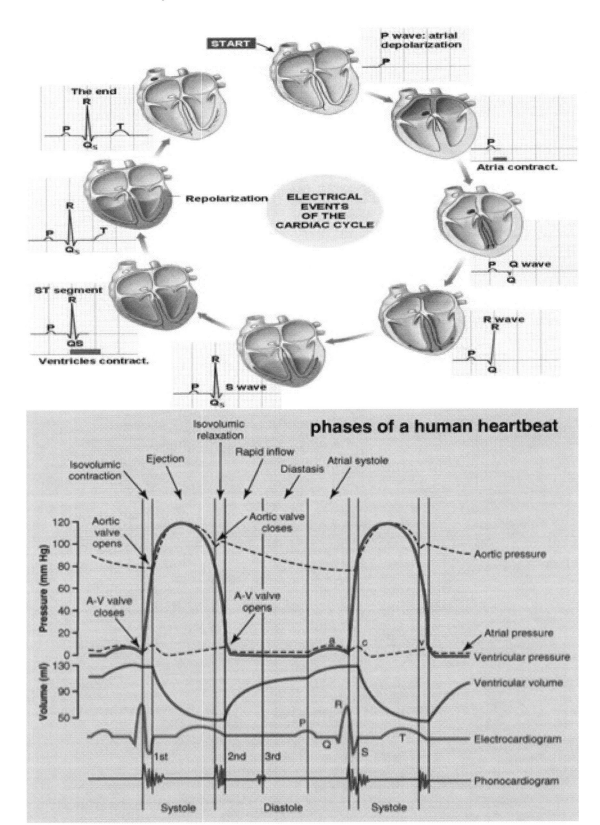

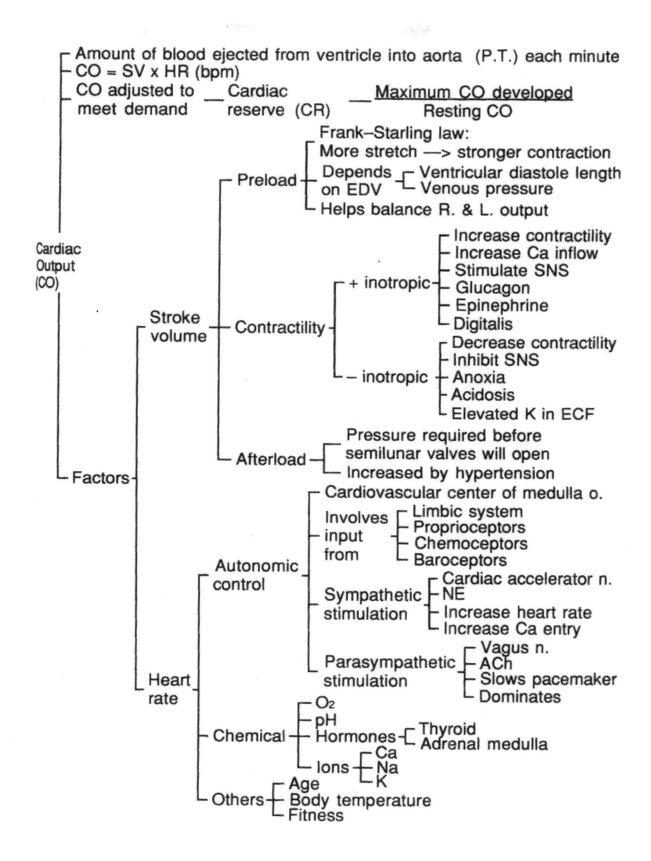

Cardiac Output (CO)
- Amount of blood ejected from ventricle into aorta (P.T.) each minute
- CO = SV x HR (bpm)
- CO adjusted to meet demand — Cardiac reserve (CR) — $\dfrac{\text{Maximum CO developed}}{\text{Resting CO}}$
- Factors
  - Stroke volume
    - Preload
      - Frank–Starling law:
      - More stretch —> stronger contraction
      - Depends on EDV
        - Ventricular diastole length
        - Venous pressure
      - Helps balance R. & L. output
    - Contractility
      - + inotropic
        - Increase contractility
        - Increase Ca inflow
        - Stimulate SNS
        - Glucagon
        - Epinephrine
        - Digitalis
      - − inotropic
        - Decrease contractility
        - Inhibit SNS
        - Anoxia
        - Acidosis
        - Elevated K in ECF
    - Afterload
      - Pressure required before semilunar valves will open
      - Increased by hypertension
  - Heart rate
    - Autonomic control
      - Cardiovascular center of medulla o.
      - Involves input from
        - Limbic system
        - Proprioceptors
        - Chemoceptors
        - Baroceptors
      - Sympathetic stimulation
        - Cardiac accelerator n.
        - NE
        - Increase heart rate
        - Increase Ca entry
      - Parasympathetic stimulation
        - Vagus n.
        - ACh
        - Slows pacemaker
        - Dominates
    - Chemical
      - O_2
      - pH
      - Hormones
        - Thyroid
        - Adrenal medulla
      - Ions
        - Ca
        - Na
        - K
    - Others
      - Age
      - Body temperature
      - Fitness

15

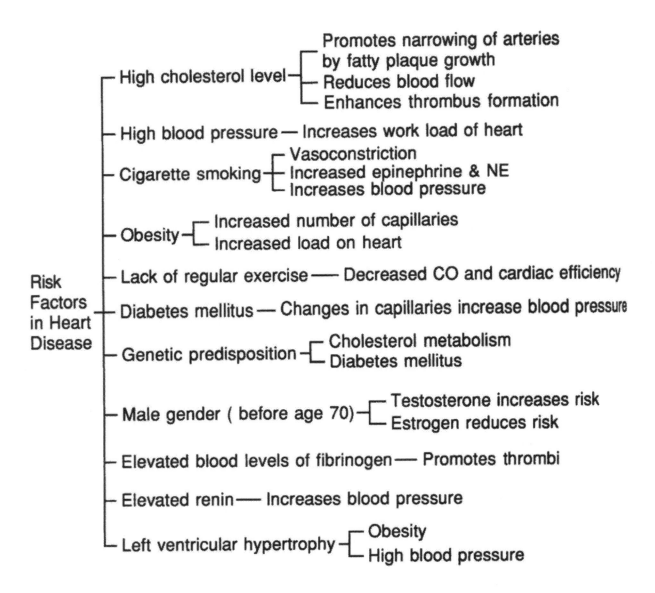

Risk Factors in Heart Disease

- High cholesterol level
  - Promotes narrowing of arteries by fatty plaque growth
  - Reduces blood flow
  - Enhances thrombus formation
- High blood pressure — Increases work load of heart
- Cigarette smoking
  - Vasoconstriction
  - Increased epinephrine & NE
  - Increases blood pressure
- Obesity
  - Increased number of capillaries
  - Increased load on heart
- Lack of regular exercise — Decreased CO and cardiac efficiency
- Diabetes mellitus — Changes in capillaries increase blood pressure
- Genetic predisposition
  - Cholesterol metabolism
  - Diabetes mellitus
- Male gender (before age 70)
  - Testosterone increases risk
  - Estrogen reduces risk
- Elevated blood levels of fibrinogen — Promotes thrombi
- Elevated renin — Increases blood pressure
- Left ventricular hypertrophy
  - Obesity
  - High blood pressure

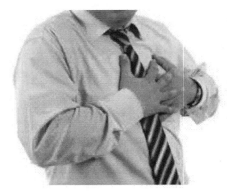
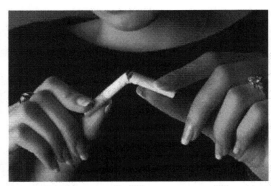

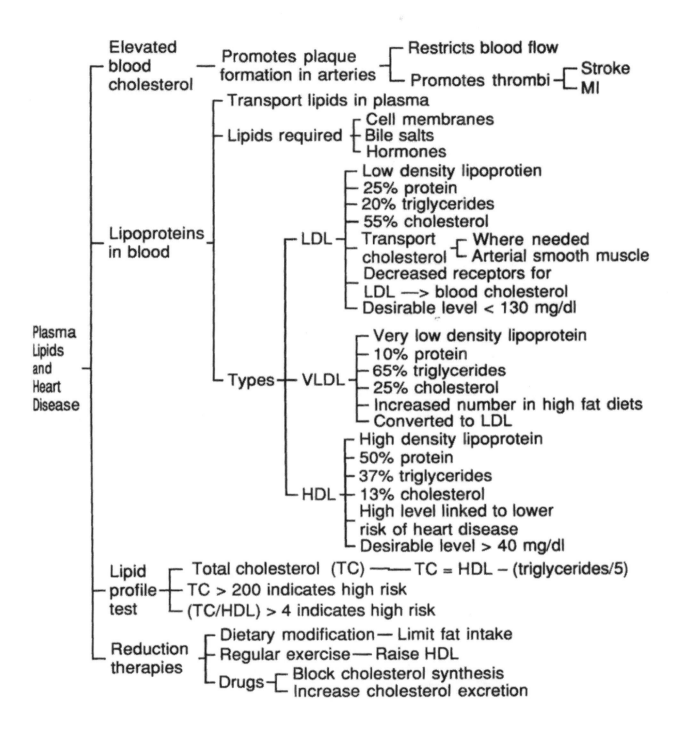

Plasma Lipids and Heart Disease

- Elevated blood cholesterol — Promotes plaque formation in arteries
  - Restricts blood flow
  - Promotes thrombi
    - Stroke
    - MI
- Lipoproteins in blood
  - Transport lipids in plasma
  - Lipids required
    - Cell membranes
    - Bile salts
    - Hormones
  - Types
    - LDL
      - Low density lipoprotien
      - 25% protein
      - 20% triglycerides
      - 55% cholesterol
      - Transport cholesterol
        - Where needed
        - Arterial smooth muscle
      - Decreased receptors for LDL —> blood cholesterol
      - Desirable level < 130 mg/dl
    - VLDL
      - Very low density lipoprotein
      - 10% protein
      - 65% triglycerides
      - 25% cholesterol
      - Increased number in high fat diets
      - Converted to LDL
    - HDL
      - High density lipoprotein
      - 50% protein
      - 37% triglycerides
      - 13% cholesterol
      - High level linked to lower risk of heart disease
      - Desirable level > 40 mg/dl
- Lipid profile test
  - Total cholesterol (TC) —— TC = HDL – (triglycerides/5)
  - TC > 200 indicates high risk
  - (TC/HDL) > 4 indicates high risk
- Reduction therapies
  - Dietary modification — Limit fat intake
  - Regular exercise — Raise HDL
  - Drugs
    - Block cholesterol synthesis
    - Increase cholesterol excretion

17

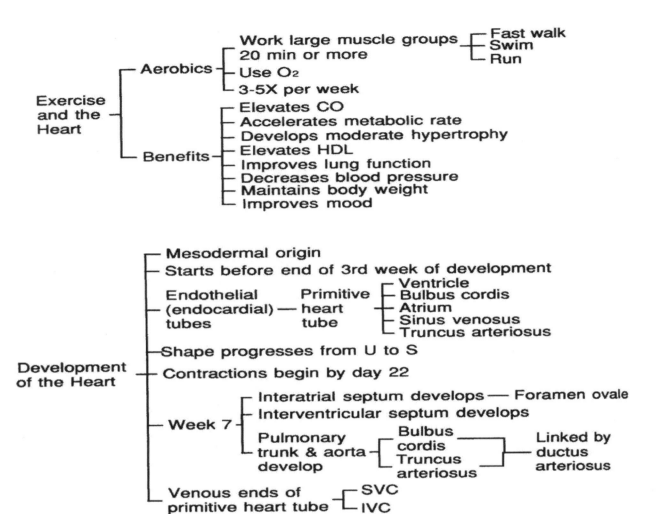

Exercise and the Heart
- Aerobics
  - Work large muscle groups
    - Fast walk
    - Swim
    - Run
  - 20 min or more
  - Use O$_2$
  - 3-5X per week
- Benefits
  - Elevates CO
  - Accelerates metabolic rate
  - Develops moderate hypertrophy
  - Elevates HDL
  - Improves lung function
  - Decreases blood pressure
  - Maintains body weight
  - Improves mood

Development of the Heart
- Mesodermal origin
- Starts before end of 3rd week of development
- Endothelial (endocardial) tubes — Primitive heart tube
  - Ventricle
  - Bulbus cordis
  - Atrium
  - Sinus venosus
  - Truncus arteriosus
- Shape progresses from U to S
- Contractions begin by day 22
- Week 7
  - Interatrial septum develops — Foramen ovale
  - Interventricular septum develops
  - Pulmonary trunk & aorta develop
    - Bulbus cordis
    - Truncus arteriosus
    - Linked by ductus arteriosus
- Venous ends of primitive heart tube
  - SVC
  - IVC

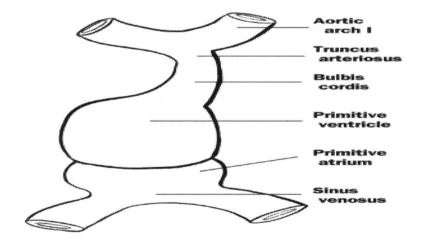

- Aortic arch I
- Truncus arteriosus
- Bulbis cordis
- Primitive ventricle
- Primitive atrium
- Sinus venosus

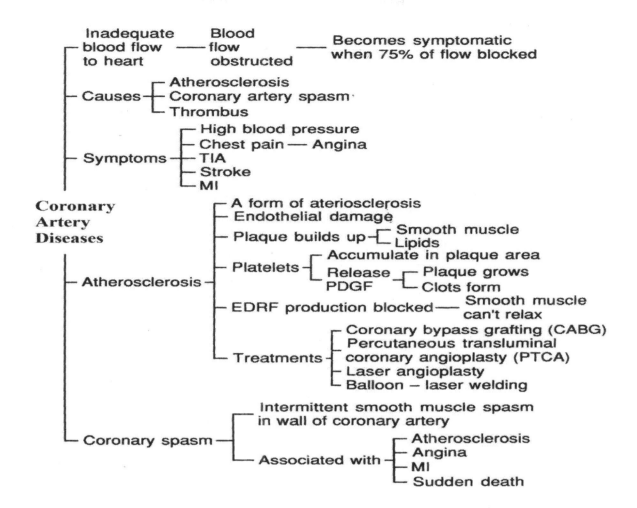

Inadequate blood flow to heart — Blood flow obstructed — Becomes symptomatic when 75% of flow blocked

Coronary Artery Diseases

- Causes
  - Atherosclerosis
  - Coronary artery spasm
  - Thrombus
- Symptoms
  - High blood pressure
  - Chest pain — Angina
  - TIA
  - Stroke
  - MI
- Atherosclerosis
  - A form of ateriosclerosis
  - Endothelial damage
  - Plaque builds up — Smooth muscle / Lipids
  - Platelets
    - Accumulate in plaque area
    - Release PDGF — Plaque grows / Clots form
  - EDRF production blocked — Smooth muscle can't relax
  - Treatments
    - Coronary bypass grafting (CABG)
    - Percutaneous transluminal coronary angioplasty (PTCA)
    - Laser angioplasty
    - Balloon — laser welding
- Coronary spasm
  - Intermittent smooth muscle spasm in wall of coronary artery
  - Associated with
    - Atherosclerosis
    - Angina
    - MI
    - Sudden death

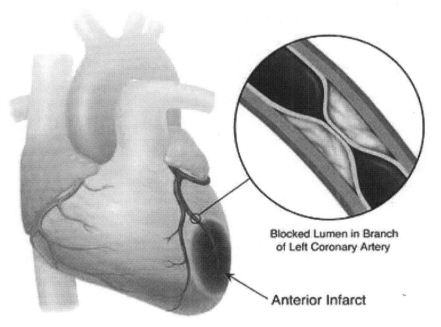

Blocked Lumen in Branch of Left Coronary Artery

Anterior Infarct

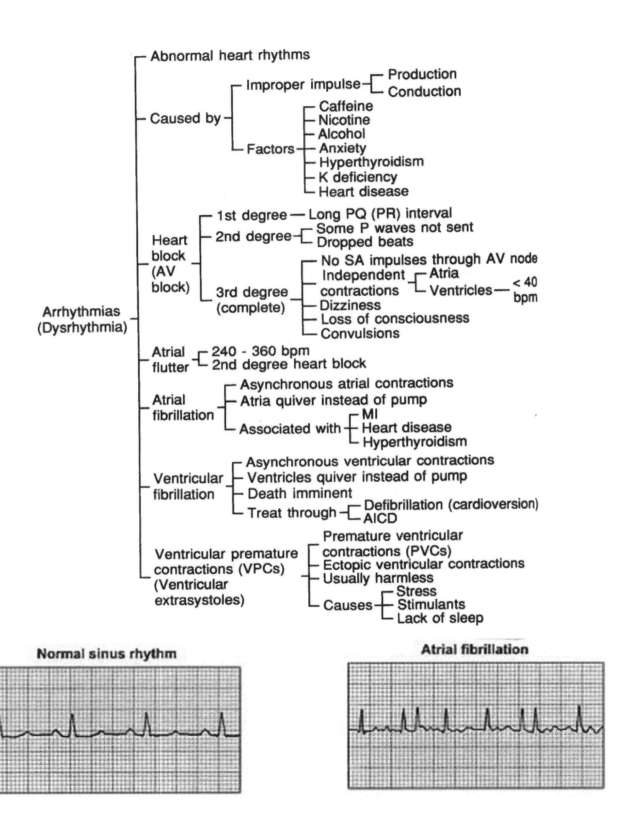

Arrhythmias (Dysrhythmia)

- Abnormal heart rhythms
- Caused by
  - Improper impulse
    - Production
    - Conduction
  - Factors
    - Caffeine
    - Nicotine
    - Alcohol
    - Anxiety
    - Hyperthyroidism
    - K deficiency
    - Heart disease
- Heart block (AV block)
  - 1st degree — Long PQ (PR) interval
  - 2nd degree
    - Some P waves not sent
    - Dropped beats
  - 3rd degree (complete)
    - No SA impulses through AV node
    - Independent contractions
      - Atria
      - Ventricles — < 40 bpm
    - Dizziness
    - Loss of consciousness
    - Convulsions
- Atrial flutter
  - 240 - 360 bpm
  - 2nd degree heart block
- Atrial fibrillation
  - Asynchronous atrial contractions
  - Atria quiver instead of pump
  - Associated with
    - MI
    - Heart disease
    - Hyperthyroidism
- Ventricular fibrillation
  - Asynchronous ventricular contractions
  - Ventricles quiver instead of pump
  - Death imminent
  - Treat through
    - Defibrillation (cardioversion)
    - AICD
- Ventricular premature contractions (VPCs) (Ventricular extrasystoles)
  - Premature ventricular contractions (PVCs)
  - Ectopic ventricular contractions
  - Usually harmless
  - Causes
    - Stress
    - Stimulants
    - Lack of sleep

Normal sinus rhythm

Atrial fibrillation

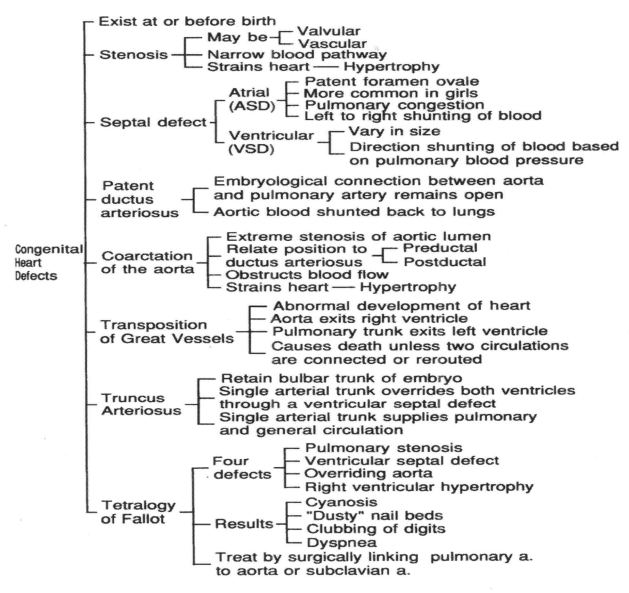

Congenital Heart Defects

- Exist at or before birth
- Stenosis
  - May be
    - Valvular
    - Vascular
  - Narrow blood pathway
  - Strains heart —— Hypertrophy
- Septal defect
  - Atrial (ASD)
    - Patent foramen ovale
    - More common in girls
    - Pulmonary congestion
    - Left to right shunting of blood
  - Ventricular (VSD)
    - Vary in size
    - Direction shunting of blood based on pulmonary blood pressure
- Patent ductus arteriosus
  - Embryological connection between aorta and pulmonary artery remains open
  - Aortic blood shunted back to lungs
- Coarctation of the aorta
  - Extreme stenosis of aortic lumen
  - Relate position to ductus arteriosus
    - Preductal
    - Postductal
  - Obstructs blood flow
  - Strains heart —— Hypertrophy
- Transposition of Great Vessels
  - Abnormal development of heart
  - Aorta exits right ventricle
  - Pulmonary trunk exits left ventricle
  - Causes death unless two circulations are connected or rerouted
- Truncus Arteriosus
  - Retain bulbar trunk of embryo
  - Single arterial trunk overrides both ventricles through a ventricular septal defect
  - Single arterial trunk supplies pulmonary and general circulation
- Tetralogy of Fallot
  - Four defects
    - Pulmonary stenosis
    - Ventricular septal defect
    - Overriding aorta
    - Right ventricular hypertrophy
  - Results
    - Cyanosis
    - "Dusty" nail beds
    - Clubbing of digits
    - Dyspnea
  - Treat by surgically linking pulmonary a. to aorta or subclavian a.

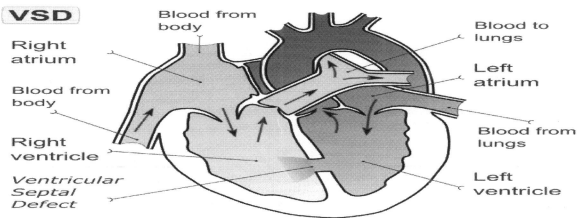

VSD

Right atrium

Blood from body

Blood from body

Right ventricle

Ventricular Septal Defect

Blood to lungs

Left atrium

Blood from lungs

Left ventricle

21

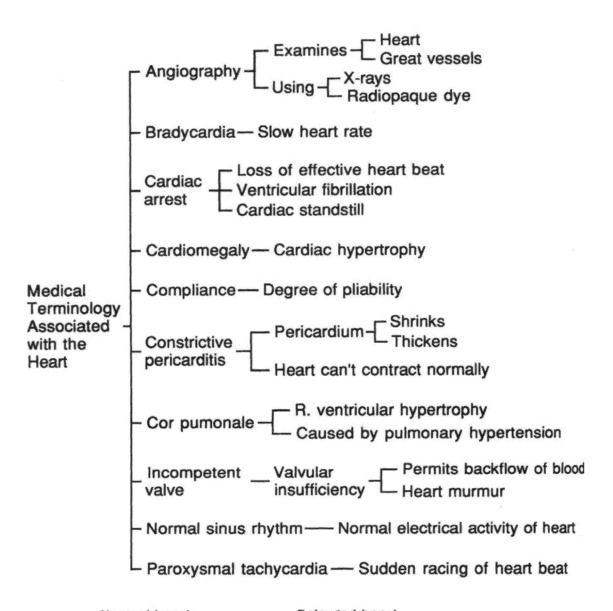

Medical Terminology Associated with the Heart

- Angiography
  - Examines
    - Heart
    - Great vessels
  - Using
    - X-rays
    - Radiopaque dye
- Bradycardia — Slow heart rate
- Cardiac arrest
  - Loss of effective heart beat
  - Ventricular fibrillation
  - Cardiac standstill
- Cardiomegaly — Cardiac hypertrophy
- Compliance — Degree of pliability
- Constrictive pericarditis
  - Pericardium
    - Shrinks
    - Thickens
  - Heart can't contract normally
- Cor pumonale
  - R. ventricular hypertrophy
  - Caused by pulmonary hypertension
- Incompetent valve — Valvular insufficiency
  - Permits backflow of blood
  - Heart murmur
- Normal sinus rhythm —— Normal electrical activity of heart
- Paroxysmal tachycardia — Sudden racing of heart beat

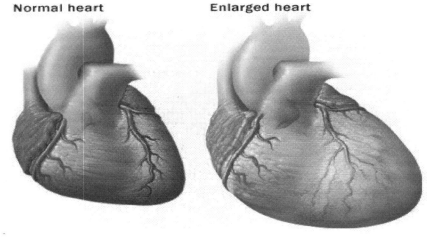

Normal heart   Enlarged heart

CHAPTER TWENTY ONE

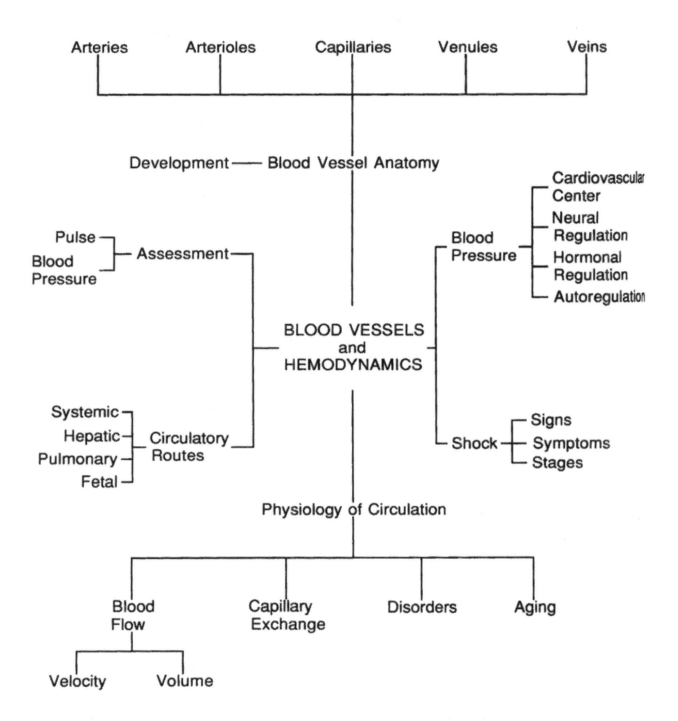

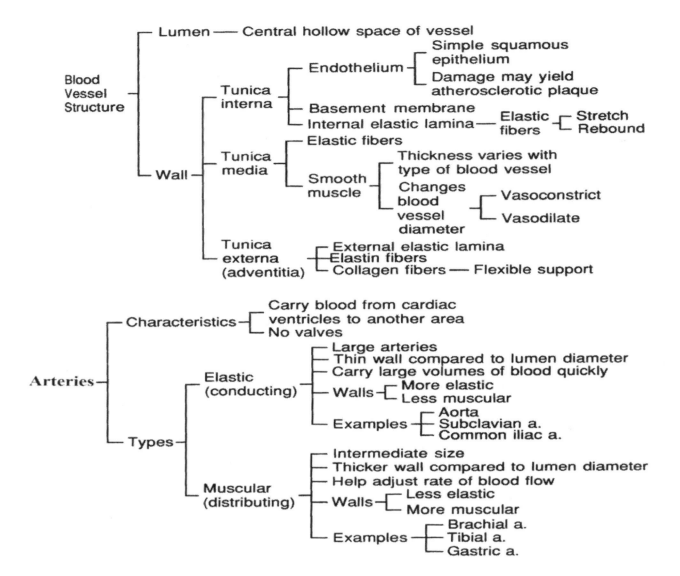

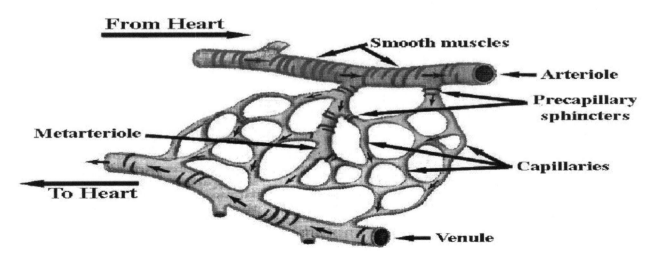

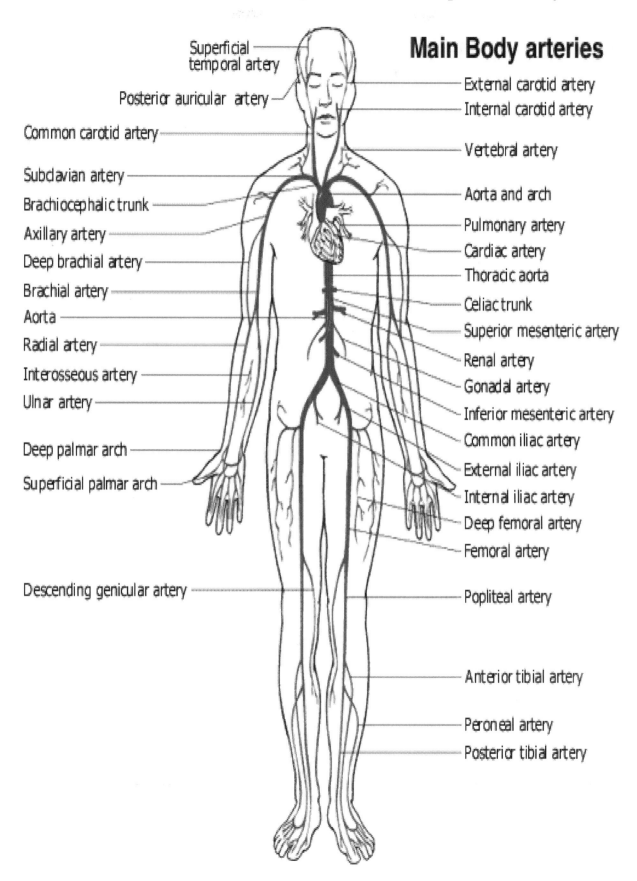

Main Body arteries

Superficial temporal artery

Posterior auricular artery

Common carotid artery

Subclavian artery

Brachiocephalic trunk

Axillary artery

Deep brachial artery

Brachial artery

Aorta

Radial artery

Interosseous artery

Ulnar artery

Deep palmar arch

Superficial palmar arch

Descending genicular artery

External carotid artery

Internal carotid artery

Vertebral artery

Aorta and arch

Pulmonary artery

Cardiac artery

Thoracic aorta

Celiac trunk

Superior mesenteric artery

Renal artery

Gonadal artery

Inferior mesenteric artery

Common iliac artery

External iliac artery

Internal iliac artery

Deep femoral artery

Femoral artery

Popliteal artery

Anterior tibial artery

Peroneal artery

Posterior tibial artery

Anastomoses
- Direct connection of 2 or more blood vessels serving area
- Occur
  - Artery to artery
  - Vein to vein
  - Arteriole to venule
- Allow collateral circulation
- End arteries
  - Do not network with other arteries
  - Damage yields necrosis of area served

Arterioles
- Nearly microscopic
- Structure varies
  - More like arteries at origin
  - More like capillaries at distal end
- Major site of blood pressure regulation — Smooth muscle controls peripheral resistance
  - Vasoconstrict — BP up
  - Vasodilate — BP down
- Metarterioles
  - Direct route through capillary bed
  - Help regulate blood flow

Capillaries
- Sites of exchange between cells and blood
  - Gases
  - Nutrients
  - Wastes
- Type & extent varies with tissue needs
- Blood flow regulated
  - Metarterioles
  - Precapillary sphincter
- Vasomotion
  - Blood flow through capillaries
  - Intermittent — 5-10 times/minute
- Materials enter/exit
  - Intracellular clefts — Pinocytotic vesicles
  - Endothelial membranes
  - Fenestrations
- Types
  - True
  - Continuous
  - Fenestrated
  - Sinusoids

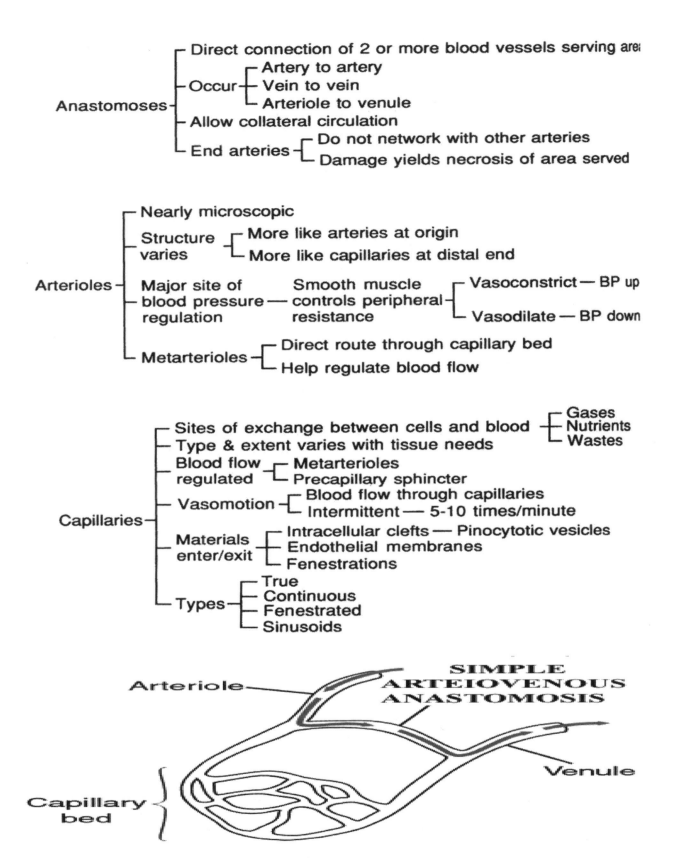

Arteriole

SIMPLE ARTEIOVENOUS ANASTOMOSIS

Venule

Capillary bed

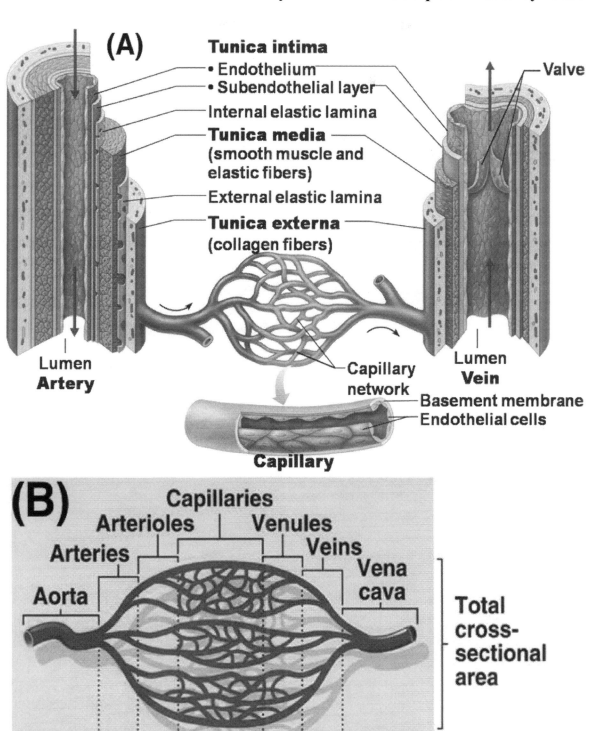

(A)

Tunica intima
- Endothelium
- Subendothelial layer

Internal elastic lamina

Tunica media
(smooth muscle and
elastic fibers)

External elastic lamina

Tunica externa
(collagen fibers)

Valve

Lumen
Artery

Capillary
network

Lumen
Vein

Basement membrane
Endothelial cells

Capillary

(B)

Capillaries

Arterioles   Venules

Arteries   Veins

Aorta   Vena
                                       cava

Total
cross-
sectional
area

Velocity of
blood flow
(mL/s)

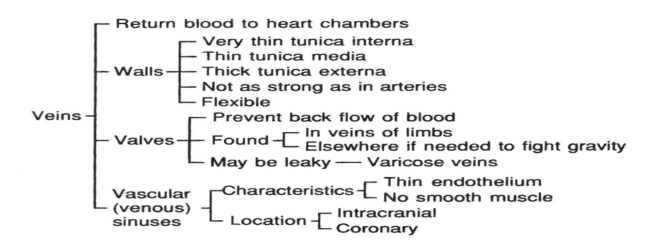

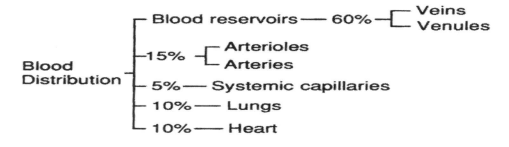

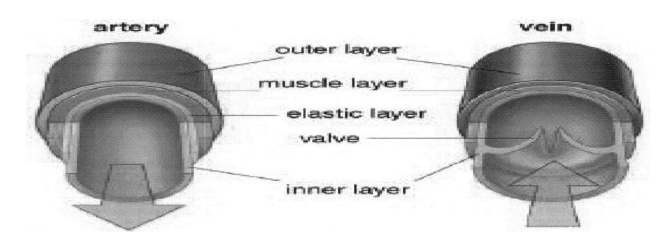

DISTRIBUTION OF BLOOD IN THE BODY AT REST

Blood flow to the major organs is represented in three ways: as a percentage of total flow, as volume per 100 grams of tissue per minute, and as an absolute rate of flow (in L/min).

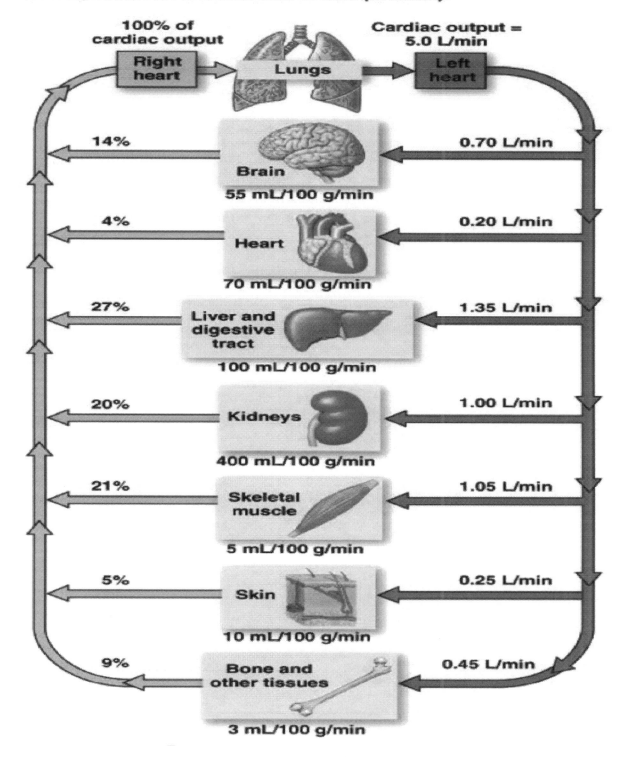

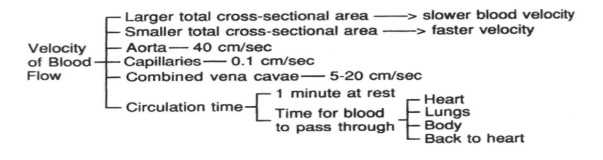

Velocity of Blood Flow
- Larger total cross-sectional area ——> slower blood velocity
- Smaller total cross-sectional area ——> faster velocity
- Aorta —— 40 cm/sec
- Capillaries —— 0.1 cm/sec
- Combined vena cavae —— 5-20 cm/sec
- Circulation time
  - 1 minute at rest
  - Time for blood to pass through
    - Heart
    - Lungs
    - Body
    - Back to heart

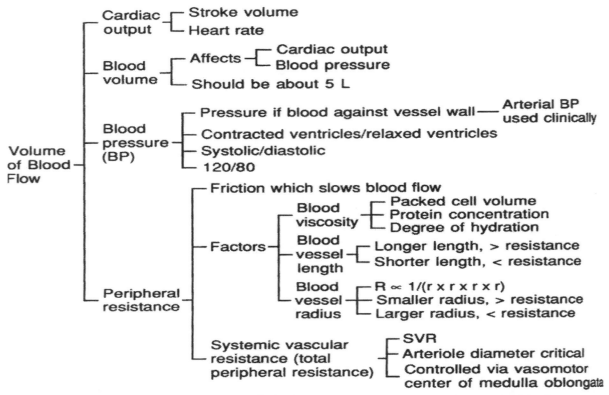

Volume of Blood Flow
- Cardiac output
  - Stroke volume
  - Heart rate
- Blood volume
  - Affects
    - Cardiac output
    - Blood pressure
  - Should be about 5 L
- Blood pressure (BP)
  - Pressure if blood against vessel wall —— Arterial BP used clinically
  - Contracted ventricles/relaxed ventricles
  - Systolic/diastolic
  - 120/80
- Peripheral resistance
  - Friction which slows blood flow
  - Factors
    - Blood viscosity
      - Packed cell volume
      - Protein concentration
      - Degree of hydration
    - Blood vessel length
      - Longer length, > resistance
      - Shorter length, < resistance
    - Blood vessel radius
      - $R \propto 1/(r \times r \times r \times r)$
      - Smaller radius, > resistance
      - Larger radius, < resistance
  - Systemic vascular resistance (total peripheral resistance)
    - SVR
    - Arteriole diameter critical
    - Controlled via vasomotor center of medulla oblongata

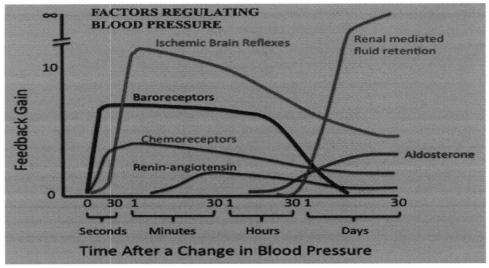

FACTORS REGULATING BLOOD PRESSURE

Ischemic Brain Reflexes
Renal mediated fluid retention
Baroreceptors
Chemoreceptors
Aldosterone
Renin-angiotensin

Feedback Gain

Time After a Change in Blood Pressure

Seconds | Minutes | Hours | Days

Blood Vessel Diameter, Cross Sectional Area, Blood Pressure And Velocity Of Blood Flow In Different Types Of Blood Vessels

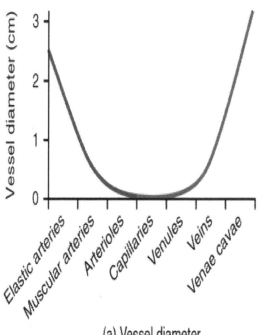

(a) Vessel diameter

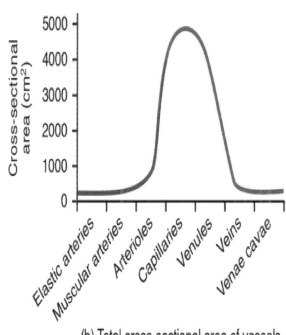

(b) Total cross-sectional area of vessels

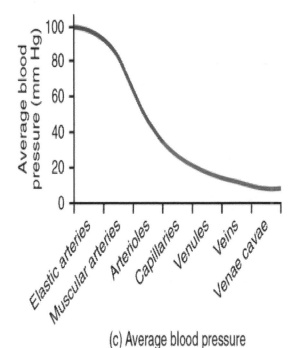

(c) Average blood pressure

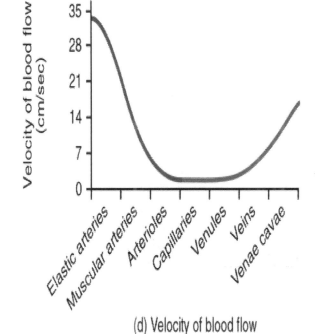

(d) Velocity of blood flow

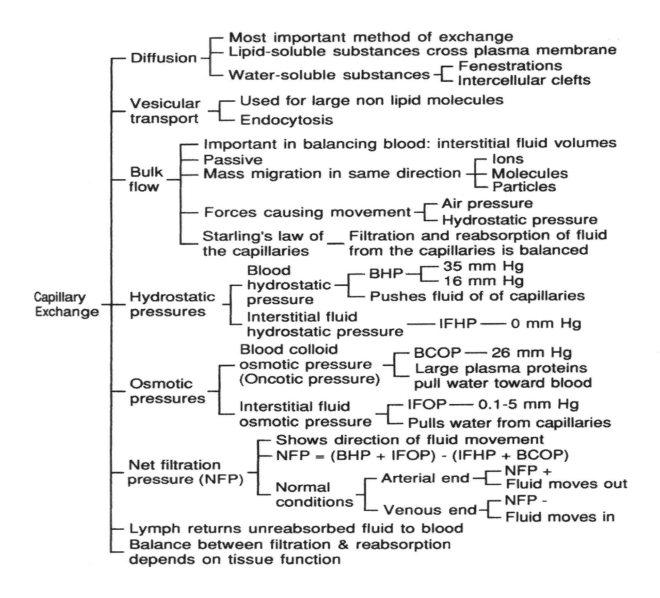

Capillary Exchange
- Diffusion
  - Most important method of exchange
  - Lipid-soluble substances cross plasma membrane
  - Water-soluble substances
    - Fenestrations
    - Intercellular clefts
- Vesicular transport
  - Used for large non lipid molecules
  - Endocytosis
- Bulk flow
  - Important in balancing blood: interstitial fluid volumes
  - Passive
  - Mass migration in same direction
    - Ions
    - Molecules
    - Particles
  - Forces causing movement
    - Air pressure
    - Hydrostatic pressure
  - Starling's law of the capillaries — Filtration and reabsorption of fluid from the capillaries is balanced
- Hydrostatic pressures
  - Blood hydrostatic pressure
    - BHP
      - 35 mm Hg
      - 16 mm Hg
    - Pushes fluid of of capillaries
  - Interstitial fluid hydrostatic pressure — IFHP — 0 mm Hg
- Osmotic pressures
  - Blood colloid osmotic pressure (Oncotic pressure)
    - BCOP — 26 mm Hg
    - Large plasma proteins pull water toward blood
  - Interstitial fluid osmotic pressure
    - IFOP — 0.1-5 mm Hg
    - Pulls water from capillaries
- Net filtration pressure (NFP)
  - Shows direction of fluid movement
  - NFP = (BHP + IFOP) - (IFHP + BCOP)
  - Normal conditions
    - Arterial end
      - NFP +
      - Fluid moves out
    - Venous end
      - NFP -
      - Fluid moves in
- Lymph returns unreabsorbed fluid to blood
- Balance between filtration & reabsorption depends on tissue function

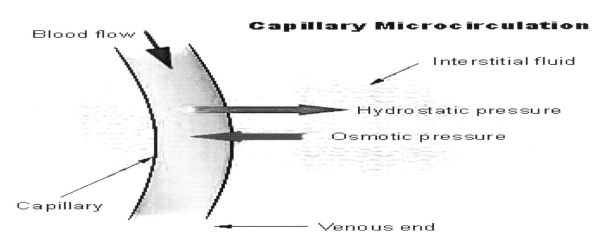

Capillary Microcirculation

Blood flow

Interstitial fluid

Hydrostatic pressure

Osmotic pressure

Capillary

Venous end

The primary function of capillaries is to allow the exchange of materials between the blood and tissue cells

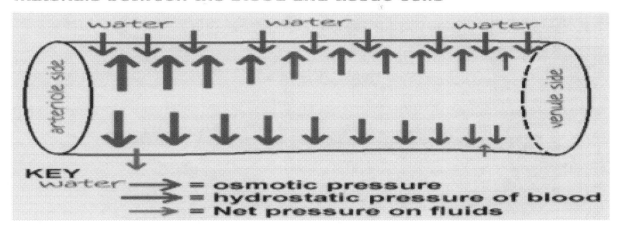

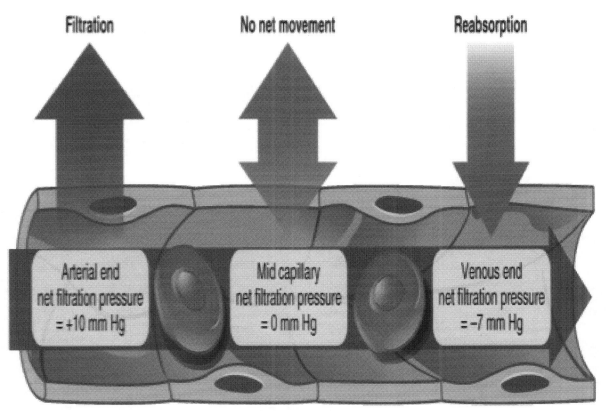

Filtration   No net movement   Reabsorption

Arterial end net filtration pressure = +10 mm Hg	Mid capillary net filtration pressure = 0 mm Hg	Venous end net filtration pressure = –7 mm Hg

Fluid exits capillary since capillary hydrostatic pressure (35 mm Hg) is greater than blood colloidal osmotic pressure (25 mm Hg)	No net movement of fluid since capillary hydrostatic pressure (25 mm Hg) = blood colloidal osmotic pressure (25 mm Hg)	Fluid re-enters capillary since capillary hydrostatic pressure (18 mm Hg) is less than blood colloidal osmotic pressure (25 mm Hg)

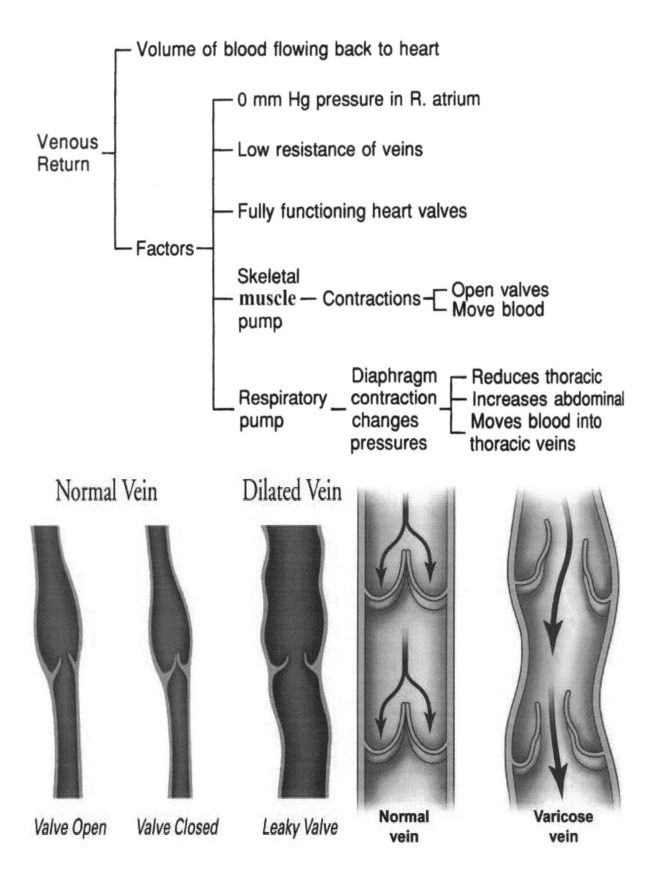

Volume of blood flowing back to heart

Venous Return

Factors
- 0 mm Hg pressure in R. atrium
- Low resistance of veins
- Fully functioning heart valves
- Skeletal **muscle** pump — Contractions — Open valves / Move blood
- Respiratory pump — Diaphragm contraction changes pressures — Reduces thoracic / Increases abdominal / Moves blood into thoracic veins

Normal Vein

Dilated Vein

Valve Open   Valve Closed   Leaky Valve   **Normal vein**   **Varicose vein**

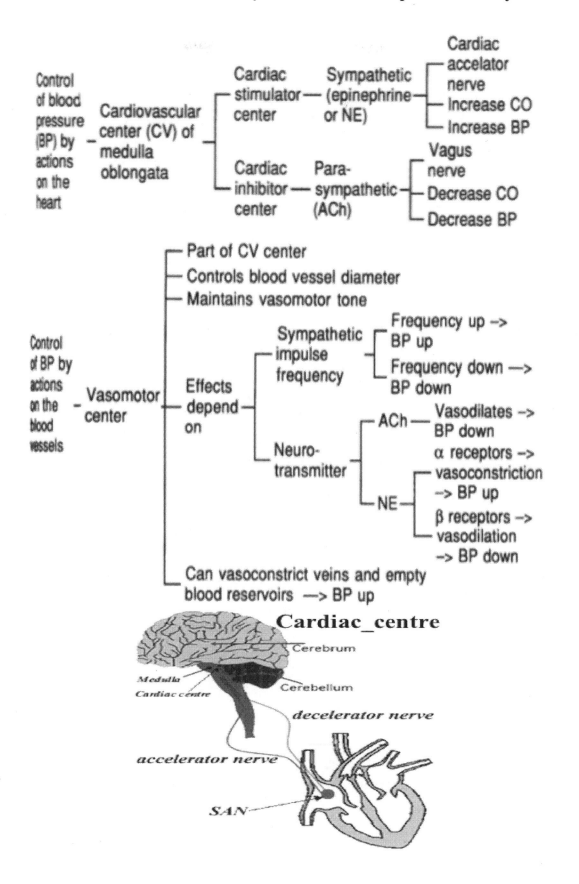

Control of blood pressure (BP) by actions on the heart — Cardiovascular center (CV) of medulla oblongata

Cardiac stimulator center — Sympathetic (epinephrine or NE)
- Cardiac accelator nerve
- Increase CO
- Increase BP

Cardiac inhibitor center — Para-sympathetic (ACh)
- Vagus nerve
- Decrease CO
- Decrease BP

Control of BP by actions on the blood vessels — Vasomotor center
- Part of CV center
- Controls blood vessel diameter
- Maintains vasomotor tone
- Effects depend on
  - Sympathetic impulse frequency
    - Frequency up –> BP up
    - Frequency down —> BP down
  - Neuro-transmitter
    - ACh — Vasodilates –> BP down
    - NE
      - α receptors –> vasoconstriction –> BP up
      - β receptors –> vasodilation –> BP down
- Can vasoconstrict veins and empty blood reservoirs —> BP up

Cardiac_centre

Cerebrum
Medulla
Cardiac centre
Cerebellum
decelerator nerve
accelerator nerve
SAN

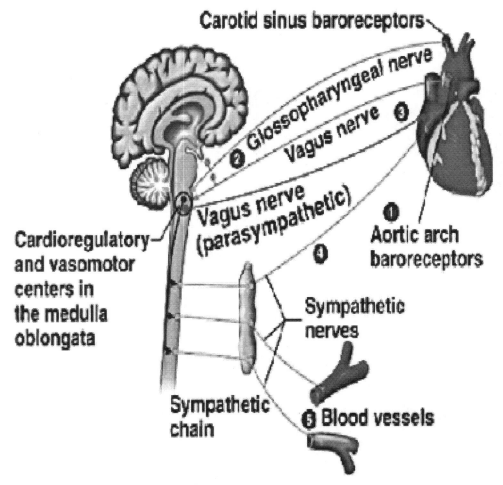

Carotid sinus baroreceptors

Glossopharyngeal nerve

❷ Glossopharyngeal nerve

Vagus nerve ❸

Vagus nerve (parasympathetic)

Cardioregulatory and vasomotor centers in the medulla oblongata

Aortic arch baroreceptors ❶

❹

Sympathetic nerves

Sympathetic chain

❺ Blood vessels

Cardiac Output Regulation

* Pumping ability of the heart is a function of the beats per minute and the volume of blood ejected per beat.

* CO = SV x HR

* Total blood volume averages about 5.5 liters.

* Each ventricle pumps the equivalent amount of blood.

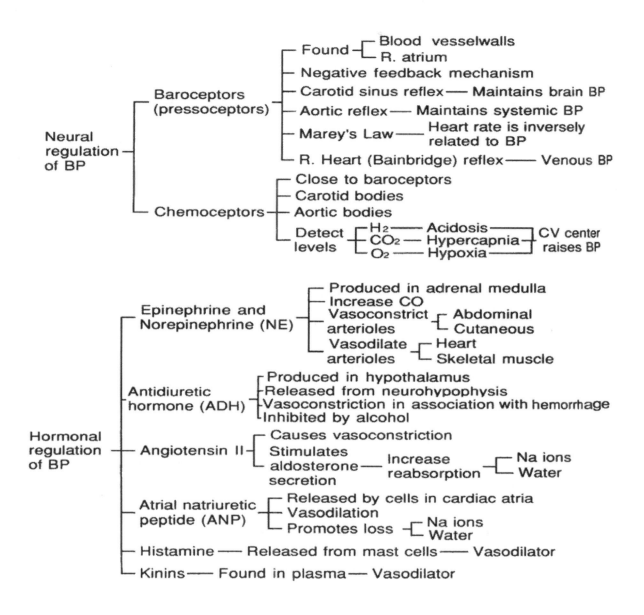

Neural regulation of BP
- Baroceptors (pressoceptors)
  - Found
    - Blood vessel walls
    - R. atrium
  - Negative feedback mechanism
  - Carotid sinus reflex —— Maintains brain BP
  - Aortic reflex —— Maintains systemic BP
  - Marey's Law —— Heart rate is inversely related to BP
  - R. Heart (Bainbridge) reflex —— Venous BP
- Chemoceptors
  - Close to baroceptors
  - Carotid bodies
  - Aortic bodies
  - Detect levels
    - H_2 —— Acidosis
    - CO_2 —— Hypercapnia
    - O_2 —— Hypoxia
    - CV center raises BP

Hormonal regulation of BP
- Epinephrine and Norepinephrine (NE)
  - Produced in adrenal medulla
  - Increase CO
  - Vasoconstrict arterioles
    - Abdominal
    - Cutaneous
  - Vasodilate arterioles
    - Heart
    - Skeletal muscle
- Antidiuretic hormone (ADH)
  - Produced in hypothalamus
  - Released from neurohypophysis
  - Vasoconstriction in association with hemorrhage
  - Inhibited by alcohol
- Angiotensin II
  - Causes vasoconstriction
  - Stimulates aldosterone secretion —— Increase reabsorption
    - Na ions
    - Water
- Atrial natriuretic peptide (ANP)
  - Released by cells in cardiac atria
  - Vasodilation
  - Promotes loss
    - Na ions
    - Water
- Histamine —— Released from mast cells —— Vasodilator
- Kinins —— Found in plasma —— Vasodilator

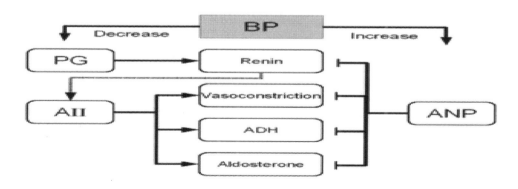

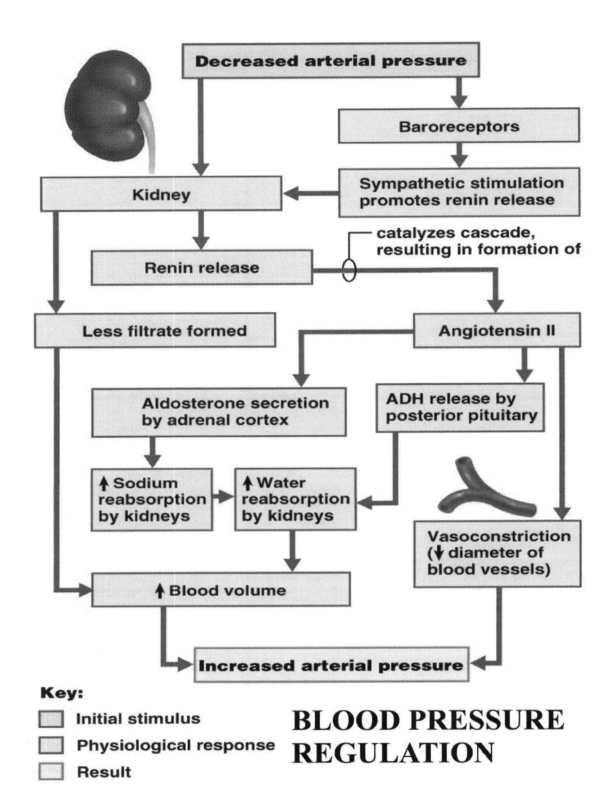

Key:

☐ Initial stimulus

☐ Physiological response

☐ Result

BLOOD PRESSURE REGULATION

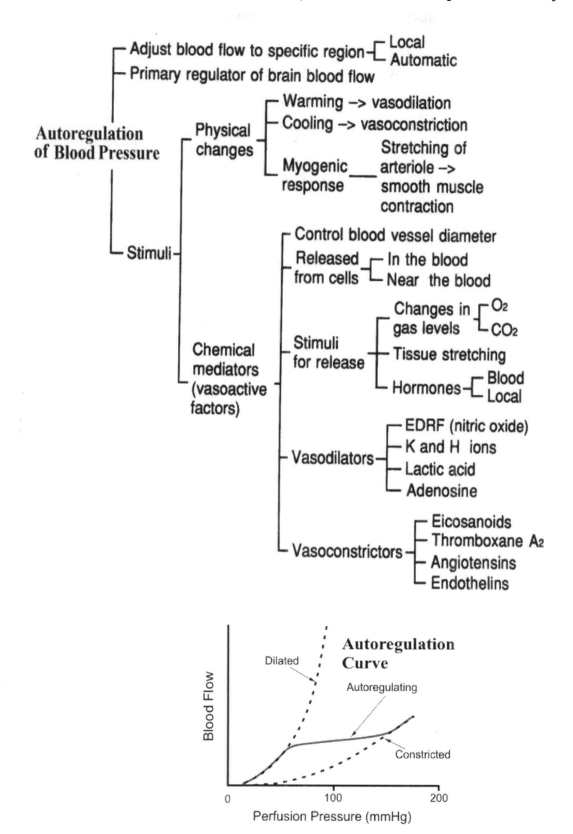

Autoregulation of Blood Pressure
- Adjust blood flow to specific region
  - Local
  - Automatic
- Primary regulator of brain blood flow
- Stimuli
  - Physical changes
    - Warming –> vasodilation
    - Cooling –> vasoconstriction
    - Myogenic response — Stretching of arteriole –> smooth muscle contraction
  - Chemical mediators (vasoactive factors)
    - Control blood vessel diameter
    - Released from cells
      - In the blood
      - Near the blood
    - Stimuli for release
      - Changes in gas levels
        - O_2
        - CO_2
      - Tissue stretching
      - Hormones
        - Blood
        - Local
    - Vasodilators
      - EDRF (nitric oxide)
      - K and H ions
      - Lactic acid
      - Adenosine
    - Vasoconstrictors
      - Eicosanoids
      - Thromboxane A_2
      - Angiotensins
      - Endothelins

Autoregulation Curve

Blood Flow (y-axis)

Dilated

Autoregulating

Constricted

Perfusion Pressure (mmHg) (x-axis): 0, 100, 200

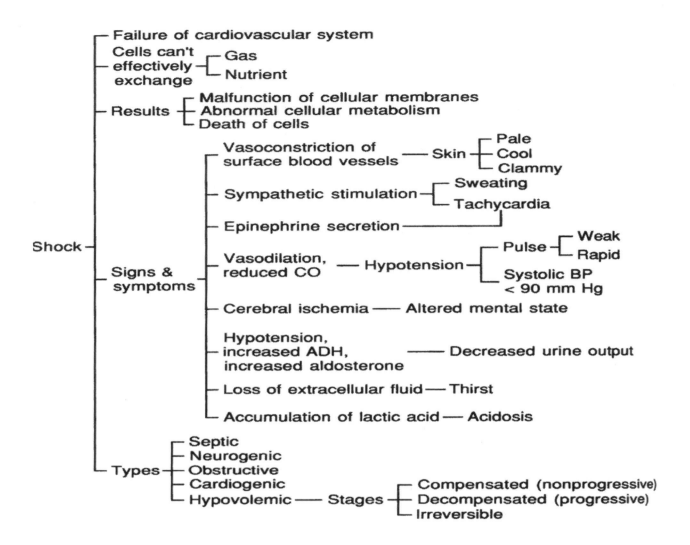

Shock
- Failure of cardiovascular system
- Cells can't effectively exchange
  - Gas
  - Nutrient
- Results
  - Malfunction of cellular membranes
  - Abnormal cellular metabolism
  - Death of cells
- Signs & symptoms
  - Vasoconstriction of surface blood vessels — Skin
    - Pale
    - Cool
    - Clammy
  - Sympathetic stimulation
    - Sweating
    - Tachycardia
  - Epinephrine secretion
  - Vasodilation, reduced CO — Hypotension
    - Pulse
      - Weak
      - Rapid
    - Systolic BP < 90 mm Hg
  - Cerebral ischemia — Altered mental state
  - Hypotension, increased ADH, increased aldosterone — Decreased urine output
  - Loss of extracellular fluid — Thirst
  - Accumulation of lactic acid — Acidosis
- Types
  - Septic
  - Neurogenic
  - Obstructive
  - Cardiogenic
  - Hypovolemic — Stages
    - Compensated (nonprogressive)
    - Decompensated (progressive)
    - Irreversible

- Place the victim in shock position
- Keep the person warm and comfortable
- Turn the victim's head to one side if neck injury is not suspected

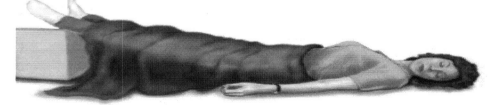

ADAM.

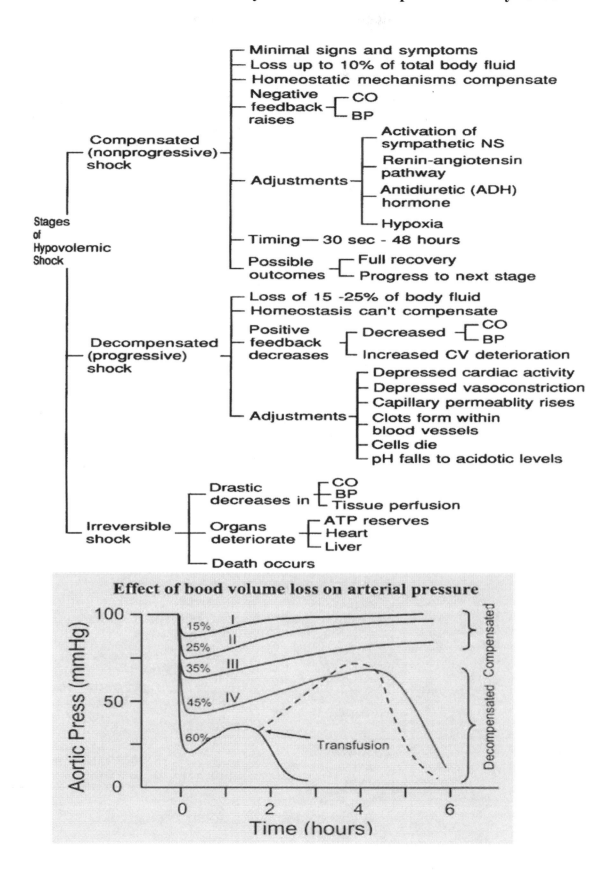

Stages of Hypovolemic Shock

Compensated (nonprogressive) shock
- Minimal signs and symptoms
- Loss up to 10% of total body fluid
- Homeostatic mechanisms compensate
- Negative feedback raises
  - CO
  - BP
- Adjustments
  - Activation of sympathetic NS
  - Renin-angiotensin pathway
  - Antidiuretic (ADH) hormone
  - Hypoxia
- Timing — 30 sec - 48 hours
- Possible outcomes
  - Full recovery
  - Progress to next stage

Decompensated (progressive) shock
- Loss of 15 -25% of body fluid
- Homeostasis can't compensate
- Positive feedback decreases
  - Decreased
    - CO
    - BP
  - Increased CV deterioration
- Adjustments
  - Depressed cardiac activity
  - Depressed vasoconstriction
  - Capillary permeablity rises
  - Clots form within blood vessels
  - Cells die
  - pH falls to acidotic levels

Irreversible shock
- Drastic decreases in
  - CO
  - BP
  - Tissue perfusion
- Organs deteriorate
  - ATP reserves
  - Heart
  - Liver
- Death occurs

Effect of bood volume loss on arterial pressure

Aortic Press (mmHg) vs Time (hours)

100
15% I
25% II
35% III
45% IV
60%
50
Transfusion
0

Time (hours): 0   2   4   6

Compensated
Decompensated

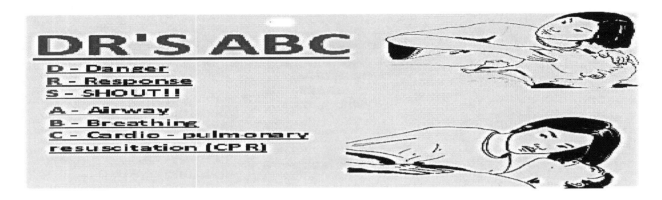

DR'S ABC

D - Danger
R - Response
S - SHOUT!!

A - Airway
B - Breathing
C - Cardio - pulmonary resuscitation (CPR)

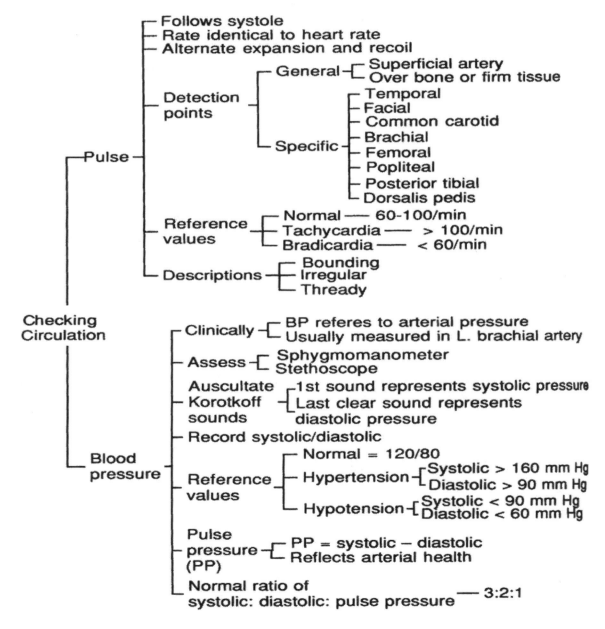

Checking Circulation

- Pulse
  - Follows systole
  - Rate identical to heart rate
  - Alternate expansion and recoil
  - Detection points
    - General
      - Superficial artery
      - Over bone or firm tissue
    - Specific
      - Temporal
      - Facial
      - Common carotid
      - Brachial
      - Femoral
      - Popliteal
      - Posterior tibial
      - Dorsalis pedis
  - Reference values
    - Normal — 60-100/min
    - Tachycardia — > 100/min
    - Bradicardia — < 60/min
  - Descriptions
    - Bounding
    - Irregular
    - Thready

- Blood pressure
  - Clinically
    - BP referes to arterial pressure
    - Usually measured in L. brachial artery
  - Assess
    - Sphygmomanometer
    - Stethoscope
  - Auscultate Korotkoff sounds
    - 1st sound represents systolic pressure
    - Last clear sound represents diastolic pressure
  - Record systolic/diastolic
  - Reference values
    - Normal = 120/80
    - Hypertension
      - Systolic > 160 mm Hg
      - Diastolic > 90 mm Hg
    - Hypotension
      - Systolic < 90 mm Hg
      - Diastolic < 60 mm Hg
  - Pulse pressure (PP)
    - PP = systolic − diastolic
    - Reflects arterial health
  - Normal ratio of systolic: diastolic: pulse pressure — 3:2:1

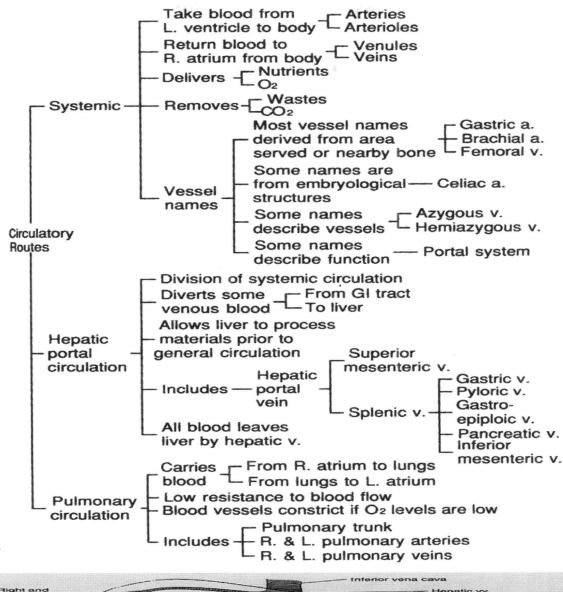

- Circulatory Routes
  - Systemic
    - Take blood from L. ventricle to body
      - Arteries
      - Arterioles
    - Return blood to R. atrium from body
      - Venules
      - Veins
    - Delivers
      - Nutrients
      - O_2
    - Removes
      - Wastes
      - CO_2
    - Vessel names
      - Most vessel names derived from area served or nearby bone
        - Gastric a.
        - Brachial a.
        - Femoral v.
      - Some names are from embryological structures — Celiac a.
      - Some names describe vessels
        - Azygous v.
        - Hemiazygous v.
      - Some names describe function — Portal system
  - Hepatic portal circulation
    - Division of systemic circulation
    - Diverts some venous blood
      - From GI tract
      - To liver
    - Allows liver to process materials prior to general circulation
    - Includes — Hepatic portal vein
      - Superior mesenteric v.
      - Splenic v.
        - Gastric v.
        - Pyloric v.
        - Gastro-epiploic v.
        - Pancreatic v.
        - Inferior mesenteric v.
    - All blood leaves liver by hepatic v.
  - Pulmonary circulation
    - Carries blood
      - From R. atrium to lungs
      - From lungs to L. atrium
    - Low resistance to blood flow
    - Blood vessels constrict if O_2 levels are low
    - Includes
      - Pulmonary trunk
      - R. & L. pulmonary arteries
      - R. & L. pulmonary veins

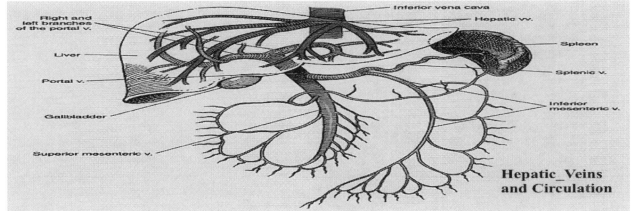

Right and left branches of the portal v.
Liver
Portal v.
Gallbladder
Superior mesenteric v.
Inferior vena cava
Hepatic vv.
Spleen
Splenic v.
Inferior mesenteric v.

Hepatic_Veins and Circulation

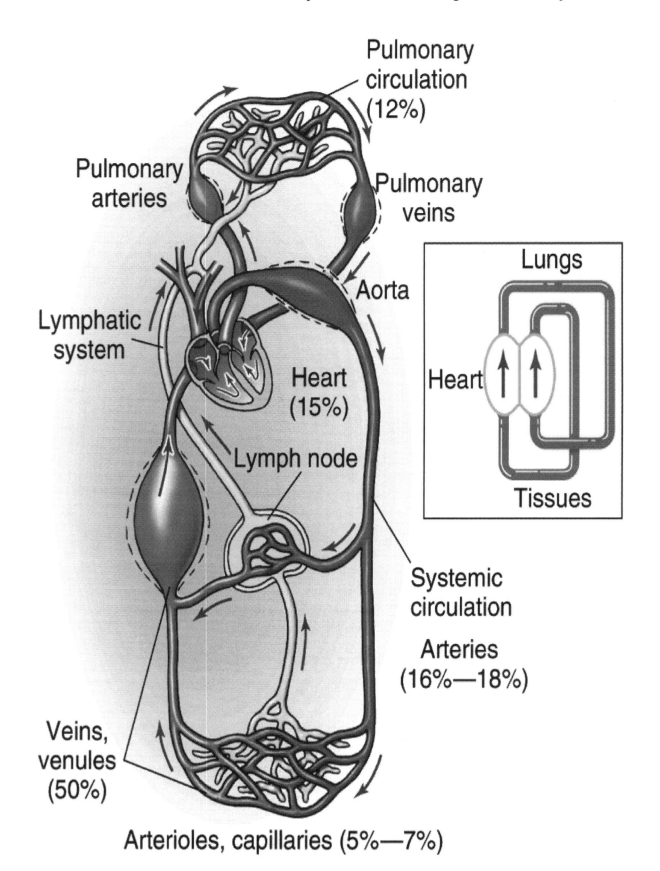

Pulmonary
circulation
(12%)

Pulmonary
arteries

Pulmonary
veins

Lymphatic
system

Aorta

Heart
(15%)

Lymph node

Lungs

Heart

Tissues

Systemic
circulation

Arteries
(16%—18%)

Veins,
venules
(50%)

Arterioles, capillaries (5%—7%)

CHAPTER TWENTY TWO

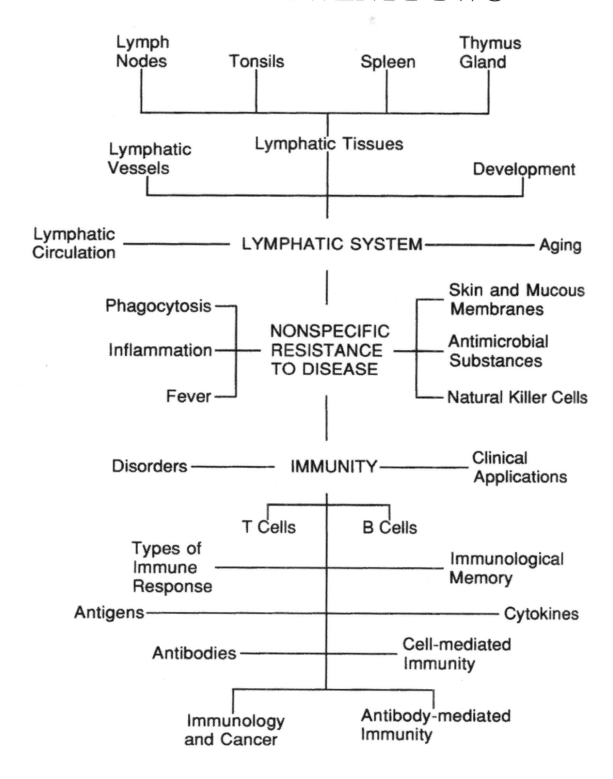

Lymph Nodes   Tonsils   Spleen   Thymus Gland

Lymphatic Tissues

Lymphatic Vessels

Development

Lymphatic Circulation —— LYMPHATIC SYSTEM —— Aging

Phagocytosis

Inflammation

Fever

NONSPECIFIC RESISTANCE TO DISEASE

Skin and Mucous Membranes

Antimicrobial Substances

Natural Killer Cells

Disorders —— IMMUNITY —— Clinical Applications

T Cells   B Cells

Types of Immune Response —— Immunological Memory

Antigens —— Cytokines

Antibodies —— Cell-mediated Immunity

Immunology and Cancer   Antibody-mediated Immunity

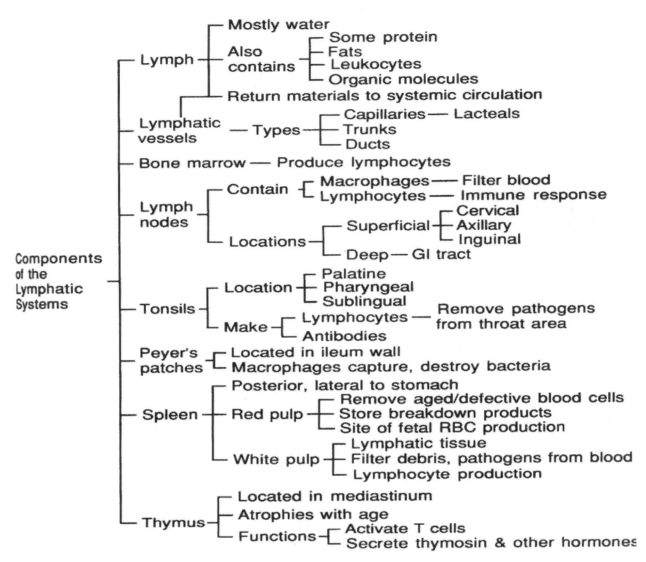

Components of the Lymphatic Systems
- Lymph
  - Mostly water
  - Also contains
    - Some protein
    - Fats
    - Leukocytes
    - Organic molecules
  - Return materials to systemic circulation
- Lymphatic vessels — Types
  - Capillaries — Lacteals
  - Trunks
  - Ducts
- Bone marrow — Produce lymphocytes
- Lymph nodes
  - Contain
    - Macrophages — Filter blood
    - Lymphocytes — Immune response
  - Locations
    - Superficial
      - Cervical
      - Axillary
      - Inguinal
    - Deep — GI tract
- Tonsils
  - Location
    - Palatine
    - Pharyngeal
    - Sublingual
  - Make
    - Lymphocytes — Remove pathogens from throat area
    - Antibodies
- Peyer's patches
  - Located in ileum wall
  - Macrophages capture, destroy bacteria
- Spleen
  - Posterior, lateral to stomach
  - Red pulp
    - Remove aged/defective blood cells
    - Store breakdown products
    - Site of fetal RBC production
  - White pulp
    - Lymphatic tissue
    - Filter debris, pathogens from blood
    - Lymphocyte production
- Thymus
  - Located in mediastinum
  - Atrophies with age
  - Functions
    - Activate T cells
    - Secrete thymosin & other hormones

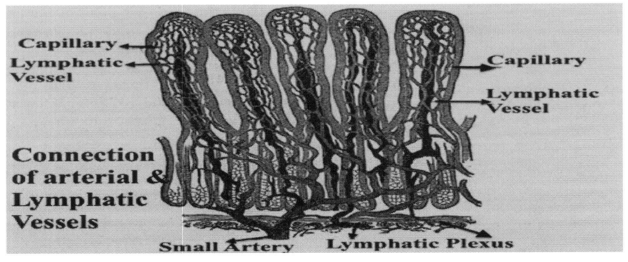

Connection of arterial & Lymphatic Vessels

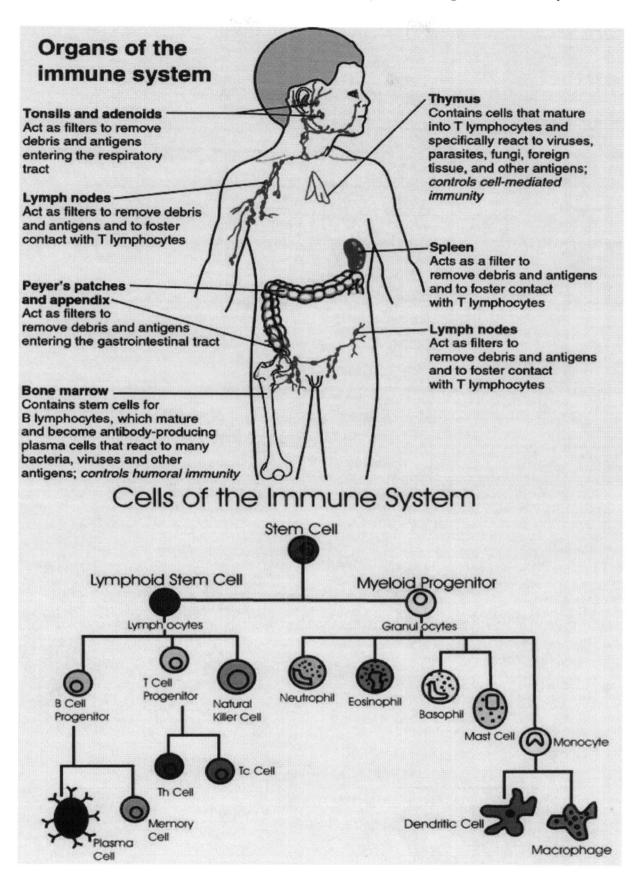

Organs of the immune system

Tonsils and adenoids
Act as filters to remove debris and antigens entering the respiratory tract

Lymph nodes
Act as filters to remove debris and antigens and to foster contact with T lymphocytes

Peyer's patches and appendix
Act as filters to remove debris and antigens entering the gastrointestinal tract

Bone marrow
Contains stem cells for B lymphocytes, which mature and become antibody-producing plasma cells that react to many bacteria, viruses and other antigens; *controls humoral immunity*

Thymus
Contains cells that mature into T lymphocytes and specifically react to viruses, parasites, fungi, foreign tissue, and other antigens; *controls cell-mediated immunity*

Spleen
Acts as a filter to remove debris and antigens and to foster contact with T lymphocytes

Lymph nodes
Act as filters to remove debris and antigens and to foster contact with T lymphocytes

Cells of the Immune System

Stem Cell

Lymphoid Stem Cell

Myeloid Progenitor

Lymphocytes

Granulocytes

B Cell Progenitor

T Cell Progenitor

Natural Killer Cell

Neutrophil

Eosinophil

Basophil

Mast Cell

Monocyte

Th Cell

Tc Cell

Plasma Cell

Memory Cell

Dendritic Cell

Macrophage

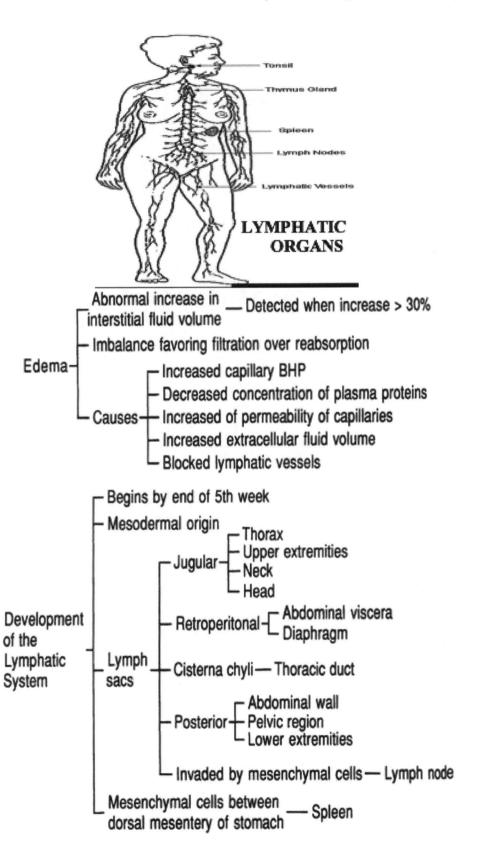

LYMPHATIC ORGANS

- Tonsil
- Thymus Gland
- Spleen
- Lymph Nodes
- Lymphatic Vessels

Edema
- Abnormal increase in interstitial fluid volume — Detected when increase > 30%
- Imbalance favoring filtration over reabsorption
- Causes
  - Increased capillary BHP
  - Decreased concentration of plasma proteins
  - Increased of permeability of capillaries
  - Increased extracellular fluid volume
  - Blocked lymphatic vessels

Development of the Lymphatic System
- Begins by end of 5th week
- Mesodermal origin
- Lymph sacs
  - Jugular
    - Thorax
    - Upper extremities
    - Neck
    - Head
  - Retroperitonal
    - Abdominal viscera
    - Diaphragm
  - Cisterna chyli — Thoracic duct
  - Posterior
    - Abdominal wall
    - Pelvic region
    - Lower extremities
  - Invaded by mesenchymal cells — Lymph node
- Mesenchymal cells between dorsal mesentery of stomach — Spleen

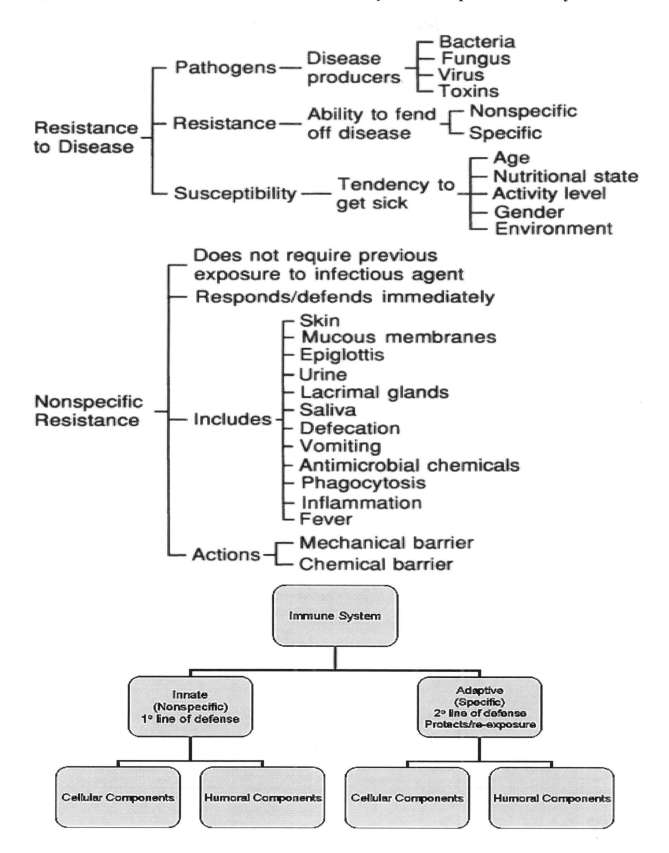

Nonspecific and Specific Immune Defense System

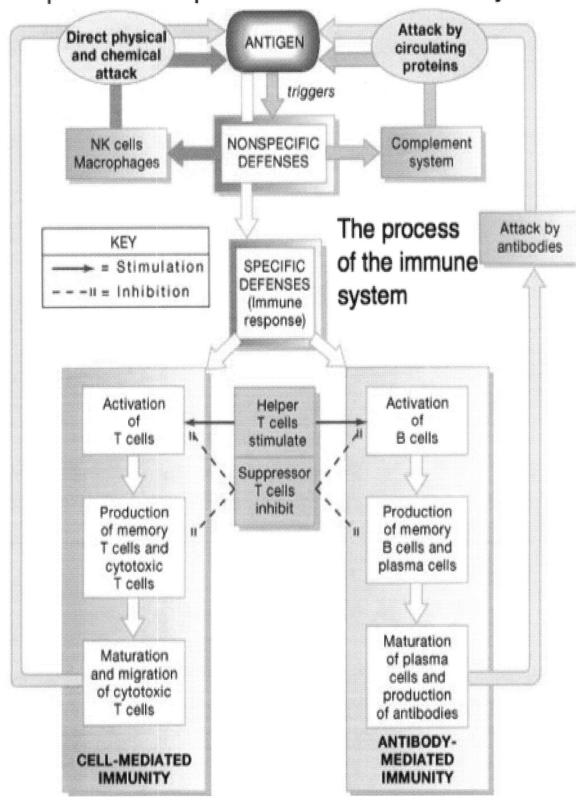

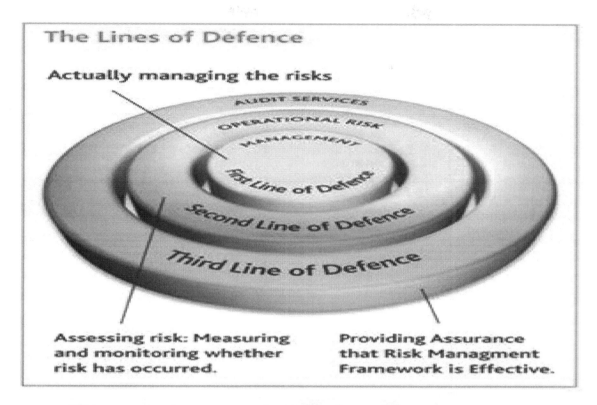

First Lines of Defence

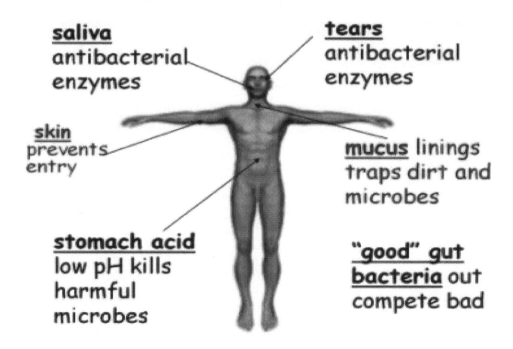

saliva antibacterial enzymes

tears antibacterial enzymes

skin prevents entry

mucus linings traps dirt and microbes

stomach acid low pH kills harmful microbes

"good" gut bacteria out compete bad

Mechanical Barriers to Disease
- Skin
  - Involved components — Epidermis / Hair
  - Mechanism — Pathogens can't get in / Shedding removes surface pathogens
  - Pathogens commonly found on skin — Staphylococcus / Tinea
- Mucous membranes
  - Line all cavities that open to exterior
  - Produce mucous — Hairs trap / Cilia move — Particles and pathogens
- Epiglottis — Prevents entry of objects (other than gases) into lower respiratory tract
- Lacrimal apparatus — Makes and drains tears / Washes eye surface
- Salivary glands — Produce saliva / Dilutes pathogens / Washes oral cavity & contents
- Urine — Flow cleanses urethra
- Vaginal secretions — Cleanses vagina
- Defecation — Eliminates pathogens
- Emesis — Expels pathogens

Chemical Barriers to Disease
- Sebum — Unsaturated fatty acids inhibit growth of — Bacteria / Fungi
- Perspiration — Wash pathogens away
- Lysozyme
  - Digest bacterial walls
  - Found in — Sweat / Tears / Saliva / Nasal secretions / Tissue fluid
- Hyaluronic acid — Slows spread of localized infections and their toxins
- Acidic pH — Destroys bacteria & toxins / Found — Skin / Gastric juice / Vaginal secretions

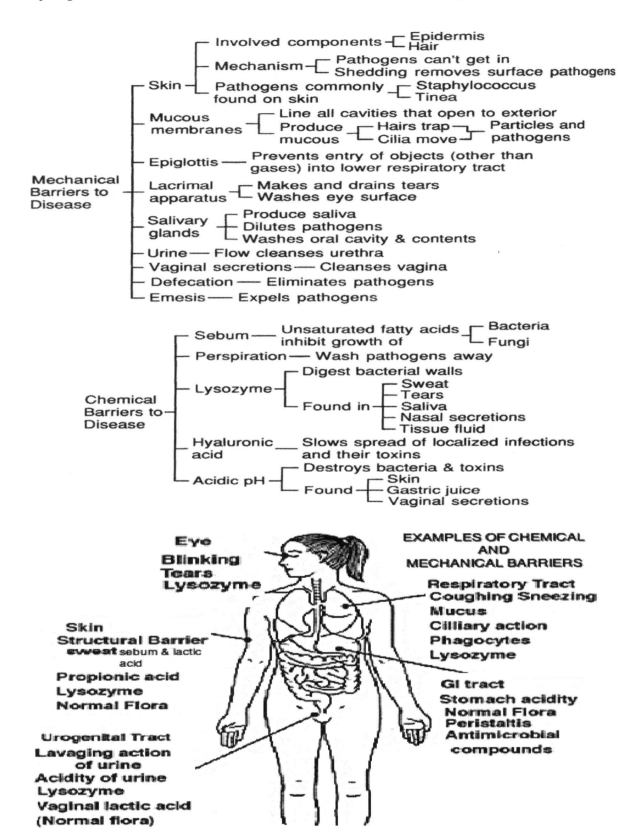

Eye
Blinking
Tears
Lysozyme

EXAMPLES OF CHEMICAL AND MECHANICAL BARRIERS

Respiratory Tract
Coughing Sneezing
Mucus
Cilliary action
Phagocytes
Lysozyme

Skin
Structural Barrier
sweat sebum & lactic acid
Propionic acid
Lysozyme
Normal Flora

GI tract
Stomach acidity
Normal Flora
Peristaltis
Antimicrobial compounds

Urogenital Tract
Lavaging action of urine
Acidity of urine
Lysozyme
Vaginal lactic acid
(Normal flora)

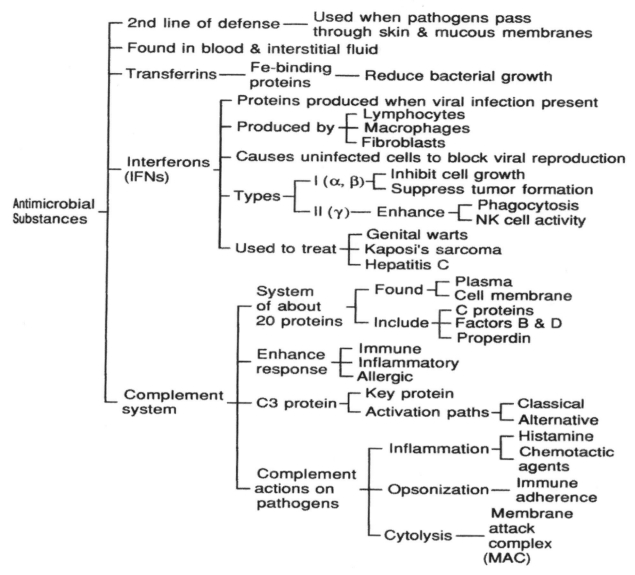

Antimicrobial Substances
- 2nd line of defense — Used when pathogens pass through skin & mucous membranes
- Found in blood & interstitial fluid
- Transferrins — Fe-binding proteins — Reduce bacterial growth
- Interferons (IFNs)
  - Proteins produced when viral infection present
  - Produced by
    - Lymphocytes
    - Macrophages
    - Fibroblasts
  - Causes uninfected cells to block viral reproduction
  - Types
    - I (α, β)
      - Inhibit cell growth
      - Suppress tumor formation
    - II (γ) — Enhance
      - Phagocytosis
      - NK cell activity
  - Used to treat
    - Genital warts
    - Kaposi's sarcoma
    - Hepatitis C
- Complement system
  - System of about 20 proteins
    - Found
      - Plasma
      - Cell membrane
    - Include
      - C proteins
      - Factors B & D
      - Properdin
  - Enhance response
    - Immune
    - Inflammatory
    - Allergic
  - C3 protein
    - Key protein
    - Activation paths
      - Classical
      - Alternative
  - Complement actions on pathogens
    - Inflammation
      - Histamine
      - Chemotactic agents
    - Opsonization — Immune adherence
    - Cytolysis — Membrane attack complex (MAC)

Interferons are molecules made by virus infected cells. They protect neighbouring cells from virus infection

Interferons

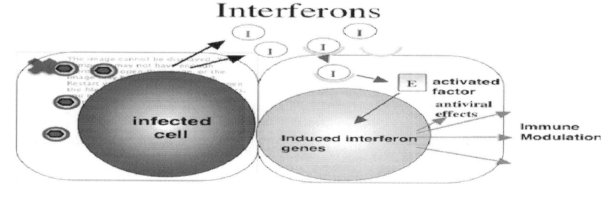

Human Nonspecific Defenses

DEFENSIVE MECHANISM	FUNCTION
Surface barriers	
Skin	Prevents entry of pathogens and foreign substances
Acid secretions	Inhibit bacterial growth on skin
Mucus	Prevents entry of pathogens; produces defensins that kill pathogens
Mucous secretions	Trap bacteria and other pathogens in digestive and respiratory tracts
Nasal hairs	Filter bacteria in nasal passages
Cilia	Move mucus and trapped materials away from respiratory passages
Gastric juice	Concentrated HCl and proteases destroy pathogens in stomach
Acid in vagina	Limits growth of fungi and bacteria in female reproductive tract
Tears, saliva	Lubricate and cleanse; contain lysozyme, which destroys bacteria

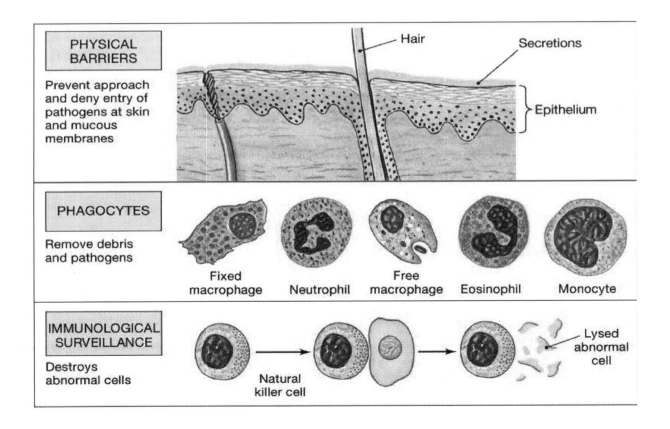

PHYSICAL BARRIERS

Prevent approach and deny entry of pathogens at skin and mucous membranes

Hair   Secretions   Epithelium

PHAGOCYTES

Remove debris and pathogens

Fixed macrophage   Neutrophil   Free macrophage   Eosinophil   Monocyte

IMMUNOLOGICAL SURVEILLANCE

Destroys abnormal cells

Natural killer cell   Lysed abnormal cell

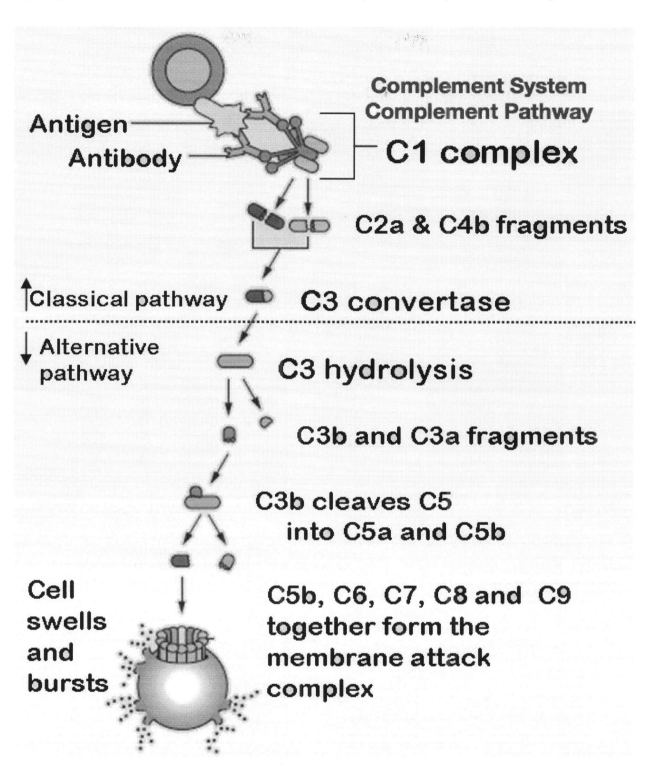

Antigen

Antibody

Complement System
Complement Pathway

C1 complex

C2a & C4b fragments

Classical pathway   **C3 convertase**

Alternative
pathway   **C3 hydrolysis**

C3b and C3a fragments

C3b cleaves C5
into C5a and C5b

Cell
swells
and
bursts

C5b, C6, C7, C8 and C9
together form the
membrane attack
complex

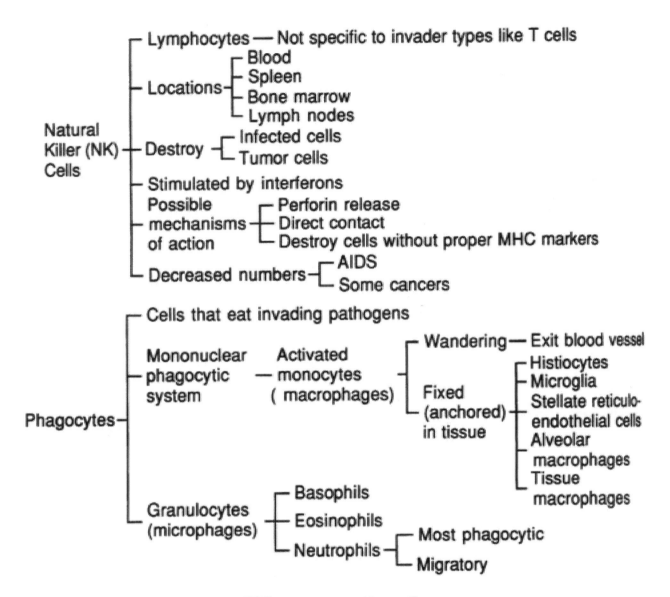

Natural Killer (NK) Cells
- Lymphocytes — Not specific to invader types like T cells
- Locations
  - Blood
  - Spleen
  - Bone marrow
  - Lymph nodes
- Destroy
  - Infected cells
  - Tumor cells
- Stimulated by interferons
- Possible mechanisms of action
  - Perforin release
  - Direct contact
  - Destroy cells without proper MHC markers
- Decreased numbers
  - AIDS
  - Some cancers

Phagocytes
- Cells that eat invading pathogens
- Mononuclear phagocytic system — Activated monocytes (macrophages)
  - Wandering — Exit blood vessel
  - Fixed (anchored) in tissue
    - Histiocytes
    - Microglia
    - Stellate reticulo-endothelial cells
    - Alveolar macrophages
    - Tissue macrophages
- Granulocytes (microphages)
  - Basophils
  - Eosinophils
  - Neutrophils
    - Most phagocytic
    - Migratory

Phagocytosis
microbe taken up by endocytosis and destroyed by within a phagolysosome

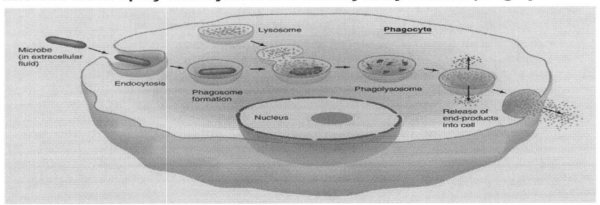

Microbe (in extracellular fluid) — Endocytosis — Phagosome formation — Lysosome — Phagolysosome — Phagocyte — Release of end-products into cell — Nucleus

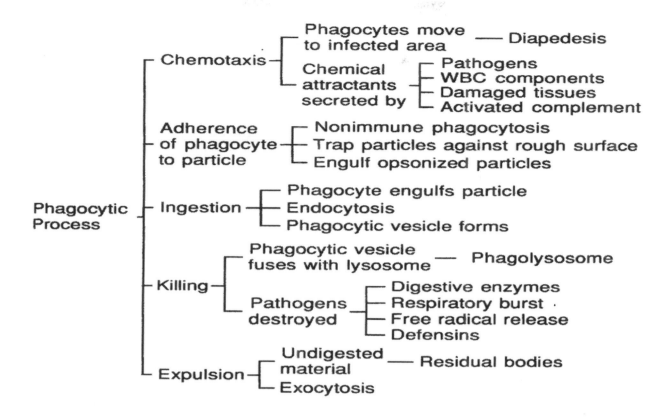

Phagocytic Process
- Chemotaxis
  - Phagocytes move to infected area — Diapedesis
  - Chemical attractants secreted by
    - Pathogens
    - WBC components
    - Damaged tissues
    - Activated complement
- Adherence of phagocyte to particle
  - Nonimmune phagocytosis
  - Trap particles against rough surface
  - Engulf opsonized particles
- Ingestion
  - Phagocyte engulfs particle
  - Endocytosis
  - Phagocytic vesicle forms
- Killing
  - Phagocytic vesicle fuses with lysosome — Phagolysosome
  - Pathogens destroyed
    - Digestive enzymes
    - Respiratory burst
    - Free radical release
    - Defensins
- Expulsion
  - Undigested material — Residual bodies
  - Exocytosis

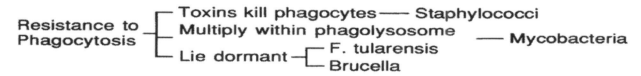

Resistance to Phagocytosis
- Toxins kill phagocytes — Staphylococci
- Multiply within phagolysosome — Mycobacteria
- Lie dormant
  - F. tularensis
  - Brucella

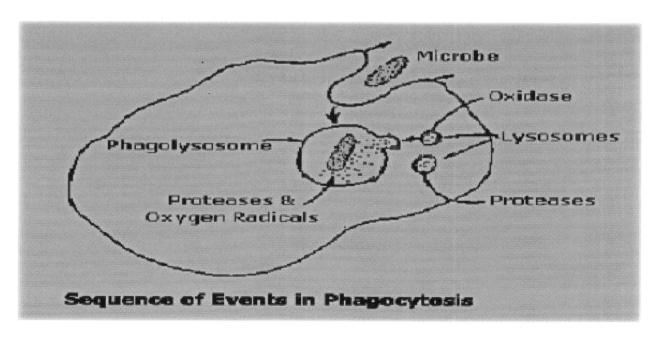

Sequence of Events in Phagocytosis

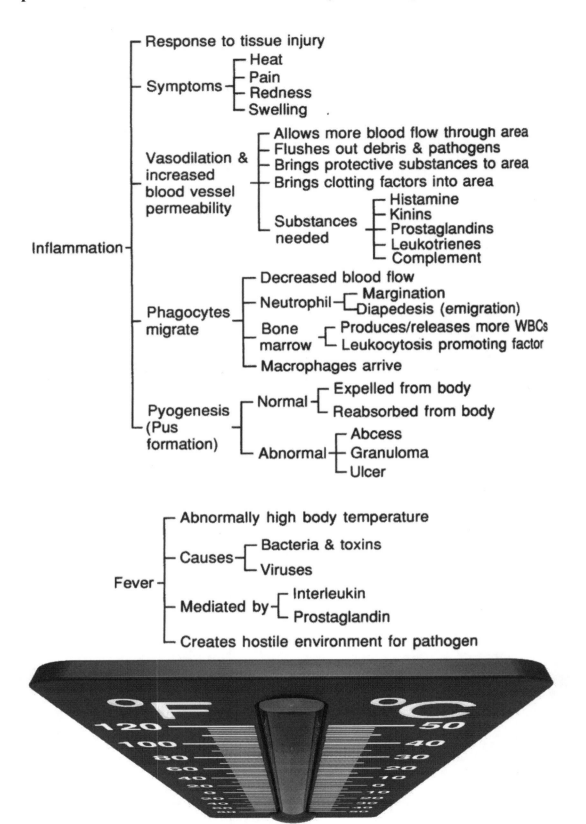

Inflammation
- Response to tissue injury
- Symptoms
  - Heat
  - Pain
  - Redness
  - Swelling
- Vasodilation & increased blood vessel permeability
  - Allows more blood flow through area
  - Flushes out debris & pathogens
  - Brings protective substances to area
  - Brings clotting factors into area
  - Substances needed
    - Histamine
    - Kinins
    - Prostaglandins
    - Leukotrienes
    - Complement
- Phagocytes migrate
  - Decreased blood flow
  - Neutrophil
    - Margination
    - Diapedesis (emigration)
  - Bone marrow
    - Produces/releases more WBCs
    - Leukocytosis promoting factor
  - Macrophages arrive
- Pyogenesis (Pus formation)
  - Normal
    - Expelled from body
    - Reabsorbed from body
  - Abnormal
    - Abcess
    - Granuloma
    - Ulcer

Fever
- Abnormally high body temperature
- Causes
  - Bacteria & toxins
  - Viruses
- Mediated by
  - Interleukin
  - Prostaglandin
- Creates hostile environment for pathogen

IFLAMATION

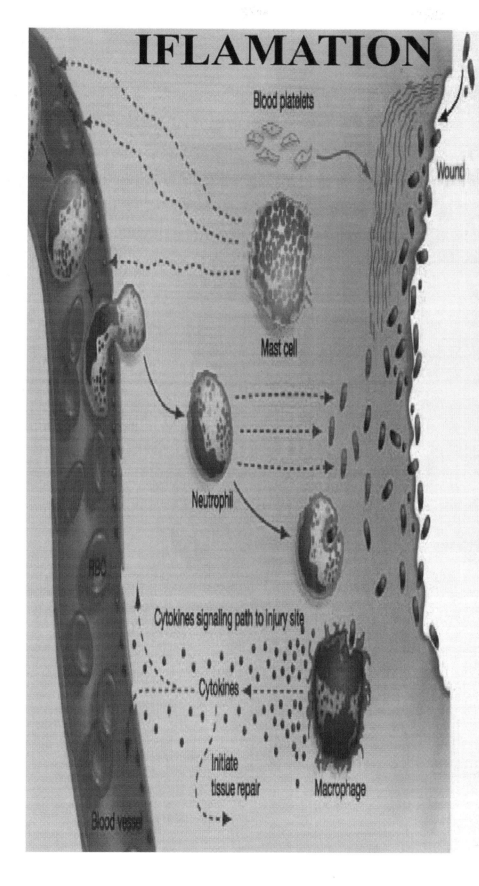

Blood platelets

Wound

Mast cell

Neutrophil

Cytokines signaling path to injury site

Cytokines

Initiate tissue repair

Macrophage

Blood vessel

RBC

1. Bacteria and other pathogens enter wound.

2. Platelets from blood release blood-clotting proteins at wound site.

3. Mast cells secrete factors that mediate vasodilation and vascular constriction. Delivery of blood, plasma, and cells to injured area increases.

4. Neutrophils secrete factors that kill and degrade pathogens.

5. Neutrophils and macrophages remove pathogens by phagocytosis.

6. Macrophages secrete hormones called cytokines that attract immune system cells to the site and activate cells involved in tissue repair.

7. Inflammatory response continues until the foreign material is eliminated and the wound is repaired.

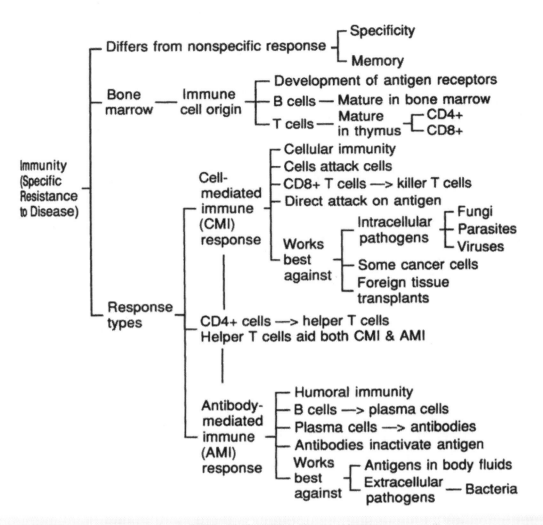

Innate *vs* adaptive immunity

	INNATE(NONSPECIFIC)	ADAPTIVE(SPECIFIC)
self / non-self discrimination	present, reaction is against foreign	present, reaction is against foreign
lag phase	absent, reponse is immediate	present, response takes at least a few days
specificity	limited, the same response is mounted to a wide variety of agents	high, the response is directed only to the agents that initiated it.
diversity	limited, hence limited specificity	extensive, and resulting in a wide range of antigen receptors.
memory	absent, subsequent exposures to agent generate the same response	present, subsequent exposures to the same agent induce amplified reponses

Basic model of human adaptive immunity
MHC ➤ major histocompatibility complex, CTL ➤ cytotoxic T lymphocytes

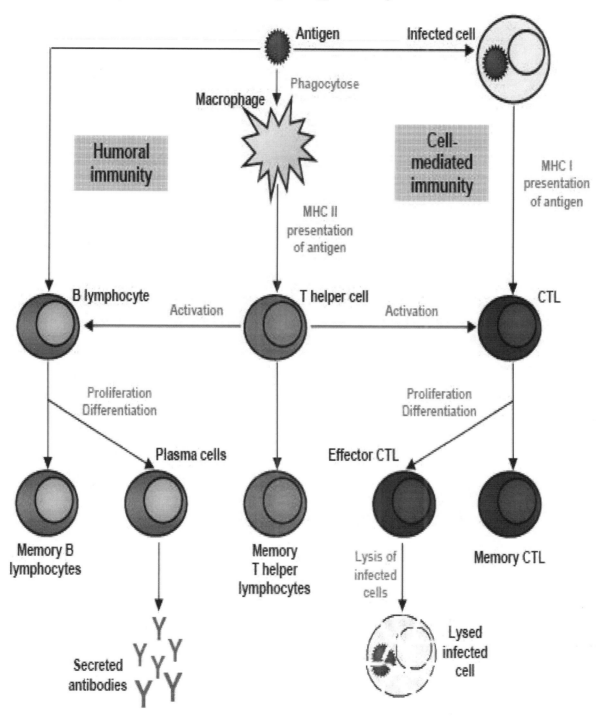

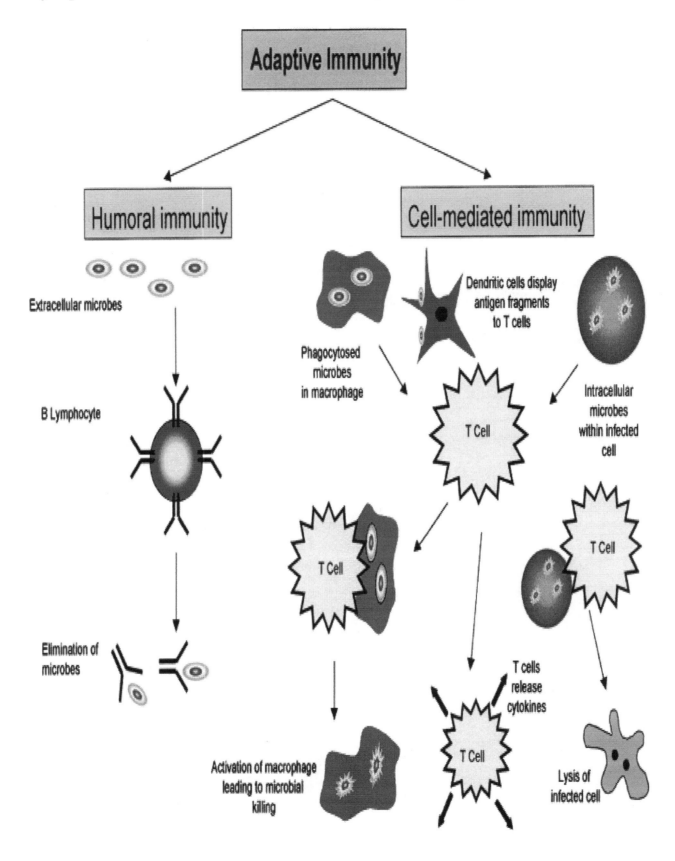

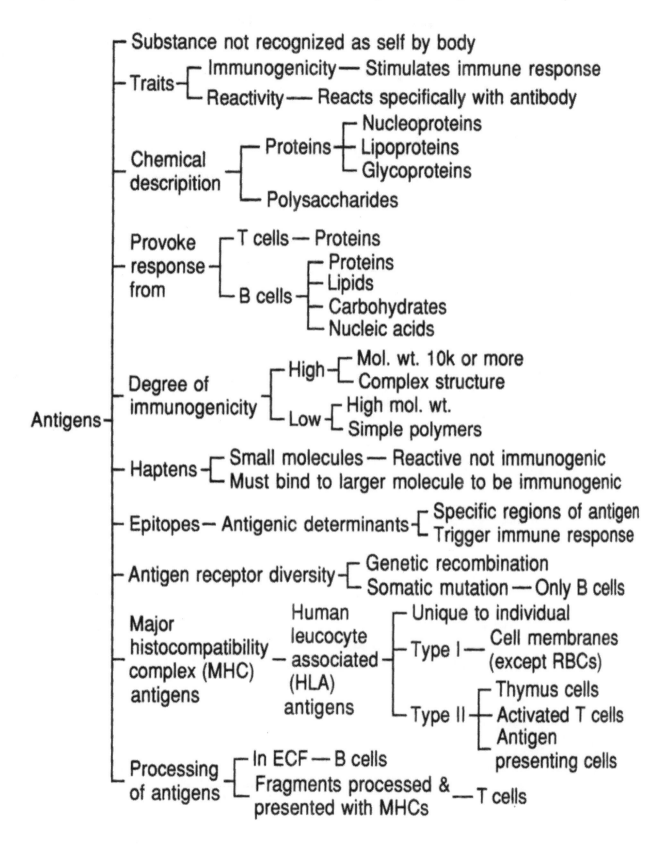

Antigens
- Traits
  - Substance not recognized as self by body
  - Immunogenicity — Stimulates immune response
  - Reactivity — Reacts specifically with antibody
- Chemical description
  - Proteins
    - Nucleoproteins
    - Lipoproteins
    - Glycoproteins
  - Polysaccharides
- Provoke response from
  - T cells — Proteins
  - B cells
    - Proteins
    - Lipids
    - Carbohydrates
    - Nucleic acids
- Degree of immunogenicity
  - High
    - Mol. wt. 10k or more
    - Complex structure
  - Low
    - High mol. wt.
    - Simple polymers
- Haptens
  - Small molecules — Reactive not immunogenic
  - Must bind to larger molecule to be immunogenic
- Epitopes — Antigenic determinants
  - Specific regions of antigen
  - Trigger immune response
- Antigen receptor diversity
  - Genetic recombination
  - Somatic mutation — Only B cells
- Major histocompatibility complex (MHC) antigens — Human leucocyte associated (HLA) antigens
  - Unique to individual
  - Type I — Cell membranes (except RBCs)
  - Type II
    - Thymus cells
    - Activated T cells
    - Antigen presenting cells
- Processing of antigens
  - In ECF — B cells
  - Fragments processed & presented with MHCs — T cells

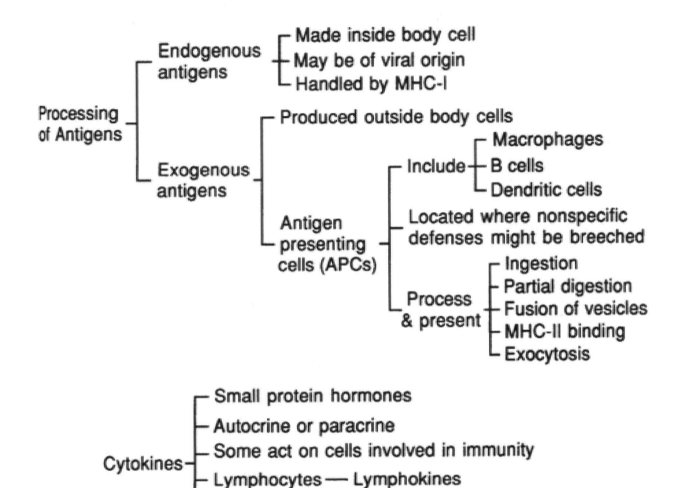

Processing of Antigens
- Endogenous antigens
  - Made inside body cell
  - May be of viral origin
  - Handled by MHC-I
- Exogenous antigens
  - Produced outside body cells
  - Antigen presenting cells (APCs)
    - Include
      - Macrophages
      - B cells
      - Dendritic cells
    - Located where nonspecific defenses might be breeched
    - Process & present
      - Ingestion
      - Partial digestion
      - Fusion of vesicles
      - MHC-II binding
      - Exocytosis

Cytokines
- Small protein hormones
- Autocrine or paracrine
- Some act on cells involved in immunity
- Lymphocytes — Lymphokines
- Monocytes Macrophages — Monokines

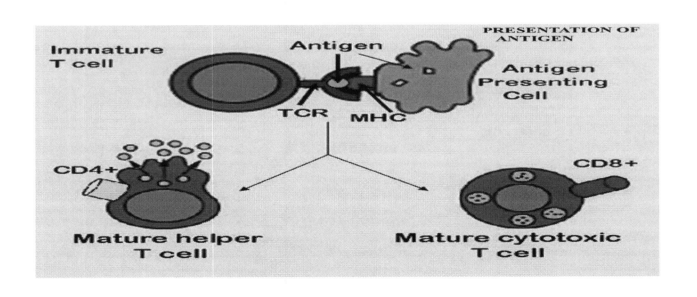

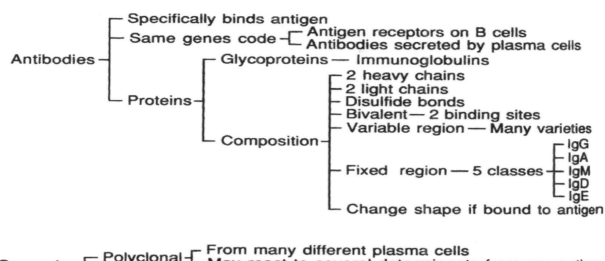

Antibodies
- Specifically binds antigen
- Same genes code
  - Antigen receptors on B cells
  - Antibodies secreted by plasma cells
- Proteins
  - Glycoproteins — Immunoglobulins
  - Composition
    - 2 heavy chains
    - 2 light chains
    - Disulfide bonds
    - Bivalent — 2 binding sites
    - Variable region — Many varieties
    - Fixed region — 5 classes
      - IgG
      - IgA
      - IgM
      - IgD
      - IgE
    - Change shape if bound to antigen

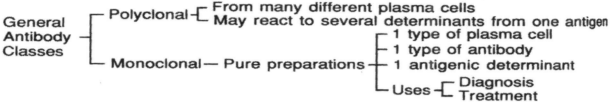

General Antibody Classes
- Polyclonal
  - From many different plasma cells
  - May react to several determinants from one antigen
- Monoclonal — Pure preparations
  - 1 type of plasma cell
  - 1 type of antibody
  - 1 antigenic determinant
  - Uses
    - Diagnosis
    - Treatment

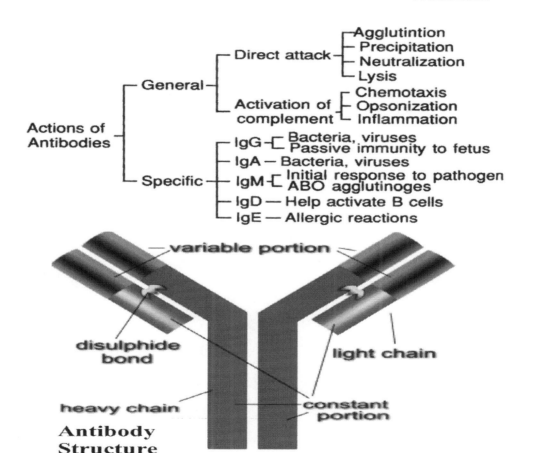

Actions of Antibodies
- General
  - Direct attack
    - Agglutintion
    - Precipitation
    - Neutralization
    - Lysis
  - Activation of complement
    - Chemotaxis
    - Opsonization
    - Inflammation
- Specific
  - IgG
    - Bacteria, viruses
    - Passive immunity to fetus
  - IgA — Bacteria, viruses
  - IgM
    - Initial response to pathogen
    - ABO agglutinoges
  - IgD — Help activate B cells
  - IgE — Allergic reactions

variable portion

disulphide bond

light chain

heavy chain

constant portion

Antibody Structure

Actions of Antibodies

Antibodies may inhibit infection by (a) preventing the antigen from binding its target, (b) tagging a pathogen for destruction by macrophages or neutrophils, or (c) activating the complement cascade.

(a) Neutralization Antibodies prevent a virus or toxic protein from binding their target.

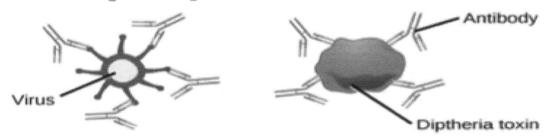

Virus

Antibody

Diptheria toxin

(b) Opsonization A pathogen tagged by antibodies is consumed by a macrophage or neutrophil.

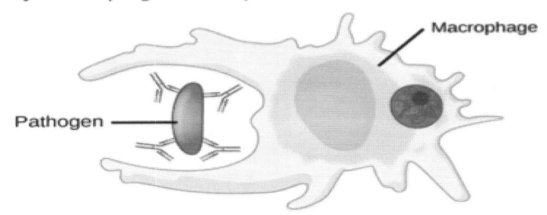

Macrophage

Pathogen

(c) Complement activation Antibodies attached to the surface of a pathogen cell activate the complement system.

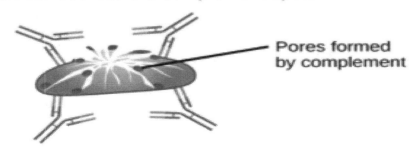

Pores formed by complement

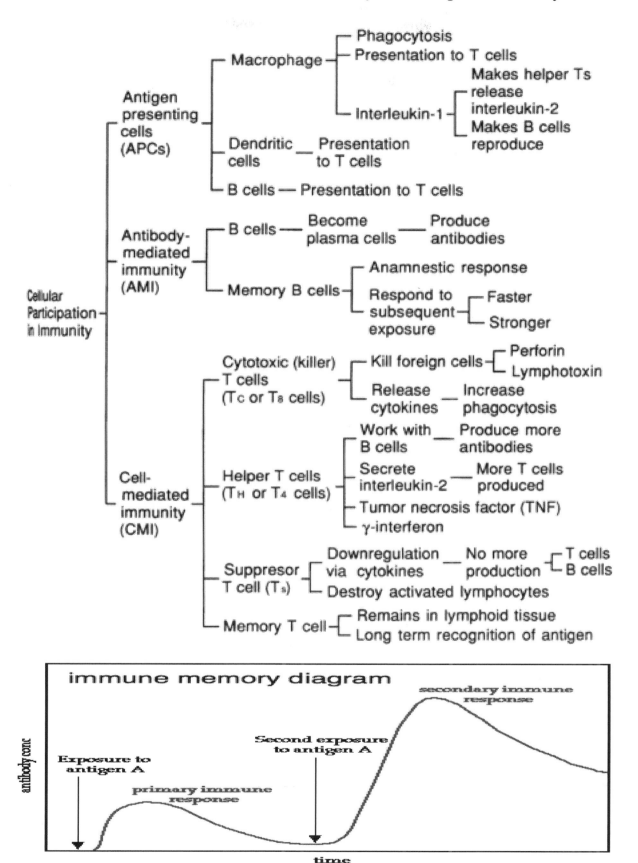

Cellular Participation in Immunity

- Antigen presenting cells (APCs)
  - Macrophage
    - Phagocytosis
    - Presentation to T cells
    - Interleukin-1
      - Makes helper Ts release interleukin-2
      - Makes B cells reproduce
  - Dendritic cells — Presentation to T cells
  - B cells — Presentation to T cells
- Antibody-mediated immunity (AMI)
  - B cells — Become plasma cells — Produce antibodies
  - Memory B cells
    - Anamnestic response
    - Respond to subsequent exposure
      - Faster
      - Stronger
- Cell-mediated immunity (CMI)
  - Cytotoxic (killer) T cells (Tc or T8 cells)
    - Kill foreign cells
      - Perforin
      - Lymphotoxin
    - Release cytokines — Increase phagocytosis
  - Helper T cells (TH or T4 cells)
    - Work with B cells — Produce more antibodies
    - Secrete interleukin-2 — More T cells produced
    - Tumor necrosis factor (TNF)
    - γ-interferon
  - Suppressor T cell (Ts)
    - Downregulation via cytokines — No more production
      - T cells
      - B cells
    - Destroy activated lymphocytes
  - Memory T cell
    - Remains in lymphoid tissue
    - Long term recognition of antigen

immune memory diagram

antibody conc

Exposure to antigen A

primary immune response

Second exposure to antigen A

secondary immune response

time

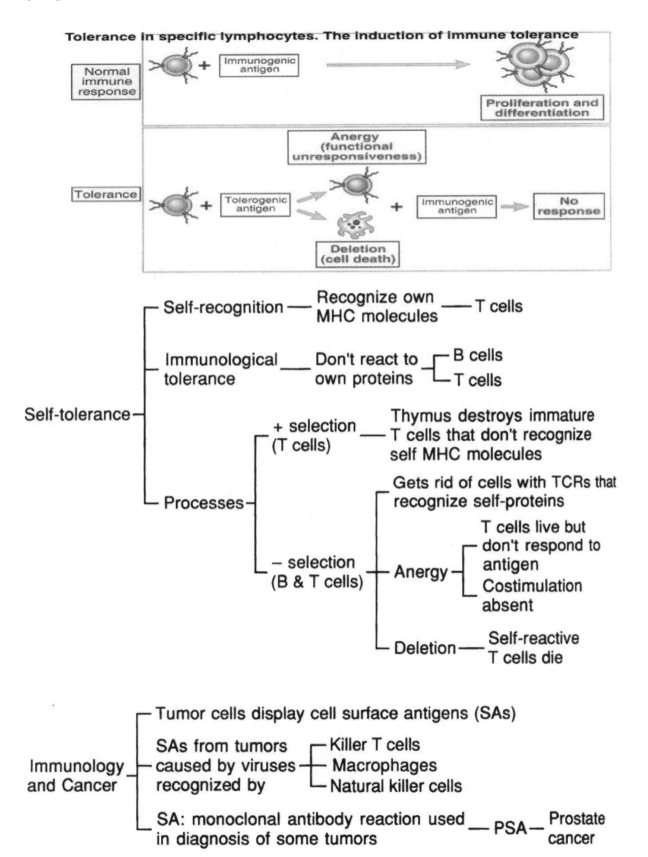

Tolerance in specific lymphocytes. The induction of immune tolerance

Normal immune response

+ Immunogenic antigen → Proliferation and differentiation

Tolerance

+ Tolerogenic antigen → Anergy (functional unresponsiveness) / Deletion (cell death) + Immunogenic antigen → No response

Self-tolerance
- Self-recognition — Recognize own MHC molecules — T cells
- Immunological tolerance — Don't react to own proteins — B cells / T cells
- Processes
  - + selection (T cells) — Thymus destroys immature T cells that don't recognize self MHC molecules
  - – selection (B & T cells)
    - Gets rid of cells with TCRs that recognize self-proteins
    - Anergy — T cells live but don't respond to antigen / Costimulation absent
    - Deletion — Self-reactive T cells die

Immunology and Cancer
- Tumor cells display cell surface antigens (SAs)
- SAs from tumors caused by viruses recognized by — Killer T cells / Macrophages / Natural killer cells
- SA: monoclonal antibody reaction used in diagnosis of some tumors — PSA — Prostate cancer

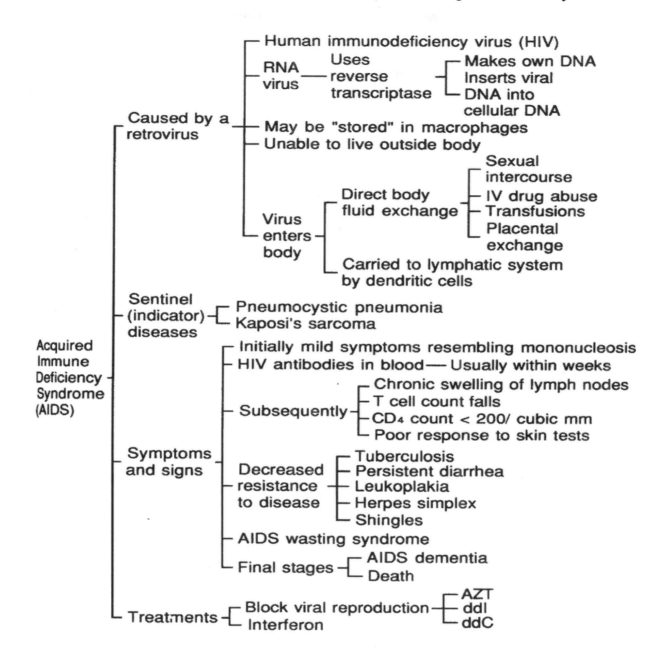

Acquired Immune Deficiency Syndrome (AIDS)

- Caused by a retrovirus
  - RNA virus — Uses reverse transcriptase
    - Human immunodeficiency virus (HIV)
    - Makes own DNA
    - Inserts viral DNA into cellular DNA
  - May be "stored" in macrophages
  - Unable to live outside body
  - Virus enters body
    - Direct body fluid exchange
      - Sexual intercourse
      - IV drug abuse
      - Transfusions
      - Placental exchange
    - Carried to lymphatic system by dendritic cells
- Sentinel (indicator) diseases
  - Pneumocystic pneumonia
  - Kaposi's sarcoma
- Symptoms and signs
  - Initially mild symptoms resembling mononucleosis
  - HIV antibodies in blood — Usually within weeks
  - Subsequently
    - Chronic swelling of lymph nodes
    - T cell count falls
    - CD_4 count < 200/ cubic mm
    - Poor response to skin tests
  - Decreased resistance to disease
    - Tuberculosis
    - Persistent diarrhea
    - Leukoplakia
    - Herpes simplex
    - Shingles
  - AIDS wasting syndrome
  - Final stages
    - AIDS dementia
    - Death
- Treatments
  - Block viral reproduction
    - AZT
    - ddI
    - ddC
  - Interferon

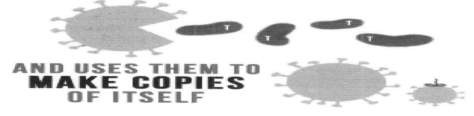

What is HIV or AIDS?
HIV ATTACKS YOUR T-CELLS
AND USES THEM TO MAKE COPIES OF ITSELF

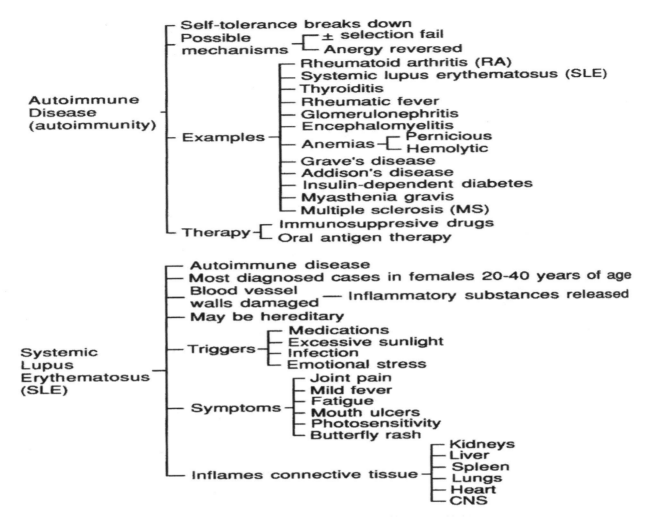

Autoimmune Disease (autoimmunity)
- Possible mechanisms
  - Self-tolerance breaks down
  - ± selection fail
  - Anergy reversed
- Examples
  - Rheumatoid arthritis (RA)
  - Systemic lupus erythematosus (SLE)
  - Thyroiditis
  - Rheumatic fever
  - Glomerulonephritis
  - Encephalomyelitis
  - Anemias
    - Pernicious
    - Hemolytic
  - Grave's disease
  - Addison's disease
  - Insulin-dependent diabetes
  - Myasthenia gravis
  - Multiple sclerosis (MS)
- Therapy
  - Immunosuppresive drugs
  - Oral antigen therapy

Systemic Lupus Erythematosus (SLE)
- Autoimmune disease
- Most diagnosed cases in females 20-40 years of age
- Blood vessel walls damaged — Inflammatory substances released
- May be hereditary
- Triggers
  - Medications
  - Excessive sunlight
  - Infection
  - Emotional stress
- Symptoms
  - Joint pain
  - Mild fever
  - Fatigue
  - Mouth ulcers
  - Photosensitivity
  - Butterfly rash
- Inflames connective tissue
  - Kidneys
  - Liver
  - Spleen
  - Lungs
  - Heart
  - CNS

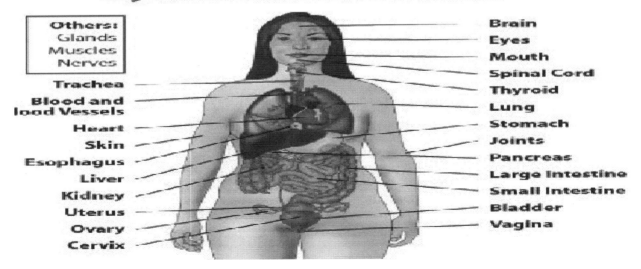

Body Parts That Can Be Affected by Autoimmune Diseases

Others:
Glands
Muscles
Nerves

Trachea
Blood and Blood Vessels
Heart
Skin
Esophagus
Liver
Kidney
Uterus
Ovary
Cervix

Brain
Eyes
Mouth
Spinal Cord
Thyroid
Lung
Stomach
Joints
Pancreas
Large Intestine
Small Intestine
Bladder
Vagina

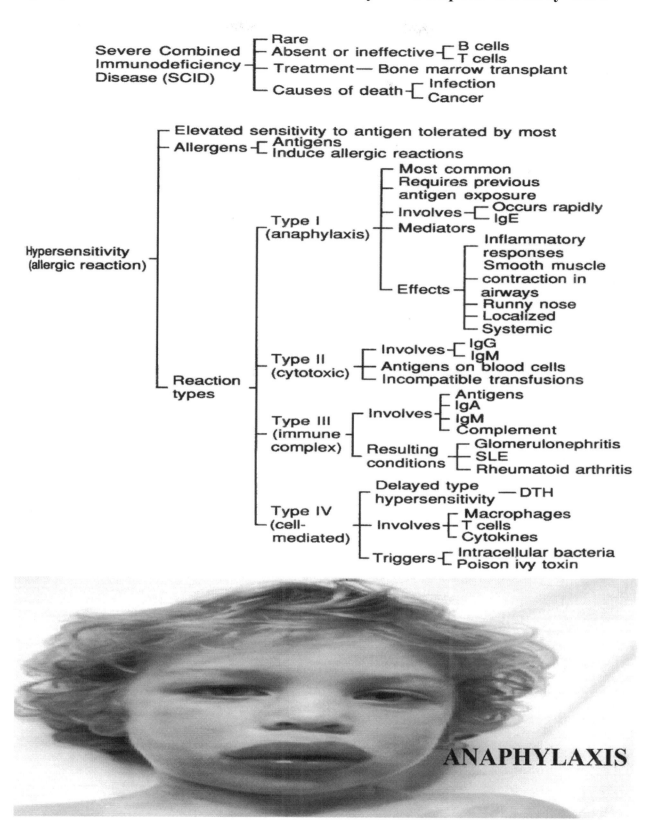

Severe Combined Immunodeficiency Disease (SCID)
- Rare
- Absent or ineffective
  - B cells
  - T cells
- Treatment — Bone marrow transplant
- Causes of death
  - Infection
  - Cancer

Hypersensitivity (allergic reaction)
- Elevated sensitivity to antigen tolerated by most
- Allergens
  - Antigens
  - Induce allergic reactions
- Reaction types
  - Type I (anaphylaxis)
    - Most common
    - Requires previous antigen exposure
    - Involves
      - Occurs rapidly
      - IgE
    - Mediators
    - Effects
      - Inflammatory responses
      - Smooth muscle contraction in airways
      - Runny nose
      - Localized
      - Systemic
  - Type II (cytotoxic)
    - Involves
      - IgG
      - IgM
    - Antigens on blood cells
    - Incompatible transfusions
  - Type III (immune complex)
    - Involves
      - Antigens
      - IgA
      - IgM
      - Complement
    - Resulting conditions
      - Glomerulonephritis
      - SLE
      - Rheumatoid arthritis
  - Type IV (cell-mediated)
    - Delayed type hypersensitivity — DTH
    - Involves
      - Macrophages
      - T cells
      - Cytokines
    - Triggers
      - Intracellular bacteria
      - Poison ivy toxin

ANAPHYLAXIS

TYPES OF HYPERSENSITIVITY (ALLERGIC REACTION)

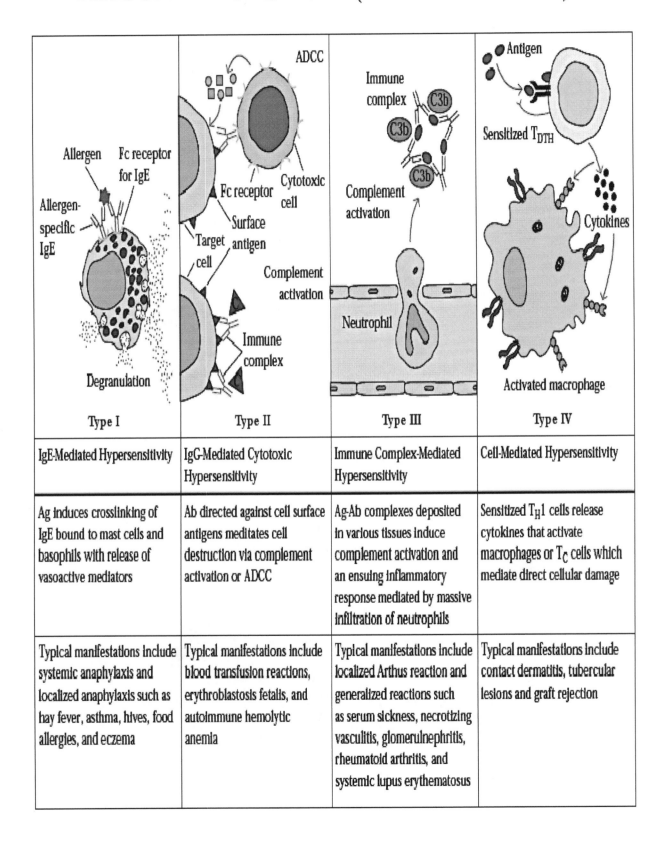

Allergen Fc receptor for IgE Allergen-specific IgE Degranulation **Type I**	ADCC Fc receptor Cytotoxic cell Surface antigen Target cell Complement activation Immune complex **Type II**	Immune complex C3b C3b C3b Complement activation Neutrophil **Type III**	Antigen Sensitized T$_{DTH}$ Cytokines Activated macrophage **Type IV**
IgE-Mediated Hypersensitivity	IgG-Mediated Cytotoxic Hypersensitivity	Immune Complex-Mediated Hypersensitivity	Cell-Mediated Hypersensitivity
Ag induces crosslinking of IgE bound to mast cells and basophils with release of vasoactive mediators	Ab directed against cell surface antigens mediates cell destruction via complement activation or ADCC	Ag-Ab complexes deposited in various tissues induce complement activation and an ensuing inflammatory response mediated by massive infiltration of neutrophils	Sensitized T$_H$1 cells release cytokines that activate macrophages or T$_C$ cells which mediate direct cellular damage
Typical manifestations include systemic anaphylaxis and localized anaphylaxis such as hay fever, asthma, hives, food allergies, and eczema	Typical manifestations include blood transfusion reactions, erythroblastosis fetalis, and autoimmune hemolytic anemia	Typical manifestations include localized Arthus reaction and generalized reactions such as serum sickness, necrotizing vasculitis, glomerulnephritis, rheumatoid arthritis, and systemic lupus erythematosus	Typical manifestations include contact dermatitis, tubercular lesions and graft rejection

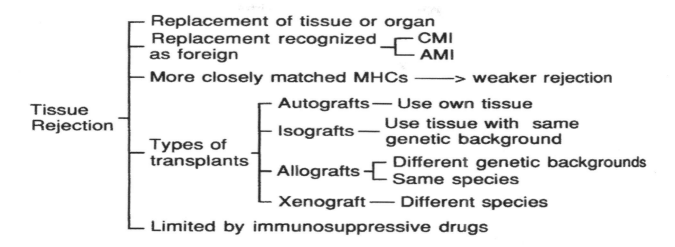

Tissue Rejection
- Replacement of tissue or organ
- Replacement recognized as foreign
  - CMI
  - AMI
- More closely matched MHCs ——> weaker rejection
- Types of transplants
  - Autografts — Use own tissue
  - Isografts — Use tissue with same genetic background
  - Allografts
    - Different genetic backgrounds
    - Same species
  - Xenograft — Different species
- Limited by immunosuppressive drugs

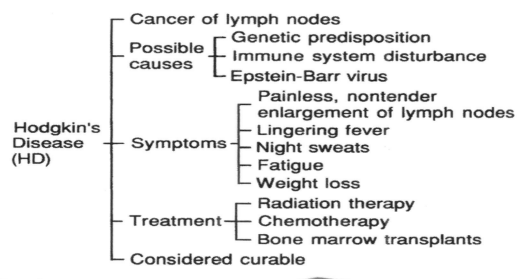

Hodgkin's Disease (HD)
- Cancer of lymph nodes
- Possible causes
  - Genetic predisposition
  - Immune system disturbance
  - Epstein-Barr virus
- Symptoms
  - Painless, nontender enlargement of lymph nodes
  - Lingering fever
  - Night sweats
  - Fatigue
  - Weight loss
- Treatment
  - Radiation therapy
  - Chemotherapy
  - Bone marrow transplants
- Considered curable

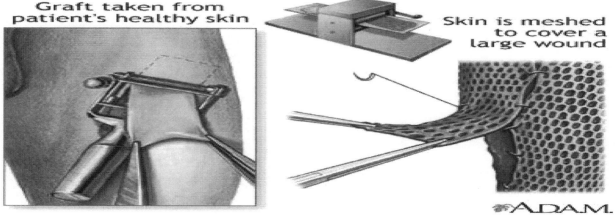

Graft taken from patient's healthy skin

Skin is meshed to cover a large wound

®ADAM.

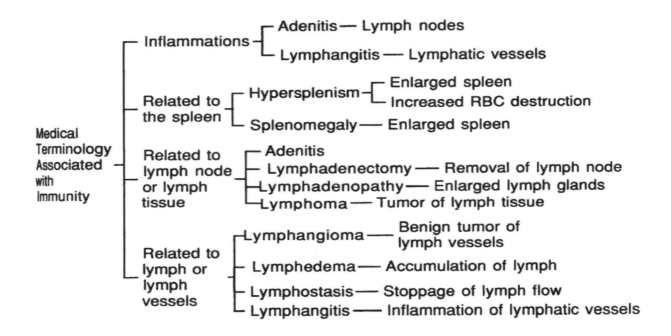

Inflammation in skin cancer

Shows that adaptive immune cells called B cells produce the signal that kindles inflammation in the epidermal layer of the skin. One model of how this might work is that a molecule (antigen) present in the tumors environment stimulates the B cells to release antibodies that target innate immune cells (such as neutrophils, macrophages and mast cells), which set up and maintain inflammation. Once activated, the innate cells release factors (triangles) that can promote growth and spreading of the tumor

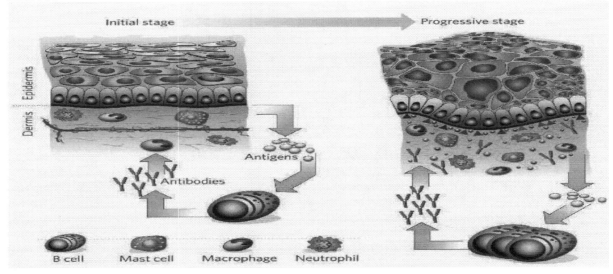

CHAPTER TWENTY THREE

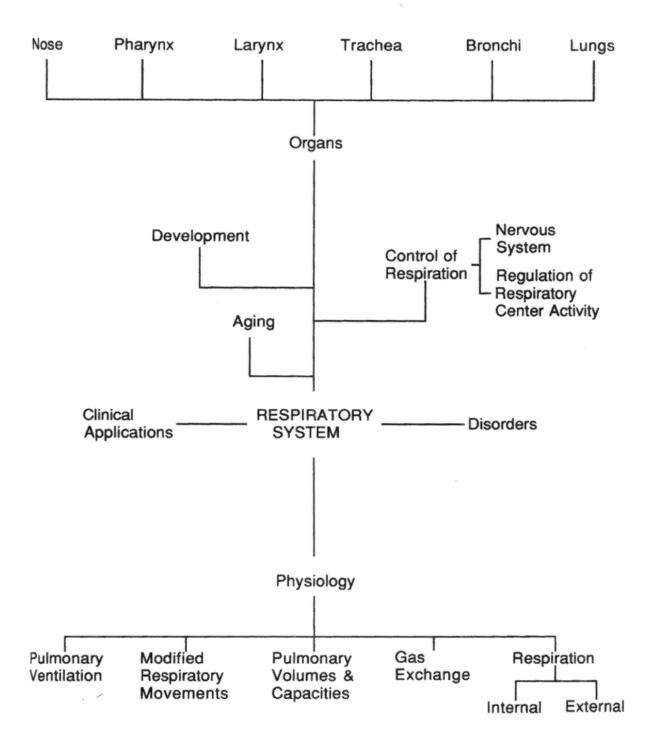

Nose   Pharynx   Larynx   Trachea   Bronchi   Lungs

Organs

Development

Control of Respiration
- Nervous System
- Regulation of Respiratory Center Activity

Aging

Clinical Applications   RESPIRATORY SYSTEM   Disorders

Physiology

Pulmonary Ventilation   Modified Respiratory Movements   Pulmonary Volumes & Capacities   Gas Exchange   Respiration

Internal   External

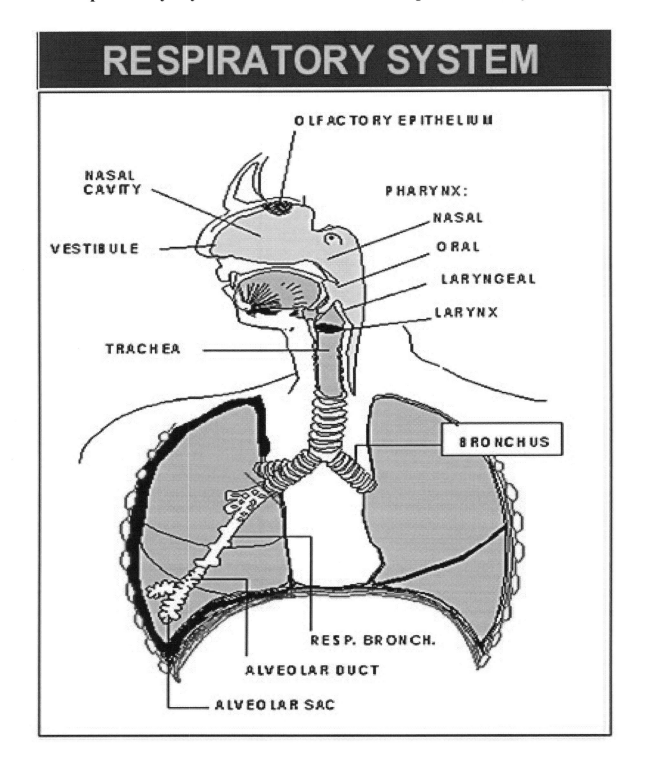

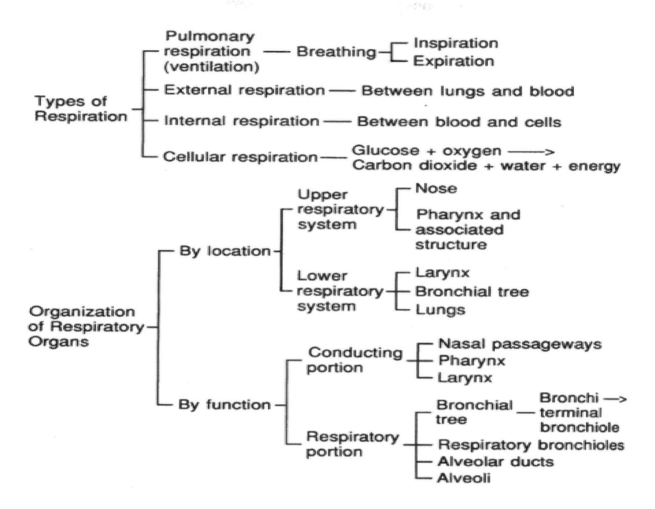

Types of Respiration
- Pulmonary respiration (ventilation) — Breathing
  - Inspiration
  - Expiration
- External respiration — Between lungs and blood
- Internal respiration — Between blood and cells
- Cellular respiration — Glucose + oxygen ——> Carbon dioxide + water + energy

Organization of Respiratory Organs
- By location
  - Upper respiratory system
    - Nose
    - Pharynx and associated structure
  - Lower respiratory system
    - Larynx
    - Bronchial tree
    - Lungs
- By function
  - Conducting portion
    - Nasal passageways
    - Pharynx
    - Larynx
  - Respiratory portion
    - Bronchial tree — Bronchi ——> terminal bronchiole
    - Respiratory bronchioles
    - Alveolar ducts
    - Alveoli

The Respiratory Tree

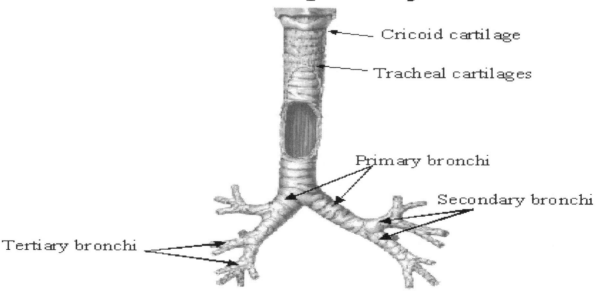

- Cricoid cartilage
- Tracheal cartilages
- Primary bronchi
- Secondary bronchi
- Tertiary bronchi

	THE RESPIRATORY TREE ZONING	Number of tubes in branch
	Name of branches	
Conducting zone	Trachea	1
	Bronchi	2
		4
		8
	Bronchioles	16
		32
	Terminal bronchioles	6×10^4
Respiratory zone	Respiratory bronchioles	5×10^5
	Alveolar ducts	
	Alveolar sacs	8×10^6

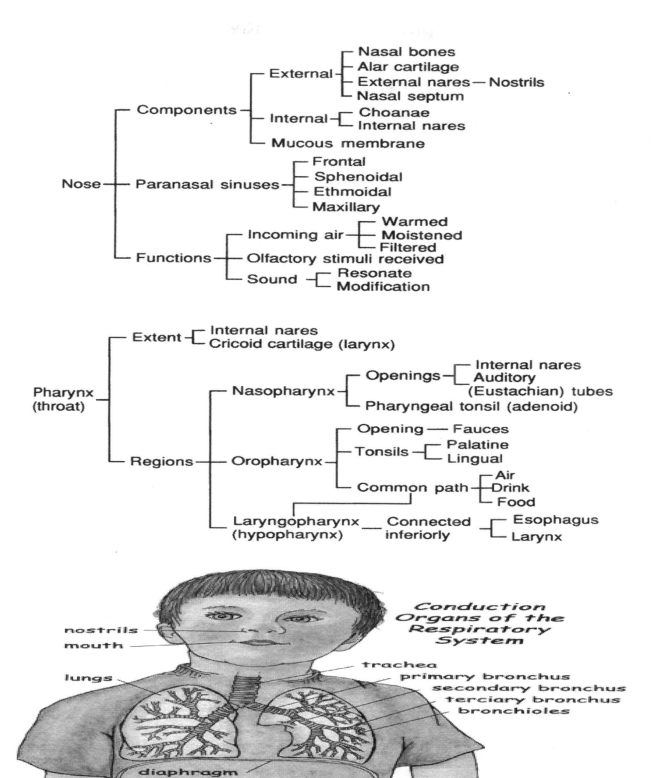

Nose
- Components
  - External
    - Nasal bones
    - Alar cartilage
    - External nares — Nostrils
    - Nasal septum
  - Internal
    - Choanae
    - Internal nares
  - Mucous membrane
- Paranasal sinuses
  - Frontal
  - Sphenoidal
  - Ethmoidal
  - Maxillary
- Functions
  - Incoming air
    - Warmed
    - Moistened
    - Filtered
  - Olfactory stimuli received
  - Sound
    - Resonate
    - Modification

Pharynx (throat)
- Extent
  - Internal nares
  - Cricoid cartilage (larynx)
- Regions
  - Nasopharynx
    - Openings
      - Internal nares
      - Auditory (Eustachian) tubes
    - Pharyngeal tonsil (adenoid)
  - Oropharynx
    - Opening — Fauces
    - Tonsils
      - Palatine
      - Lingual
    - Common path
      - Air
      - Drink
      - Food
  - Laryngopharynx (hypopharynx) — Connected inferiorly
    - Esophagus
    - Larynx

Conduction Organs of the Respiratory System

- nostrils
- mouth
- lungs
- trachea
- primary bronchus
- secondary bronchus
- terciary bronchus
- bronchioles
- diaphragm

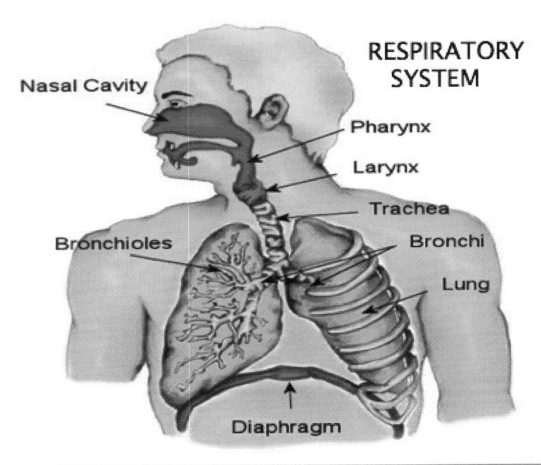

RESPIRATORY SYSTEM

Nasal Cavity

Pharynx

Larynx

Trachea

Bronchioles

Bronchi

Lung

Diaphragm

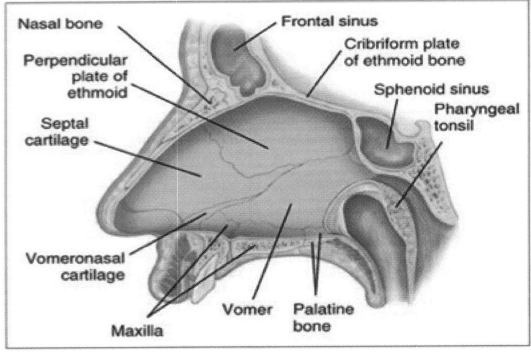

Nasal bone

Frontal sinus

Perpendicular plate of ethmoid

Cribriform plate of ethmoid bone

Sphenoid sinus

Pharyngeal tonsil

Septal cartilage

Vomeronasal cartilage

Maxilla

Vomer

Palatine bone

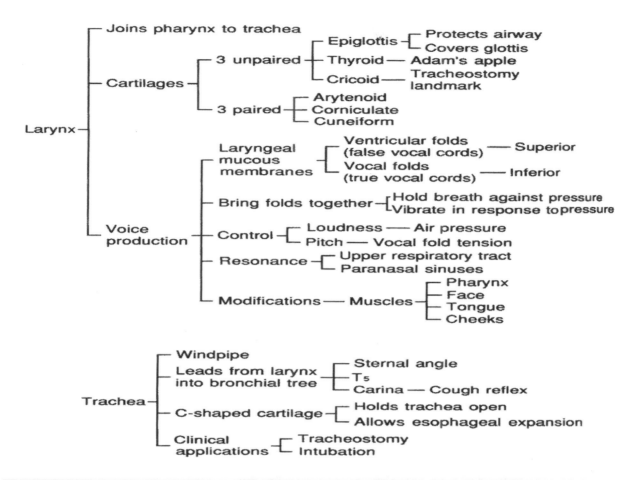

- Larynx
  - Joins pharynx to trachea
  - Cartilages
    - 3 unpaired
      - Epiglottis
        - Protects airway
        - Covers glottis
      - Thyroid — Adam's apple
      - Cricoid — Tracheostomy landmark
    - 3 paired
      - Arytenoid
      - Corniculate
      - Cuneiform
  - Voice production
    - Laryngeal mucous membranes
      - Ventricular folds (false vocal cords) — Superior
      - Vocal folds (true vocal cords) — Inferior
    - Bring folds together
      - Hold breath against pressure
      - Vibrate in response to pressure
    - Control
      - Loudness — Air pressure
      - Pitch — Vocal fold tension
    - Resonance
      - Upper respiratory tract
      - Paranasal sinuses
    - Modifications — Muscles
      - Pharynx
      - Face
      - Tongue
      - Cheeks

- Trachea
  - Windpipe
  - Leads from larynx into bronchial tree
    - Sternal angle
    - T5
    - Carina — Cough reflex
  - C-shaped cartilage
    - Holds trachea open
    - Allows esophageal expansion
  - Clinical applications
    - Tracheostomy
    - Intubation

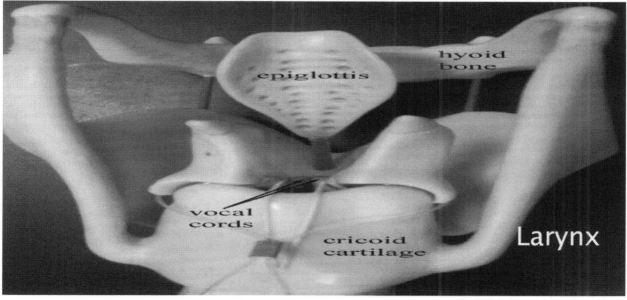

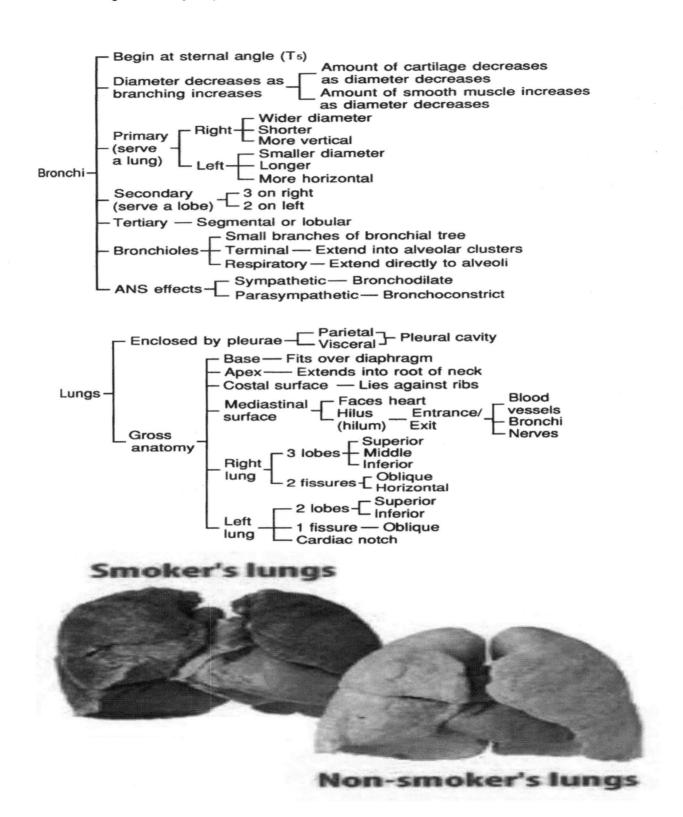

Bronchi
- Begin at sternal angle (T5)
- Diameter decreases as branching increases
  - Amount of cartilage decreases as diameter decreases
  - Amount of smooth muscle increases as diameter decreases
- Primary (serve a lung)
  - Right
    - Wider diameter
    - Shorter
    - More vertical
  - Left
    - Smaller diameter
    - Longer
    - More horizontal
- Secondary (serve a lobe)
  - 3 on right
  - 2 on left
- Tertiary — Segmental or lobular
- Bronchioles
  - Small branches of bronchial tree
  - Terminal — Extend into alveolar clusters
  - Respiratory — Extend directly to alveoli
- ANS effects
  - Sympathetic — Bronchodilate
  - Parasympathetic — Bronchoconstrict

Lungs
- Enclosed by pleurae
  - Parietal
  - Visceral
  - Pleural cavity
- Gross anatomy
  - Base — Fits over diaphragm
  - Apex — Extends into root of neck
  - Costal surface — Lies against ribs
  - Mediastinal surface
    - Faces heart
    - Hilus (hilum) — Entrance/Exit
      - Blood vessels
      - Bronchi
      - Nerves
  - Right lung
    - 3 lobes
      - Superior
      - Middle
      - Inferior
    - 2 fissures
      - Oblique
      - Horizontal
  - Left lung
    - 2 lobes
      - Superior
      - Inferior
    - 1 fissure — Oblique
    - Cardiac notch

Smoker's lungs

Non-smoker's lungs

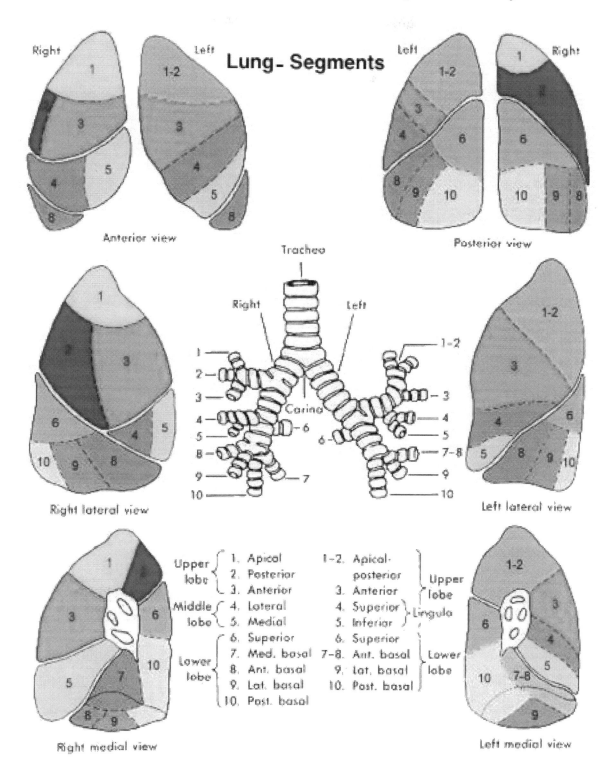

Lung - Segments

Upper lobe	1. Apical	1-2. Apical-posterior	Upper lobe
	2. Posterior	3. Anterior	
	3. Anterior		
Middle lobe	4. Lateral	4. Superior	Lingula
	5. Medial	5. Inferior	
Lower lobe	6. Superior	6. Superior	Lower lobe
	7. Med. basal	7-8. Ant. basal	
	8. Ant. basal	9. Lat. basal	
	9. Lat. basal	10. Post. basal	
	10. Post. basal		

Anterior view · Posterior view · Right lateral view · Left lateral view · Right medial view · Left medial view · Trachea · Carina

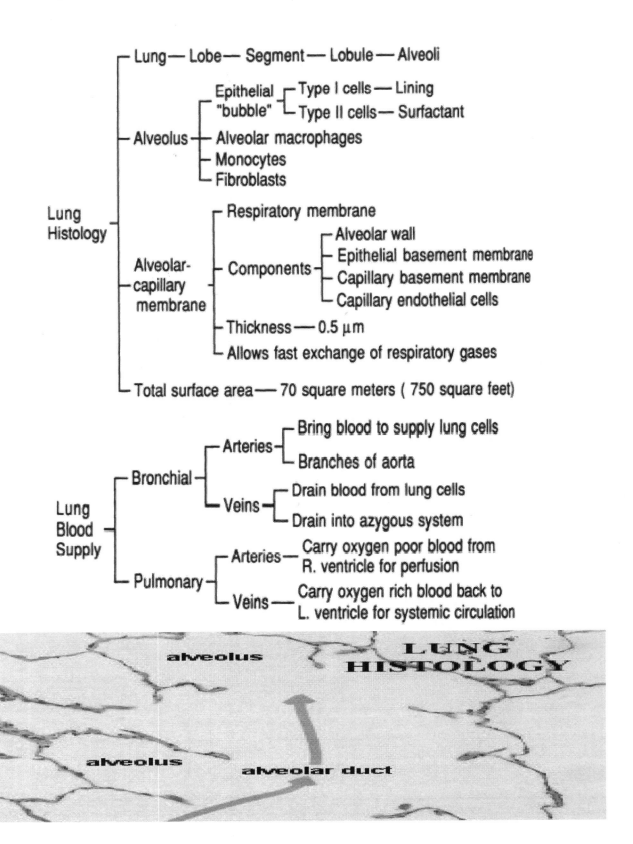

Lung Histology

- Lung — Lobe — Segment — Lobule — Alveoli
- Alveolus
  - Epithelial "bubble"
    - Type I cells — Lining
    - Type II cells — Surfactant
  - Alveolar macrophages
  - Monocytes
  - Fibroblasts
- Alveolar-capillary membrane
  - Respiratory membrane
  - Components
    - Alveolar wall
    - Epithelial basement membrane
    - Capillary basement membrane
    - Capillary endothelial cells
  - Thickness — 0.5 μm
  - Allows fast exchange of respiratory gases
- Total surface area — 70 square meters (750 square feet)

Lung Blood Supply

- Bronchial
  - Arteries
    - Bring blood to supply lung cells
    - Branches of aorta
  - Veins
    - Drain blood from lung cells
    - Drain into azygous system
- Pulmonary
  - Arteries — Carry oxygen poor blood from R. ventricle for perfusion
  - Veins — Carry oxygen rich blood back to L. ventricle for systemic circulation

LUNG HISTOLOGY

alveolus

alveolus

alveolar duct

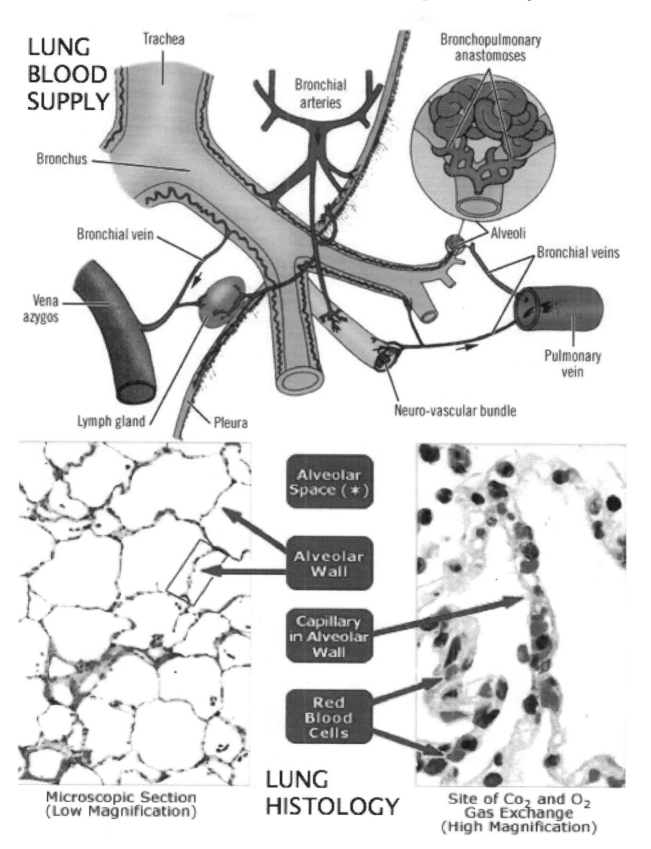

LUNG
BLOOD
SUPPLY

Trachea

Bronchopulmonary
anastomoses

Bronchial
arteries

Bronchus

Alveoli

Bronchial vein

Bronchial veins

Vena
azygos

Pulmonary
vein

Lymph gland

Pleura

Neuro-vascular bundle

Alveolar
Space (*)

Alveolar
Wall

Capillary
in Alveolar
Wall

Red
Blood
Cells

Microscopic Section
(Low Magnification)

LUNG
HISTOLOGY

Site of CO_2 and O_2
Gas Exchange
(High Magnification)

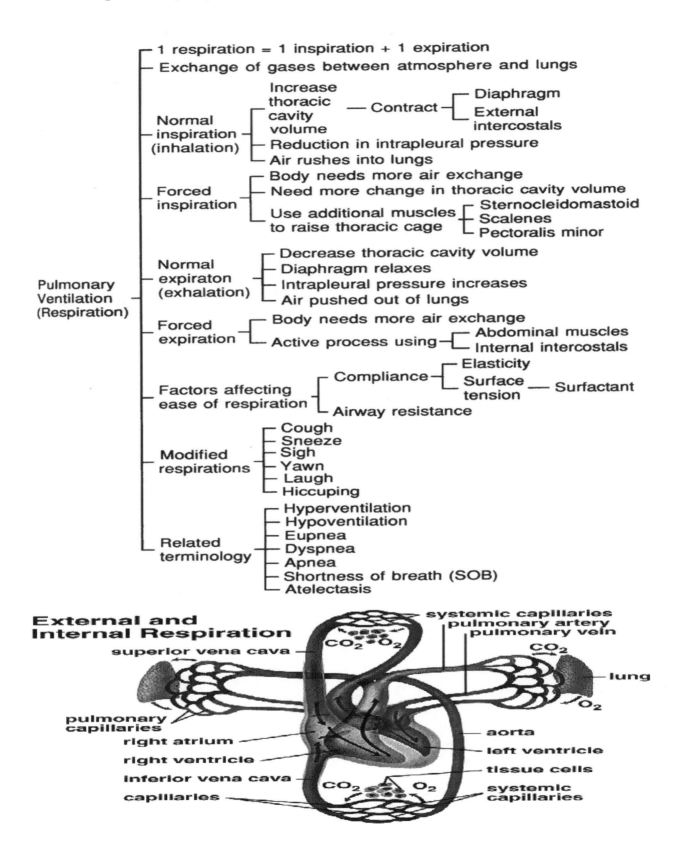

Pulmonary Ventilation (Respiration)

- 1 respiration = 1 inspiration + 1 expiration
- Exchange of gases between atmosphere and lungs

Normal inspiration (inhalation)
- Increase thoracic cavity volume — Contract — Diaphragm / External intercostals
- Reduction in intrapleural pressure
- Air rushes into lungs

Forced inspiration
- Body needs more air exchange
- Need more change in thoracic cavity volume
- Use additional muscles to raise thoracic cage — Sternocleidomastoid / Scalenes / Pectoralis minor

Normal expiraton (exhalation)
- Decrease thoracic cavity volume
- Diaphragm relaxes
- Intrapleural pressure increases
- Air pushed out of lungs

Forced expiration
- Body needs more air exchange
- Active process using — Abdominal muscles / Internal intercostals

Factors affecting ease of respiration
- Compliance — Elasticity / Surface tension — Surfactant
- Airway resistance

Modified respirations
- Cough
- Sneeze
- Sigh
- Yawn
- Laugh
- Hiccuping

Related terminology
- Hyperventilation
- Hypoventilation
- Eupnea
- Dyspnea
- Apnea
- Shortness of breath (SOB)
- Atelectasis

External and Internal Respiration

systemic capillaries
pulmonary artery
pulmonary vein
superior vena cava
CO_2 O_2
CO_2
lung
O_2
pulmonary capillaries
right atrium
right ventricle
inferior vena cava
capillaries
CO_2 O_2
aorta
left ventricle
tissue cells
systemic capillaries

PULMONARY VENTILATION(RESPIRATION)

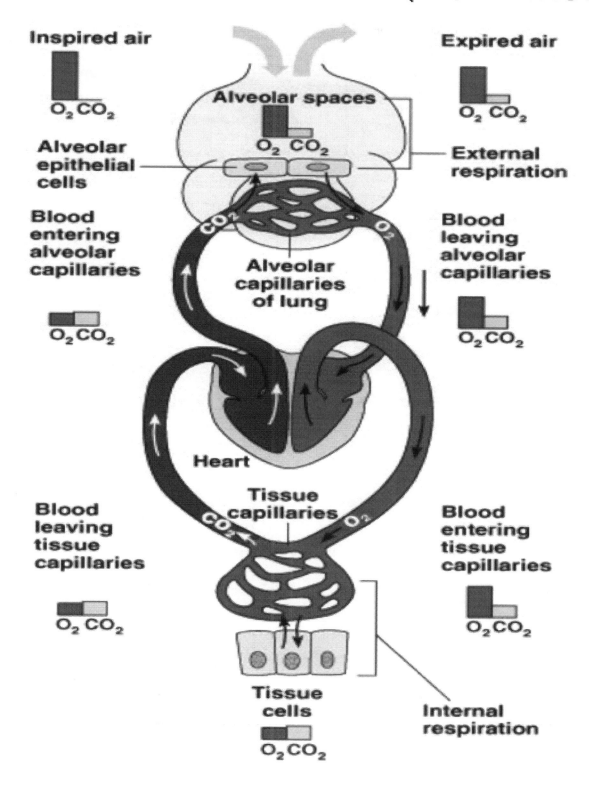

Inspired air
O_2 CO_2

Expired air
O_2 CO_2

Alveolar spaces
O_2 CO_2

Alveolar epithelial cells

External respiration

Blood entering alveolar capillaries
O_2 CO_2

Alveolar capillaries of lung

Blood leaving alveolar capillaries
O_2 CO_2

Heart

Blood leaving tissue capillaries
O_2 CO_2

Tissue capillaries

Blood entering tissue capillaries
O_2 CO_2

Tissue cells
O_2 CO_2

Internal respiration

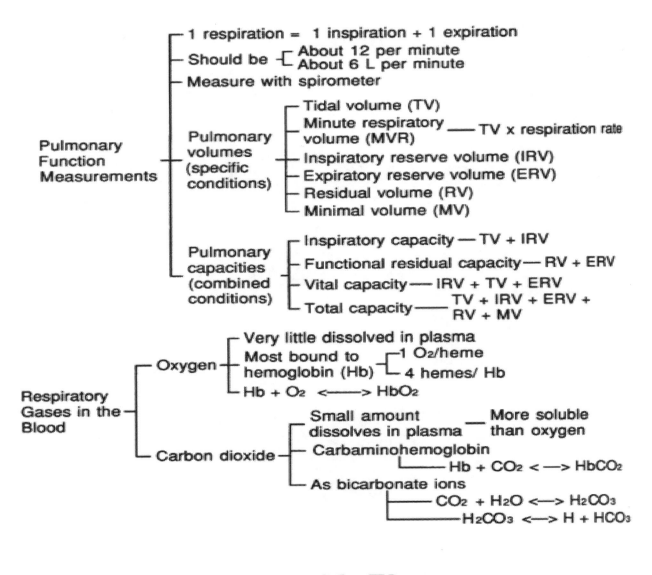

29Nov2012 _____ 23:50 RESULT OF ARTERIAL
Sample Type_____ Art BLOOD GAS ANALYSIS
                    ON AIR
At 37C   NORMAL VALUES
pH_____ 7.48   (7.35-7.45)

pCO2_____ 2.9 kPa   (4.9-6.1)

pO2_____ 15.5 kPa   (10-13.1)

Cl_____ 100 mM   (95-105)

Na_____ 142 mM   (135-145)

K_____ 3.2 mM   (3.5-5.0)

HCO3_____ 17 mM   (22-28)

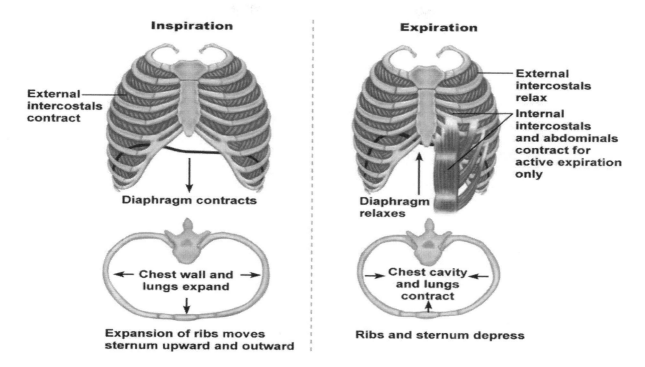

Inspiration

External intercostals contract

Diaphragm contracts

Chest wall and lungs expand

Expansion of ribs moves sternum upward and outward

Expiration

External intercostals relax

Internal intercostals and abdominals contract for active expiration only

Diaphragm relaxes

Chest cavity and lungs contract

Ribs and sternum depress

A spirometer tracing showing lung volumes and capacities.

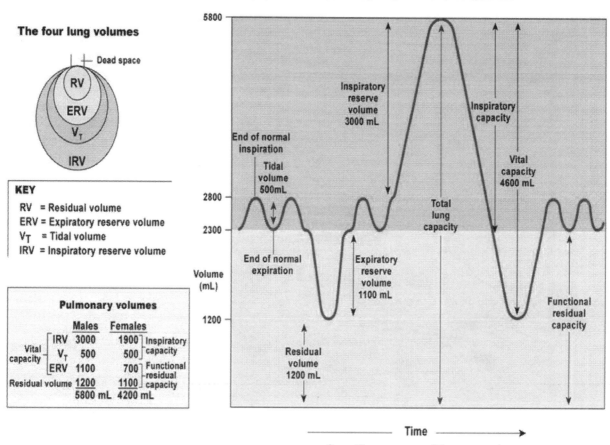

The four lung volumes

Dead space

RV

ERV

V_T

IRV

KEY

RV = Residual volume
ERV = Expiratory reserve volume
V_T = Tidal volume
IRV = Inspiratory reserve volume

Pulmonary volumes				
		Males	Females	
Vital capacity	IRV	3000	1900	Inspiratory capacity
	V_T	500	500	
	ERV	1100	700	Functional residual capacity
Residual volume		1200	1100	
		5800 mL	4200 mL	

Volume (mL)

5800

2800
2300

1200

Inspiratory reserve volume 3000 mL

End of normal inspiration

Tidal volume 500mL

End of normal expiration

Expiratory reserve volume 1100 mL

Residual volume 1200 mL

Total lung capacity

Inspiratory capacity

Vital capacity 4600 mL

Functional residual capacity

Time

Capacities are sums of 2 or more volumes.

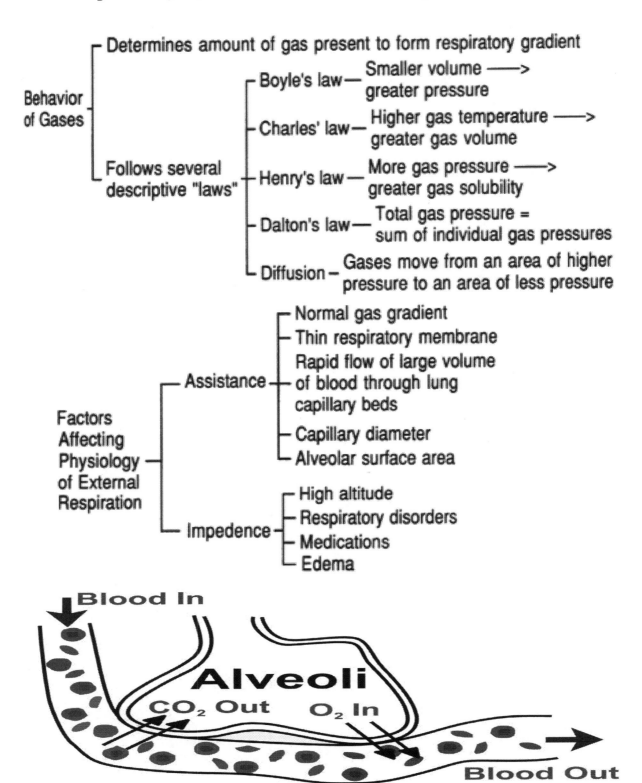

Behavior of Gases
- Determines amount of gas present to form respiratory gradient
- Follows several descriptive "laws"
  - Boyle's law — Smaller volume ——> greater pressure
  - Charles' law — Higher gas temperature ——> greater gas volume
  - Henry's law — More gas pressure ——> greater gas solubility
  - Dalton's law — Total gas pressure = sum of individual gas pressures
  - Diffusion — Gases move from an area of higher pressure to an area of less pressure

Factors Affecting Physiology of External Respiration
- Assistance
  - Normal gas gradient
  - Thin respiratory membrane
  - Rapid flow of large volume of blood through lung capillary beds
  - Capillary diameter
  - Alveolar surface area
- Impedence
  - High altitude
  - Respiratory disorders
  - Medications
  - Edema

Blood In

Alveoli

CO_2 Out O_2 In

Blood Out

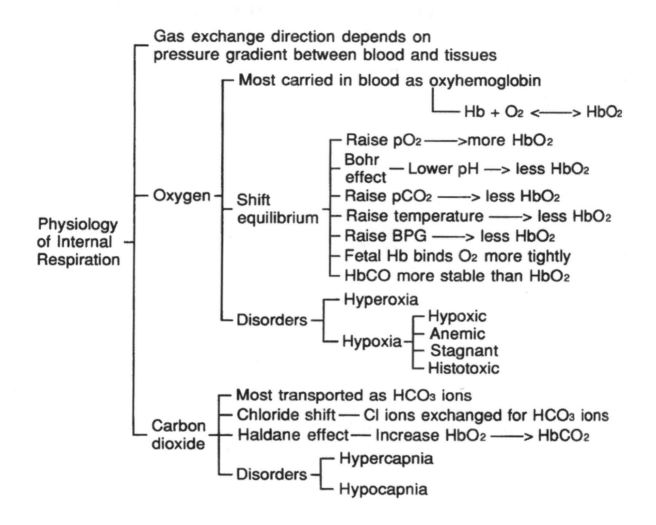

Physiology of Internal Respiration
- Gas exchange direction depends on pressure gradient between blood and tissues
- Oxygen
  - Most carried in blood as oxyhemoglobin
    - $Hb + O_2 \longleftrightarrow HbO_2$
  - Shift equilibrium
    - Raise $pO_2 \longrightarrow$ more HbO_2
    - Bohr effect — Lower pH $\longrightarrow$ less HbO_2
    - Raise $pCO_2 \longrightarrow$ less HbO_2
    - Raise temperature $\longrightarrow$ less HbO_2
    - Raise BPG $\longrightarrow$ less HbO_2
    - Fetal Hb binds O_2 more tightly
    - HbCO more stable than HbO_2
  - Disorders
    - Hyperoxia
    - Hypoxia
      - Hypoxic
      - Anemic
      - Stagnant
      - Histotoxic
- Carbon dioxide
  - Most transported as HCO_3 ions
  - Chloride shift — Cl ions exchanged for HCO_3 ions
  - Haldane effect — Increase $HbO_2 \longrightarrow HbCO_2$
  - Disorders
    - Hypercapnia
    - Hypocapnia

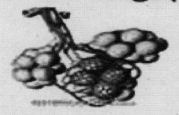
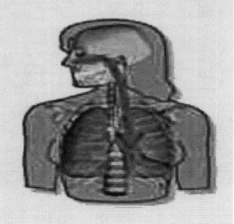

External vs. Internal Respiration

- **External = at the level of the lungs (alveoli)**

- **Internal = at the level of the REST OF THE BODY**

EXTERNAL & INTERNAL RESPIRATION

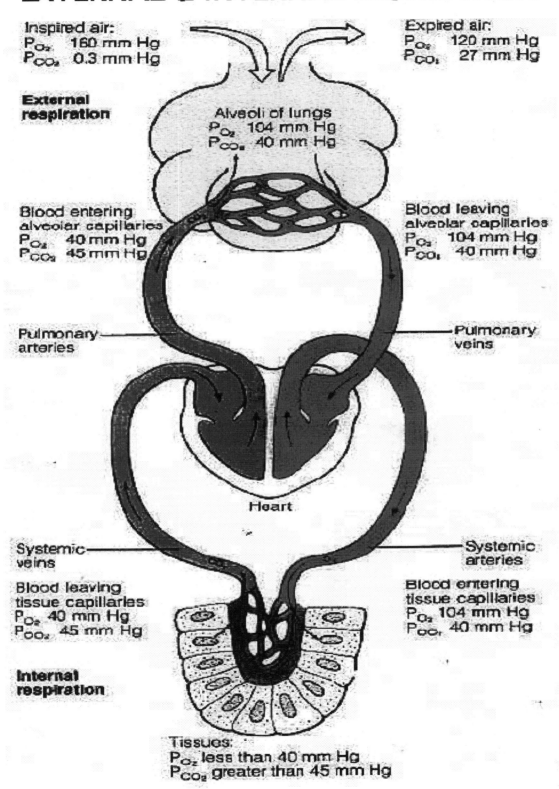

Inspired air:
P$_{O_2}$ 160 mm Hg
P$_{CO_2}$ 0.3 mm Hg

Expired air:
P$_{O_2}$ 120 mm Hg
P$_{CO_2}$ 27 mm Hg

External respiration

Alveoli of lungs
P$_{O_2}$ 104 mm Hg
P$_{CO_2}$ 40 mm Hg

Blood entering
alveolar capillaries
P$_{O_2}$ 40 mm Hg
P$_{CO_2}$ 45 mm Hg

Blood leaving
alveolar capillaries
P$_{O_2}$ 104 mm Hg
P$_{CO_2}$ 40 mm Hg

Pulmonary arteries

Pulmonary veins

Heart

Systemic veins

Systemic arteries

Blood leaving
tissue capillaries
P$_{O_2}$ 40 mm Hg
P$_{CO_2}$ 45 mm Hg

Blood entering
tissue capillaries
P$_{O_2}$ 104 mm Hg
P$_{CO_2}$ 40 mm Hg

Internal respiration

Tissues:
P$_{O_2}$ less than 40 mm Hg
P$_{CO_2}$ greater than 45 mm Hg

Gas Exchange in the Lungs

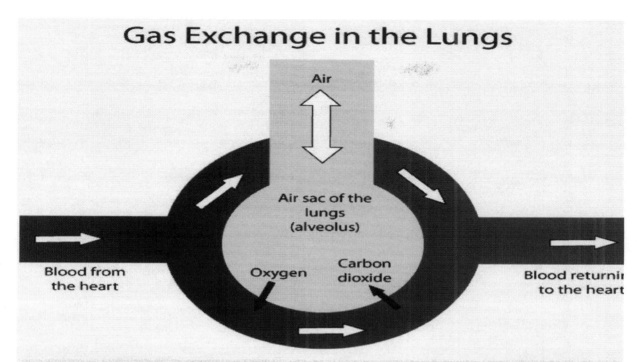

This is a simple representation of blood flowing through a capillary next to the alveolar-capillary membrane of an alveolus (for more about the rest of these structures see the distal respiratory tree).

The blood corpuscles that carry carbon dioxide and/or oxygen in the blood deliver carbon dioxide to the alveolus because the concentration of carbon dioxide is higher in the incoming blood than in the alveolus filled with freshly inhaled air.

As the carbon dixoide leaves the blood corpuscles they are "re-filled" with oxygen supplied by the oxygen in the alveolus because the concentration of oxygen is higher in the freshly inhaled air in the alveolus than in the incoming blood.

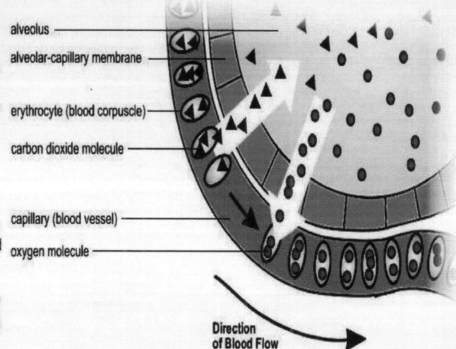

The exchange of gases between the alveoli and the blood occurs by diffusion of the gases through the tissues and is driven by the tendency for equalisation of pressures of the gases on each side of the alveolar-capillary membrane, as well as the tendency for fluids to diffuse from high- to lower- concentrations (when free to do so). The extremely large* total surface area of alveoli in the lungs makes this process extremely efficient, and therefore also very fast.

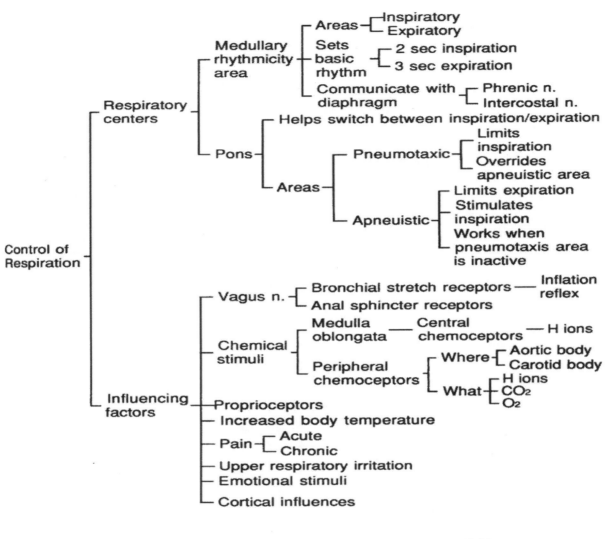

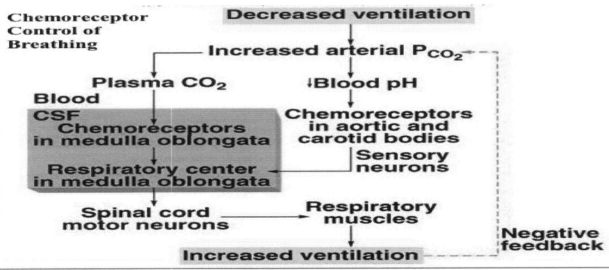

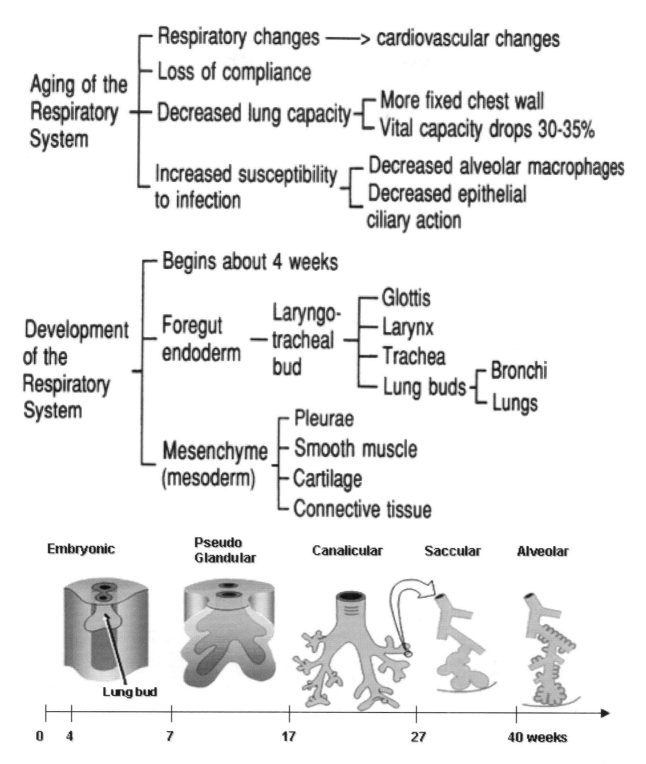

Aging of the Respiratory System
- Respiratory changes ——> cardiovascular changes
- Loss of compliance
- Decreased lung capacity
  - More fixed chest wall
  - Vital capacity drops 30-35%
- Increased susceptibility to infection
  - Decreased alveolar macrophages
  - Decreased epithelial ciliary action

Development of the Respiratory System
- Begins about 4 weeks
- Foregut endoderm — Laryngo-tracheal bud
  - Glottis
  - Larynx
  - Trachea
  - Lung buds
    - Bronchi
    - Lungs
- Mesenchyme (mesoderm)
  - Pleurae
  - Smooth muscle
  - Cartilage
  - Connective tissue

Embryonic   Pseudo Glandular   Canalicular   Saccular   Alveolar

Lung bud

0   4   7   17   27   40 weeks

The stages of pulmonary development

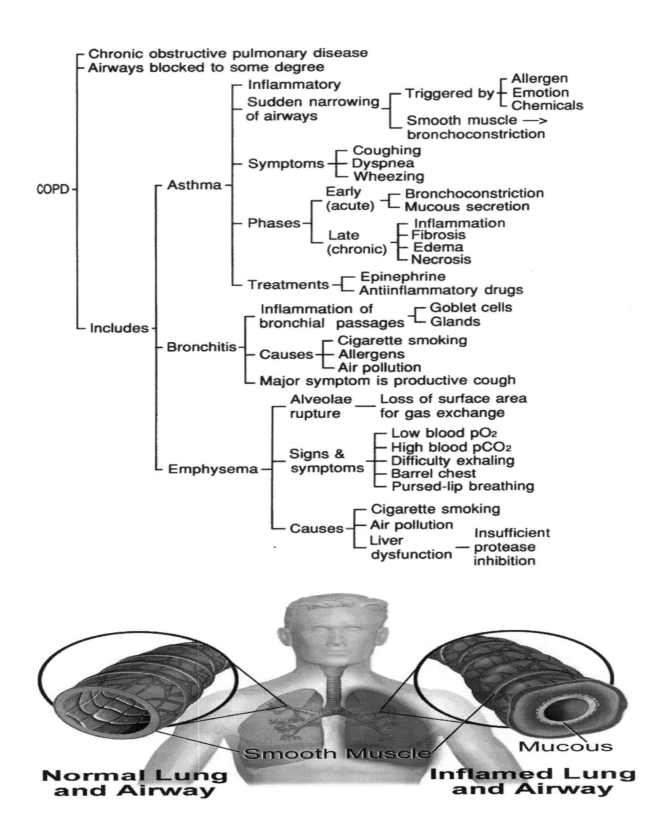

COPD
- Chronic obstructive pulmonary disease
- Airways blocked to some degree
- Includes
  - Asthma
    - Inflammatory
    - Sudden narrowing of airways
      - Triggered by
        - Allergen
        - Emotion
        - Chemicals
      - Smooth muscle —> bronchoconstriction
    - Symptoms
      - Coughing
      - Dyspnea
      - Wheezing
    - Phases
      - Early (acute)
        - Bronchoconstriction
        - Mucous secretion
      - Late (chronic)
        - Inflammation
        - Fibrosis
        - Edema
        - Necrosis
    - Treatments
      - Epinephrine
      - Antiinflammatory drugs
  - Bronchitis
    - Inflammation of bronchial passages
      - Goblet cells
      - Glands
    - Causes
      - Cigarette smoking
      - Allergens
      - Air pollution
    - Major symptom is productive cough
  - Emphysema
    - Alveolae rupture — Loss of surface area for gas exchange
    - Signs & symptoms
      - Low blood pO_2
      - High blood pCO_2
      - Difficulty exhaling
      - Barrel chest
      - Pursed-lip breathing
    - Causes
      - Cigarette smoking
      - Air pollution
      - Liver dysfunction — Insufficient protease inhibition

Smooth Muscle   Mucous

Normal Lung and Airway   Inflamed Lung and Airway

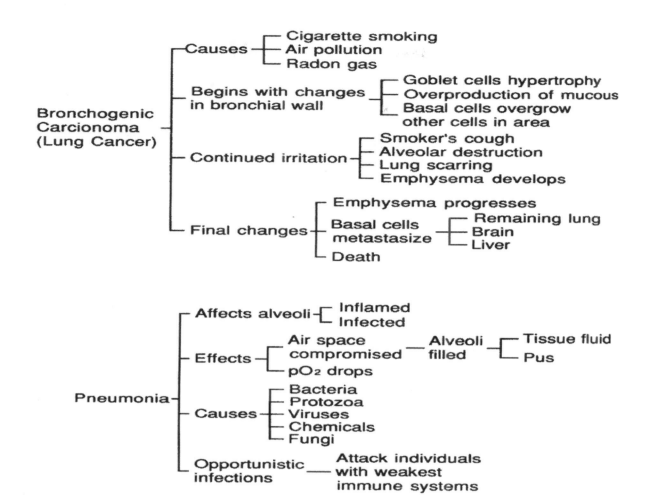

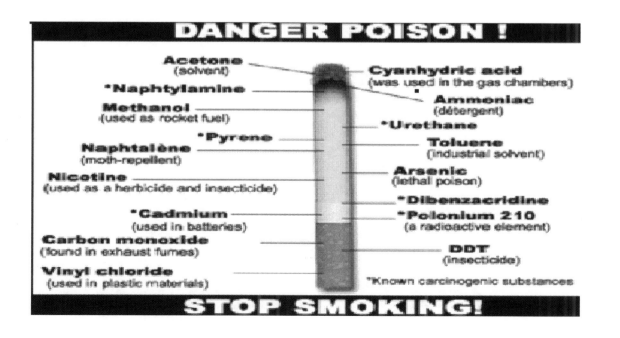

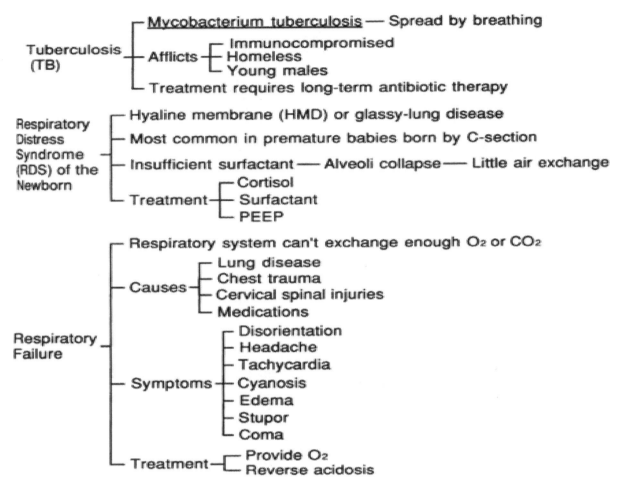

Tuberculosis (TB)
- Mycobacterium tuberculosis — Spread by breathing
- Afflicts
  - Immunocompromised
  - Homeless
  - Young males
- Treatment requires long-term antibiotic therapy

Respiratory Distress Syndrome (RDS) of the Newborn
- Hyaline membrane (HMD) or glassy-lung disease
- Most common in premature babies born by C-section
- Insufficient surfactant — Alveoli collapse — Little air exchange
- Treatment
  - Cortisol
  - Surfactant
  - PEEP

Respiratory Failure
- Respiratory system can't exchange enough O_2 or CO_2
- Causes
  - Lung disease
  - Chest trauma
  - Cervical spinal injuries
  - Medications
- Symptoms
  - Disorientation
  - Headache
  - Tachycardia
  - Cyanosis
  - Edema
  - Stupor
  - Coma
- Treatment
  - Provide O_2
  - Reverse acidosis

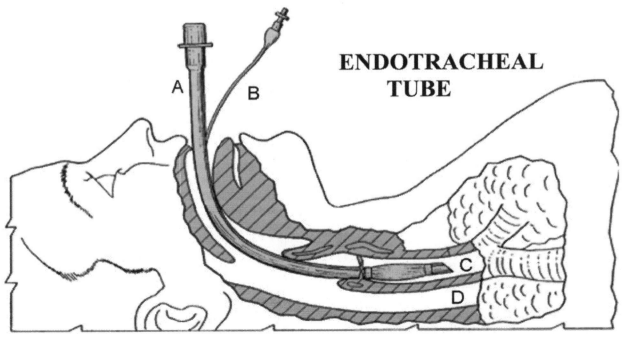

ENDOTRACHEAL TUBE

A
B
C
D

Sudden Infant Death Syndrome (SIDS)
- Crib death — Most often
  - Between ages 1 week —> 1 year
  - Otherwise healthy infants
- Possible causes
  - Post-viral syndrome
  - Laryngospasm
  - Malfunction of respiratory center — Use sleep monitors; disrupt apnea

Coryza
- Common cold
- Caused by rhinoviruses
- Symptoms
  - Sneezing
  - Runny nose
  - Congestion
  - Nonproductive cough

Influenza
- Viral illness
- Fever
- Muscular aches
- Headache
- Cold symptoms

Pulmonary Embolism
- Obstruction in pulmonary arterial circulation
- Types of emboli
  - Blood clot
  - Fat
  - Air
- Risk factors
  - Bed confinement
  - Fractures
  - Malignancy
  - Pregnancy
  - Smoking
  - Oral contraceptives
- Signs & symptoms
  - Sudden dyspnea
  - Chest pain
  - Hemoptysis
- Treatment
  - Anticoagulant therapy
  - Bedrest
  - Analgesia
  - O_2

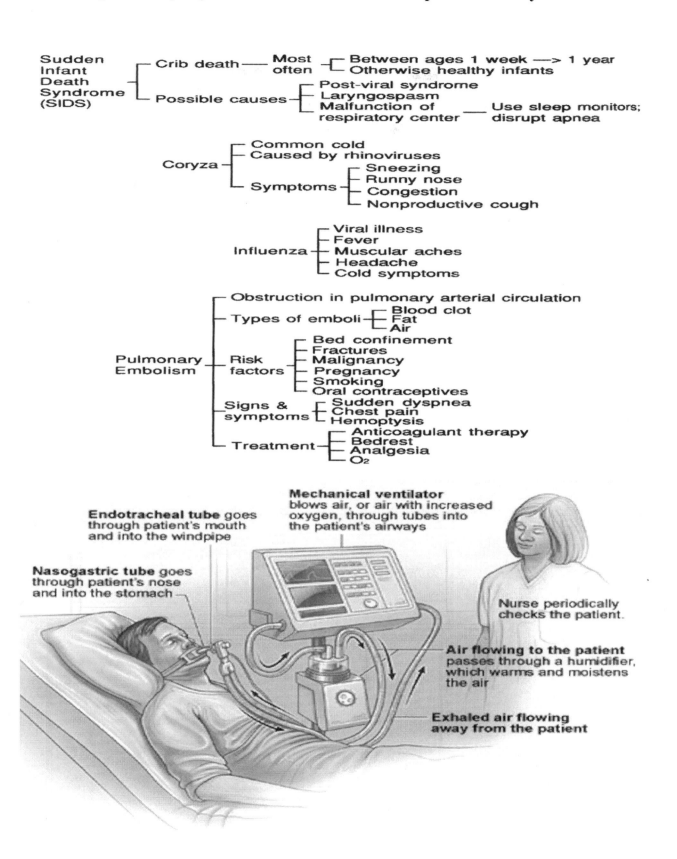

Endotracheal tube goes through patient's mouth and into the windpipe

Mechanical ventilator blows air, or air with increased oxygen, through tubes into the patient's airways

Nasogastric tube goes through patient's nose and into the stomach

Nurse periodically checks the patient.

Air flowing to the patient passes through a humidifier, which warms and moistens the air

Exhaled air flowing away from the patient

Pulmonary Edema
- Interstitial fluid accumulates
  - Alveoli
  - Interstitial spaces
- Origins
  - Pulmonary — Leaky capillaries
  - Cardiac — Higher capillary pressure
- Symptoms
  - Dyspnea
  - Wheezing
  - Tachypnea
  - Feeling of suffocation
  - Pallor
  - Diaphoresis
- Treatment
  - O_2
  - Acid-base correction
  - Mechanical ventilation

Cystic Fibrosis (CF)
- Congenital
  - Error in Cl ion movement
  - Affects mostly Caucasians
- Affects secretory epithelia
  - Respiratory tract
  - Pancreatic ducts
  - Salivary glands
  - Sweat glands
- Signs & symptoms
  - Very salty sweat
  - Pancreatic duct blockage — Malnutrition
  - Respiratory tract blockage
    - Trapped mucous
    - Scarring of airways
- Treatment
  - Percussion
  - Ventilation support
  - Modified diet

Smoke Inhalation Injury
- Components
  - Limited O_2 availability
    - CO
    - CN
  - Heat damage to upper respiratory tract
  - Chemical damage to lungs
    - Acids
    - Aldehydes
- Signs & symptoms
  - Confusion
  - Coma
  - Cardiac arrest
  - Acidosis
  - Dyspnea
  - Hypoxemia
  - Bronchopneumonia
  - Atelectasis
- Treatment
  - O_2
  - Suction
  - Bronchodilators
  - Fluid therapy

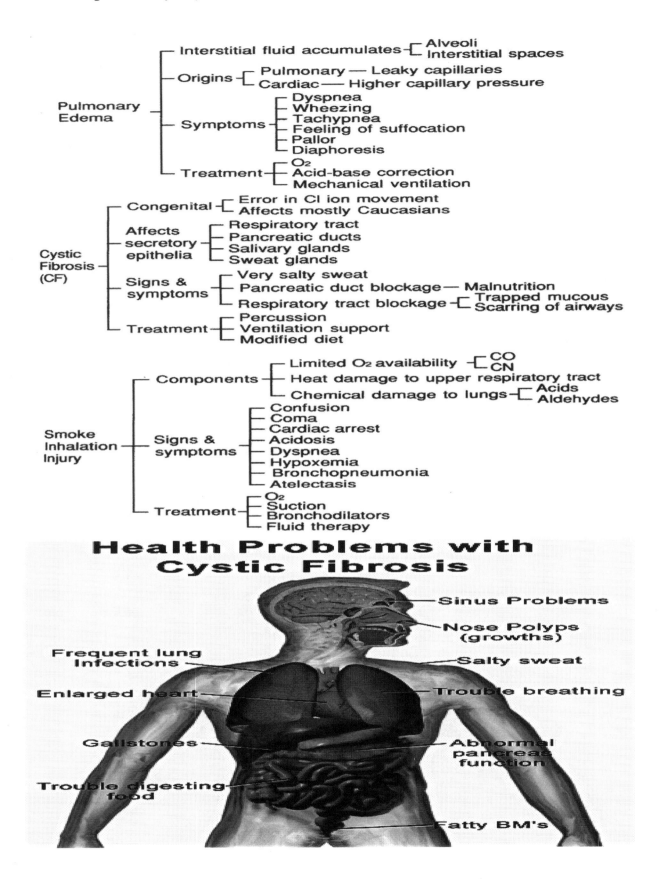

Health Problems with Cystic Fibrosis

- Sinus Problems
- Nose Polyps (growths)
- Frequent lung Infections
- Salty sweat
- Enlarged heart
- Trouble breathing
- Gallstones
- Abnormal pancreas function
- Trouble digesting food
- Fatty BM's

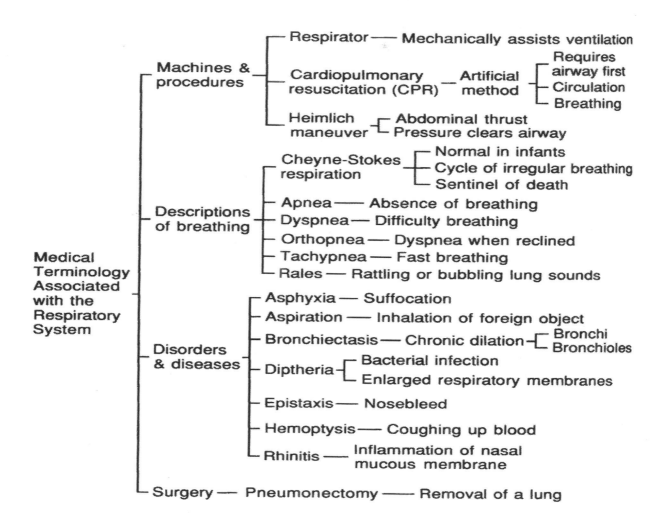

Medical Terminology Associated with the Respiratory System

- Machines & procedures
  - Respirator —— Mechanically assists ventilation
  - Cardiopulmonary resuscitation (CPR) — Artificial method
    - Requires airway first
    - Circulation
    - Breathing
  - Heimlich maneuver
    - Abdominal thrust
    - Pressure clears airway
- Descriptions of breathing
  - Cheyne-Stokes respiration
    - Normal in infants
    - Cycle of irregular breathing
    - Sentinel of death
  - Apnea —— Absence of breathing
  - Dyspnea — Difficulty breathing
  - Orthopnea —— Dyspnea when reclined
  - Tachypnea —— Fast breathing
  - Rales — Rattling or bubbling lung sounds
- Disorders & diseases
  - Asphyxia — Suffocation
  - Aspiration —— Inhalation of foreign object
  - Bronchiectasis —— Chronic dilation
    - Bronchi
    - Bronchioles
  - Diptheria
    - Bacterial infection
    - Enlarged respiratory membranes
  - Epistaxis —— Nosebleed
  - Hemoptysis —— Coughing up blood
  - Rhinitis —— Inflammation of nasal mucous membrane
- Surgery — Pneumonectomy —— Removal of a lung

orthopnea

form of dyspnea in which the person can breathe comfortably only when standing or sitting erect; associated with asthma and emphysema and angina pectoris

CHAPTER TWENTY FOUR

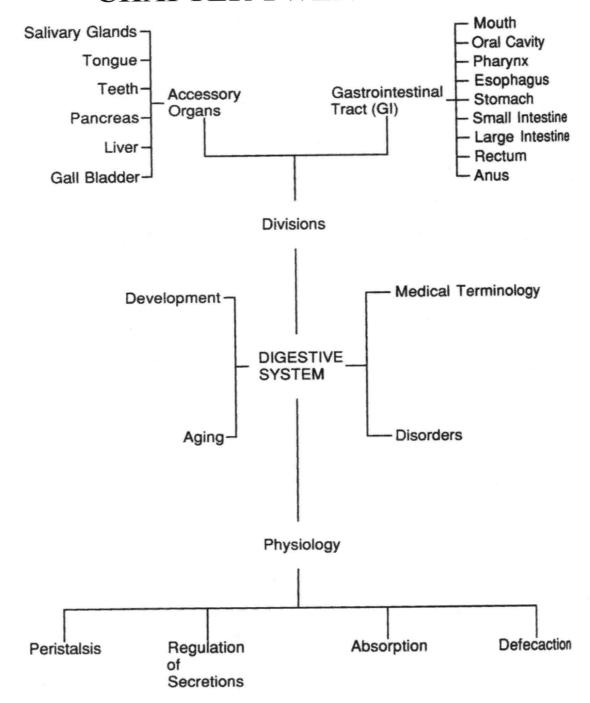

Salivary Glands
Tongue
Teeth
Pancreas
Liver
Gall Bladder

Accessory Organs

Gastrointestinal Tract (GI)

Mouth
Oral Cavity
Pharynx
Esophagus
Stomach
Small Intestine
Large Intestine
Rectum
Anus

Divisions

Development

Aging

DIGESTIVE SYSTEM

Medical Terminology

Disorders

Physiology

Peristalsis

Regulation of Secretions

Absorption

Defecaction

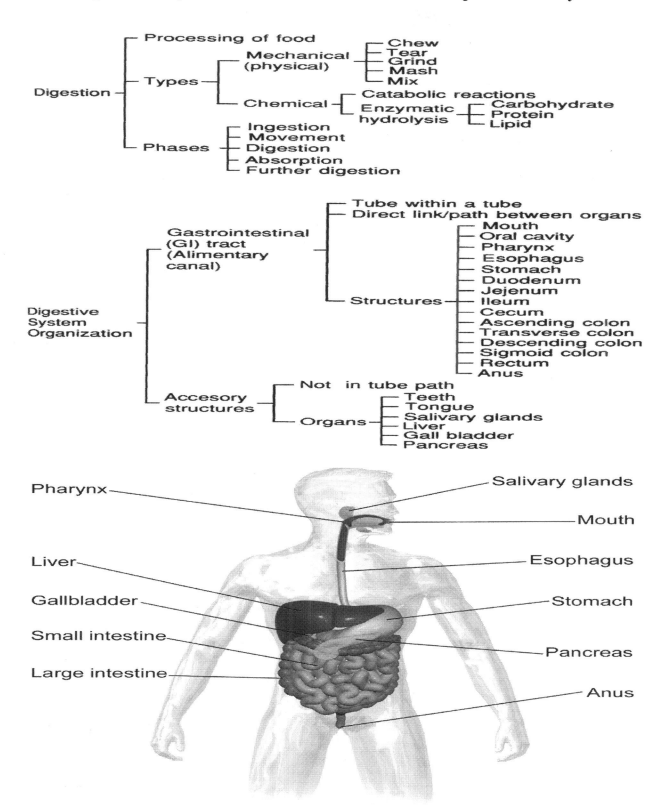

Digestion ─┬─ Processing of food
           ├─ Types ─┬─ Mechanical (physical) ─┬─ Chew
           │   │   ├─ Tear
           │   │   ├─ Grind
           │   │   ├─ Mash
           │   │   └─ Mix
           │   └─ Chemical ─┬─ Catabolic reactions
           │   └─ Enzymatic hydrolysis ─┬─ Carbohydrate
           │   ├─ Protein
           │   └─ Lipid
           └─ Phases ─┬─ Ingestion
                      ├─ Movement
                      ├─ Digestion
                      ├─ Absorption
                      └─ Further digestion

Digestive System Organization ─┬─ Gastrointestinal (GI) tract (Alimentary canal) ─┬─ Tube within a tube
                                │   ├─ Direct link/path between organs
                                │   └─ Structures ─┬─ Mouth
                                │   ├─ Oral cavity
                                │   ├─ Pharynx
                                │   ├─ Esophagus
                                │   ├─ Stomach
                                │   ├─ Duodenum
                                │   ├─ Jejenum
                                │   ├─ Ileum
                                │   ├─ Cecum
                                │   ├─ Ascending colon
                                │   ├─ Transverse colon
                                │   ├─ Descending colon
                                │   ├─ Sigmoid colon
                                │   ├─ Rectum
                                │   └─ Anus
                                └─ Accesory structures ─┬─ Not in tube path
                                                        └─ Organs ─┬─ Teeth
                                                                   ├─ Tongue
                                                                   ├─ Salivary glands
                                                                   ├─ Liver
                                                                   ├─ Gall bladder
                                                                   └─ Pancreas

Pharynx —

Liver —

Gallbladder —

Small intestine —

Large intestine —

Salivary glands

Mouth

Esophagus

Stomach

Pancreas

Anus

The Components of the Digestive System

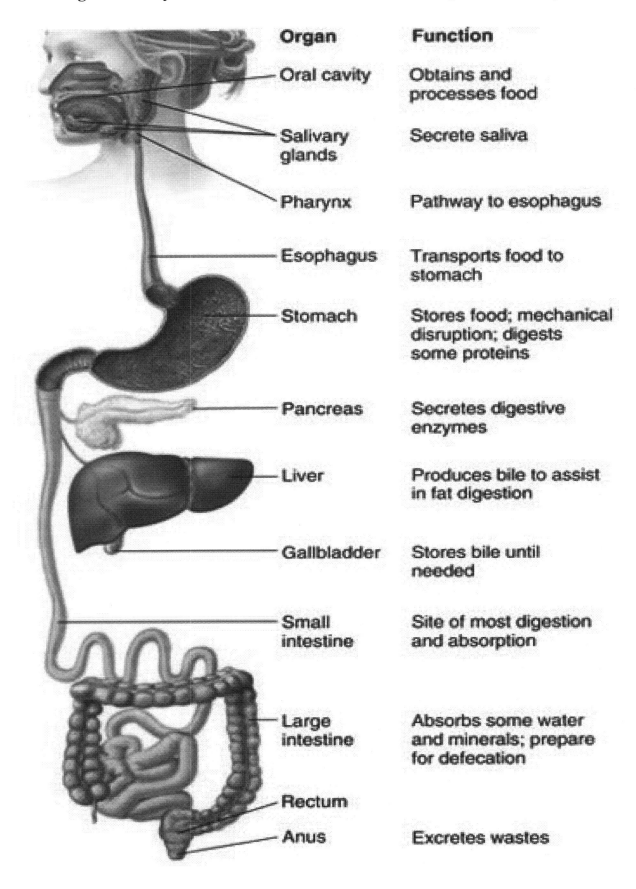

Organ	Function
Oral cavity	Obtains and processes food
Salivary glands	Secrete saliva
Pharynx	Pathway to esophagus
Esophagus	Transports food to stomach
Stomach	Stores food; mechanical disruption; digests some proteins
Pancreas	Secretes digestive enzymes
Liver	Produces bile to assist in fat digestion
Gallbladder	Stores bile until needed
Small intestine	Site of most digestion and absorption
Large intestine	Absorbs some water and minerals; prepare for defecation
Rectum	
Anus	Excretes wastes

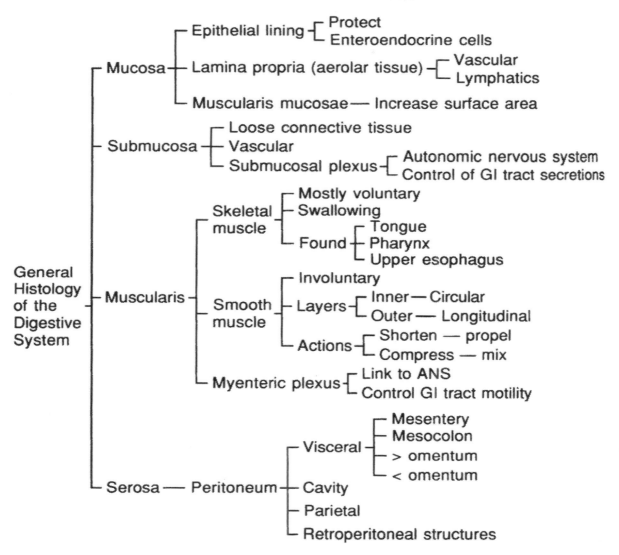

General Histology of the Digestive System
- Mucosa
  - Epithelial lining
    - Protect
    - Enteroendocrine cells
  - Lamina propria (aerolar tissue)
    - Vascular
    - Lymphatics
  - Muscularis mucosae — Increase surface area
- Submucosa
  - Loose connective tissue
  - Vascular
  - Submucosal plexus
    - Autonomic nervous system
    - Control of GI tract secretions
- Muscularis
  - Skeletal muscle
    - Mostly voluntary
    - Swallowing
    - Found
      - Tongue
      - Pharynx
      - Upper esophagus
  - Smooth muscle
    - Involuntary
    - Layers
      - Inner — Circular
      - Outer — Longitudinal
    - Actions
      - Shorten — propel
      - Compress — mix
  - Myenteric plexus
    - Link to ANS
    - Control GI tract motility
- Serosa — Peritoneum
  - Visceral
    - Mesentery
    - Mesocolon
    - > omentum
    - < omentum
  - Cavity
  - Parietal
  - Retroperitoneal structures

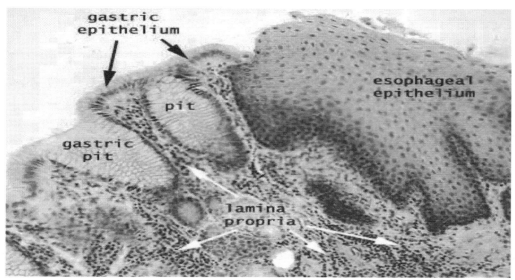

gastric epithelium

esophageal epithelium

pit

gastric pit

lamina propria

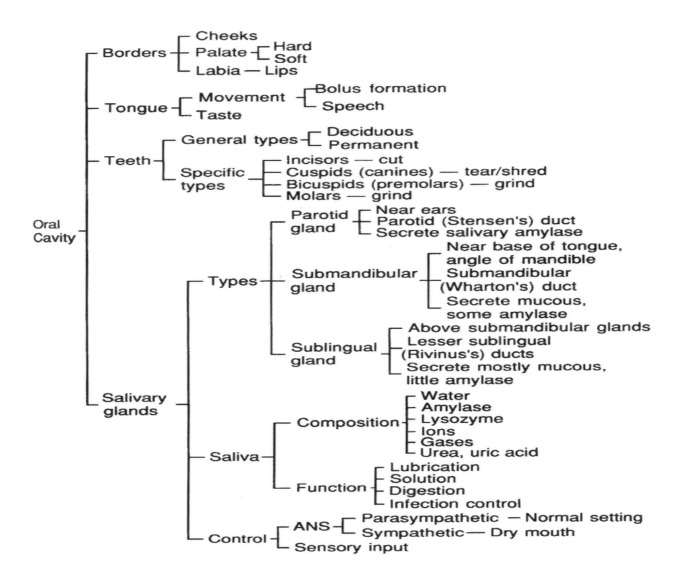

- Oral Cavity
  - Borders
    - Cheeks
    - Palate
      - Hard
      - Soft
    - Labia — Lips
  - Tongue
    - Movement
      - Bolus formation
      - Speech
    - Taste
  - Teeth
    - General types
      - Deciduous
      - Permanent
    - Specific types
      - Incisors — cut
      - Cuspids (canines) — tear/shred
      - Bicuspids (premolars) — grind
      - Molars — grind
  - Salivary glands
    - Types
      - Parotid gland
        - Near ears
        - Parotid (Stensen's) duct
        - Secrete salivary amylase
      - Submandibular gland
        - Near base of tongue, angle of mandible
        - Submandibular (Wharton's) duct
        - Secrete mucous, some amylase
      - Sublingual gland
        - Above submandibular glands
        - Lesser sublingual (Rivinus's) ducts
        - Secrete mostly mucous, little amylase
    - Saliva
      - Composition
        - Water
        - Amylase
        - Lysozyme
        - Ions
        - Gases
        - Urea, uric acid
      - Function
        - Lubrication
        - Solution
        - Digestion
        - Infection control
    - Control
      - ANS
        - Parasympathetic — Normal setting
        - Sympathetic — Dry mouth
      - Sensory input

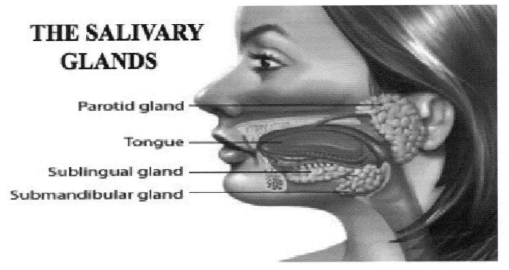

THE SALIVARY GLANDS

- Parotid gland
- Tongue
- Sublingual gland
- Submandibular gland

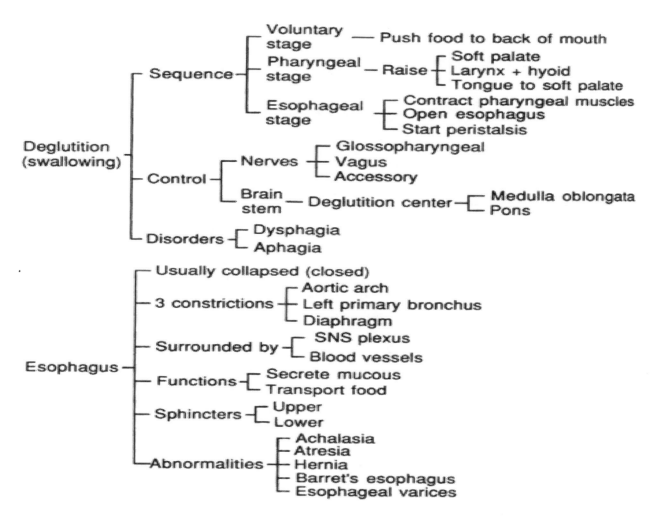

Deglutition (swallowing)
- Sequence
  - Voluntary stage — Push food to back of mouth
  - Pharyngeal stage — Raise
    - Soft palate
    - Larynx + hyoid
    - Tongue to soft palate
  - Esophageal stage
    - Contract pharyngeal muscles
    - Open esophagus
    - Start peristalsis
- Control
  - Nerves
    - Glossopharyngeal
    - Vagus
    - Accessory
  - Brain stem — Deglutition center
    - Medulla oblongata
    - Pons
- Disorders
  - Dysphagia
  - Aphagia

Esophagus
- Usually collapsed (closed)
- 3 constrictions
  - Aortic arch
  - Left primary bronchus
  - Diaphragm
- Surrounded by
  - SNS plexus
  - Blood vessels
- Functions
  - Secrete mucous
  - Transport food
- Sphincters
  - Upper
  - Lower
- Abnormalities
  - Achalasia
  - Atresia
  - Hernia
  - Barret's esophagus
  - Esophageal varices

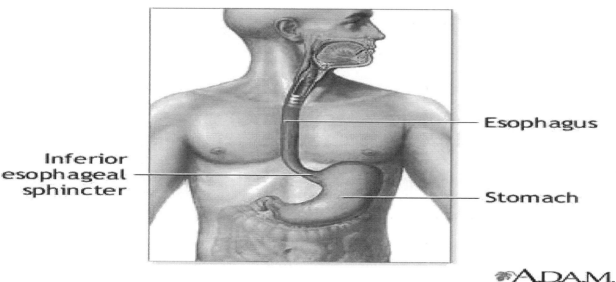

Inferior esophageal sphincter

Esophagus

Stomach

✦ADAM.

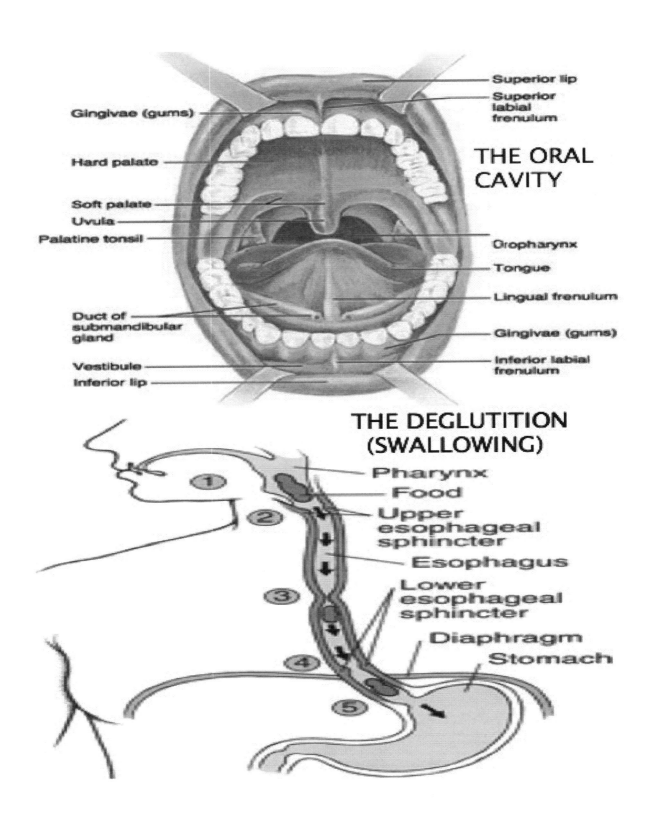

Gingivae (gums)

Hard palate

Soft palate

Uvula

Palatine tonsil

Duct of
submandibular
gland

Vestibule

Inferior lip

Superior lip

Superior
labial
frenulum

THE ORAL
CAVITY

Oropharynx

Tongue

Lingual frenulum

Gingivae (gums)

Inferior labial
frenulum

THE DEGLUTITION
(SWALLOWING)

Pharynx

Food

Upper
esophageal
sphincter

Esophagus

Lower
esophageal
sphincter

Diaphragm

Stomach

Stomach
- Usually "J"-shaped
- Left side, anterior to spleen
- Mucous membrane
  - G cells —— Make gastrin
  - Goblet cells — Make mucous
  - Gastric pit ___ Oxyntic gland ___ Parietal cells —— Make HCl
  - Chief cells — Zymogenic cells
    - Pepsin
    - Gastric lipase
- 3 muscle layers
  - Oblique
  - Circular
  - Longitudinal
- Regions
  - Cardiac sphincter
  - Fundus
  - Antrum (pylorus)
  - Pyloric sphincter
- Vascular
- Inner surface thrown into folds — Rugae
- Contains enzymes that work best at pH 1-2
- Functions
  - Mix food
  - Reservoir
  - Start digestion of
    - Protein
    - Nucleic acids
    - Fats
  - Activates some enzymes
  - Destroy some bacteria
  - Makes intrinsic factor —— B_{12} absorption
  - Destroys some bacteria
  - Absorbs
    - Alcohol
    - Water
    - Lipophilic acid
    - B_{12}

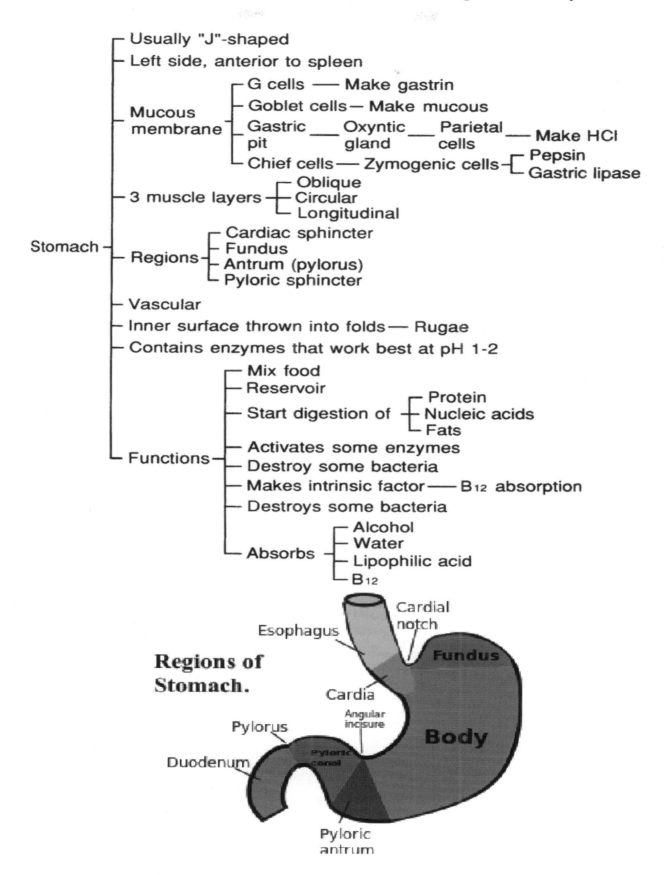

Regions of Stomach.

Esophagus

Cardial notch

Fundus

Cardia

Angular incisure

Pylorus

Pyloric canal

Body

Duodenum

Pyloric antrum

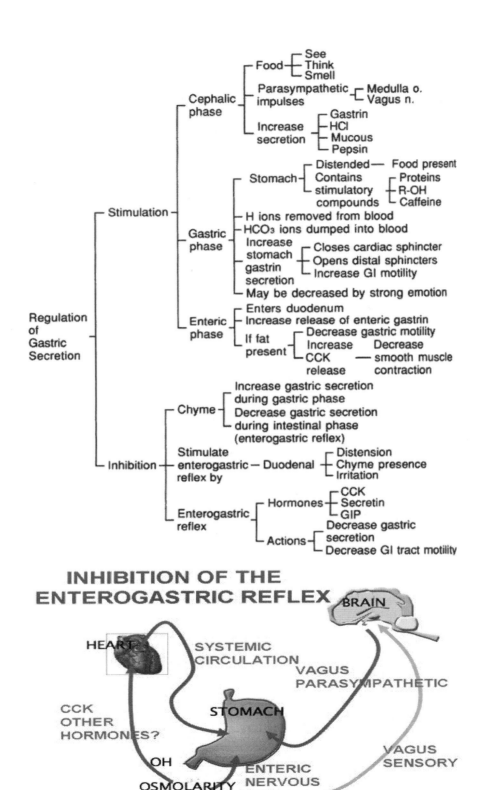

```
                                    ┌── See
                        ┌── Food ───┼── Think
                        │           └── Smell
           ┌── Cephalic ┤ Parasympathetic ──┬── Medulla o.
           │    phase   │ impulses           └── Vagus n.
           │            │           ┌── Gastrin
           │            └── Increase┤── HCl
           │                secretion── Mucous
           │                        └── Pepsin
           │                        ┌── Distended ─── Food present
           │              ┌── Stomach┤── Contains      ┌── Proteins
           │              │          │   stimulatory ──┤── R-OH
┌── Stimulation ─┤          │          └── compounds    └── Caffeine
│          │              ├── H ions removed from blood
│          │              ├── HCO₃ ions dumped into blood
│          │   ┌── Gastric┤── Increase    ┌── Closes cardiac sphincter
│          │   │   phase  │   stomach     │── Opens distal sphincters
│          │   │          │   gastrin ────┤── Increase GI motility
│          │   │          │   secretion
│          │   │          └── May be decreased by strong emotion
│          │   │          ┌── Enters duodenum
│          │   └── Enteric├── Increase release of enteric gastrin
│          │       phase  │           ┌── Decrease gastric motility
│          │              └── If fat ──┤── Increase      Decrease
│          │                  present  └── CCK      ─── smooth muscle
│          │                              release        contraction
```

Regulation of Gastric Secretion — Stimulation

```
           ┌── Chyme ──┬── Increase gastric secretion
           │           │   during gastric phase
           │           └── Decrease gastric secretion
           │               during intestinal phase
           │               (enterogastric reflex)
           │   Stimulate              ┌── Distension
└── Inhibition ─┤── enterogastric ── Duodenal ┤── Chyme presence
           │   reflex by             └── Irritation
           │              ┌── Hormones ┬── CCK
           │              │            │── Secretin
           └── Enterogastric┤          └── GIP
               reflex       │          ┌── Decrease gastric
                            └── Actions┤   secretion
                                       └── Decrease GI tract motility
```

INHIBITION OF THE ENTEROGASTRIC REFLEX

BRAIN

HEART

SYSTEMIC CIRCULATION

VAGUS PARASYMPATHETIC

CCK OTHER HORMONES?

STOMACH

OH

OSMOLARITY FAT

ENTERIC NERVOUS

VAGUS SENSORY

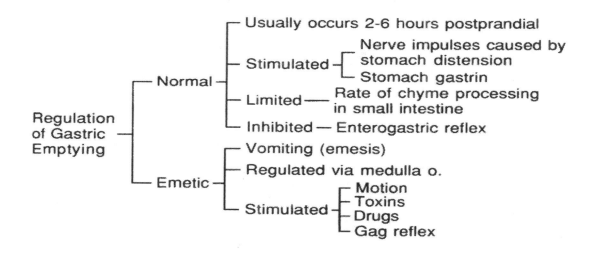

Regulation of Gastric Emptying
- Normal
  - Usually occurs 2-6 hours postprandial
  - Stimulated
    - Nerve impulses caused by stomach distension
    - Stomach gastrin
  - Limited — Rate of chyme processing in small intestine
  - Inhibited — Enterogastric reflex
- Emetic
  - Vomiting (emesis)
  - Regulated via medulla o.
  - Stimulated
    - Motion
    - Toxins
    - Drugs
    - Gag reflex

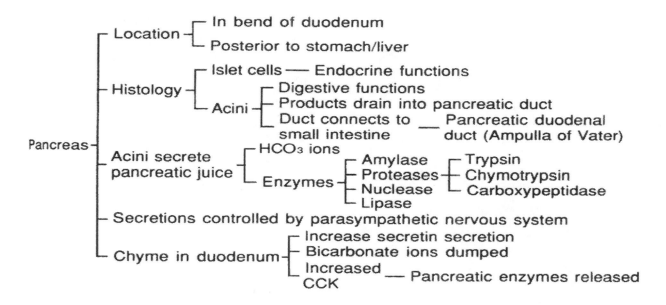

Pancreas
- Location
  - In bend of duodenum
  - Posterior to stomach/liver
- Histology
  - Islet cells — Endocrine functions
  - Acini
    - Digestive functions
    - Products drain into pancreatic duct
    - Duct connects to small intestine — Pancreatic duodenal duct (Ampulla of Vater)
- Acini secrete pancreatic juice
  - HCO_3 ions
  - Enzymes
    - Amylase
    - Proteases
      - Trypsin
      - Chymotrypsin
      - Carboxypeptidase
    - Nuclease
    - Lipase
- Secretions controlled by parasympathetic nervous system
- Chyme in duodenum
  - Increase secretin secretion
  - Bicarbonate ions dumped
  - Increased CCK — Pancreatic enzymes released

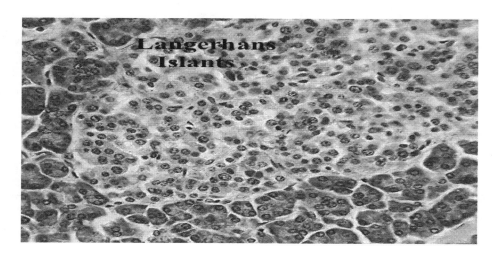

Langerhans Islants

(a) Pancreas and duodenum (b) Histological section through the pancreas, Acini cells, intercalated, intralobular, interlobular, pancreatic ducts

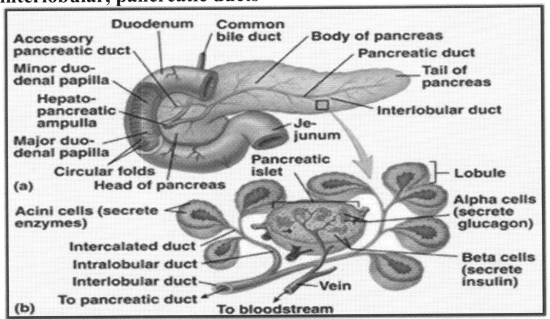

Duodenum and ifs relation to pancreases, liver and gallbladder

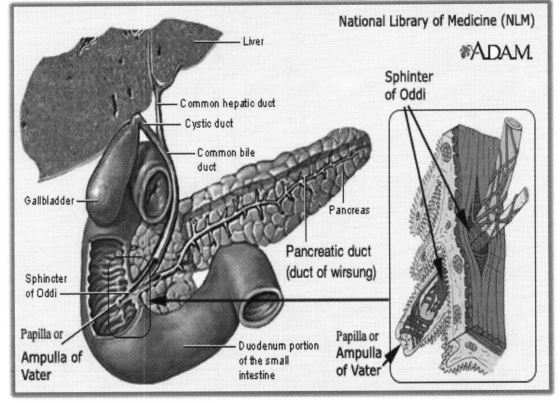

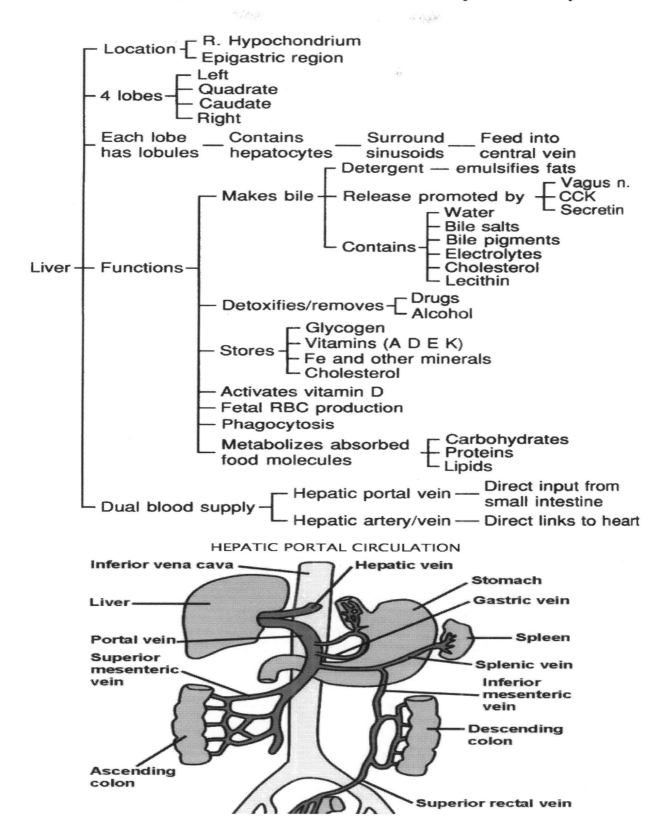

Liver
- Location
  - R. Hypochondrium
  - Epigastric region
- 4 lobes
  - Left
  - Quadrate
  - Caudate
  - Right
- Each lobe has lobules — Contains hepatocytes — Surround sinusoids — Feed into central vein
- Functions
  - Makes bile
    - Detergent — emulsifies fats
    - Release promoted by
      - Vagus n.
      - CCK
      - Secretin
    - Contains
      - Water
      - Bile salts
      - Bile pigments
      - Electrolytes
      - Cholesterol
      - Lecithin
  - Detoxifies/removes
    - Drugs
    - Alcohol
  - Stores
    - Glycogen
    - Vitamins (A D E K)
    - Fe and other minerals
    - Cholesterol
  - Activates vitamin D
  - Fetal RBC production
  - Phagocytosis
  - Metabolizes absorbed food molecules
    - Carbohydrates
    - Proteins
    - Lipids
- Dual blood supply
  - Hepatic portal vein — Direct input from small intestine
  - Hepatic artery/vein — Direct links to heart

HEPATIC PORTAL CIRCULATION

- Inferior vena cava
- Hepatic vein
- Stomach
- Gastric vein
- Liver
- Spleen
- Portal vein
- Splenic vein
- Superior mesenteric vein
- Inferior mesenteric vein
- Descending colon
- Ascending colon
- Superior rectal vein

Nutrient
Metabolism
in the
Liver
- Carbohydrate metabolism
  - Raise blood sugar
    - Gluconeogenesis
    - Glycogenolysis
  - Lower blood sugar
    - Glycolysis
    - Glycogenesis
- Lipid metabolism
  - β - oxidation
  - Ketogenesis
  - Lipogenesis
  - Stores fats
  - Cholesterol
    - Synthesis
    - Breakdown
- Protein metabolism
  - Deamination
  - Transamination
  - $NH_3 \longrightarrow NH_4$
  - Synthesis
    - Plasma proteins
    - Heparin

Gall Bladder
- Lies in fossa under quadrate lobe of liver
- Bile
  - Concentration
  - Storage & release
- Contains smooth muscle — Forces bile out after meal
- Hepatopancreatic ampulla (sphincter of Oddi)
  - Closed — Empty small intestine — Bile stored
  - Open — Full small intestine — Bile secreted

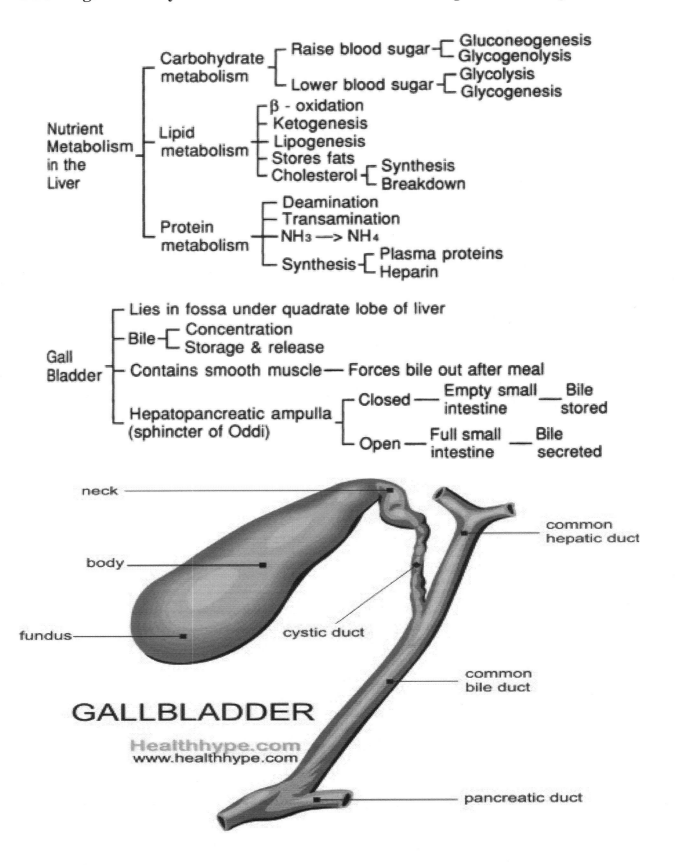

GALLBLADDER

neck

body

fundus

cystic duct

common hepatic duct

common bile duct

pancreatic duct

Healthhype.com
www.healthhype.com

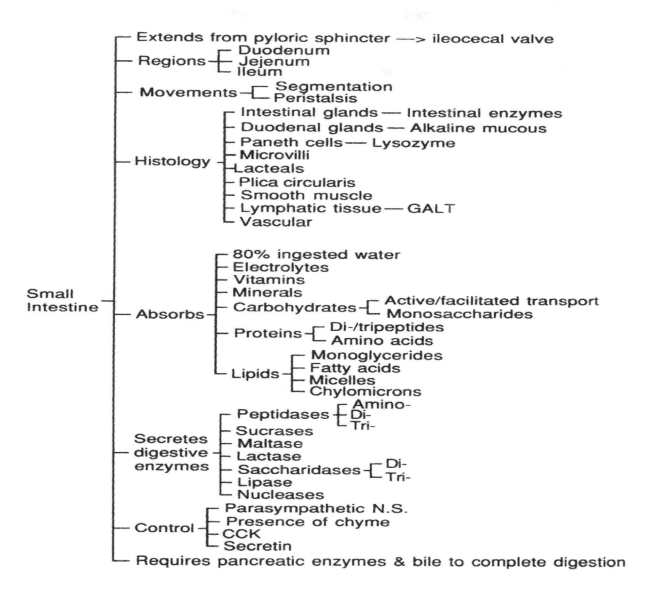

- Small Intestine
  - Extends from pyloric sphincter —> ileocecal valve
  - Regions
    - Duodenum
    - Jejenum
    - Ileum
  - Movements
    - Segmentation
    - Peristalsis
  - Histology
    - Intestinal glands — Intestinal enzymes
    - Duodenal glands — Alkaline mucous
    - Paneth cells — Lysozyme
    - Microvilli
    - Lacteals
    - Plica circularis
    - Smooth muscle
    - Lymphatic tissue — GALT
    - Vascular
  - Absorbs
    - 80% ingested water
    - Electrolytes
    - Vitamins
    - Minerals
    - Carbohydrates
      - Active/facilitated transport
      - Monosaccharides
    - Proteins
      - Di-/tripeptides
      - Amino acids
    - Lipids
      - Monoglycerides
      - Fatty acids
      - Micelles
      - Chylomicrons
  - Secretes digestive enzymes
    - Peptidases
      - Amino-
      - Di-
      - Tri-
    - Sucrases
    - Maltase
    - Lactase
    - Saccharidases
      - Di-
      - Tri-
    - Lipase
    - Nucleases
  - Control
    - Parasympathetic N.S.
    - Presence of chyme
    - CCK
    - Secretin
  - Requires pancreatic enzymes & bile to complete digestion

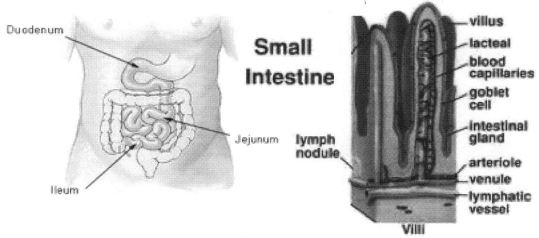

Small Intestine

Duodenum

Jejunum

Ileum

- villus
- lacteal
- blood capillaries
- goblet cell
- intestinal gland
- arteriole
- venule
- lymphatic vessel

lymph nodule

Villi

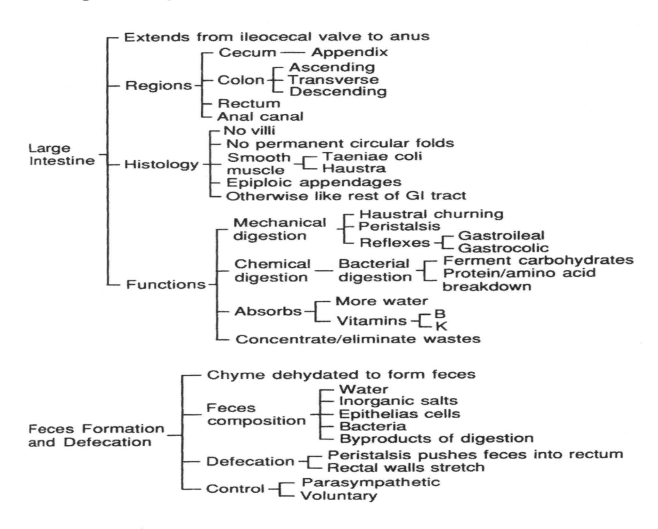

Large Intestine
- Extends from ileocecal valve to anus
- Regions
  - Cecum — Appendix
  - Colon
    - Ascending
    - Transverse
    - Descending
  - Rectum
  - Anal canal
- Histology
  - No villi
  - No permanent circular folds
  - Smooth muscle
    - Taeniae coli
    - Haustra
  - Epiploic appendages
  - Otherwise like rest of GI tract
- Functions
  - Mechanical digestion
    - Haustral churning
    - Peristalsis
    - Reflexes
      - Gastroileal
      - Gastrocolic
  - Chemical digestion — Bacterial digestion
    - Ferment carbohydrates
    - Protein/amino acid breakdown
  - Absorbs
    - More water
    - Vitamins
      - B
      - K
  - Concentrate/eliminate wastes

Feces Formation and Defecation
- Chyme dehydated to form feces
- Feces composition
  - Water
  - Inorganic salts
  - Epithelias cells
  - Bacteria
  - Byproducts of digestion
- Defecation
  - Peristalsis pushes feces into rectum
  - Rectal walls stretch
- Control
  - Parasympathetic
  - Voluntary

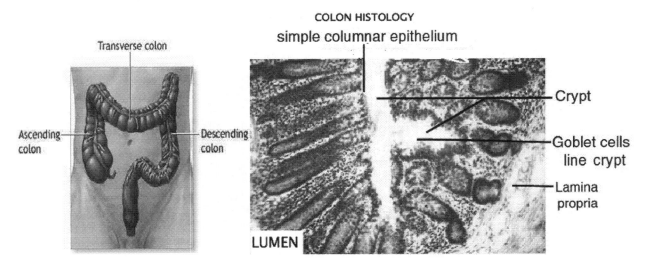

Transverse colon

Ascending colon

Descending colon

COLON HISTOLOGY
simple columnar epithelium

Crypt

Goblet cells line crypt

Lamina propria

LUMEN

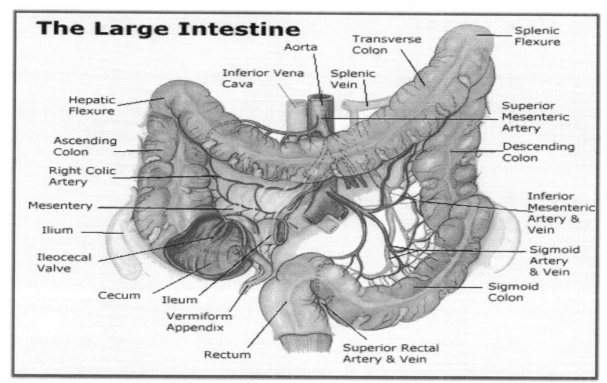

Ingested Fluid, salivary, gastric, pancreatic and intestinal secretions and or absorption: Net egested about 200 cc fluids daily

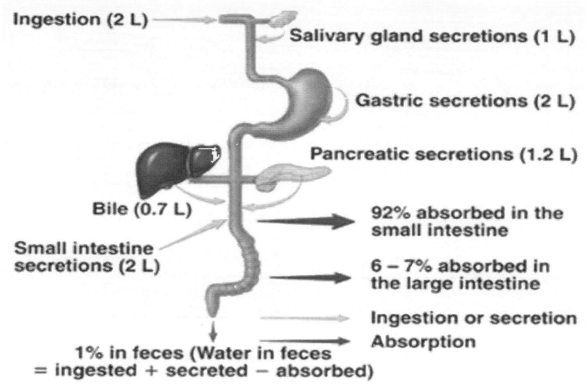

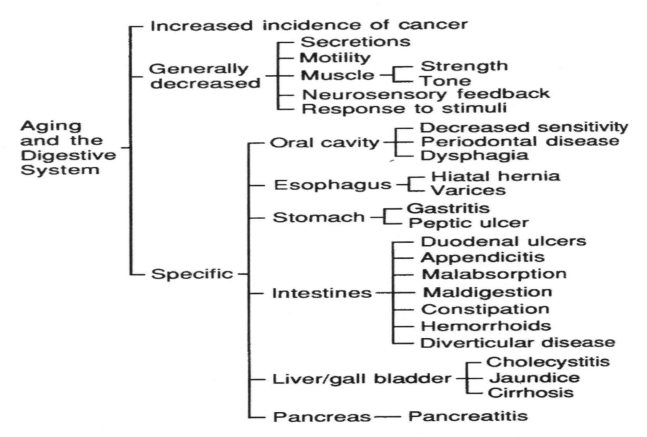

How does aging affect the digestive system?

As we age, the digestive process becomes less efficient.
- In the mouth, food may not be properly broken down due to missing teeth or gum problems as well as lowered saliva production
- The lower sphincter that regulates the flow of food from the esophagus into the stomach, can weaken resulting in reflux, a back flowing of food or acid (heartburn)
- Loss of muscle tone causes food to move more slowly along the digestive tract
- The stomach becomes less elastic and cannot hold as much food
- The production of acids and enzymes declines. A decline in the production of lactase, an enzyme that digests dairy products can lead to lactose intolerance, a condition that causes bloating and gas when milk products are consumed

Development

Begins 2 weeks post-conception
- Endoderm
  - Cavity = primitive gut
  - Layer
    - Epithelial lining
    - Glands
- Mesoderm
  - Smooth muscle
  - Connective tissue

End of 3rd week
- Foregut — Ectoderm — Stomodeum — Oral cavity
- Midgut — Attached to yolk sac until 5th week
- Hindgut — Ectoderm — Proctodeum — Anus

Foregut derivatives
- Oral cavity
- Esophagus
- Stomach
- Part of duodenum
- Endoderm
  - Salivary glands
  - Liver
  - Gall bladder
  - Pancreas

Midgut derivatives
- Rest of duodenum
- Jejenum
- Ileum
- Cecum
- Appendix
- Ascending colon
- Most of transverse colon

Hindgut
- Rest of transverse colon
- Sigmoid colon
- Rectum

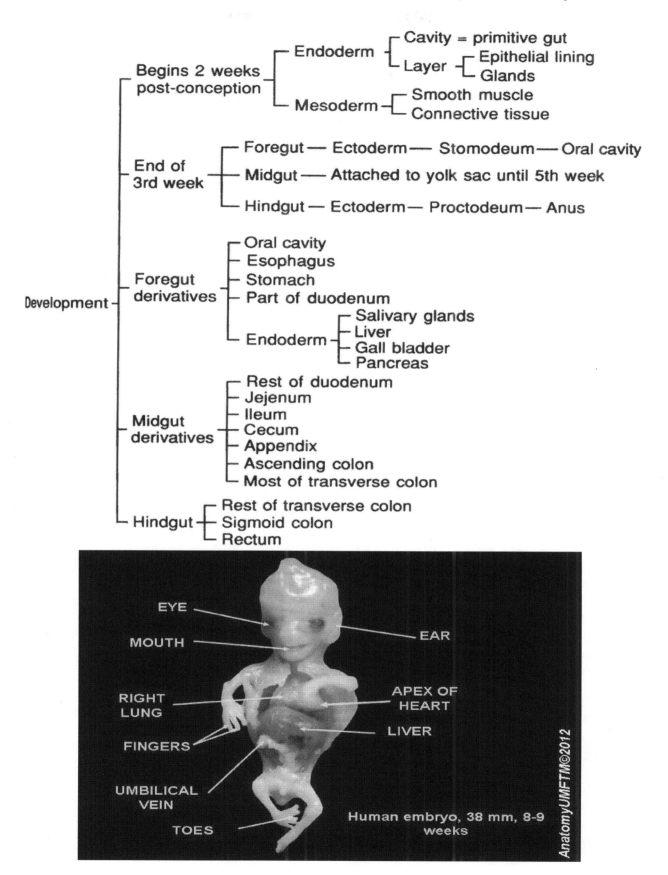

EYE

MOUTH

EAR

RIGHT LUNG

APEX OF HEART

FINGERS

LIVER

UMBILICAL VEIN

TOES

Human embryo, 38 mm, 8-9 weeks

AnatomyUMFTM©2012

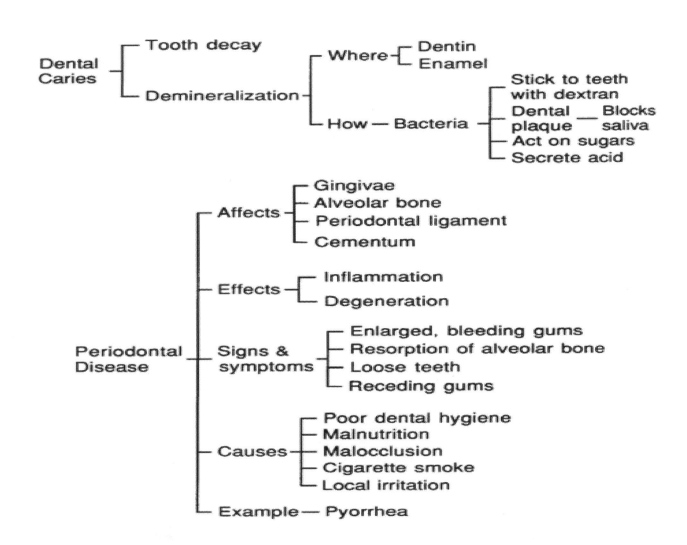

Dental Caries
- Tooth decay
- Demineralization
  - Where
    - Dentin
    - Enamel
  - How — Bacteria
    - Stick to teeth with dextran
    - Dental plaque — Blocks saliva
    - Act on sugars
    - Secrete acid

Periodontal Disease
- Affects
  - Gingivae
  - Alveolar bone
  - Periodontal ligament
  - Cementum
- Effects
  - Inflammation
  - Degeneration
- Signs & symptoms
  - Enlarged, bleeding gums
  - Resorption of alveolar bone
  - Loose teeth
  - Receding gums
- Causes
  - Poor dental hygiene
  - Malnutrition
  - Malocclusion
  - Cigarette smoke
  - Local irritation
- Example — Pyorrhea

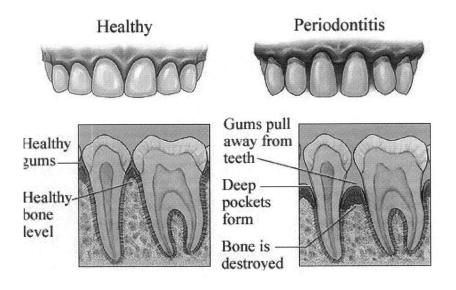

Healthy   Periodontitis

Healthy gums
Healthy bone level

Gums pull away from teeth
Deep pockets form
Bone is destroyed

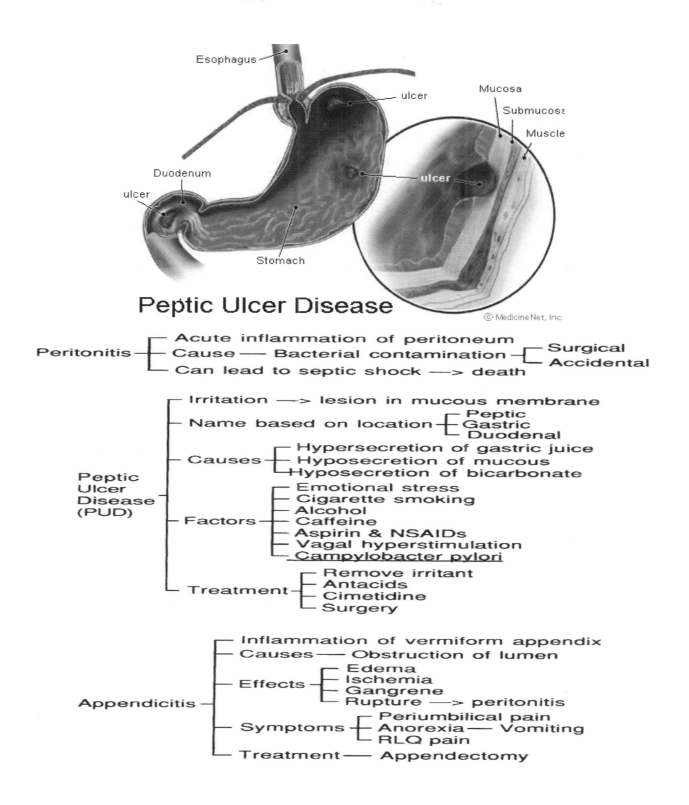

Peptic Ulcer Disease

Peritonitis
- Acute inflammation of peritoneum
- Cause — Bacterial contamination
  - Surgical
  - Accidental
- Can lead to septic shock —> death

Peptic Ulcer Disease (PUD)
- Irritation —> lesion in mucous membrane
- Name based on location
  - Peptic
  - Gastric
  - Duodenal
- Causes
  - Hypersecretion of gastric juice
  - Hyposecretion of mucous
  - Hyposecretion of bicarbonate
- Factors
  - Emotional stress
  - Cigarette smoking
  - Alcohol
  - Caffeine
  - Aspirin & NSAIDs
  - Vagal hyperstimulation
  - Campylobacter pylori
- Treatment
  - Remove irritant
  - Antacids
  - Cimetidine
  - Surgery

Appendicitis
- Inflammation of vermiform appendix
- Causes — Obstruction of lumen
- Effects
  - Edema
  - Ischemia
  - Gangrene
  - Rupture —> peritonitis
- Symptoms
  - Periumbilical pain
  - Anorexia — Vomiting
  - RLQ pain
- Treatment — Appendectomy

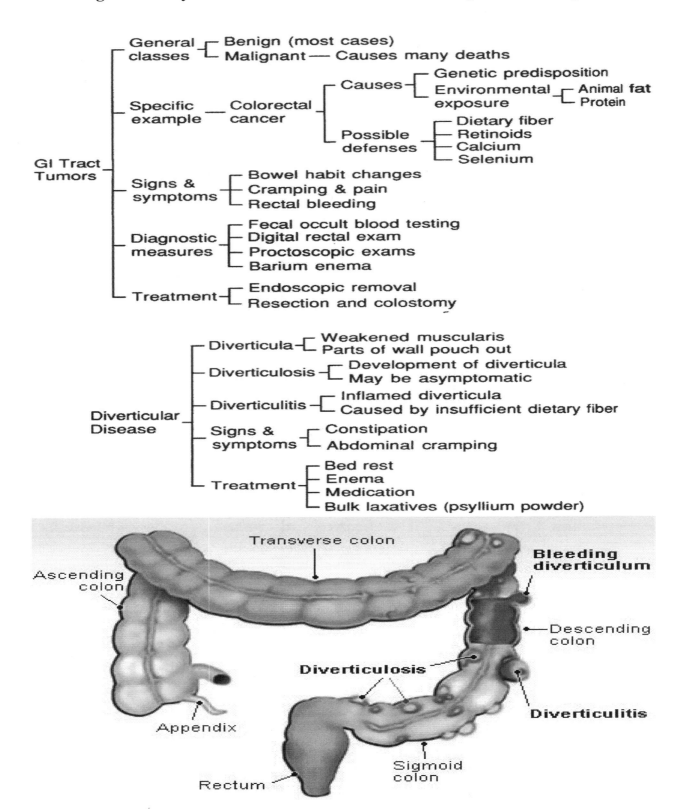

GI Tract Tumors
- General classes
  - Benign (most cases)
  - Malignant — Causes many deaths
- Specific example — Colorectal cancer
  - Causes
    - Genetic predisposition
    - Environmental exposure
      - Animal fat
      - Protein
  - Possible defenses
    - Dietary fiber
    - Retinoids
    - Calcium
    - Selenium
- Signs & symptoms
  - Bowel habit changes
  - Cramping & pain
  - Rectal bleeding
- Diagnostic measures
  - Fecal occult blood testing
  - Digital rectal exam
  - Proctoscopic exams
  - Barium enema
- Treatment
  - Endoscopic removal
  - Resection and colostomy

Diverticular Disease
- Diverticula
  - Weakened muscularis
  - Parts of wall pouch out
- Diverticulosis
  - Development of diverticula
  - May be asymptomatic
- Diverticulitis
  - Inflamed diverticula
  - Caused by insufficient dietary fiber
- Signs & symptoms
  - Constipation
  - Abdominal cramping
- Treatment
  - Bed rest
  - Enema
  - Medication
  - Bulk laxatives (psyllium powder)

Transverse colon

Bleeding diverticulum

Ascending colon

Descending colon

Diverticulosis

Diverticulitis

Appendix

Sigmoid colon

Rectum

Diverticular Disease

Cirrhosis
- Liver
  - Enlarged
  - Scarred
- Caused by chronic inflammation
  - Hepatitis
  - Environmental exposure
    - Toxins
    - Alcohol
    - Parasites
- Signs & symptoms
  - Chronic illness
  - Jaundice
  - Lower extremity edema
  - Uncontrolled bleeding
  - Increased sensitivity to medication

Hepatitis
- Inflammation of liver
- Causes
  - Viruses
  - Drugs
  - Chemicals
- Types
  - Hepatitis A (infectious)
    - Type A virus
    - Transmitted by fecal-oral route
    - Flu-like symptoms
    - Recovery
      - 4 - 6 weeks
      - No permanent liver damage
  - Hepatitis B (serum)
    - Type B virus
    - Transmission
      - Sexual intercourse
      - Transfusions
      - IV drug use
      - Saliva
      - Tears
    - Infected individuals act as carrier
    - At risk for cirrhosis
    - Vaccine available
  - Hepatitis C (non-A, non-B)
    - Viral transmission, not type A or B
    - May cause
      - Cirrhosis
      - Liver cancer
    - Transmitted like type B
    - Causes much of transfusion associated hepatitis

Hepatitis B_replication.

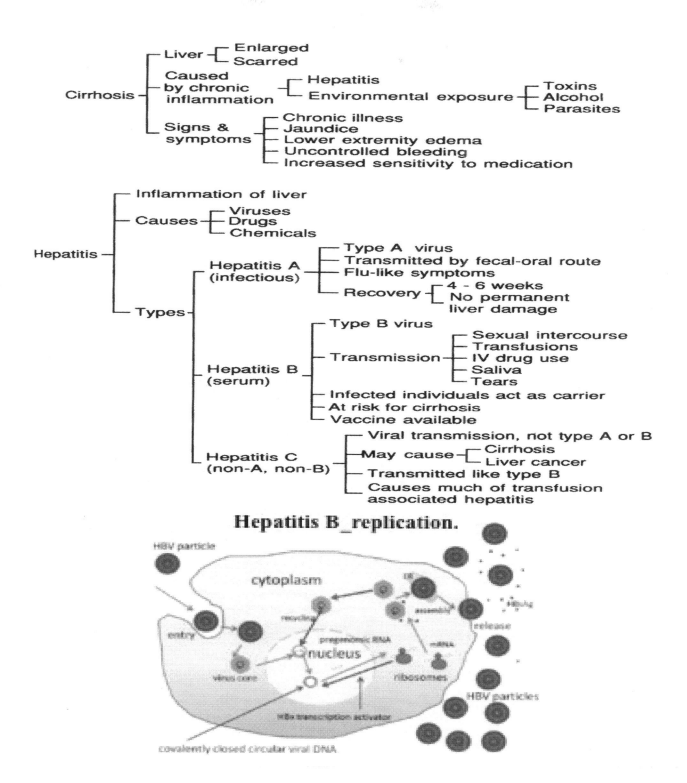

Various Digestive System Diseases

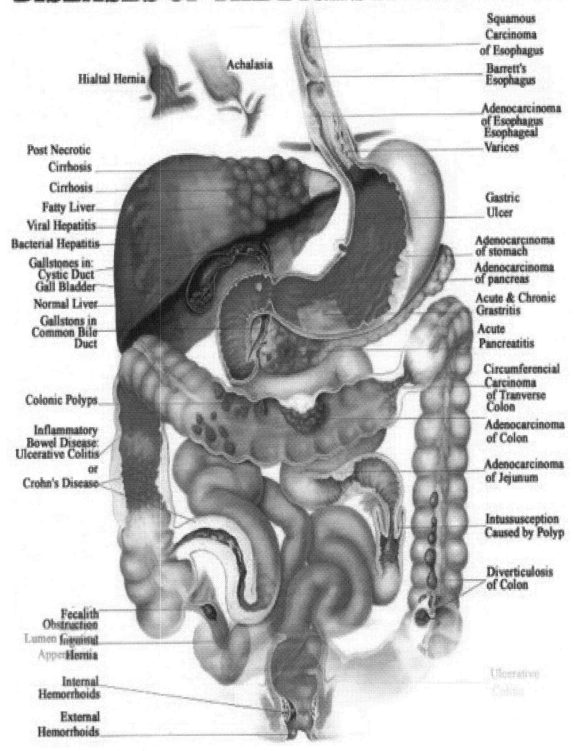

DISEASES OF THE DIGESTIVE SYSTEM

Hialtal Hernia

Achalasia

Squamous Carcinoma of Esophagus

Barrett's Esophagus

Adenocarcinoma of Esophagus Esophageal Varices

Post Necrotic Cirrhosis

Cirrhosis

Fatty Liver

Viral Hepatitis

Bacterial Hepatitis

Gallstones in: Cystic Duct Gall Bladder

Normal Liver

Gallstons in Common Bile Duct

Gastric Ulcer

Adenocarcinoma of stomach

Adenocarcinoma of pancreas

Acute & Chronic Grastritis

Acute Pancreatitis

Colonic Polyps

Inflammatory Bowel Disease: Ulcerative Colitis or Crohn's Disease

Circumferencial Carcinoma of Tranverse Colon

Adenocarcinoma of Colon

Adenocarcinoma of Jejunum

Intussusception Caused by Polyp

Diverticulosis of Colon

Fecalith Obstruction

Lumen Inguinal Appe Hernia

Internal Hemorrhoids

External Hemorrhoids

Ulcerative Colitis

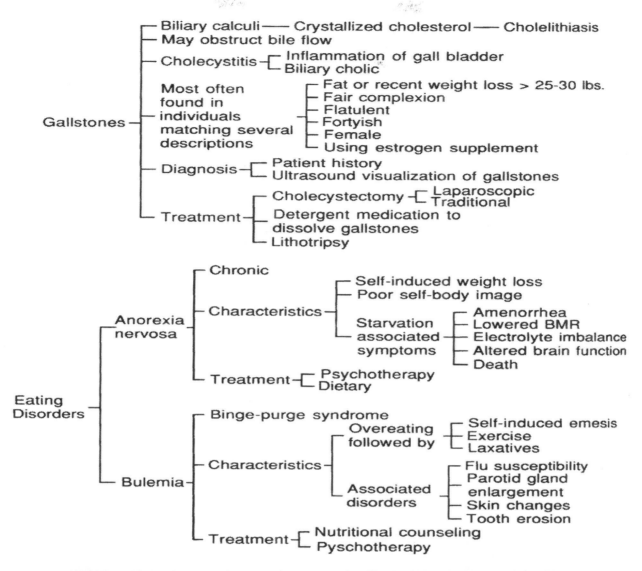

- **Gallstones**
  - Biliary calculi —— Crystallized cholesterol —— Cholelithiasis
  - May obstruct bile flow
  - Cholecystitis
    - Inflammation of gall bladder
    - Biliary cholic
  - Most often found in individuals matching several descriptions
    - Fat or recent weight loss > 25-30 lbs.
    - Fair complexion
    - Flatulent
    - Fortyish
    - Female
    - Using estrogen supplement
  - Diagnosis
    - Patient history
    - Ultrasound visualization of gallstones
  - Treatment
    - Cholecystectomy
      - Laparoscopic
      - Traditional
    - Detergent medication to dissolve gallstones
    - Lithotripsy

- **Eating Disorders**
  - Anorexia nervosa
    - Chronic
    - Characteristics
      - Self-induced weight loss
      - Poor self-body image
      - Starvation associated symptoms
        - Amenorrhea
        - Lowered BMR
        - Electrolyte imbalance
        - Altered brain function
        - Death
    - Treatment
      - Psychotherapy
      - Dietary
  - Bulemia
    - Binge-purge syndrome
    - Characteristics
      - Overeating followed by
        - Self-induced emesis
        - Exercise
        - Laxatives
      - Associated disorders
        - Flu susceptibility
        - Parotid gland enlargement
        - Skin changes
        - Tooth erosion
    - Treatment
      - Nutritional counseling
      - Pyschotherapy

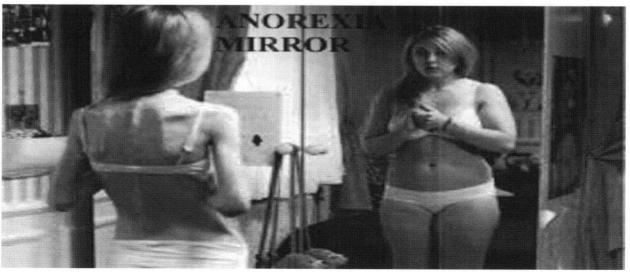

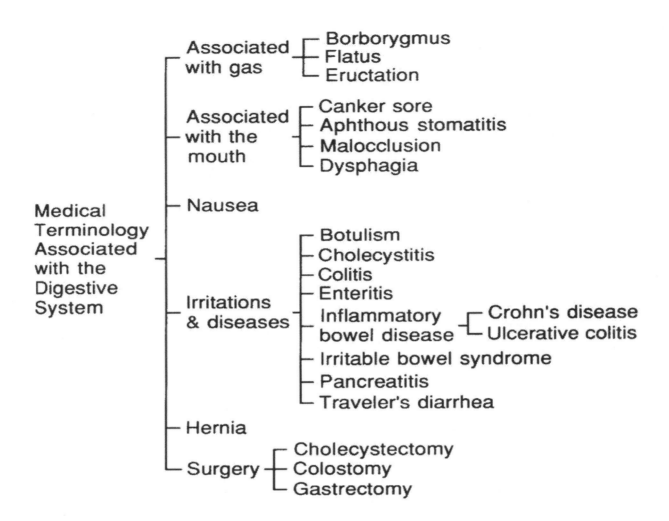

- Medical Terminology Associated with the Digestive System
  - Associated with gas
    - Borborygmus
    - Flatus
    - Eructation
  - Associated with the mouth
    - Canker sore
    - Aphthous stomatitis
    - Malocclusion
    - Dysphagia
  - Nausea
  - Irritations & diseases
    - Botulism
    - Cholecystitis
    - Colitis
    - Enteritis
    - Inflammatory bowel disease
      - Crohn's disease
      - Ulcerative colitis
    - Irritable bowel syndrome
    - Pancreatitis
    - Traveler's diarrhea
  - Hernia
  - Surgery
    - Cholecystectomy
    - Colostomy
    - Gastrectomy

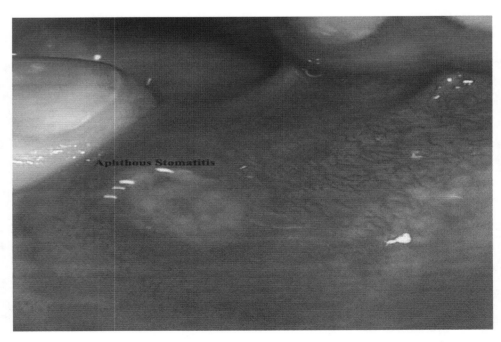

Aphthous Stomatitis

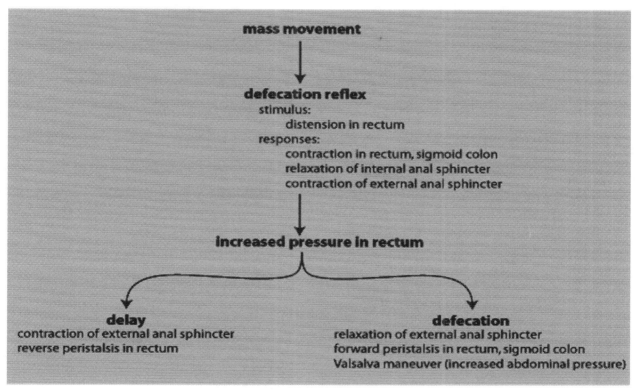

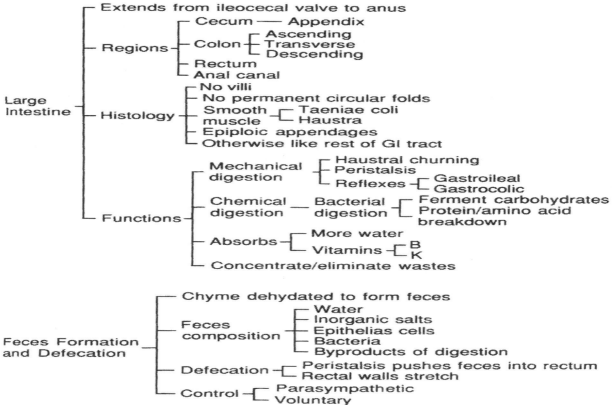

Bristol Stool Chart

Type 1		Separate hard lumps, like nuts (hard to pass)
Type 2		Sausage-shaped but lumpy
Type 3		Like a sausage but with cracks on its surface
Type 4		Like a sausage or snake, smooth and soft
Type 5		Soft blobs with clear-cut edges (passed easily)
Type 6		Fluffy pieces with ragged edges, a mushy stool
Type 7		Watery, no solid pieces. **Entirely Liquid**

CHAPTER TWENTY FIVE

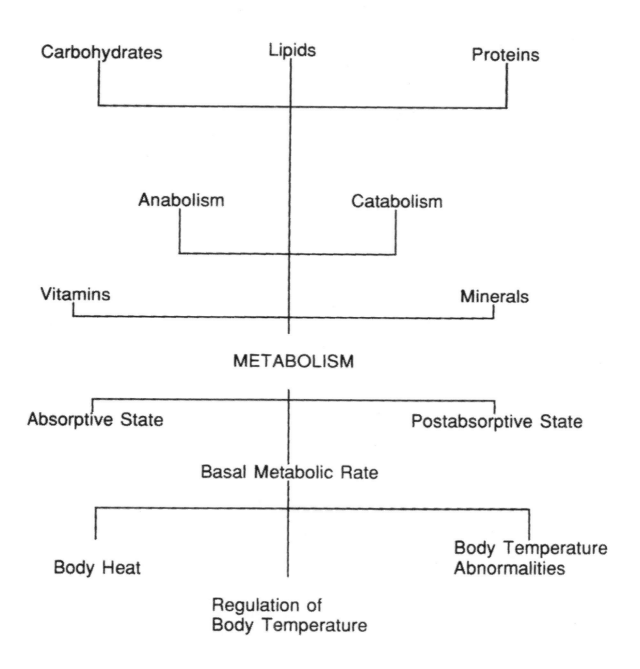

Carbohydrates   Lipids   Proteins

Anabolism   Catabolism

Vitamins   Minerals

METABOLISM

Absorptive State   Postabsorptive State

Basal Metabolic Rate

Body Heat   Body Temperature
                                           Abnormalities

Regulation of
Body Temperature

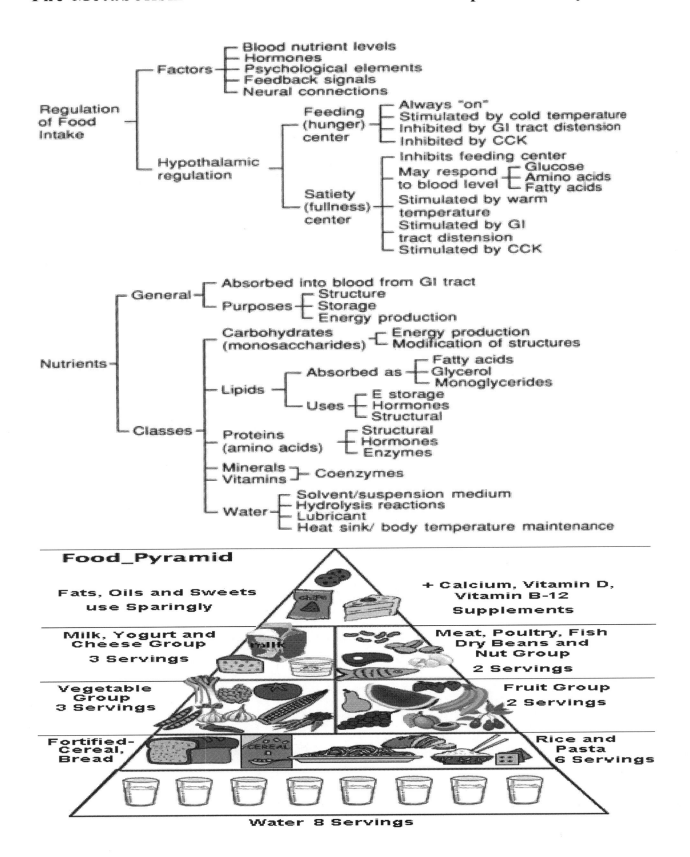

Regulation of Food Intake
- Factors
  - Blood nutrient levels
  - Hormones
  - Psychological elements
  - Feedback signals
  - Neural connections
- Hypothalamic regulation
  - Feeding (hunger) center
    - Always "on"
    - Stimulated by cold temperature
    - Inhibited by GI tract distension
    - Inhibited by CCK
  - Satiety (fullness) center
    - Inhibits feeding center
    - May respond to blood level
      - Glucose
      - Amino acids
      - Fatty acids
    - Stimulated by warm temperature
    - Stimulated by GI tract distension
    - Stimulated by CCK

Nutrients
- General
  - Absorbed into blood from GI tract
  - Purposes
    - Structure
    - Storage
    - Energy production
- Classes
  - Carbohydrates (monosaccharides)
    - Energy production
    - Modification of structures
  - Lipids
    - Absorbed as
      - Fatty acids
      - Glycerol
      - Monoglycerides
    - Uses
      - E storage
      - Hormones
      - Structural
  - Proteins (amino acids)
    - Structural
    - Hormones
    - Enzymes
  - Minerals / Vitamins
    - Coenzymes
  - Water
    - Solvent/suspension medium
    - Hydrolysis reactions
    - Lubricant
    - Heat sink/ body temperature maintenance

Food_Pyramid

Fats, Oils and Sweets use Sparingly

+ Calcium, Vitamin D, Vitamin B-12 Supplements

Milk, Yogurt and Cheese Group 3 Servings

Meat, Poultry, Fish Dry Beans and Nut Group 2 Servings

Vegetable Group 3 Servings

Fruit Group 2 Servings

Fortified-Cereal, Bread

Rice and Pasta 6 Servings

Water 8 Servings

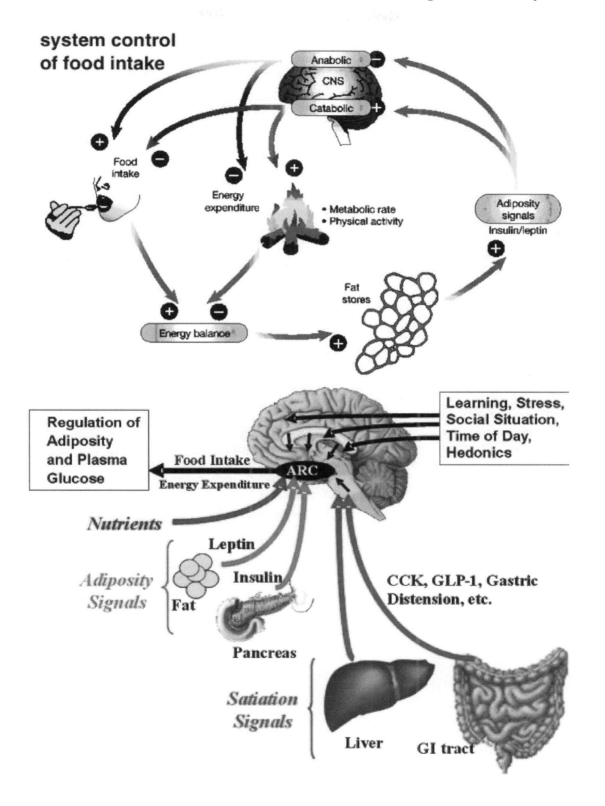

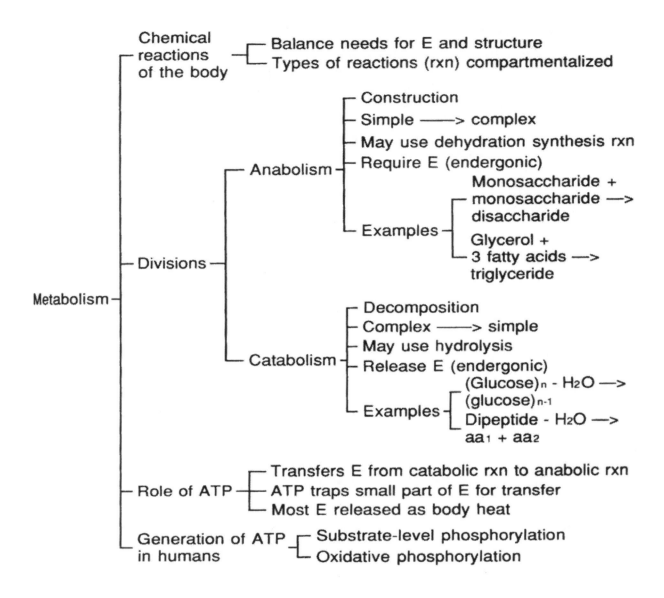

Metabolism ─
- Chemical reactions of the body
  - Balance needs for E and structure
  - Types of reactions (rxn) compartmentalized
- Divisions
  - Anabolism
    - Construction
    - Simple ──> complex
    - May use dehydration synthesis rxn
    - Require E (endergonic)
    - Examples
      - Monosaccharide + monosaccharide ──> disaccharide
      - Glycerol + 3 fatty acids ──> triglyceride
  - Catabolism
    - Decomposition
    - Complex ──> simple
    - May use hydrolysis
    - Release E (endergonic)
    - Examples
      - $(Glucose)_n - H_2O$ ──> $(glucose)_{n-1}$
      - $Dipeptide - H_2O$ ──> $aa_1 + aa_2$
- Role of ATP
  - Transfers E from catabolic rxn to anabolic rxn
  - ATP traps small part of E for transfer
  - Most E released as body heat
- Generation of ATP in humans
  - Substrate-level phosphorylation
  - Oxidative phosphorylation

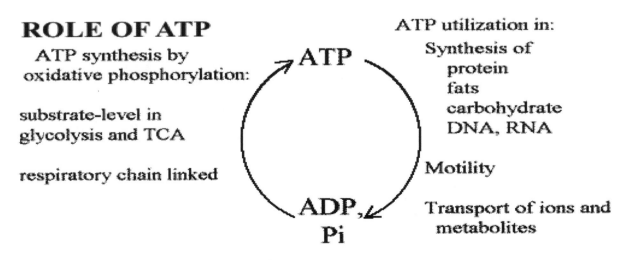

ROLE OF ATP

ATP synthesis by oxidative phosphorylation:

substrate-level in glycolysis and TCA

respiratory chain linked

ATP utilization in:

Synthesis of
protein
fats
carbohydrate
DNA, RNA

Motility

Transport of ions and metabolites

ATP

ADP, Pi

Metabolism- (A) Catabolic Reactions break down large; Complex Molecules to provide smaller Molecules and Energy (ATP). (B) Anabolic Reactions use ATP Energy to build larger Molecules from smaller building blocks

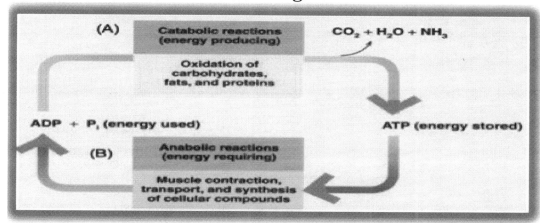

Comparison of Catabolism and Anabolism

		Catabolism	Anabolism
Descriptors of the Overall Process	Purpose	Energy generation	Formation of useful compounds
	Nature of the Process	Oxidative, degradative	Reductive, synthetic
	Energetics	Yields energy	Uses energy
Descriptors of the Chemical Participants	Types of Starting Materials	Highly variable, often complex	Relatively few, simple structures
	Types of Final Products	Relatively few, simple structures	Highly variable, often complex
	Typical Coenzyme/ Cosubstrate Transformations	ADP ----> ATP NAD+ ----> NADH	ATP---> ADP or AMP NADPH ---> NADP$^+$

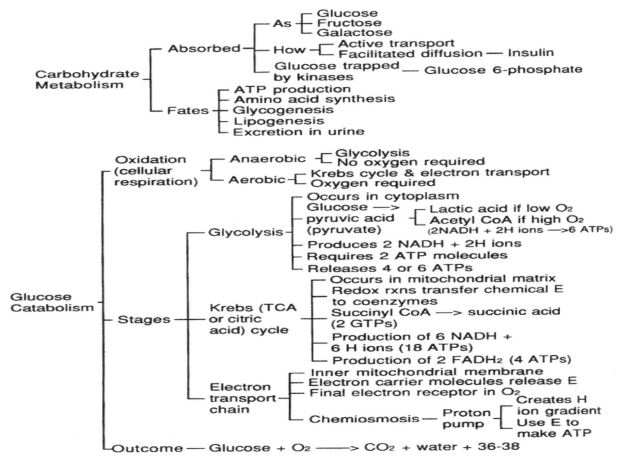

Carbohydrate Metabolism
- Absorbed
  - As
    - Glucose
    - Fructose
    - Galactose
  - How
    - Active transport
    - Facilitated diffusion — Insulin
  - Glucose trapped by kinases — Glucose 6-phosphate
- Fates
  - ATP production
  - Amino acid synthesis
  - Glycogenesis
  - Lipogenesis
  - Excretion in urine

Glucose Catabolism
- Oxidation (cellular respiration)
  - Anaerobic
    - Glycolysis
    - No oxygen required
  - Aerobic
    - Krebs cycle & electron transport
    - Oxygen required
- Stages
  - Glycolysis
    - Occurs in cytoplasm
    - Glucose —> pyruvic acid (pyruvate)
      - Lactic acid if low O_2
      - Acetyl CoA if high O_2 (2NADH + 2H ions —>6 ATPs)
    - Produces 2 NADH + 2H ions
    - Requires 2 ATP molecules
    - Releases 4 or 6 ATPs
  - Krebs (TCA or citric acid) cycle
    - Occurs in mitochondrial matrix
    - Redox rxns transfer chemical E to coenzymes
    - Succinyl CoA —> succinic acid (2 GTPs)
    - Production of 6 NADH + 6 H ions (18 ATPs)
    - Production of 2 $FADH_2$ (4 ATPs)
  - Electron transport chain
    - Inner mitochondrial membrane
    - Electron carrier molecules release E
    - Final electron receptor in O_2
    - Chemiosmosis — Proton pump
      - Creates H ion gradient
      - Use E to make ATP
- Outcome — Glucose + O_2 ——> CO_2 + water + 36-38

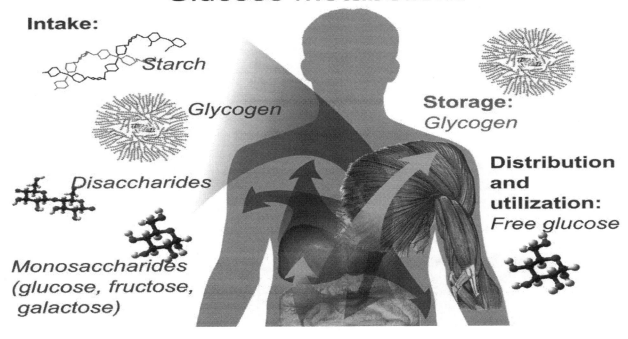

Glucose metabolism

Intake:
Starch

Glycogen

Disaccharides

Monosaccharides (glucose, fructose, galactose)

Storage: *Glycogen*

Distribution and utilization: *Free glucose*

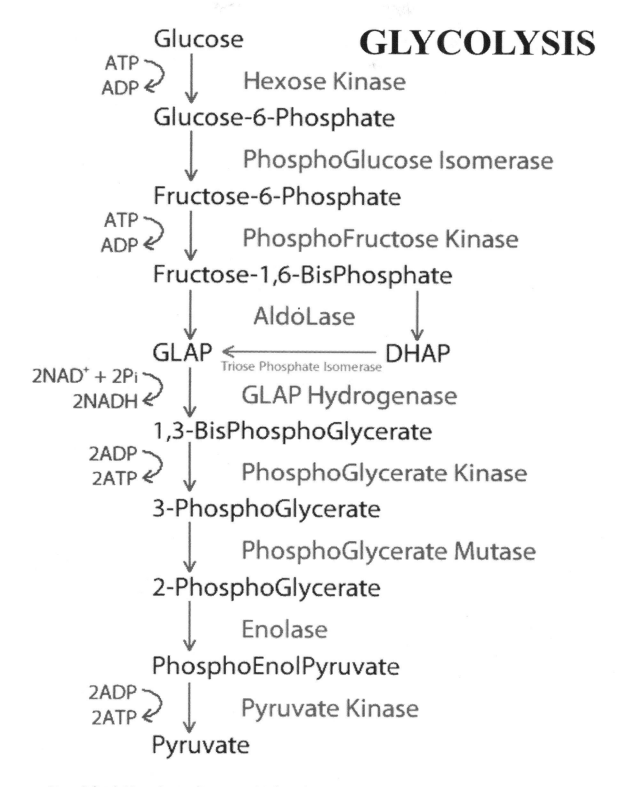

Glucose   **GLYCOLYSIS**

ATP ⌐
ADP ↙   Hexose Kinase

Glucose-6-Phosphate

PhosphoGlucose Isomerase

Fructose-6-Phosphate

ATP ⌐
ADP ↙   PhosphoFructose Kinase

Fructose-1,6-BisPhosphate

AldóLase

GLAP ← DHAP
Triose Phosphate Isomerase

$2NAD^+ + 2Pi$ ⌐
2NADH ↙   GLAP Hydrogenase

1,3-BisPhosphoGlycerate

2ADP ⌐
2ATP ↙   PhosphoGlycerate Kinase

3-PhosphoGlycerate

PhosphoGlycerate Mutase

2-PhosphoGlycerate

Enolase

PhosphoEnolPyruvate

2ADP ⌐
2ATP ↙   Pyruvate Kinase

Pyruvate

Simplified Glycolysis diagram. Molecule names contain extra capitals to illustrate
components. 21/02/2010 followchemistry.wordpress.com

CARBOHYDRATES ARE A. MONOSACCHARIDES, B. DISACCHARIDES & C. POLYSACCHARIDES

Depending on the availability of oxygen, pyruvic acid may be converted to lactic acid or may enter the Krebs cycle.

Glucose → 2 pyruvic acid → 2 lactic acid (anaerobic pathway)

Or goes aerobically

Glucose → 2 pyruvic acid → Krebs cycle (aerobic pathway)

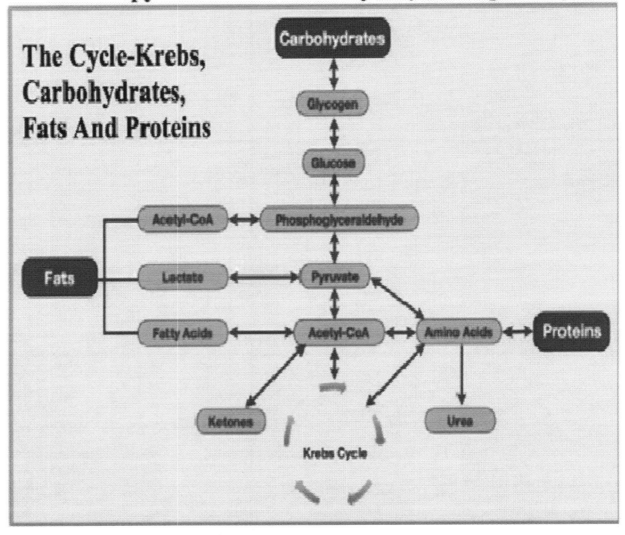

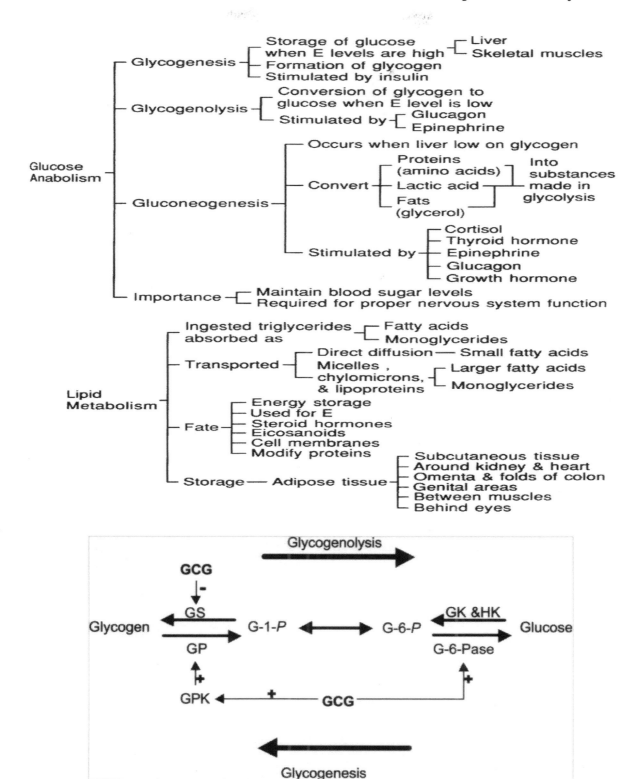

Glucose Anabolism
- Glycogenesis
  - Storage of glucose when E levels are high
    - Liver
    - Skeletal muscles
  - Formation of glycogen
  - Stimulated by insulin
- Glycogenolysis
  - Conversion of glycogen to glucose when E level is low
  - Stimulated by
    - Glucagon
    - Epinephrine
- Gluconeogenesis
  - Occurs when liver low on glycogen
  - Convert
    - Proteins (amino acids)
    - Lactic acid
    - Fats (glycerol)
    - Into substances made in glycolysis
  - Stimulated by
    - Cortisol
    - Thyroid hormone
    - Epinephrine
    - Glucagon
    - Growth hormone
- Importance
  - Maintain blood sugar levels
  - Required for proper nervous system function

Lipid Metabolism
- Ingested triglycerides absorbed as
  - Fatty acids
  - Monoglycerides
- Transported
  - Direct diffusion — Small fatty acids
  - Micelles, chylomicrons, & lipoproteins
    - Larger fatty acids
    - Monoglycerides
- Fate
  - Energy storage
  - Used for E
  - Steroid hormones
  - Eicosanoids
  - Cell membranes
  - Modify proteins
- Storage — Adipose tissue
  - Subcutaneous tissue
  - Around kidney & heart
  - Omenta & folds of colon
  - Genital areas
  - Between muscles
  - Behind eyes

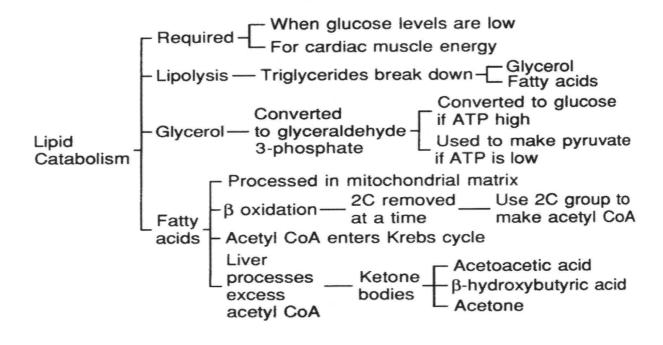

Lipid Catabolism
- Required
  - When glucose levels are low
  - For cardiac muscle energy
- Lipolysis — Triglycerides break down
  - Glycerol
  - Fatty acids
- Glycerol — Converted to glyceraldehyde 3-phosphate
  - Converted to glucose if ATP high
  - Used to make pyruvate if ATP is low
- Fatty acids
  - Processed in mitochondrial matrix
  - β oxidation — 2C removed at a time — Use 2C group to make acetyl CoA
  - Acetyl CoA enters Krebs cycle
  - Liver processes excess acetyl CoA — Ketone bodies
    - Acetoacetic acid
    - β-hydroxybutyric acid
    - Acetone

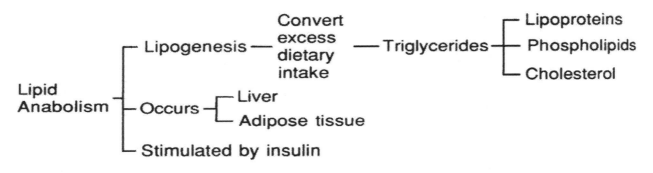

Lipid Anabolism
- Lipogenesis — Convert excess dietary intake — Triglycerides
  - Lipoproteins
  - Phospholipids
  - Cholesterol
- Occurs
  - Liver
  - Adipose tissue
- Stimulated by insulin

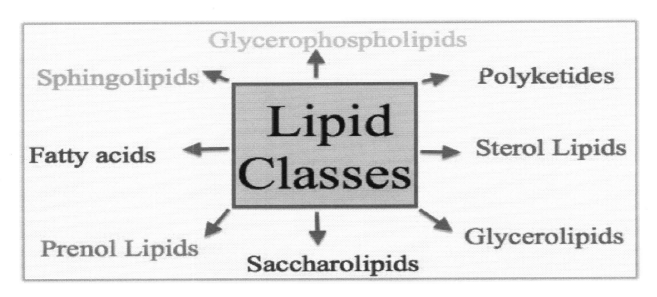

Glycerophospholipids

Sphingolipids

Polyketides

Fatty acids

Lipid Classes

Sterol Lipids

Prenol Lipids

Saccharolipids

Glycerolipids

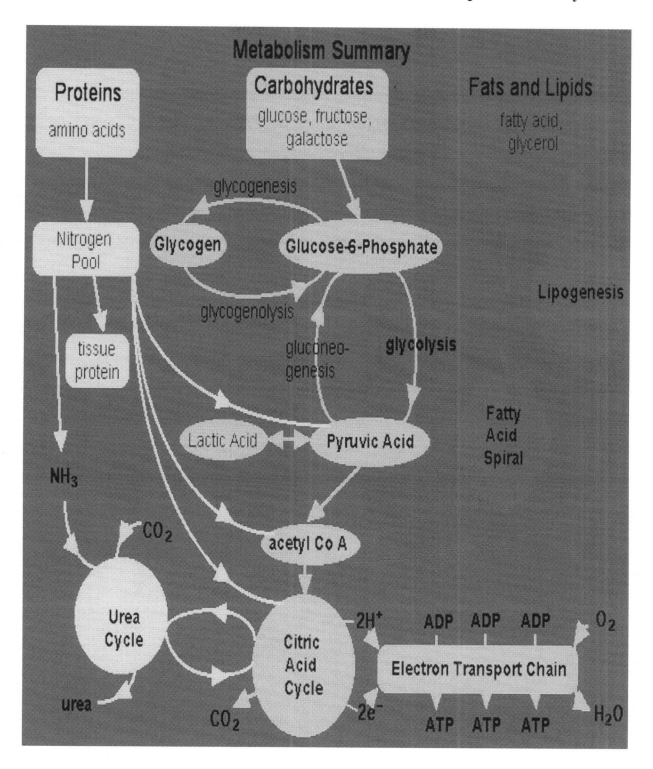

Metabolism Summary

Proteins
amino acids

Carbohydrates
glucose, fructose,
galactose

Fats and Lipids
fatty acid,
glycerol

glycogenesis

Nitrogen
Pool

Glycogen

Glucose-6-Phosphate

Lipogenesis

glycogenolysis

tissue
protein

gluconeo-
genesis

glycolysis

NH_3

Lactic Acid

Pyruvic Acid

Fatty
Acid
Spiral

CO_2

acetyl Co A

Urea
Cycle

Citric
Acid
Cycle

$2H^+$

ADP　ADP　ADP

O_2

Electron Transport Chain

urea

CO_2

$2e^-$

ATP　ATP　ATP

H_2O

Protein Metabolism
- Proteins —> amino acids
- Amino acids —— Absorbed into blood
  - Active transport
  - Through intestinal wall
- Excess converted, not stored
  - Gluconeogenesis
  - Lipogenesis
  - ATP production
- Uses
  - Enzymes
  - Transport molecules
  - Antibodies
  - Contractile elements
  - Structure
  - Hormones

Protein Catabolism
- Body recycles amino acids from catabolized proteins
- Conversion of amino acids by liver
  - Occurs when other E sources are low
  - Processes
    - Deamination
    - Decarboxylation
    - Dehydrogenation
- Amino acids enter cells by active transport
  - Insulin
  - Growth hormone

Protein Anabolism
- Formation of peptide bonds
- Links amino acids together in protein
- Occurs in most cells
- Influenced by hormones
  - Growth hormone
  - Thyroid hormones
  - Insulin
- Dietary protein level critical
  - Pregnancy
  - Growth
  - Repair
- General classes of amino acids used
  - Essential
  - Nonessential —— Transamination rxn

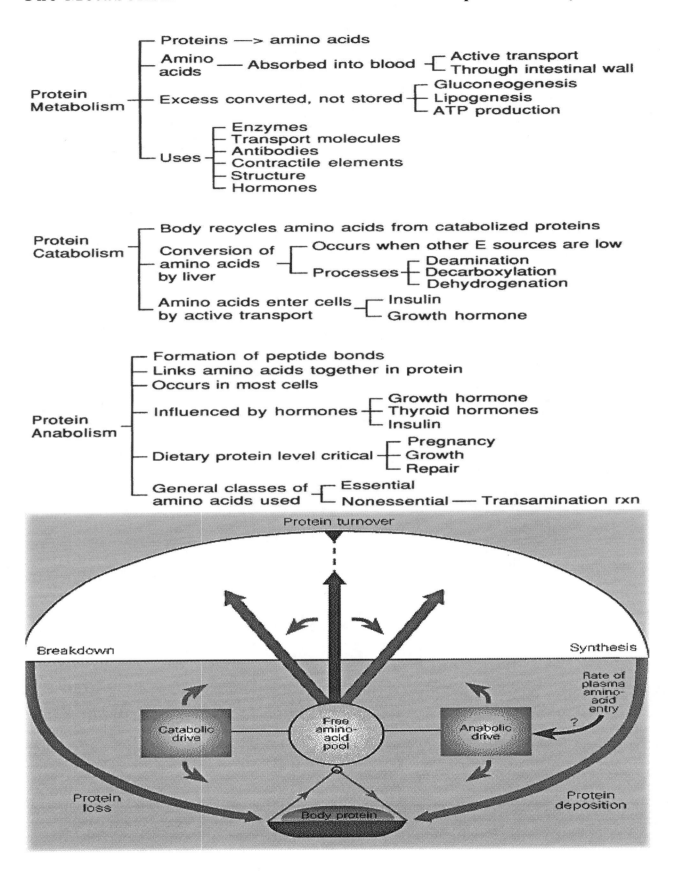

Protein and Amino Acid Metabolism

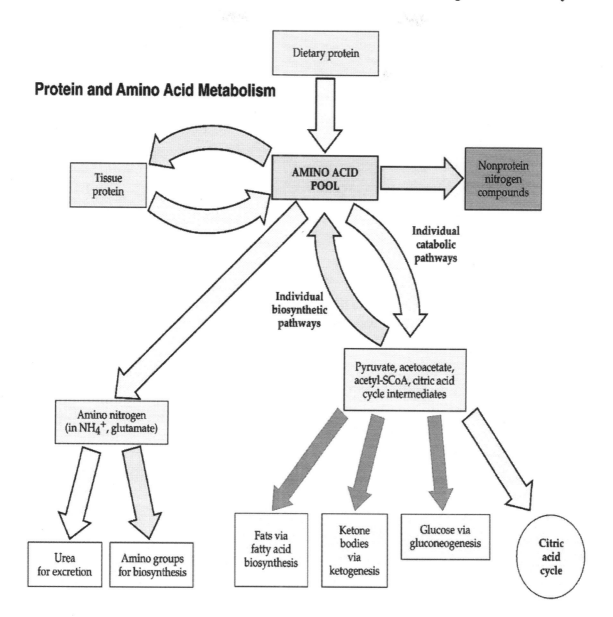

PROTEIN DEGRADATION

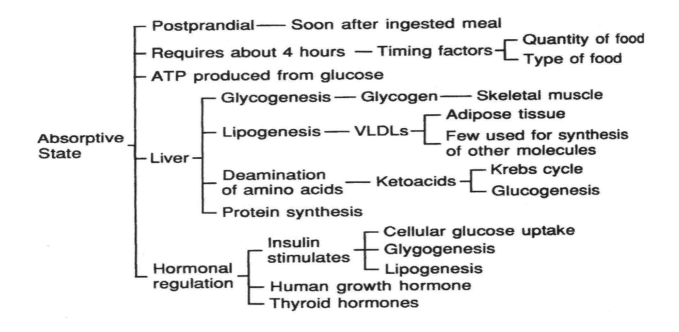

Absorptive State
- Postprandial — Soon after ingested meal
- Requires about 4 hours — Timing factors
  - Quantity of food
  - Type of food
- ATP produced from glucose
- Liver
  - Glycogenesis — Glycogen — Skeletal muscle
  - Lipogenesis — VLDLs
    - Adipose tissue
    - Few used for synthesis of other molecules
  - Deamination of amino acids — Ketoacids
    - Krebs cycle
    - Glucogenesis
  - Protein synthesis
- Hormonal regulation
  - Insulin stimulates
    - Cellular glucose uptake
    - Glygogenesis
    - Lipogenesis
  - Human growth hormone
  - Thyroid hormones

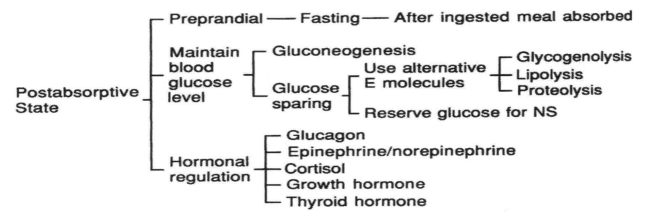

Postabsorptive State
- Preprandial — Fasting — After ingested meal absorbed
- Maintain blood glucose level
  - Gluconeogenesis
  - Glucose sparing
    - Use alternative E molecules
      - Glycogenolysis
      - Lipolysis
      - Proteolysis
    - Reserve glucose for NS
- Hormonal regulation
  - Glucagon
  - Epinephrine/norepinephrine
  - Cortisol
  - Growth hormone
  - Thyroid hormone

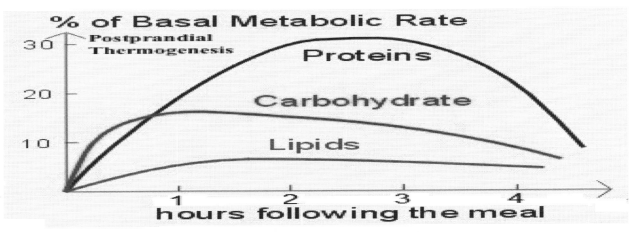

% of Basal Metabolic Rate

Postprandial Thermogenesis

Proteins

Carbohydrate

Lipids

hours following the meal

Summary of Metabolism

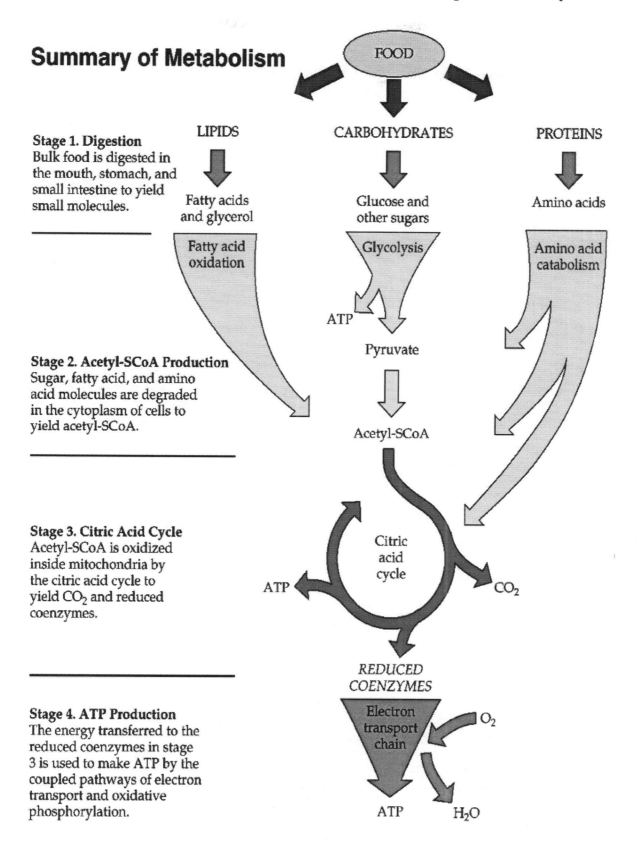

Stage 1. Digestion
Bulk food is digested in the mouth, stomach, and small intestine to yield small molecules.

Stage 2. Acetyl-SCoA Production
Sugar, fatty acid, and amino acid molecules are degraded in the cytoplasm of cells to yield acetyl-SCoA.

Stage 3. Citric Acid Cycle
Acetyl-SCoA is oxidized inside mitochondria by the citric acid cycle to yield CO_2 and reduced coenzymes.

Stage 4. ATP Production
The energy transferred to the reduced coenzymes in stage 3 is used to make ATP by the coupled pathways of electron transport and oxidative phosphorylation.

FOOD

LIPIDS   CARBOHYDRATES   PROTEINS

Fatty acids and glycerol   Glucose and other sugars   Amino acids

Fatty acid oxidation   Glycolysis   Amino acid catabolism

ATP

Pyruvate

Acetyl-SCoA

Citric acid cycle

ATP CO_2

REDUCED COENZYMES

Electron transport chain O_2

ATP H_2O

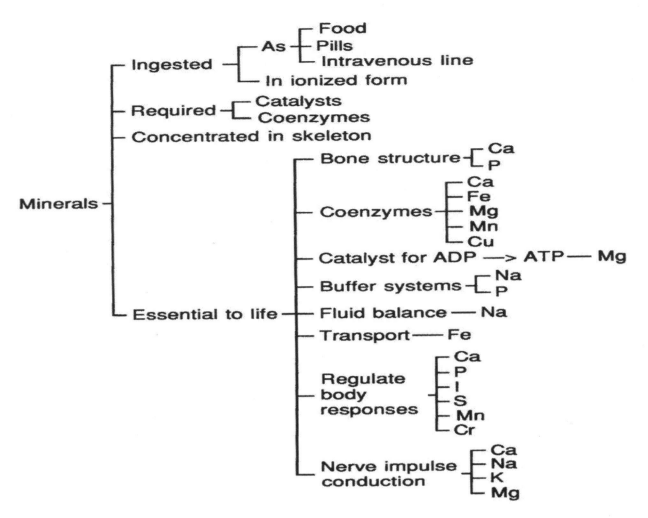

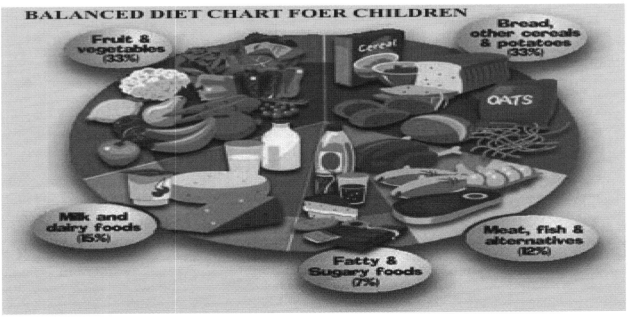

BALANCED DIET CHART FOER CHILDREN

Fruit & vegetables (33%)

Bread, other cereals & potatoes (33%)

Milk and dairy foods (15%)

Fatty & Sugary foods (7%)

Meat, fish & alternatives (12%)

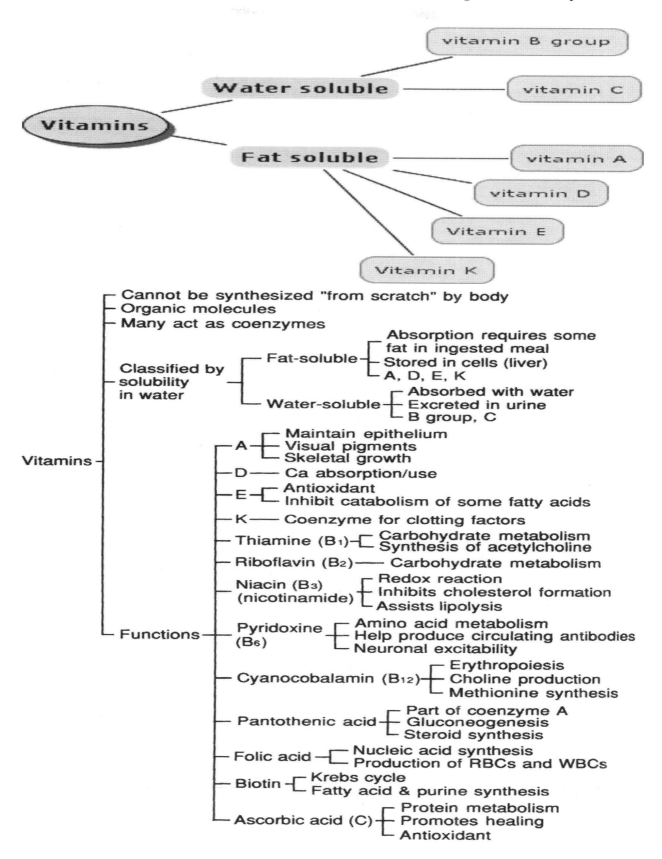

THE MINERAL CHART

Mineral	RDA/AI		Best Sources	Functions
	Men	Women		
Calcium	1,000mg	1,000mg	Milk and milk products	Strong bones, teeth, muscle tissue; regulates heart beat, muscle action, and nerve function; blood clotting
Chromium	35ug	25ug	Corn oil, clams, whole-grain cereals, brewer's yeast	Glucose metabolism (energy); increases effectiveness of insulin
Copper	900ug	900ug	Oysters, nuts, organ meats, legumes	Formation of red blood cells; bone growth and health; works with vitamin C to form elastin
Fluoride	4mg	3mg	Fluorinated water, teas, marine fish	Stimulates bone formation; inhibits or even reverses dental caries
Iodine	150ug	150ug	Seafood, iodized salt	Component of hormone thyroxine, which controls metabolism
Iron	8mg	18mg	Meats, especially organ meats, legumes	Hemoglobin formation; improves blood quality; increases resistance to stress and disease
Magnesium	420mg	320mg	Nuts, green vegetables, whole grains	Acid/alkaline balance; important in metabolism of carbohydrates, minerals, and sugar (glucose)
Manganese	2.3mg	1.8mg	Nuts, whole grains, vegetables, fruits	Enzyme activation; carbohydrate and fat production; sex hormone production; skeletal development
Molybdenum	45ug	45ug	Legumes, grain products, nuts	Functions as a cofactor for a limited number of enzymes in humans
Phosphorus	700mg	700mg	Fish, meat, poultry, eggs, grains	Bone development; important in protein, fat, and carbohydrate utilization
Potassium	4700mg	4700mg	Lean meat, vegetables, fruits	Fluid balance; controls activity of heart muscle, nervous system, and kidneys
Selenium	55ug	55ug	Seafood, organ meats, lean meats, grains	Protects body tissues against oxidative damage from radiation, pollution, and normal metabolic processing
Zinc	11mg	8mg	Lean meats, liver, eggs, seafood, whole grains	Involved in digestion and metabolism; important in development of reproductive system; aids in healing

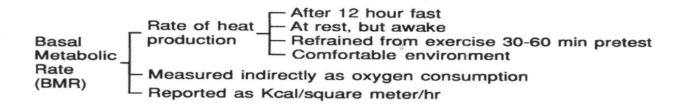

Basal Metabolic Rate (BMR)
- Rate of heat production
  - After 12 hour fast
  - At rest, but awake
  - Refrained from exercise 30-60 min pretest
  - Comfortable environment
- Measured indirectly as oxygen consumption
- Reported as Kcal/square meter/hr

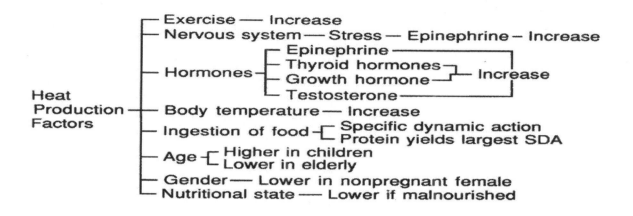

Heat Production Factors
- Exercise — Increase
- Nervous system — Stress — Epinephrine – Increase
- Hormones
  - Epinephrine
  - Thyroid hormones
  - Growth hormone
  - Testosterone
  — Increase
- Body temperature — Increase
- Ingestion of food
  - Specific dynamic action
  - Protein yields largest SDA
- Age
  - Higher in children
  - Lower in elderly
- Gender — Lower in nonpregnant female
- Nutritional state — Lower if malnourished

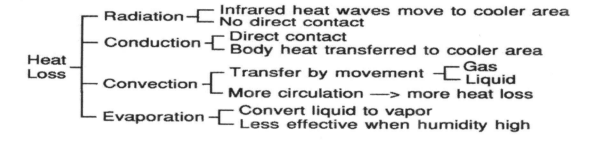

Heat Loss
- Radiation
  - Infrared heat waves move to cooler area
  - No direct contact
- Conduction
  - Direct contact
  - Body heat transferred to cooler area
- Convection
  - Transfer by movement
    - Gas
    - Liquid
  - More circulation ——> more heat loss
- Evaporation
  - Convert liquid to vapor
  - Less effective when humidity high

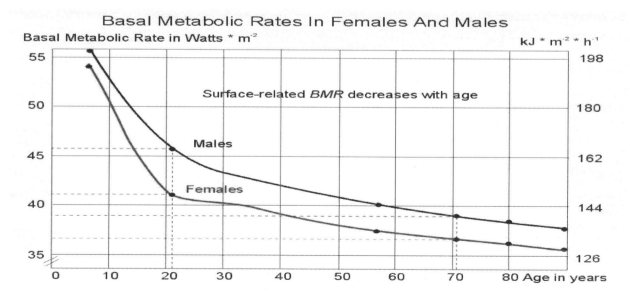

Basal Metabolic Rates In Females And Males

Basal Metabolic Rate in Watts * m⁻²   kJ * m⁻² * h⁻¹

Surface-related *BMR* decreases with age

Males

Females

Age in years

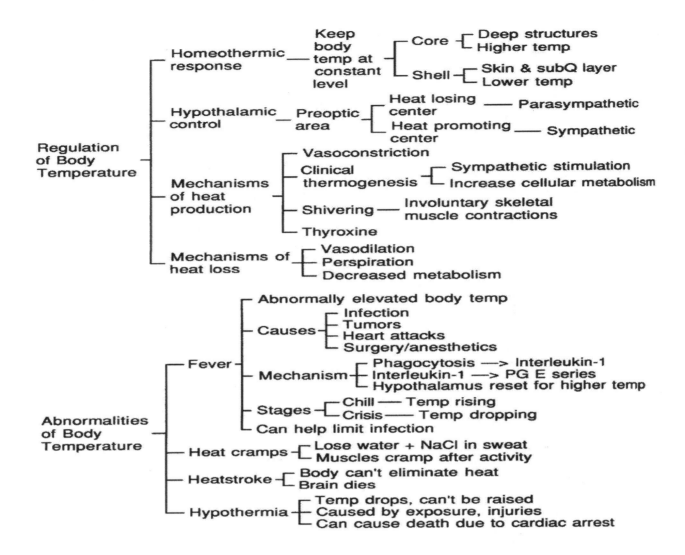

Regulation of Body Temperature
- Homeothermic response — Keep body temp at constant level
  - Core — Deep structures / Higher temp
  - Shell — Skin & subQ layer / Lower temp
- Hypothalamic control — Preoptic area
  - Heat losing center — Parasympathetic
  - Heat promoting center — Sympathetic
- Mechanisms of heat production
  - Vasoconstriction
  - Clinical thermogenesis — Sympathetic stimulation / Increase cellular metabolism
  - Shivering — Involuntary skeletal muscle contractions
  - Thyroxine
- Mechanisms of heat loss
  - Vasodilation
  - Perspiration
  - Decreased metabolism

Abnormalities of Body Temperature
- Fever
  - Abnormally elevated body temp
  - Causes
    - Infection
    - Tumors
    - Heart attacks
    - Surgery/anesthetics
  - Mechanism
    - Phagocytosis —> Interleukin-1
    - Interleukin-1 —> PG E series
    - Hypothalamus reset for higher temp
  - Stages
    - Chill — Temp rising
    - Crisis — Temp dropping
  - Can help limit infection
- Heat cramps
  - Lose water + NaCl in sweat
  - Muscles cramp after activity
- Heatstroke
  - Body can't eliminate heat
  - Brain dies
- Hypothermia
  - Temp drops, can't be raised
  - Caused by exposure, injuries
  - Can cause death due to cardiac arrest

REGULATION OF BODY TEMPERATURE

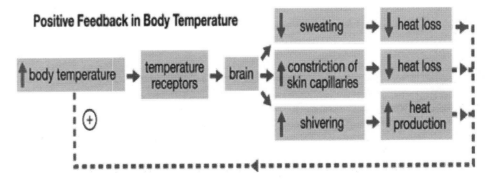

Positive Feedback in Body Temperature

↑ body temperature → temperature receptors → brain →
- ↓ sweating → ↓ heat loss →
- ↑ constriction of skin capillaries → ↓ heat loss →
- ↑ shivering → ↑ heat production →

(+)

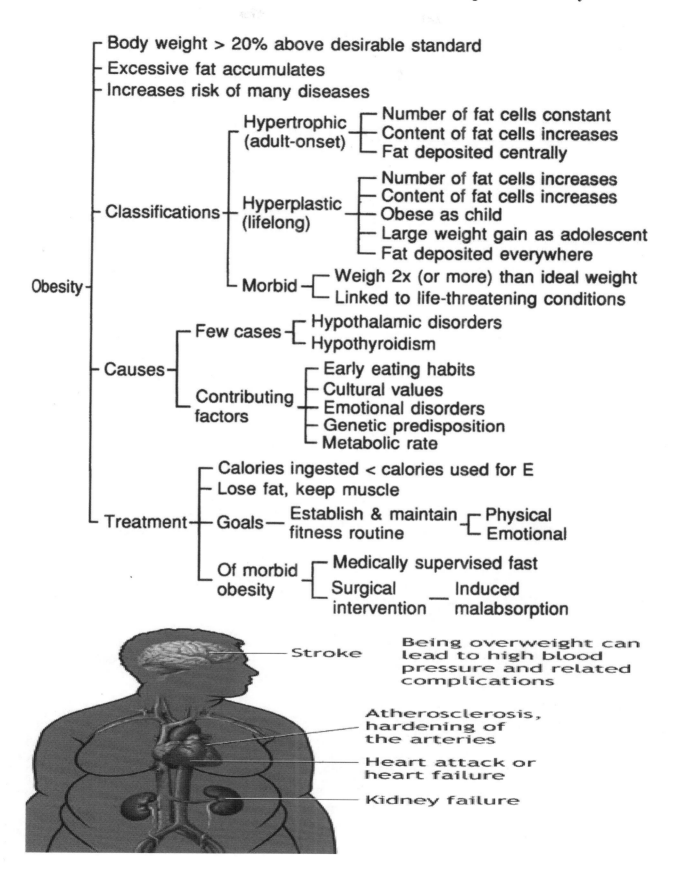

Obesity
- Body weight > 20% above desirable standard
- Excessive fat accumulates
- Increases risk of many diseases
- Classifications
  - Hypertrophic (adult-onset)
    - Number of fat cells constant
    - Content of fat cells increases
    - Fat deposited centrally
  - Hyperplastic (lifelong)
    - Number of fat cells increases
    - Content of fat cells increases
    - Obese as child
    - Large weight gain as adolescent
    - Fat deposited everywhere
  - Morbid
    - Weigh 2x (or more) than ideal weight
    - Linked to life-threatening conditions
- Causes
  - Few cases
    - Hypothalamic disorders
    - Hypothyroidism
  - Contributing factors
    - Early eating habits
    - Cultural values
    - Emotional disorders
    - Genetic predisposition
    - Metabolic rate
- Treatment
  - Calories ingested < calories used for E
  - Lose fat, keep muscle
  - Goals
    - Establish & maintain fitness routine
      - Physical
      - Emotional
  - Of morbid obesity
    - Medically supervised fast
    - Surgical intervention — Induced malabsorption

Stroke

Being overweight can lead to high blood pressure and related complications

Atherosclerosis, hardening of the arteries

Heart attack or heart failure

Kidney failure

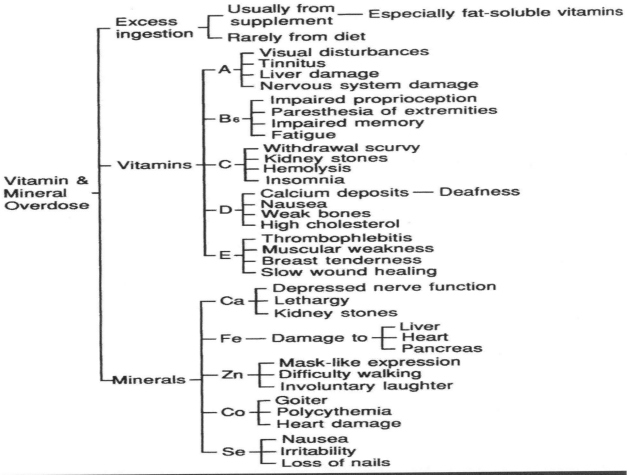

Vitamin & Mineral Overdose

- Excess ingestion
  - Usually from supplement —— Especially fat-soluble vitamins
  - Rarely from diet
- Vitamins
  - A
    - Visual disturbances
    - Tinnitus
    - Liver damage
    - Nervous system damage
  - B₆
    - Impaired proprioception
    - Paresthesia of extremities
    - Impaired memory
    - Fatigue
  - C
    - Withdrawal scurvy
    - Kidney stones
    - Hemolysis
    - Insomnia
  - D
    - Calcium deposits —— Deafness
    - Nausea
    - Weak bones
    - High cholesterol
  - E
    - Thrombophlebitis
    - Muscular weakness
    - Breast tenderness
    - Slow wound healing
- Minerals
  - Ca
    - Depressed nerve function
    - Lethargy
    - Kidney stones
  - Fe —— Damage to
    - Liver
    - Heart
    - Pancreas
  - Zn
    - Mask-like expression
    - Difficulty walking
    - Involuntary laughter
  - Co
    - Goiter
    - Polycythemia
    - Heart damage
  - Se
    - Nausea
    - Irritability
    - Loss of nails

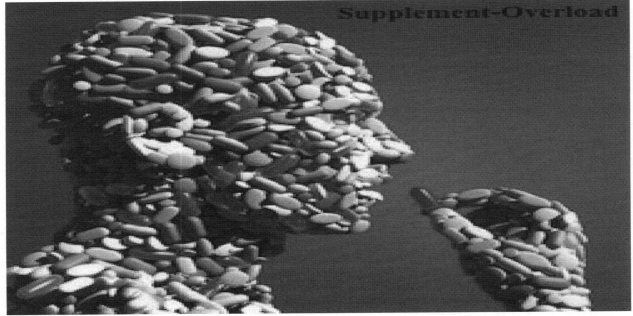

Supplement-Overload

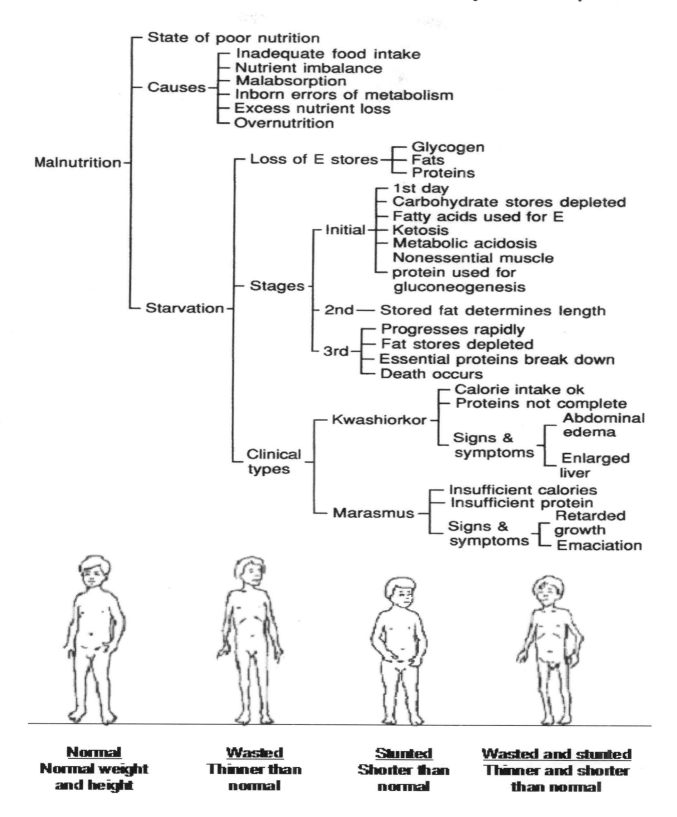

- Malnutrition
  - State of poor nutrition
  - Causes
    - Inadequate food intake
    - Nutrient imbalance
    - Malabsorption
    - Inborn errors of metabolism
    - Excess nutrient loss
    - Overnutrition
  - Starvation
    - Loss of E stores
      - Glycogen
      - Fats
      - Proteins
    - Stages
      - Initial
        - 1st day
        - Carbohydrate stores depleted
        - Fatty acids used for E
        - Ketosis
        - Metabolic acidosis
        - Nonessential muscle protein used for gluconeogenesis
      - 2nd — Stored fat determines length
      - 3rd
        - Progresses rapidly
        - Fat stores depleted
        - Essential proteins break down
        - Death occurs
    - Clinical types
      - Kwashiorkor
        - Calorie intake ok
        - Proteins not complete
        - Signs & symptoms
          - Abdominal edema
          - Enlarged liver
      - Marasmus
        - Insufficient calories
        - Insufficient protein
        - Signs & symptoms
          - Retarded growth
          - Emaciation

Normal
Normal weight and height

Wasted
Thinner than normal

Stunted
Shorter than normal

Wasted and stunted
Thinner and shorter than normal

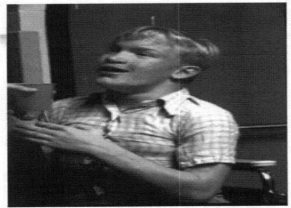
Boy with untreated PKU

Because a child with PKU lacks the normally functioning enzyme necessary to break down phenylalanine (PHE), it accumulates in the blood and body tissues.

This excess PHE can prevent normal brain development and result in mental retardation.

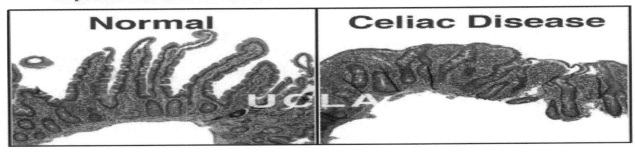

Phenylketonuria (PKU)
- Inborn metabolic error
- Missing enzyme phenylalanine hydroxylase
- Can't convert phenylalanine to tyrosine
- Phenylalanine accumulates in blood
- Neurotoxic effects can cause mental retardation
- Diagnosed by blood test at birth
- Treated by restricting dietary phenylalanine

Celiac Disease
- Gluten causes destruction of intestinal villi
- Malabsorption occurs
- Treat by limiting grain intake to rice and corn

CHAPTER TWENTY SIX

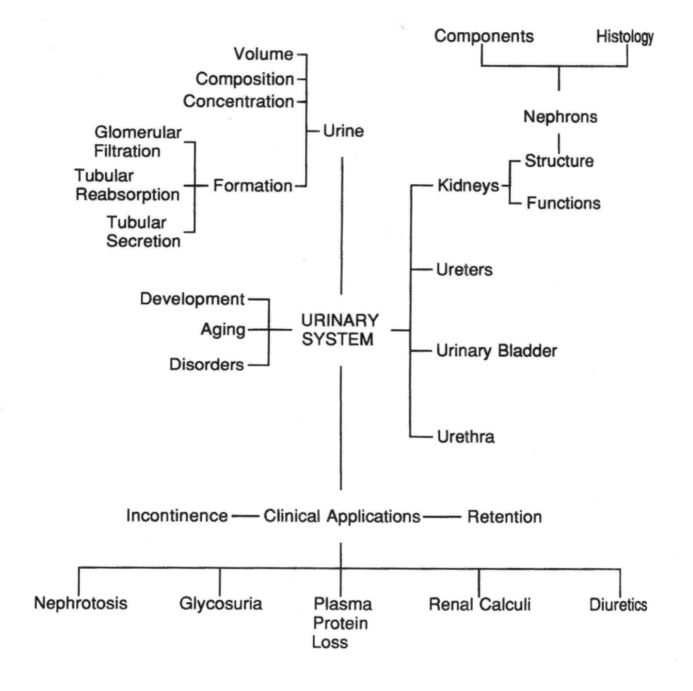

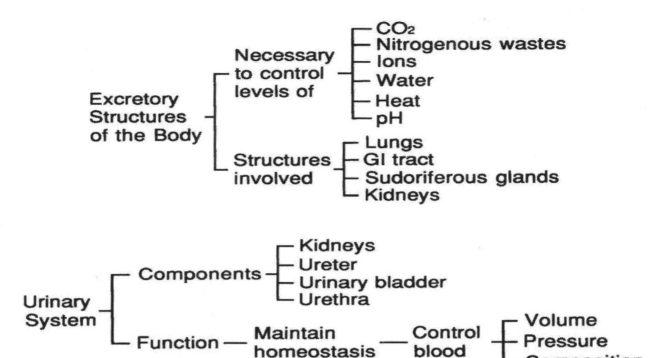

Excretory Structures of the Body
- Necessary to control levels of
  - CO₂
  - Nitrogenous wastes
  - Ions
  - Water
  - Heat
  - pH
- Structures involved
  - Lungs
  - GI tract
  - Sudoriferous glands
  - Kidneys

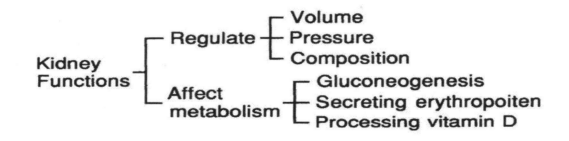

Urinary System
- Components
  - Kidneys
  - Ureter
  - Urinary bladder
  - Urethra
- Function — Maintain homeostasis — Control blood
  - Volume
  - Pressure
  - Composition

Kidney Functions
- Regulate
  - Volume
  - Pressure
  - Composition
- Affect metabolism
  - Gluconeogenesis
  - Secreting erythropoiten
  - Processing vitamin D

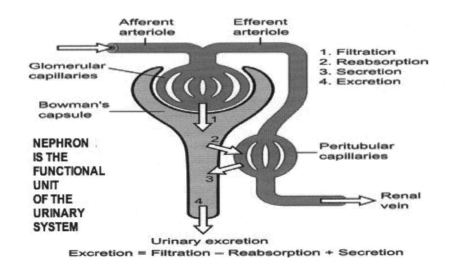

Afferent arteriole
Efferent arteriole
Glomerular capillaries
Bowman's capsule
NEPHRON IS THE FUNCTIONAL UNIT OF THE URINARY SYSTEM
1. Filtration
2. Reabsorption
3. Secretion
4. Excretion
Peritubular capillaries
Renal vein
Urinary excretion
Excretion = Filtration – Reabsorption + Secretion

URINARY SYSTEM

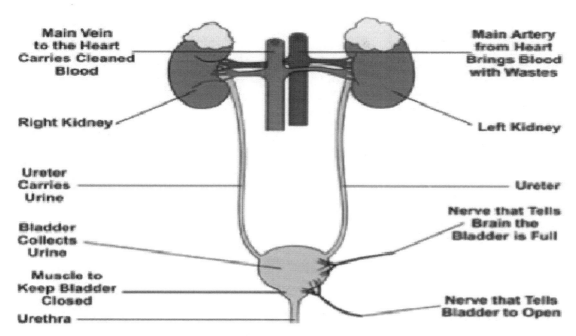

Organs of the Urinary System

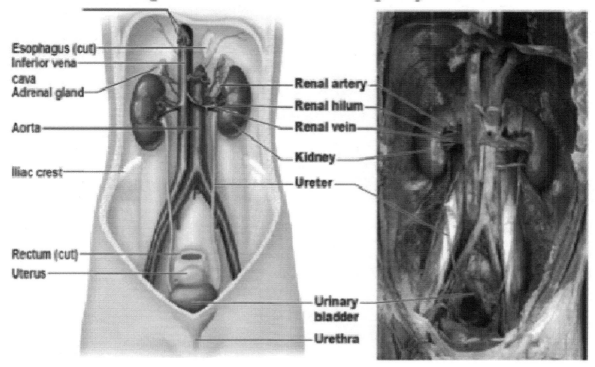

Anatomy of the Kidney
- External
  - Reddish-brown
  - Bean-shaped
  - Hilus
    - Directed toward vertebral column
    - Entry site
      - Blood vessels
      - Lymphatic vessels
      - Nerves
      - Ureter
      - Renal sinus
  - Surrounded by 3 tissue layers
    - Renal capsule
    - Adipose capsule
    - Renal fascia
  - Retroperitoneal — Posterior to parietal peritoneum
  - Usually lie
    - Just above waist
    - T_{12} - L_3
    - R. kidney lower than L.
- Internal anatomy (coronal section)
  - Outer cortex — Renal columns
  - Inner medulla — Renal pyramids — Renal papillae
  - Parenchyma = cortex + renal pyramids
  - Renal sinus — Renal pelvis — Calyces
    - Major
    - Minor

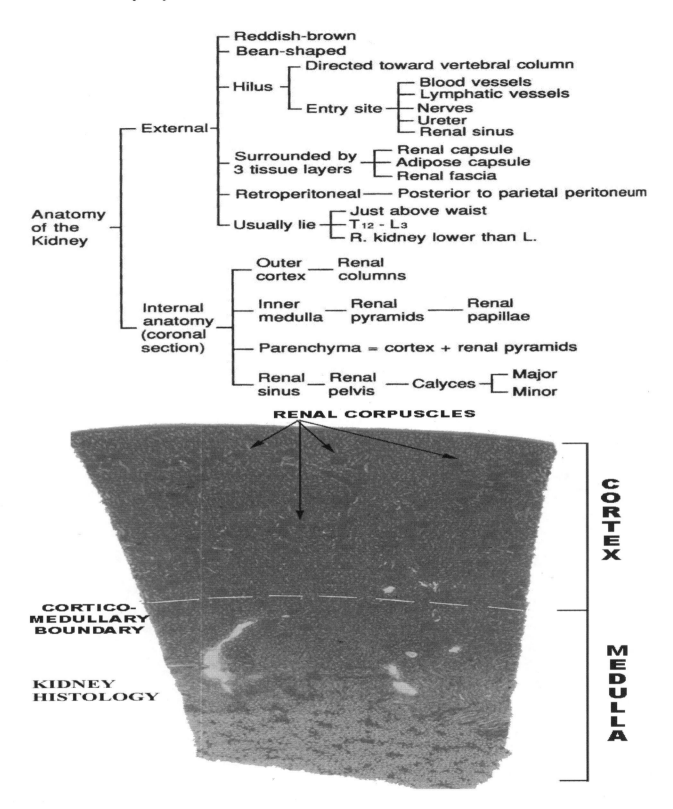

RENAL CORPUSCLES

CORTEX

CORTICO-MEDULLARY BOUNDARY

KIDNEY HISTOLOGY

MEDULLA

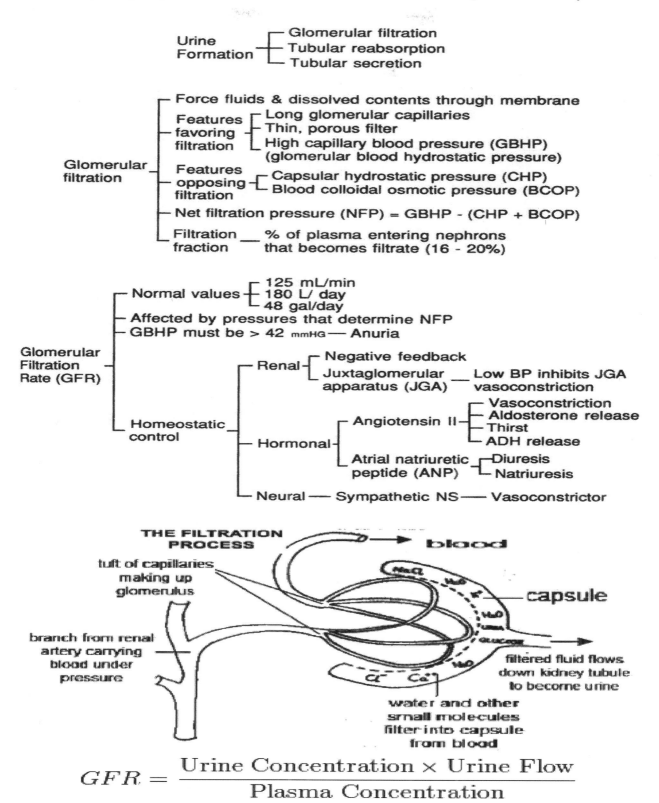

Urine
Formation
- Glomerular filtration
- Tubular reabsorption
- Tubular secretion

Glomerular filtration
- Force fluids & dissolved contents through membrane
- Features favoring filtration
  - Long glomerular capillaries
  - Thin, porous filter
  - High capillary blood pressure (GBHP) (glomerular blood hydrostatic pressure)
- Features opposing filtration
  - Capsular hydrostatic pressure (CHP)
  - Blood colloidal osmotic pressure (BCOP)
- Net filtration pressure (NFP) = GBHP - (CHP + BCOP)
- Filtration fraction — % of plasma entering nephrons that becomes filtrate (16 - 20%)

Glomerular Filtration Rate (GFR)
- Normal values
  - 125 mL/min
  - 180 L/ day
  - 48 gal/day
- Affected by pressures that determine NFP
- GBHP must be > 42 mmHG — Anuria
- Homeostatic control
  - Renal
    - Negative feedback
    - Juxtaglomerular apparatus (JGA) — Low BP inhibits JGA vasoconstriction
  - Hormonal
    - Angiotensin II
      - Vasoconstriction
      - Aldosterone release
      - Thirst
      - ADH release
    - Atrial natriuretic peptide (ANP)
      - Diuresis
      - Natriuresis
  - Neural — Sympathetic NS — Vasoconstrictor

THE FILTRATION PROCESS

tuft of capillaries making up glomerulus

blood

capsule

branch from renal artery carrying blood under pressure

filtered fluid flows down kidney tubule to become urine

water and other small molecules filter into capsule from blood

$$GFR = \frac{\text{Urine Concentration} \times \text{Urine Flow}}{\text{Plasma Concentration}}$$

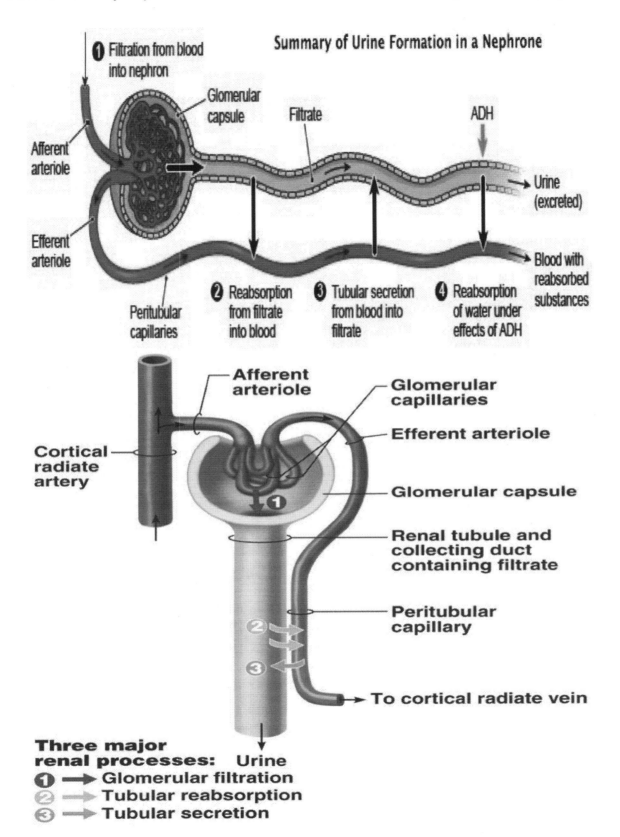

Summary of Urine Formation in a Nephrone

❶ Filtration from blood into nephron

Glomerular capsule

Filtrate

ADH

Afferent arteriole

Efferent arteriole

Urine (excreted)

Blood with reabsorbed substances

Peritubular capillaries

❷ Reabsorption from filtrate into blood

❸ Tubular secretion from blood into filtrate

❹ Reabsorption of water under effects of ADH

Afferent arteriole

Glomerular capillaries

Efferent arteriole

Cortical radiate artery

Glomerular capsule

Renal tubule and collecting duct containing filtrate

Peritubular capillary

To cortical radiate vein

Urine

Three major renal processes:

❶ ➡ **Glomerular filtration**

❷ ➡ **Tubular reabsorption**

❸ ➡ **Tubular secretion**

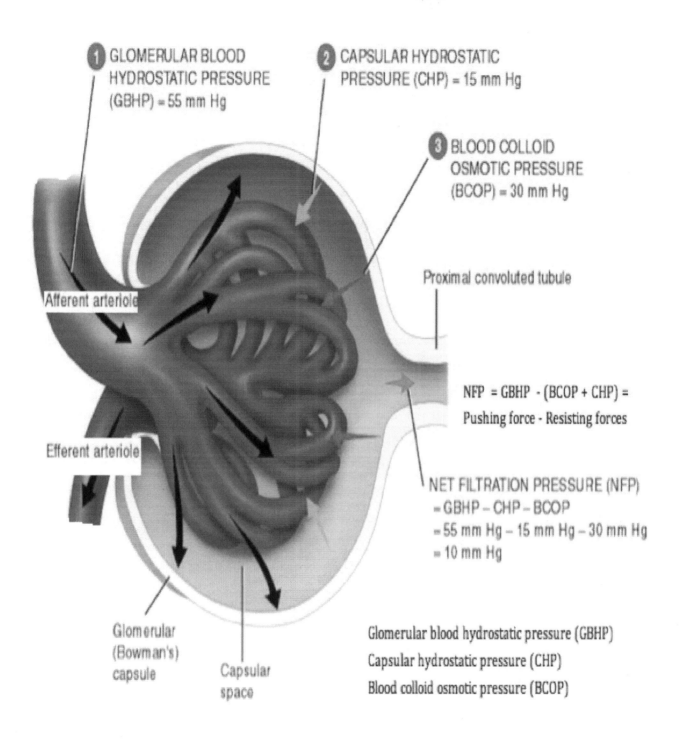

① GLOMERULAR BLOOD HYDROSTATIC PRESSURE (GBHP) = 55 mm Hg

② CAPSULAR HYDROSTATIC PRESSURE (CHP) = 15 mm Hg

③ BLOOD COLLOID OSMOTIC PRESSURE (BCOP) = 30 mm Hg

Afferent arteriole

Efferent arteriole

Proximal convoluted tubule

Glomerular (Bowman's) capsule

Capsular space

NFP = GBHP - (BCOP + CHP) =
Pushing force - Resisting forces

NET FILTRATION PRESSURE (NFP)
= GBHP - CHP - BCOP
= 55 mm Hg - 15 mm Hg - 30 mm Hg
= 10 mm Hg

Glomerular blood hydrostatic pressure (GBHP)

Capsular hydrostatic pressure (CHP)

Blood colloid osmotic pressure (BCOP)

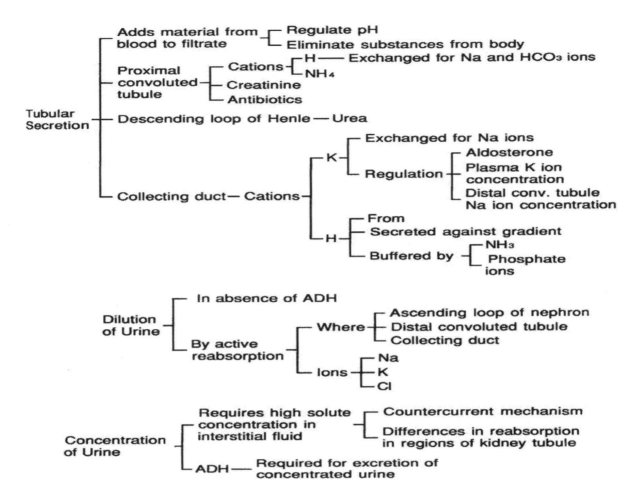

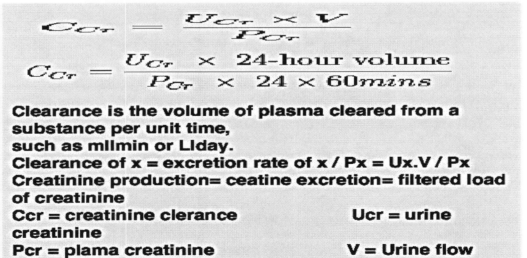

$$C_{Cr} = \frac{U_{Cr} \times V}{P_{Cr}}$$

$$C_{Cr} = \frac{U_{Cr} \times 24\text{-hour volume}}{P_{Cr} \times 24 \times 60 mins}$$

Clearance is the volume of plasma cleared from a substance per unit time,
such as ml/min or L/day.
Clearance of x = excretion rate of x / Px = Ux.V / Px
Creatinine production= ceatine excretion= filtered load of creatinine
Ccr = creatinine clerance creatinine   Ucr = urine
Pcr = plama creatinine   V = Urine flow

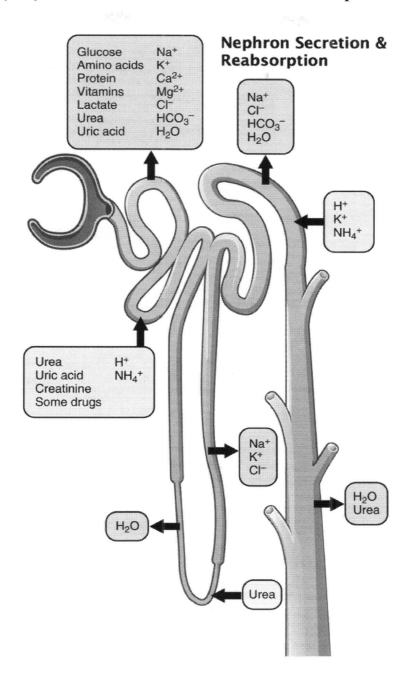

Glucose Na^+
Amino acids K^+
Protein Ca^{2+}
Vitamins Mg^{2+}
Lactate Cl^-
Urea HCO_3^-
Uric acid H_2O

Nephron Secretion & Reabsorption

Na^+
Cl^-
HCO_3^-
H_2O

H^+
K^+
NH_4^+

Urea H^+
Uric acid NH_4^+
Creatinine
Some drugs

Na^+
K^+
Cl^-

H_2O
Urea

H_2O

Urea

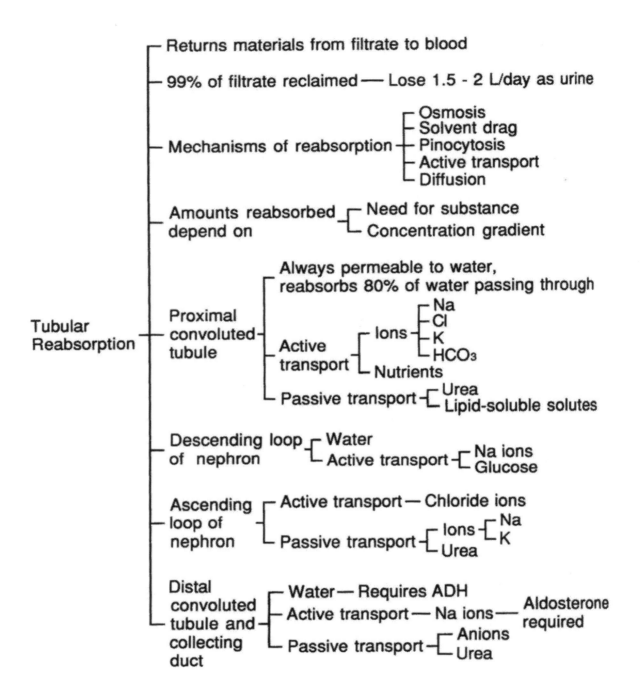

Tubular Reabsorption

- Returns materials from filtrate to blood
- 99% of filtrate reclaimed — Lose 1.5 - 2 L/day as urine
- Mechanisms of reabsorption
  - Osmosis
  - Solvent drag
  - Pinocytosis
  - Active transport
  - Diffusion
- Amounts reabsorbed depend on
  - Need for substance
  - Concentration gradient
- Proximal convoluted tubule
  - Always permeable to water, reabsorbs 80% of water passing through
  - Active transport
    - Ions
      - Na
      - Cl
      - K
      - HCO_3
    - Nutrients
  - Passive transport
    - Urea
    - Lipid-soluble solutes
- Descending loop of nephron
  - Water
  - Active transport
    - Na ions
    - Glucose
- Ascending loop of nephron
  - Active transport — Chloride ions
  - Passive transport
    - Ions
      - Na
      - K
    - Urea
- Distal convoluted tubule and collecting duct
  - Water — Requires ADH
  - Active transport — Na ions — Aldosterone required
  - Passive transport
    - Anions
    - Urea

Countercurrent Multiplier

Filtrate entering the descending limb becomes progressively more concentrated as it loses water.

Blood in the vasa recta removes water leaving the loop of Henle. **(Not Shown)**

The ascending limb pumps out Na+, K+, and Cl-, and filtrate becomes hyposmotic.

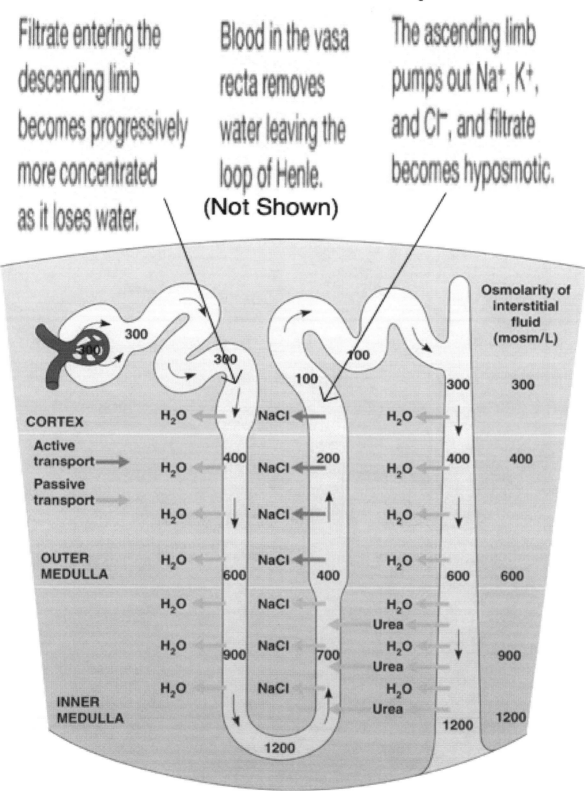

FUNCTION OF NEPHRON - URINE FORMATION

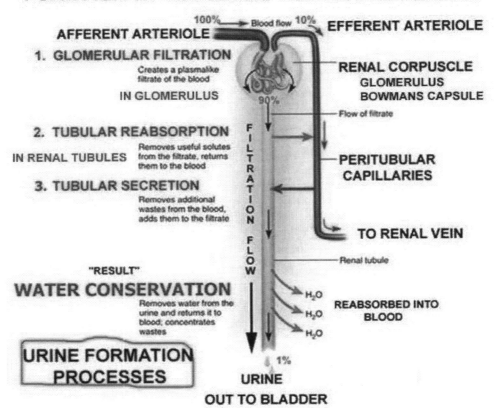

100% → Blood flow 10%

AFFERENT ARTERIOLE   **EFFERENT ARTERIOLE**

1. GLOMERULAR FILTRATION   **RENAL CORPUSCLE**
Creates a plasmalike filtrate of the blood   GLOMERULUS
IN GLOMERULUS   BOWMANS CAPSULE

90%

Flow of filtrate

2. TUBULAR REABSORPTION
IN RENAL TUBULES   Removes useful solutes from the filtrate, returns them to the blood

PERITUBULAR CAPILLARIES

3. TUBULAR SECRETION
Removes additional wastes from the blood, adds them to the filtrate

TO RENAL VEIN

Renal tubule

"RESULT"
WATER CONSERVATION
Removes water from the urine and returns it to blood; concentrates wastes

H_2O
H_2O **REABSORBED INTO BLOOD**
H_2O

URINE FORMATION PROCESSES

FILTRATION FLOW

↓ 1%
URINE
OUT TO BLADDER

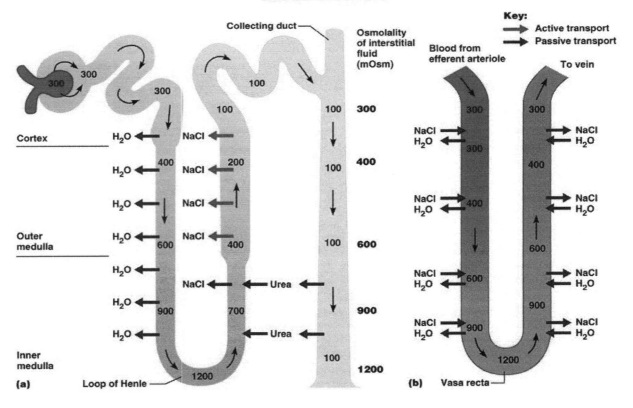

Key:
⇒ Active transport
→ Passive transport

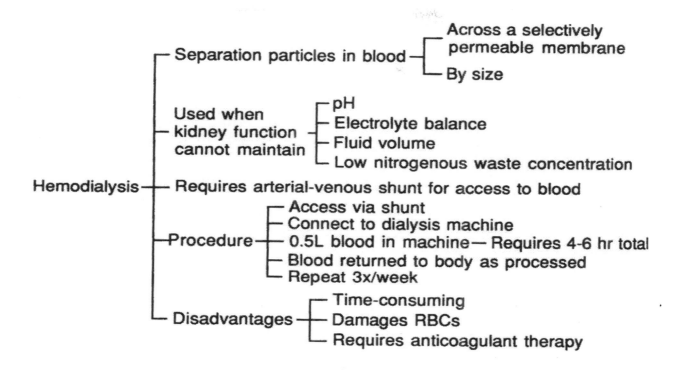

Hemodialysis
- Separation particles in blood
  - Across a selectively permeable membrane
  - By size
- Used when kidney function cannot maintain
  - pH
  - Electrolyte balance
  - Fluid volume
  - Low nitrogenous waste concentration
- Requires arterial-venous shunt for access to blood
- Procedure
  - Access via shunt
  - Connect to dialysis machine
  - 0.5L blood in machine — Requires 4-6 hr total
  - Blood returned to body as processed
  - Repeat 3x/week
- Disadvantages
  - Time-consuming
  - Damages RBCs
  - Requires anticoagulant therapy

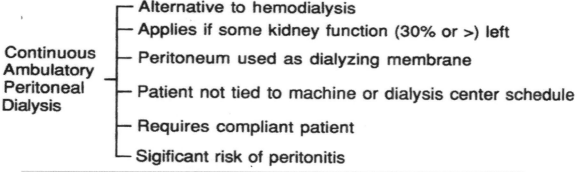

Continuous Ambulatory Peritoneal Dialysis
- Alternative to hemodialysis
- Applies if some kidney function (30% or >) left
- Peritoneum used as dialyzing membrane
- Patient not tied to machine or dialysis center schedule
- Requires compliant patient
- Sigificant risk of peritonitis

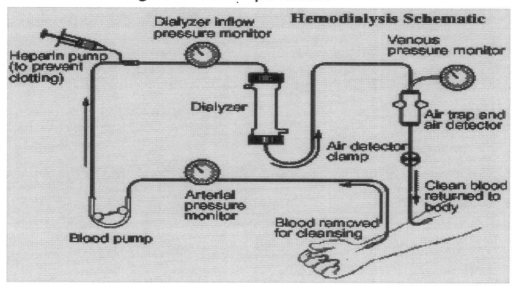

Hemodialysis Schematic

Dialyzer inflow pressure monitor

Venous pressure monitor

Heparin pump (to prevent clotting)

Dialyzer

Air trap and air detector

Air detector clamp

Arterial pressure monitor

Clean blood returned to body

Blood removed for cleansing

Blood pump

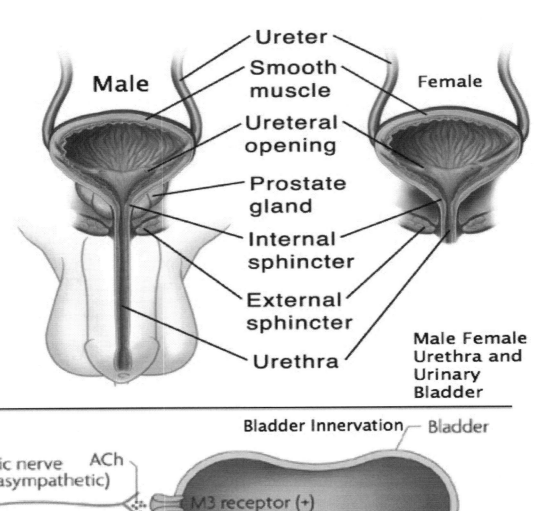

Male

Female

Ureter

Smooth muscle

Ureteral opening

Prostate gland

Internal sphincter

External sphincter

Urethra

Male Female Urethra and Urinary Bladder

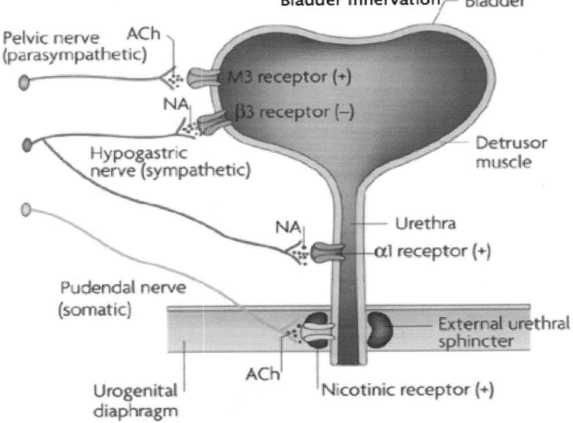

Bladder Innervation — Bladder

Pelvic nerve (parasympathetic)   ACh

M3 receptor (+)

NA

β3 receptor (−)

Hypogastric nerve (sympathetic)

Detrusor muscle

NA

Urethra

α1 receptor (+)

Pudendal nerve (somatic)

External urethral sphincter

Urogenital diaphragm

ACh

Nicotinic receptor (+)

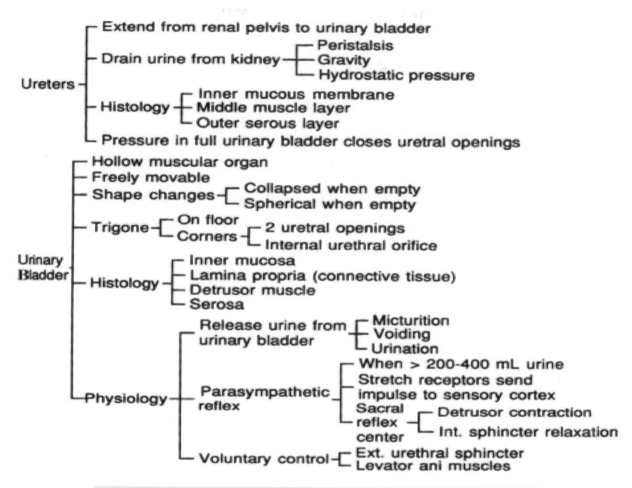

Ureters
- Extend from renal pelvis to urinary bladder
- Drain urine from kidney
  - Peristalsis
  - Gravity
  - Hydrostatic pressure
- Histology
  - Inner mucous membrane
  - Middle muscle layer
  - Outer serous layer
- Pressure in full urinary bladder closes uretral openings

Urinary Bladder
- Hollow muscular organ
- Freely movable
- Shape changes
  - Collapsed when empty
  - Spherical when empty
- Trigone
  - On floor
  - Corners
    - 2 uretral openings
    - Internal urethral orifice
- Histology
  - Inner mucosa
  - Lamina propria (connective tissue)
  - Detrusor muscle
  - Serosa
- Physiology
  - Release urine from urinary bladder
    - Micturition
    - Voiding
    - Urination
  - Parasympathetic reflex
    - When > 200-400 mL urine
    - Stretch receptors send impulse to sensory cortex
    - Sacral reflex center
      - Detrusor contraction
      - Int. sphincter relaxation
  - Voluntary control
    - Ext. urethral sphincter
    - Levator ani muscles

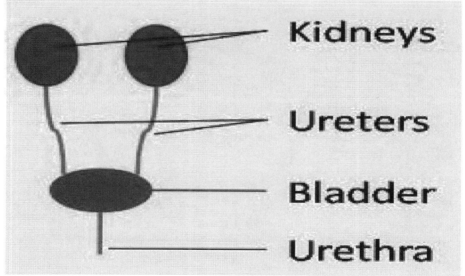

Kidneys

Ureters

Bladder

Urethra

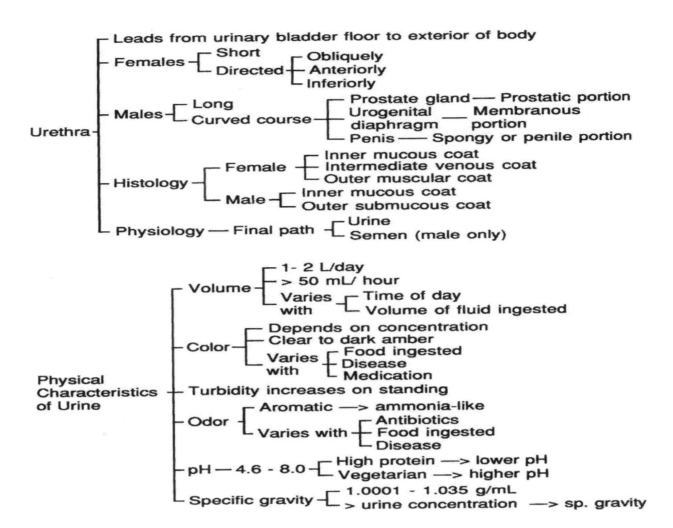

- **Urethra**
  - Leads from urinary bladder floor to exterior of body
  - **Females**
    - Short
    - Directed
      - Obliquely
      - Anteriorly
      - Inferiorly
  - **Males**
    - Long
    - Curved course
      - Prostate gland — Prostatic portion
      - Urogenital diaphragm — Membranous portion
      - Penis — Spongy or penile portion
  - **Histology**
    - Female
      - Inner mucous coat
      - Intermediate venous coat
      - Outer muscular coat
    - Male
      - Inner mucous coat
      - Outer submucous coat
  - **Physiology** — Final path
    - Urine
    - Semen (male only)

- **Physical Characteristics of Urine**
  - **Volume**
    - 1- 2 L/day
    - > 50 mL/ hour
    - Varies with
      - Time of day
      - Volume of fluid ingested
  - **Color**
    - Depends on concentration
    - Clear to dark amber
    - Varies with
      - Food ingested
      - Disease
      - Medication
  - **Turbidity** increases on standing
  - **Odor**
    - Aromatic —> ammonia-like
    - Varies with
      - Antibiotics
      - Food ingested
      - Disease
  - **pH** — 4.6 - 8.0
    - High protein —> lower pH
    - Vegetarian —> higher pH
  - **Specific gravity**
    - 1.0001 - 1.035 g/mL
    - > urine concentration —> sp. gravity

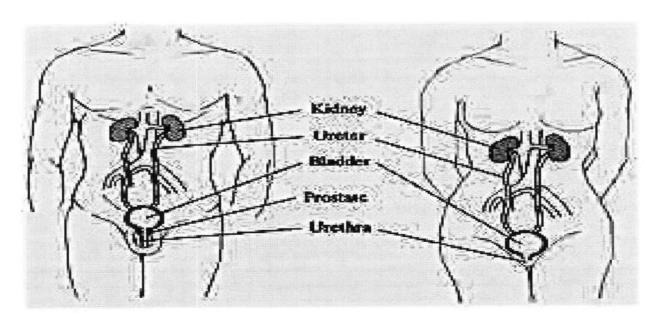

Kidney
Ureter
Bladder
Prostate
Urethra

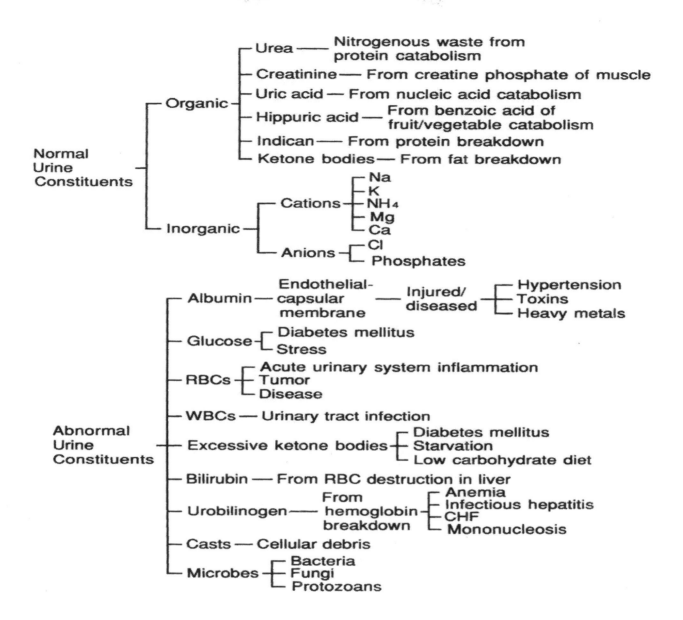

Normal Urine Constituents
- Organic
  - Urea — Nitrogenous waste from protein catabolism
  - Creatinine — From creatine phosphate of muscle
  - Uric acid — From nucleic acid catabolism
  - Hippuric acid — From benzoic acid of fruit/vegetable catabolism
  - Indican — From protein breakdown
  - Ketone bodies — From fat breakdown
- Inorganic
  - Cations
    - Na
    - K
    - NH₄
    - Mg
    - Ca
  - Anions
    - Cl
    - Phosphates

Abnormal Urine Constituents
- Albumin — Endothelial-capsular membrane — Injured/diseased
  - Hypertension
  - Toxins
  - Heavy metals
- Glucose
  - Diabetes mellitus
  - Stress
- RBCs
  - Acute urinary system inflammation
  - Tumor
  - Disease
- WBCs — Urinary tract infection
- Excessive ketone bodies
  - Diabetes mellitus
  - Starvation
  - Low carbohydrate diet
- Bilirubin — From RBC destruction in liver
- Urobilinogen — From hemoglobin breakdown
  - Anemia
  - Infectious hepatitis
  - CHF
  - Mononucleosis
- Casts — Cellular debris
- Microbes
  - Bacteria
  - Fungi
  - Protozoans

THE URINE TESTS

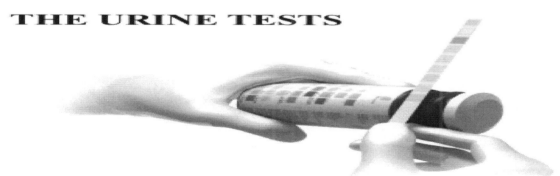

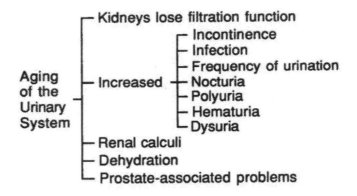

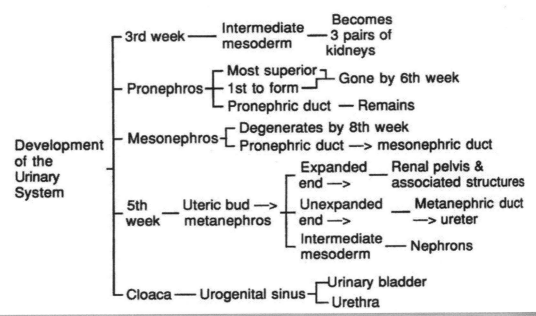

Development of Urinary system and reproductive system

1. Development of kidney and ureter

2. Development of urinary bladder and urethra

3. Abnormality in urinary system

4. Development of gonad

5. Development of reproductive tracts

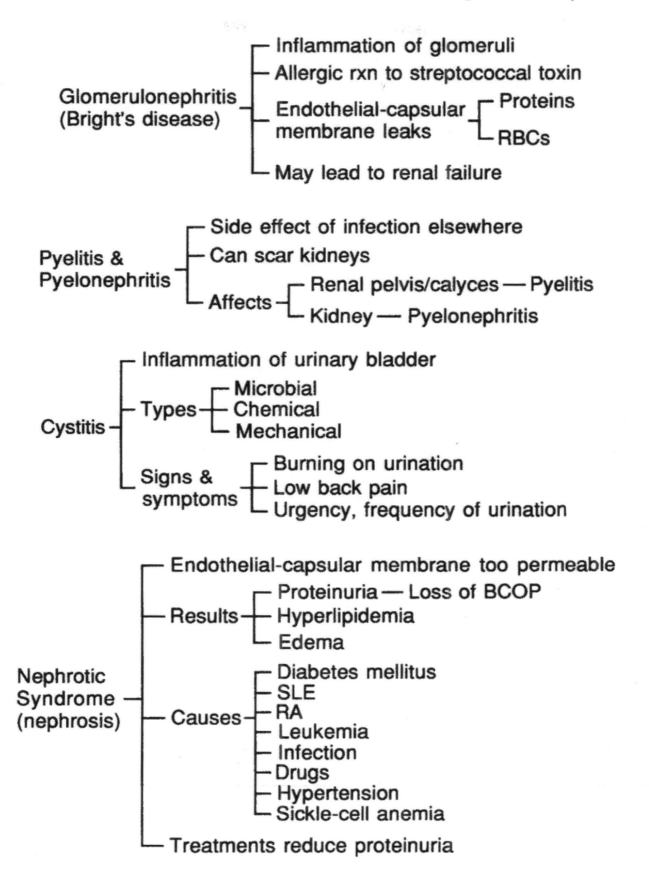

Glomerulonephritis (Bright's disease)
- Inflammation of glomeruli
- Allergic rxn to streptococcal toxin
- Endothelial-capsular membrane leaks
  - Proteins
  - RBCs
- May lead to renal failure

Pyelitis & Pyelonephritis
- Side effect of infection elsewhere
- Can scar kidneys
- Affects
  - Renal pelvis/calyces — Pyelitis
  - Kidney — Pyelonephritis

Cystitis
- Inflammation of urinary bladder
- Types
  - Microbial
  - Chemical
  - Mechanical
- Signs & symptoms
  - Burning on urination
  - Low back pain
  - Urgency, frequency of urination

Nephrotic Syndrome (nephrosis)
- Endothelial-capsular membrane too permeable
- Results
  - Proteinuria — Loss of BCOP
  - Hyperlipidemia
  - Edema
- Causes
  - Diabetes mellitus
  - SLE
  - RA
  - Leukemia
  - Infection
  - Drugs
  - Hypertension
  - Sickle-cell anemia
- Treatments reduce proteinuria

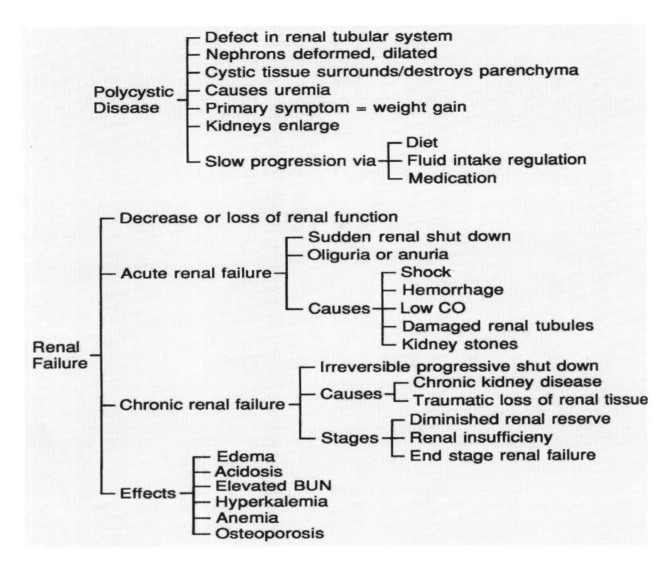

Polycystic Disease
- Defect in renal tubular system
- Nephrons deformed, dilated
- Cystic tissue surrounds/destroys parenchyma
- Causes uremia
- Primary symptom = weight gain
- Kidneys enlarge
- Slow progression via
  - Diet
  - Fluid intake regulation
  - Medication

Renal Failure
- Decrease or loss of renal function
- Acute renal failure
  - Sudden renal shut down
  - Oliguria or anuria
  - Causes
    - Shock
    - Hemorrhage
    - Low CO
    - Damaged renal tubules
    - Kidney stones
- Chronic renal failure
  - Irreversible progressive shut down
  - Causes
    - Chronic kidney disease
    - Traumatic loss of renal tissue
  - Stages
    - Diminished renal reserve
    - Renal insufficieny
    - End stage renal failure
- Effects
  - Edema
  - Acidosis
  - Elevated BUN
  - Hyperkalemia
  - Anemia
  - Osteoporosis

Polycystic Kidney Disease

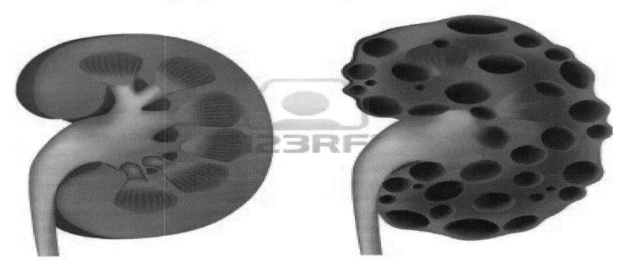

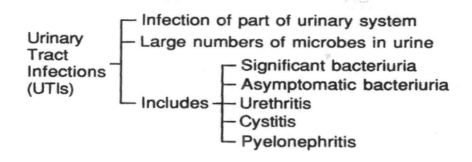

Urinary Tract Infections (UTIs)
- Infection of part of urinary system
- Large numbers of microbes in urine
- Includes
  - Significant bacteriuria
  - Asymptomatic bacteriuria
  - Urethritis
  - Cystitis
  - Pyelonephritis

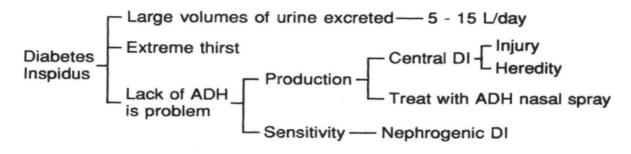

Diabetes Inspidus
- Large volumes of urine excreted —— 5 - 15 L/day
- Extreme thirst
- Lack of ADH is problem
  - Production
    - Central DI
      - Injury
      - Heredity
    - Treat with ADH nasal spray
  - Sensitivity —— Nephrogenic DI

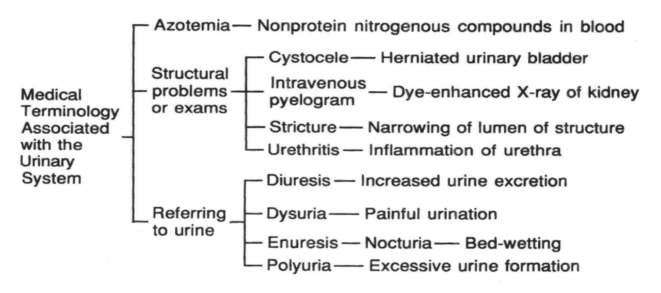

Medical Terminology Associated with the Urinary System
- Azotemia —— Nonprotein nitrogenous compounds in blood
- Structural problems or exams
  - Cystocele —— Herniated urinary bladder
  - Intravenous pyelogram —— Dye-enhanced X-ray of kidney
  - Stricture —— Narrowing of lumen of structure
  - Urethritis —— Inflammation of urethra
- Referring to urine
  - Diuresis —— Increased urine excretion
  - Dysuria —— Painful urination
  - Enuresis —— Nocturia —— Bed-wetting
  - Polyuria —— Excessive urine formation

Diabetes mellitus	Diabetes insipidus
It results from hyposecretion of insulin.	It results from hyposecretion of ADH.
Excretion of urine with sugar.	Excretion of large amounts of dilute urine.
Excessive eating.	Dehydration.

CHAPTER TWENTY SEVEN

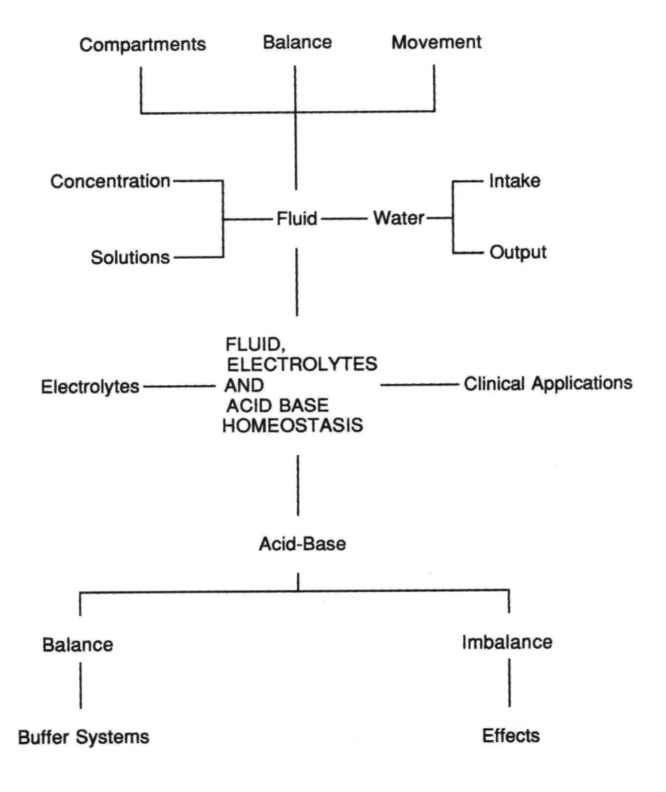

Body Fluid Compartments

Body Fluid Compartment	Volume L/100 kg body weight	
	Human	Sheep
Intracellular	50.0	31.1
Extracellular	20.0	15.5
Plasma	(5.0)	(4.9)
Interstitial	(15.0)	(10.7)
Transcellular	2.8	22.2
Alimentary tract	(1.4)	(20.0)
Other[a]	(1.4)	(2.2)
TOTAL	**72.8**	**68.8**

[a]Cerebrospinal fluid, synovial fluid, aqueous humor, and urine.

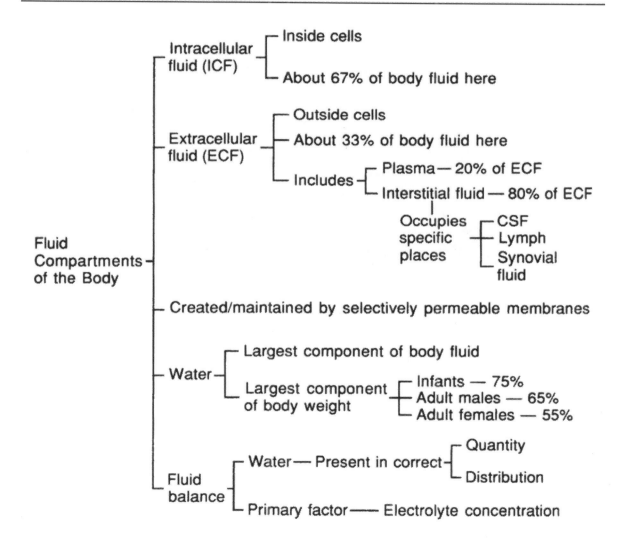

Fluid Compartments of the Body
- Intracellular fluid (ICF)
  - Inside cells
  - About 67% of body fluid here
- Extracellular fluid (ECF)
  - Outside cells
  - About 33% of body fluid here
  - Includes
    - Plasma — 20% of ECF
    - Interstitial fluid — 80% of ECF
      - Occupies specific places
        - CSF
        - Lymph
        - Synovial fluid
- Created/maintained by selectively permeable membranes
- Water
  - Largest component of body fluid
  - Largest component of body weight
    - Infants — 75%
    - Adult males — 65%
    - Adult females — 55%
- Fluid balance
  - Water — Present in correct
    - Quantity
    - Distribution
  - Primary factor —— Electrolyte concentration

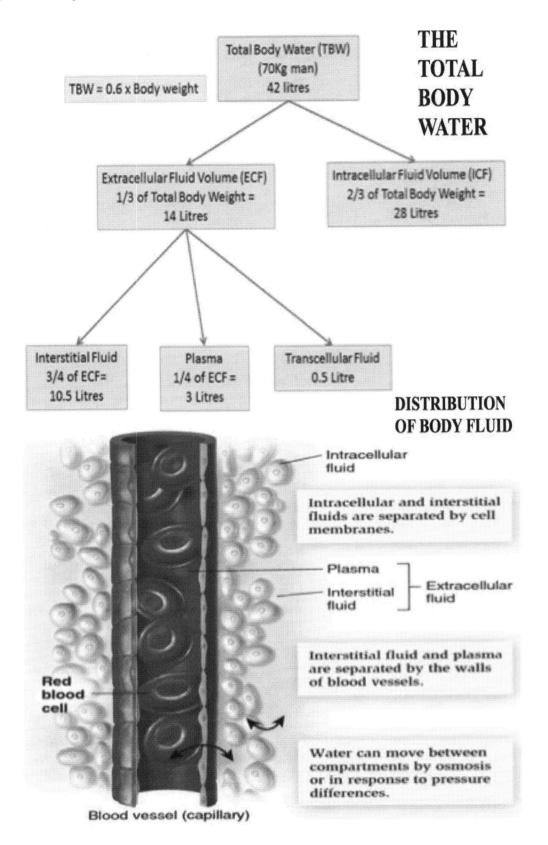

THE
TOTAL
BODY
WATER

Total Body Water (TBW)
(70Kg man)
42 litres

TBW = 0.6 x Body weight

Extracellular Fluid Volume (ECF)
1/3 of Total Body Weight =
14 Litres

Intracellular Fluid Volume (ICF)
2/3 of Total Body Weight =
28 Litres

Interstitial Fluid
3/4 of ECF=
10.5 Litres

Plasma
1/4 of ECF =
3 Litres

Transcellular Fluid
0.5 Litre

**DISTRIBUTION
OF BODY FLUID**

Intracellular
fluid

Intracellular and interstitial
fluids are separated by cell
membranes.

Plasma

Interstitial
fluid

Extracellular
fluid

Interstitial fluid and plasma
are separated by the walls
of blood vessels.

Red
blood
cell

Water can move between
compartments by osmosis
or in response to pressure
differences.

Blood vessel (capillary)

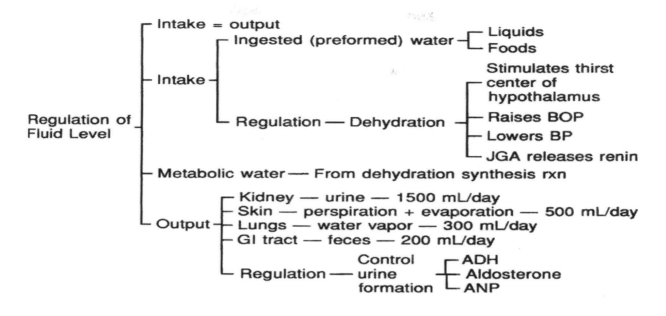

Regulation of Fluid Level
- Intake
  - Intake = output
  - Ingested (preformed) water
    - Liquids
    - Foods
  - Regulation — Dehydration
    - Stimulates thirst center of hypothalamus
    - Raises BOP
    - Lowers BP
    - JGA releases renin
- Metabolic water — From dehydration synthesis rxn
- Output
  - Kidney — urine — 1500 mL/day
  - Skin — perspiration + evaporation — 500 mL/day
  - Lungs — water vapor — 300 mL/day
  - GI tract — feces — 200 mL/day
  - Regulation — Control urine formation
    - ADH
    - Aldosterone
    - ANP

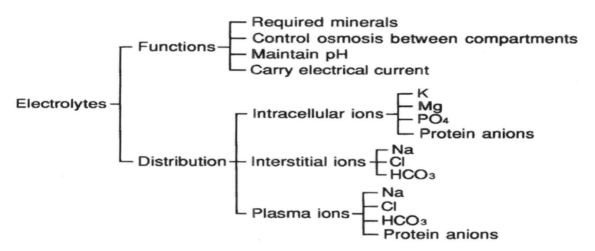

Electrolytes
- Functions
  - Required minerals
  - Control osmosis between compartments
  - Maintain pH
  - Carry electrical current
- Distribution
  - Intracellular ions
    - K
    - Mg
    - PO$_4$
    - Protein anions
  - Interstitial ions
    - Na
    - Cl
    - HCO$_3$
  - Plasma ions
    - Na
    - Cl
    - HCO$_3$
    - Protein anions

Comparison Between Electrolytes of the Extracellular and Intracellular Fluid

	Extracellular Fluid	Intracellular Fluid
Na$^+$	142 mEq/L	10 mEq/L
K$^+$	4 mEq/L	140 mEq/L
Ca^{++}	5 mEq/L	<1 mEq/L
Mg^{++}	3 mEq/L	58 mEq/L
Cl$^-$	103 mEq/L	4 mEq/L
HCO$_3$$^+$	28 mEq/L	10 mEq/L
Phosphates	4 mEq/L	75 mEq/L
SO$_4$$^{--}$	1 mEq/L	2 mEq/L
Osmolality	281 mOsm/L	281 mOsm/L

Regulation of Water Intake

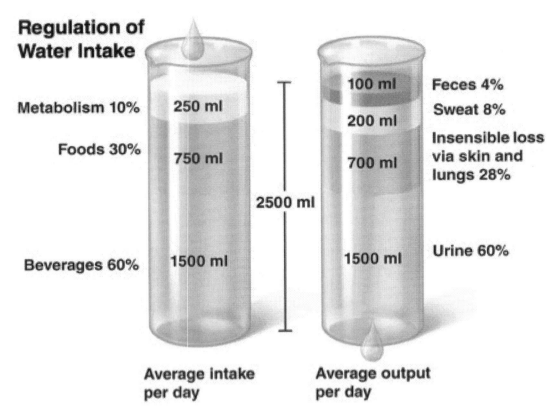

Metabolism 10%   250 ml

Foods 30%   750 ml

2500 ml

Beverages 60%   1500 ml

100 ml   Feces 4%

200 ml   Sweat 8%

700 ml   Insensible loss via skin and lungs 28%

1500 ml   Urine 60%

Average intake per day

Average output per day

Daily Water Transfer

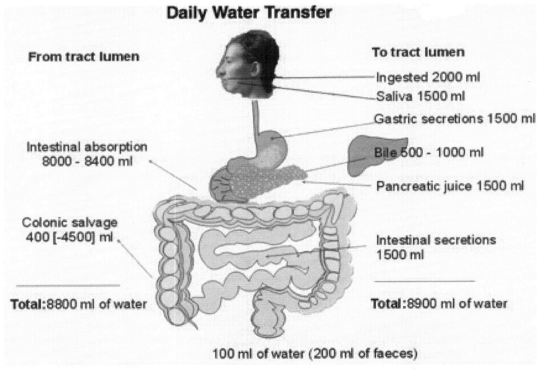

From tract lumen

To tract lumen

Ingested 2000 ml

Saliva 1500 ml

Gastric secretions 1500 ml

Intestinal absorption 8000 - 8400 ml

Bile 500 - 1000 ml

Pancreatic juice 1500 ml

Colonic salvage 400 [-4500] ml

Intestinal secretions 1500 ml

Total: 8800 ml of water

Total: 8900 ml of water

100 ml of water (200 ml of faeces)

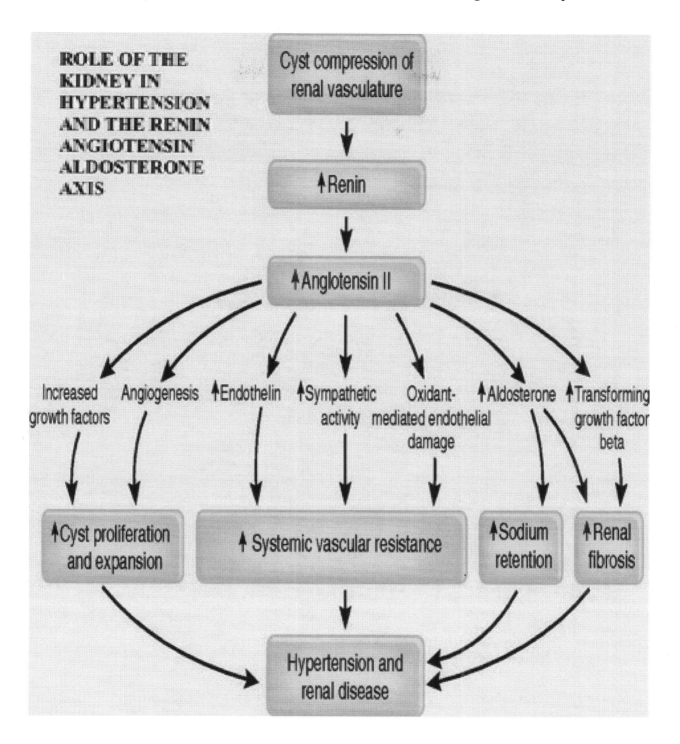

ROLE OF THE KIDNEY IN HYPERTENSION AND THE RENIN ANGIOTENSIN ALDOSTERONE AXIS

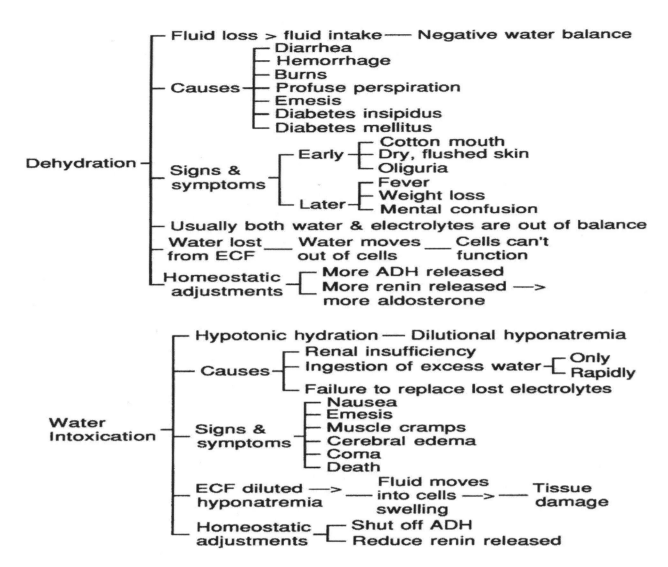

Dehydration
- Fluid loss > fluid intake — Negative water balance
- Causes
  - Diarrhea
  - Hemorrhage
  - Burns
  - Profuse perspiration
  - Emesis
  - Diabetes insipidus
  - Diabetes mellitus
- Signs & symptoms
  - Early
    - Cotton mouth
    - Dry, flushed skin
    - Oliguria
  - Later
    - Fever
    - Weight loss
    - Mental confusion
- Usually both water & electrolytes are out of balance
- Water lost from ECF — Water moves out of cells — Cells can't function
- Homeostatic adjustments
  - More ADH released
  - More renin released —> more aldosterone

Water Intoxication
- Hypotonic hydration — Dilutional hyponatremia
- Causes
  - Renal insufficiency
  - Ingestion of excess water
    - Only
    - Rapidly
  - Failure to replace lost electrolytes
- Signs & symptoms
  - Nausea
  - Emesis
  - Muscle cramps
  - Cerebral edema
  - Coma
  - Death
- ECF diluted —> hyponatremia — Fluid moves into cells —> swelling — Tissue damage
- Homeostatic adjustments
  - Shut off ADH
  - Reduce renin released

Hyperosmolar Hyponatremia

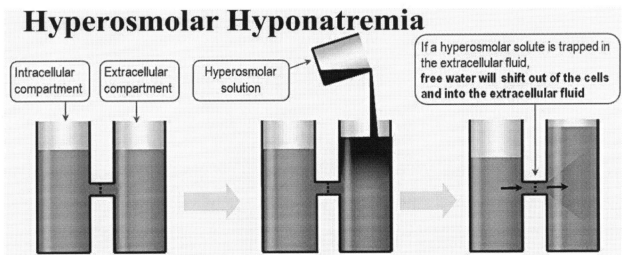

Intracellular compartment   Extracellular compartment   Hyperosmolar solution

If a hyperosmolar solute is trapped in the extracellular fluid, **free water will shift out of the cells and into the extracellular fluid**

Dehydration versus water intoxication

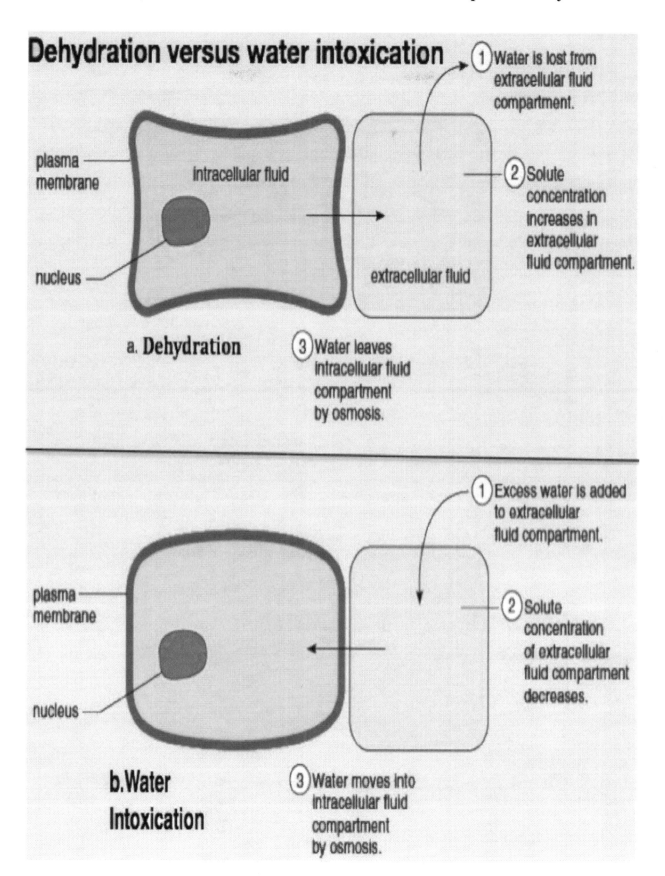

plasma membrane

intracellular fluid

nucleus

extracellular fluid

a. **Dehydration**

① Water is lost from extracellular fluid compartment.

② Solute concentration increases in extracellular fluid compartment.

③ Water leaves intracellular fluid compartment by osmosis.

plasma membrane

nucleus

b. Water Intoxication

① Excess water is added to extracellular fluid compartment.

② Solute concentration of extracellular fluid compartment decreases.

③ Water moves into intracellular fluid compartment by osmosis.

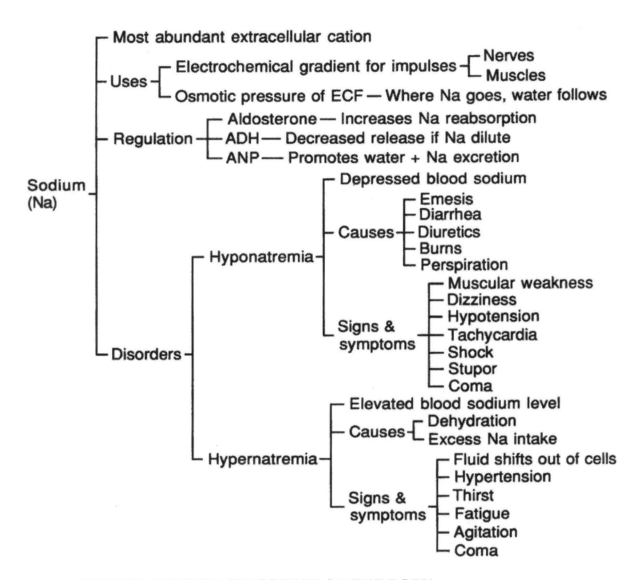

EFFECTS OF THE LOW SODIUM ON THE BODY

Sodium Plasma concentration (mEq/L)	Signs/symptoms
130-135	Asymptomatic
125-130	Nausea and malaise
115-120	Headache, lethargy, disorientation
Severe and rapidly developing	Seizure, coma, permanent brain damage, respiratory arrest, brainstem herniation, and death

Fluid and Electrolyte Balance

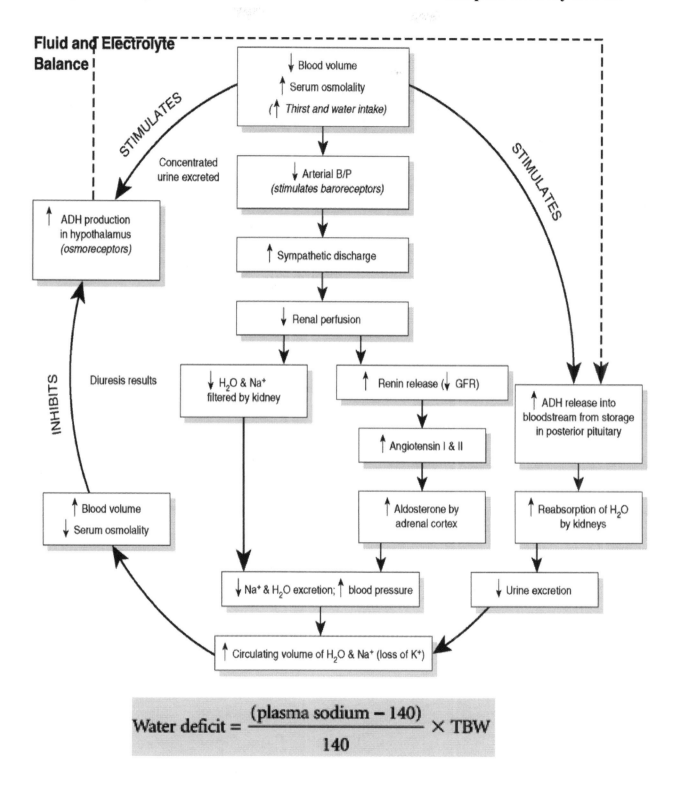

ADH production in hypothalamus *(osmoreceptors)*

STIMULATES

Concentrated urine excreted

↓ Blood volume

↑ Serum osmolality

(↑ Thirst and water intake)

↓ Arterial B/P *(stimulates baroreceptors)*

↑ Sympathetic discharge

↓ Renal perfusion

STIMULATES

INHIBITS

Diuresis results

↑ Blood volume

↓ Serum osmolality

↓ H_2O & Na^+ filtered by kidney

↑ Renin release (↓ GFR)

↑ Angiotensin I & II

↑ Aldosterone by adrenal cortex

↑ ADH release into bloodstream from storage in posterior pituitary

↑ Reabsorption of H_2O by kidneys

↓ Na^+ & H_2O excretion; ↑ blood pressure

↓ Urine excretion

↑ Circulating volume of H_2O & Na^+ (loss of K^+)

$$\text{Water deficit} = \frac{(\text{plasma sodium} - 140)}{140} \times \text{TBW}$$

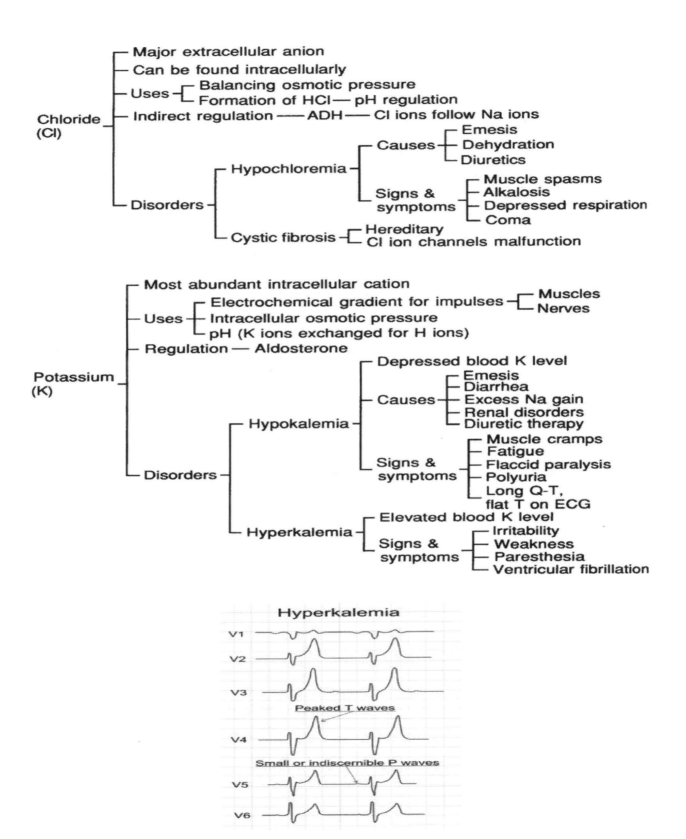

Chloride (Cl)
- Major extracellular anion
- Can be found intracellularly
- Uses
  - Balancing osmotic pressure
  - Formation of HCl — pH regulation
- Indirect regulation — ADH — Cl ions follow Na ions
- Disorders
  - Hypochloremia
    - Causes
      - Emesis
      - Dehydration
      - Diuretics
    - Signs & symptoms
      - Muscle spasms
      - Alkalosis
      - Depressed respiration
      - Coma
  - Cystic fibrosis
    - Hereditary
    - Cl ion channels malfunction

Potassium (K)
- Most abundant intracellular cation
- Uses
  - Electrochemical gradient for impulses
    - Muscles
    - Nerves
  - Intracellular osmotic pressure
  - pH (K ions exchanged for H ions)
- Regulation — Aldosterone
- Disorders
  - Hypokalemia
    - Depressed blood K level
    - Causes
      - Emesis
      - Diarrhea
      - Excess Na gain
      - Renal disorders
      - Diuretic therapy
    - Signs & symptoms
      - Muscle cramps
      - Fatigue
      - Flaccid paralysis
      - Polyuria
      - Long Q-T, flat T on ECG
  - Hyperkalemia
    - Elevated blood K level
    - Signs & symptoms
      - Irritability
      - Weakness
      - Paresthesia
      - Ventricular fibrillation

Hyperkalemia

V1
V2
V3
Peaked T waves
V4
Small or indiscernible P waves
V5
V6

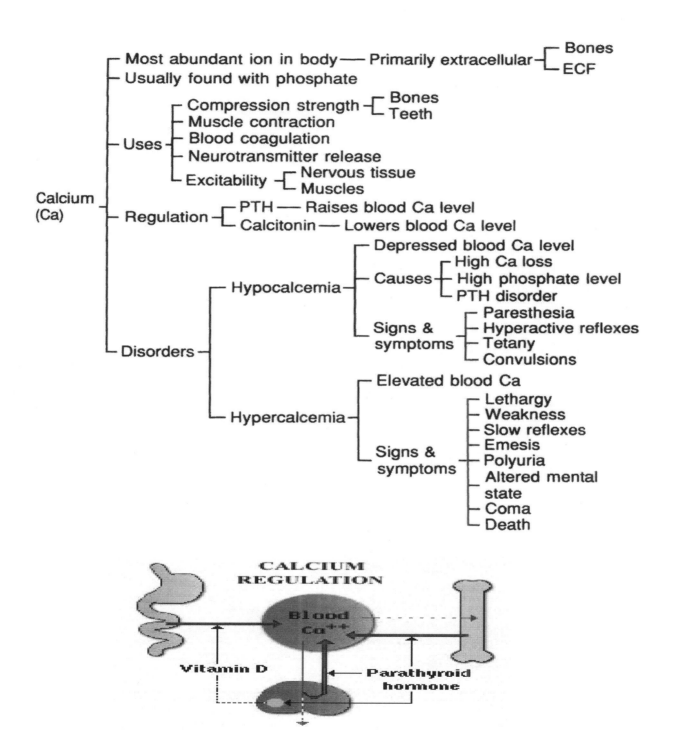

CALCIUM
REGULATION

Blood
Ca++

Vitamin D

Parathyroid
hormone

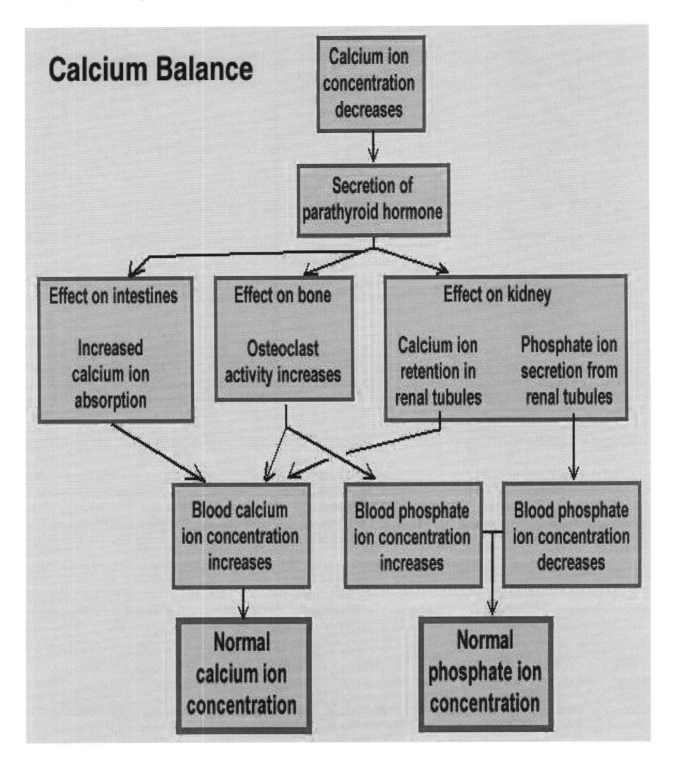

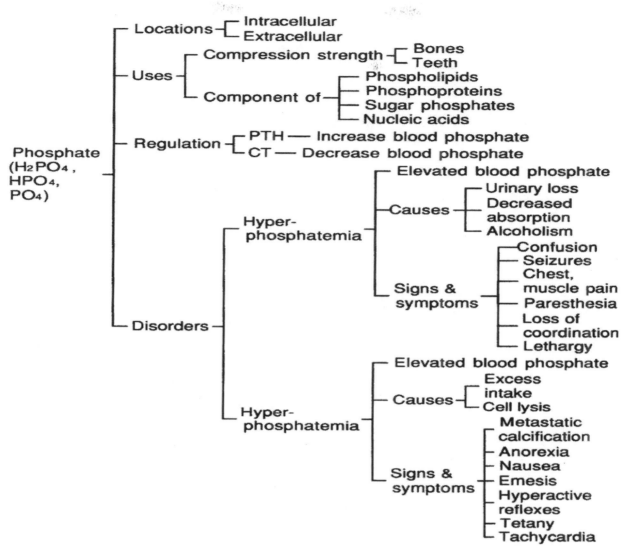

Age-Specific Normal Ranges of Blood Ionized Calcium, Total Calcium and Phosphorus

Age	Ionized Calcium (mmol/L)	Calcium (mg/dL)	Phosphorus (mg/dL)
0-5 mo	1.22-1.40	8.7-11.3	5.2-8.4
6-12 mo	1.20-1.40	8.7-11.0	5.0-7.8
1-5 y	1.22-1.32	9.4-10.8	4.5-6.5
6-12 y	1.15-1.32	9.4-10.3	3.6-5.8
13-20 y	1.12-1.30	8.8-10.2	2.3-4.5

Conversion factor for calcium and ionized calcium: mg/dL × 0.25 = mmol/L.

Conversion factor for phosphorus: mg/dL × 0.323 = mmol/L.

The Phosphate Buffer System

$$pKa = 2.1 \qquad\qquad 6.9 \qquad\qquad 12.8$$

$$H_3PO_4 \leftrightarrow H_2PO_4^{-1} + H^+ \leftrightarrow HPO_4^{-2} + H^+ \leftrightarrow PO_4^{-3} + H^+$$

3.3.2phosbuffer

① CO_2 combines with water within the type A intercalated cell, forming H_2CO_3.

② H_2CO_3 is quickly split, forming H^+ and bicarbonate ion (HCO_3^-).

③a H^+ is secreted into the filtrate by a H^+ ATPase pump.

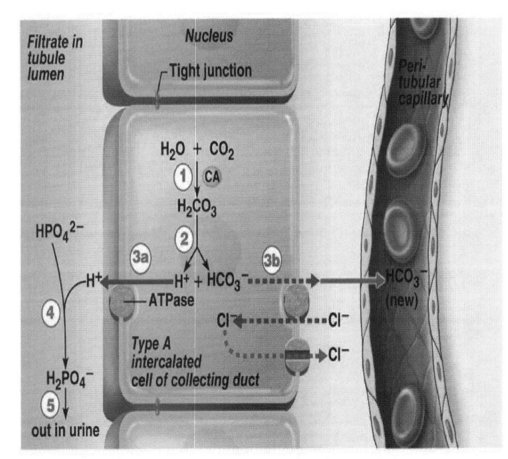

③b For each H^+ secreted, a HCO_3^- enters the peritubular capillary blood via an antiport carrier in a HCO_3^--Cl^- exchange process.

④ Secreted H^+ combines with HPO_4^{2-} in the tubular filtrate, forming $H_2PO_4^-$.

⑤ The $H_2PO_4^-$ is excreted in the urine.

→ Primary active transport
···▶ Secondary active transport
→ Simple diffusion
···▶ Facilitated diffusion

⬤ Transport protein
⊖ Ion channel
CA Carbonic anhydrase

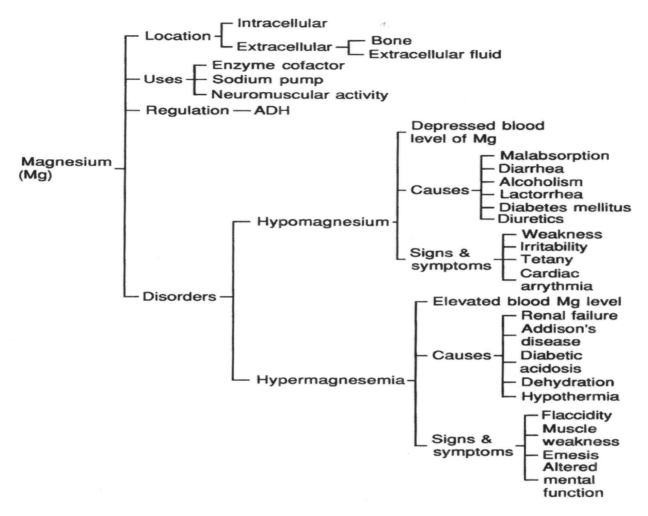

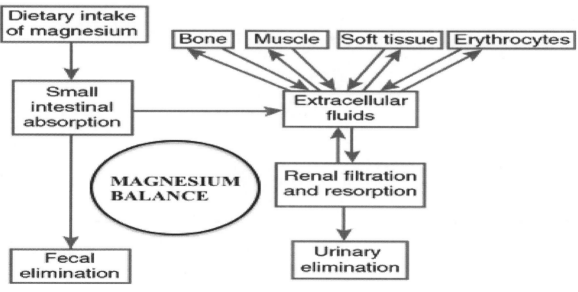

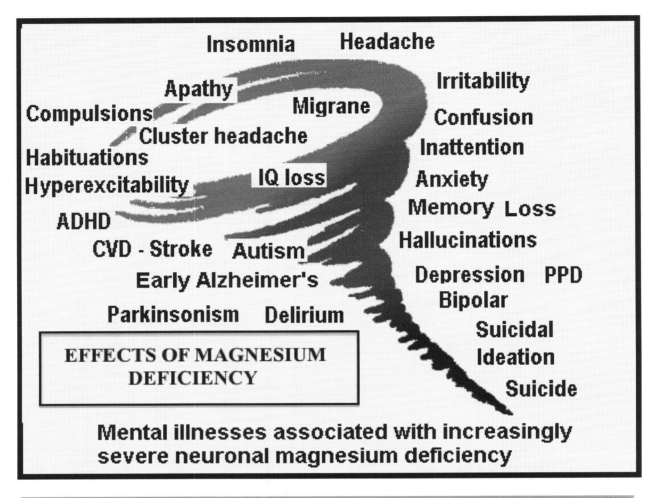

EFFECTS OF MAGNESIUM DEFICIENCY

Mental illnesses associated with increasingly severe neuronal magnesium deficiency

ELECTROCARDIOGRAPHIC CHANGES IN ELECTROLYTE IMBALANCES	
ELECTROLYTE IMBALANCE	**ELECTROCARDIOGRAPHIC CHANGES**
Hypocalcemia	Prolonged ST interval and QT interval
Hypercalcemia	Shortened ST segment Widened T wave
Hypokalemia	ST depression Shallow, flat or inverted T wave Prominent U wave
Hyperkalemia	Tall, peaked T waves Flat P waves Widened QRS complexes Prolonged PR interval
Hypomagnesemia	Tall T waves Depressed ST segment

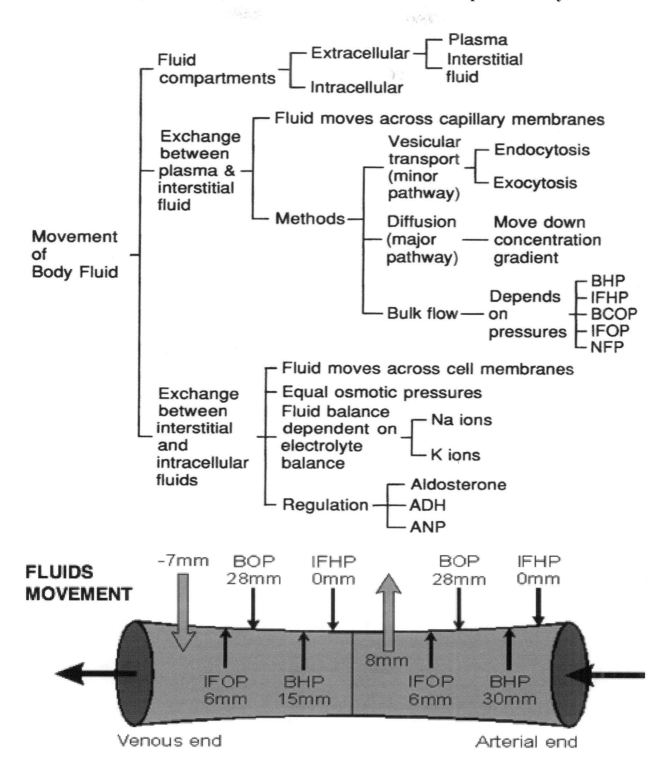

Movement of Body Fluid

- **Fluid compartments**
  - Extracellular
    - Plasma
    - Interstitial fluid
  - Intracellular

- **Exchange between plasma & interstitial fluid**
  - Fluid moves across capillary membranes
  - Methods
    - Vesicular transport (minor pathway)
      - Endocytosis
      - Exocytosis
    - Diffusion (major pathway) — Move down concentration gradient
    - Bulk flow — Depends on pressures
      - BHP
      - IFHP
      - BCOP
      - IFOP
      - NFP

- **Exchange between interstitial and intracellular fluids**
  - Fluid moves across cell membranes
  - Equal osmotic pressures
  - Fluid balance dependent on electrolyte balance
    - Na ions
    - K ions
  - Regulation
    - Aldosterone
    - ADH
    - ANP

FLUIDS MOVEMENT

-7mm   BOP 28mm   IFHP 0mm   BOP 28mm   IFHP 0mm

8mm

IFOP 6mm   BHP 15mm   IFOP 6mm   BHP 30mm

Venous end   Arterial end

BHP = Blood hydrostatic pressure
IFHP = Interstitial fluid hydrostatic pressure
BOP = Blood osmotic pressure
IFOP = Interstitial fluid osmotic pressure

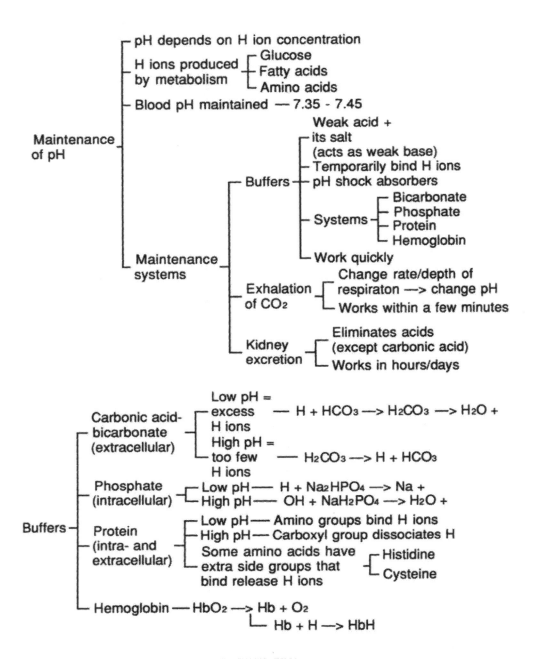

$$pH = 6.1 + \log \frac{HCO_3^-}{0.0301 \times pCO_2}$$

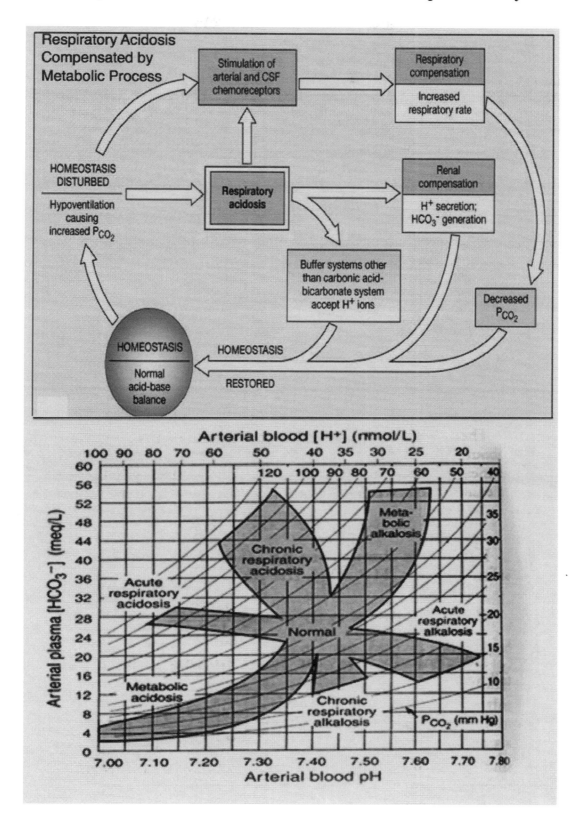

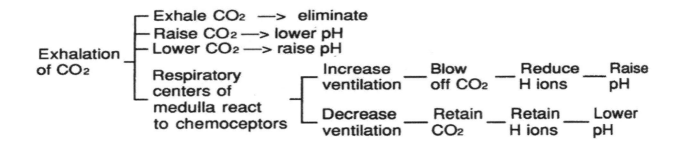

Exhalation of CO_2
- Exhale CO_2 —> eliminate
- Raise CO_2 —> lower pH
- Lower CO_2 —> raise pH
- Respiratory centers of medulla react to chemoceptors
  - Increase ventilation — Blow off CO_2 — Reduce H ions — Raise pH
  - Decrease ventilation — Retain CO_2 — Retain H ions — Lower pH

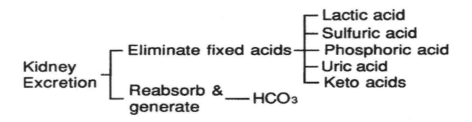

Kidney Excretion
- Eliminate fixed acids
  - Lactic acid
  - Sulfuric acid
  - Phosphoric acid
  - Uric acid
  - Keto acids
- Reabsorb & generate — HCO_3

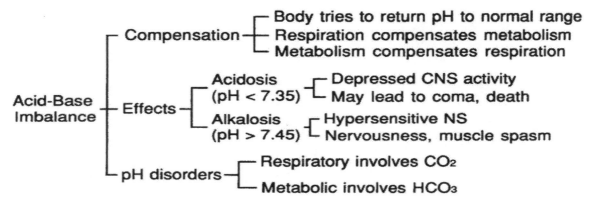

Acid-Base Imbalance
- Compensation
  - Body tries to return pH to normal range
  - Respiration compensates metabolism
  - Metabolism compensates respiration
- Effects
  - Acidosis (pH < 7.35)
    - Depressed CNS activity
    - May lead to coma, death
  - Alkalosis (pH > 7.45)
    - Hypersensitive NS
    - Nervousness, muscle spasm
- pH disorders
  - Respiratory involves CO_2
  - Metabolic involves HCO_3

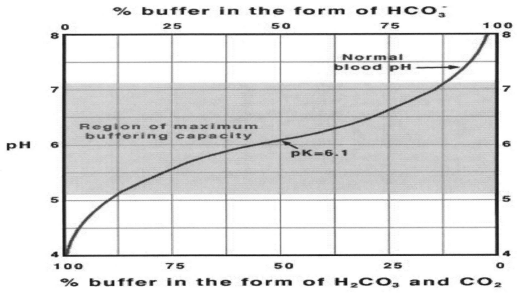

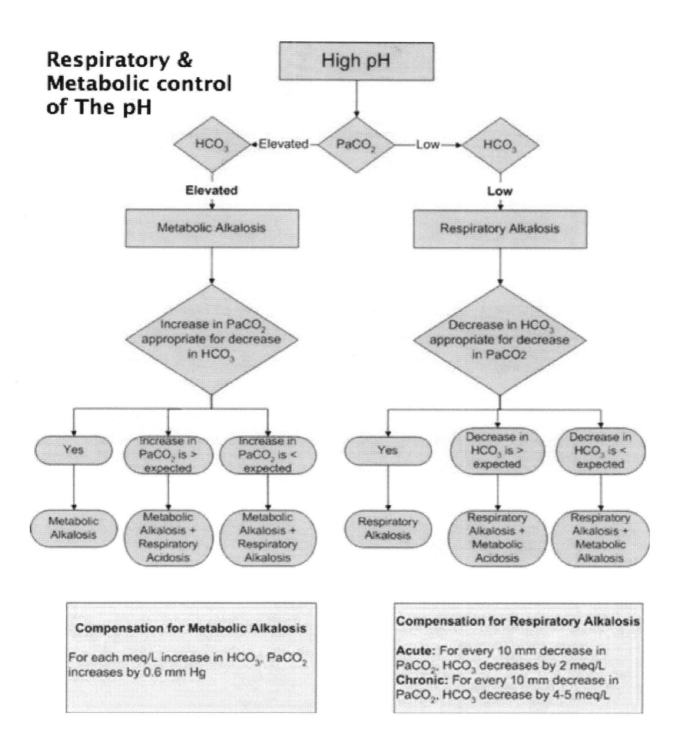

Respiratory & Metabolic control of The pH

High pH

HCO₃ ◀—Elevated— PaCO₂ —Low—▶ HCO₃

Elevated

Metabolic Alkalosis

Increase in PaCO₂ appropriate for decrease in HCO₃

- Yes → Metabolic Alkalosis
- Increase in PaCO₂ is > expected → Metabolic Alkalosis + Respiratory Acidosis
- Increase in PaCO₂ is < expected → Metabolic Alkalosis + Respiratory Alkalosis

Low

Respiratory Alkalosis

Decrease in HCO₃ appropriate for decrease in PaCO2

- Yes → Respiratory Alkalosis
- Decrease in HCO₃ is > expected → Respiratory Alkalosis + Metabolic Acidosis
- Decrease in HCO₃ is < expected → Respiratory Alkalosis + Metabolic Alkalosis

Compensation for Metabolic Alkalosis

For each meq/L increase in HCO₃, PaCO₂ increases by 0.6 mm Hg

Compensation for Respiratory Alkalosis

Acute: For every 10 mm decrease in PaCO₂, HCO₃ decreases by 2 meq/L
Chronic: For every 10 mm decrease in PaCO₂, HCO₃ decrease by 4-5 meq/L

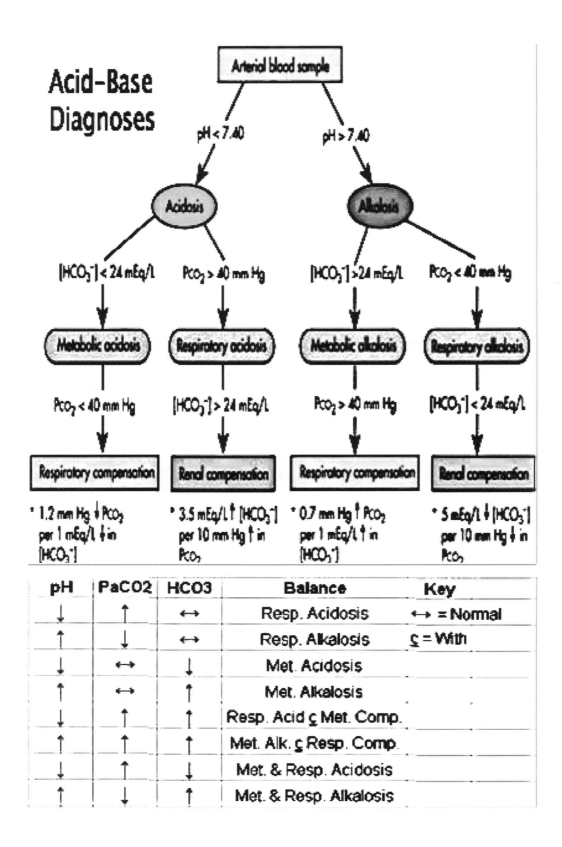

Acid-Base Diagnoses

pH	PaCO2	HCO3	Balance	Key
↓	↑	↔	Resp. Acidosis	↔ = Normal
↑	↓	↔	Resp. Alkalosis	¢ = With
↓	↔	↓	Met. Acidosis	
↑	↔	↑	Met. Alkalosis	
↓	↑	↑	Resp. Acid ¢ Met. Comp.	
↑	↑	↑	Met. Alk. ¢ Resp. Comp.	
↓	↑	↓	Met. & Resp. Acidosis	
↑	↓	↑	Met. & Resp. Alkalosis	

CHAPTER TWENTY EIGHT

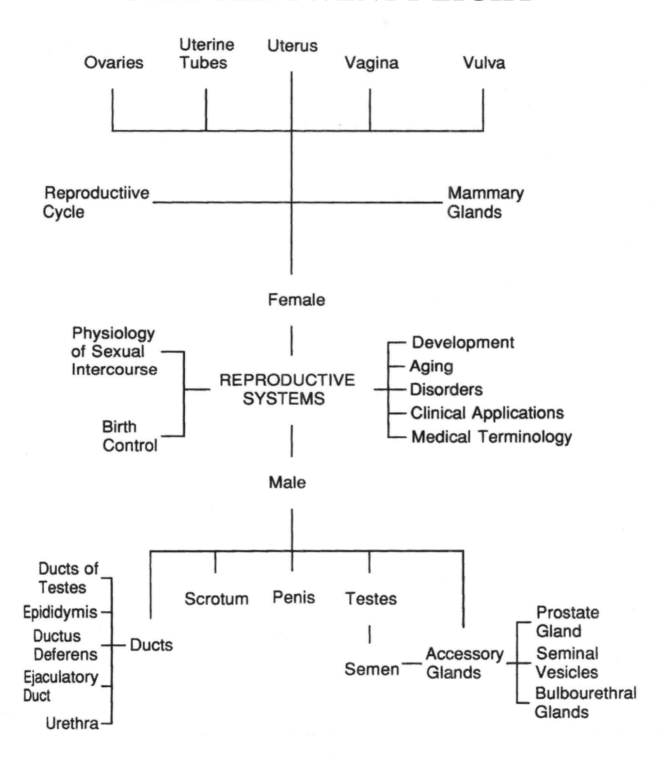

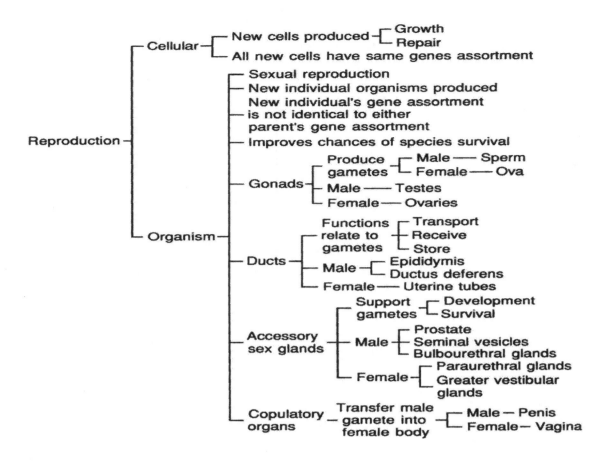

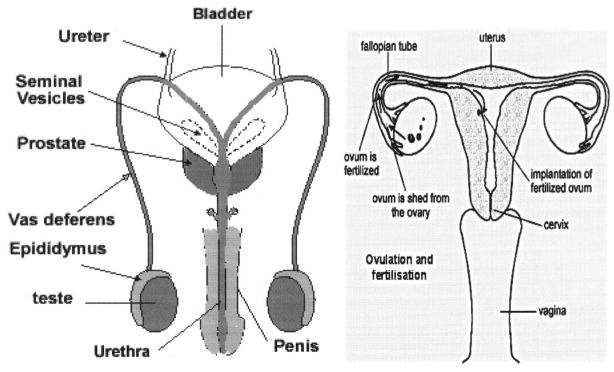

Female Reproductive System

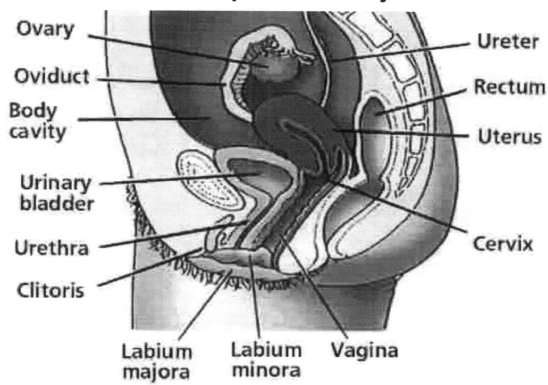

Ovary

Oviduct

Body cavity

Urinary bladder

Urethra

Clitoris

Ureter

Rectum

Uterus

Cervix

Labium majora

Labium minora

Vagina

Male Reproductive System

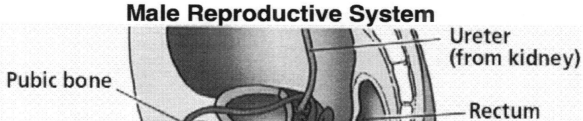

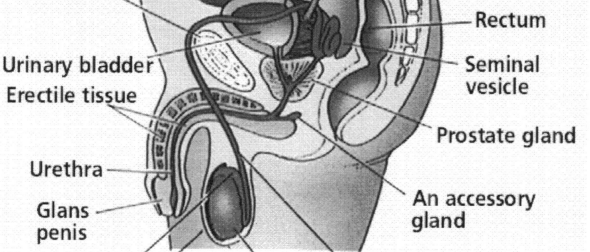

Pubic bone

Urinary bladder

Erectile tissue

Urethra

Glans penis

Epididymis

Scrotum

Testis

Vas deferens

Ureter (from kidney)

Rectum

Seminal vesicle

Prostate gland

An accessory gland

A Comparison Of Asexual Versus Sexual Reproduction

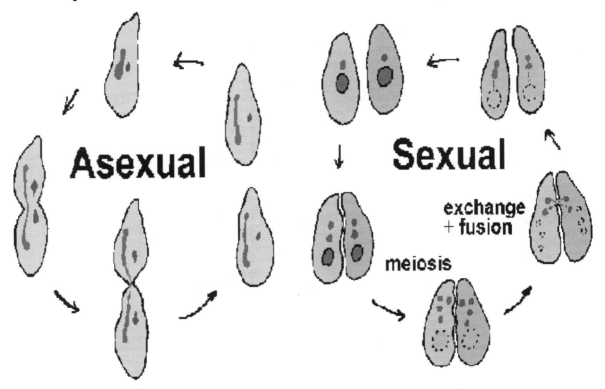

Asexual Reproduction	Sexual Reproduction
Single individual is the sole parent	Two parents give rise to offspring
Single parent passes on all its genes to its offspring	Each person passes on half its genes, to its offspring.
Offspring are genetically identical to the parent.	Offspring have a unique combination of genes inherited from both parents.
Results in a clone, or genetically identical individual. Rarely, genetic differences occur as a result of mutation, a change in DNA	Results in greater genetic variation; offspring vary genetically from their siblings and parents.

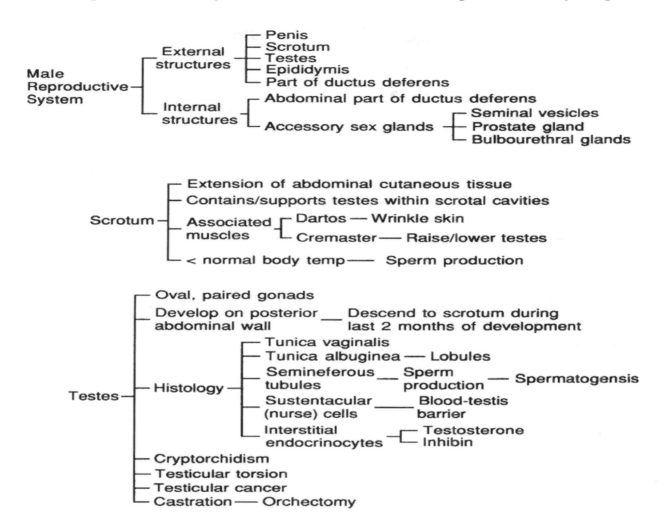

Male Reproductive System
- External structures
  - Penis
  - Scrotum
  - Testes
  - Epididymis
  - Part of ductus deferens
- Internal structures
  - Abdominal part of ductus deferens
  - Accessory sex glands
    - Seminal vesicles
    - Prostate gland
    - Bulbourethral glands

Scrotum
- Extension of abdominal cutaneous tissue
- Contains/supports testes within scrotal cavities
- Associated muscles
  - Dartos — Wrinkle skin
  - Cremaster — Raise/lower testes
- < normal body temp — Sperm production

Testes
- Oval, paired gonads
- Develop on posterior abdominal wall — Descend to scrotum during last 2 months of development
- Histology
  - Tunica vaginalis
  - Tunica albuginea — Lobules
  - Semineferous tubules — Sperm production — Spermatogensis
  - Sustentacular (nurse) cells — Blood-testis barrier
  - Interstitial endocrinocytes
    - Testosterone
    - Inhibin
- Cryptorchidism
- Testicular torsion
- Testicular cancer
- Castration — Orchectomy

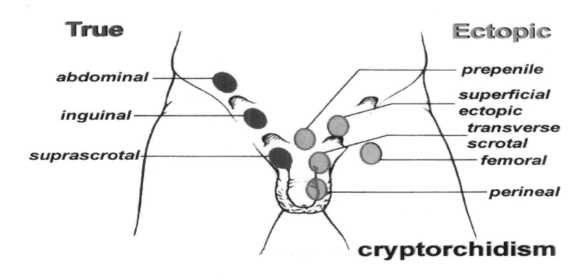

True
- abdominal
- inguinal
- suprascrotal

Ectopic
- prepenile
- superficial ectopic
- transverse scrotal
- femoral
- perineal

cryptorchidism

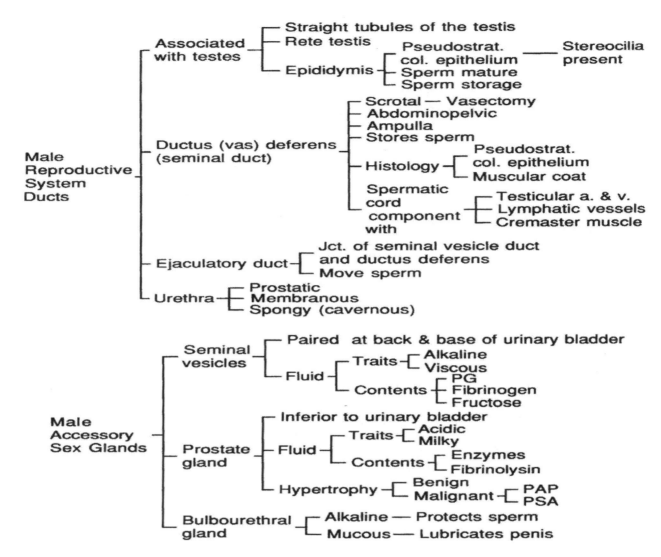

Male Reproductive System Ducts
- Associated with testes
  - Straight tubules of the testis
  - Rete testis
  - Epididymis
    - Pseudostrat. col. epithelium — Stereocilia present
    - Sperm mature
    - Sperm storage
- Ductus (vas) deferens (seminal duct)
  - Scrotal — Vasectomy
  - Abdominopelvic
  - Ampulla
  - Stores sperm
  - Histology
    - Pseudostrat. col. epithelium
    - Muscular coat
  - Spermatic cord component with
    - Testicular a. & v.
    - Lymphatic vessels
    - Cremaster muscle
- Ejaculatory duct
  - Jct. of seminal vesicle duct and ductus deferens
  - Move sperm
- Urethra
  - Prostatic
  - Membranous
  - Spongy (cavernous)

Male Accessory Sex Glands
- Seminal vesicles
  - Paired at back & base of urinary bladder
  - Fluid
    - Traits
      - Alkaline
      - Viscous
    - Contents
      - PG
      - Fibrinogen
      - Fructose
- Prostate gland
  - Inferior to urinary bladder
  - Fluid
    - Traits
      - Acidic
      - Milky
    - Contents
      - Enzymes
      - Fibrinolysin
  - Hypertrophy
    - Benign
    - Malignant
      - PAP
      - PSA
- Bulbourethral gland
  - Alkaline — Protects sperm
  - Mucous — Lubricates penis

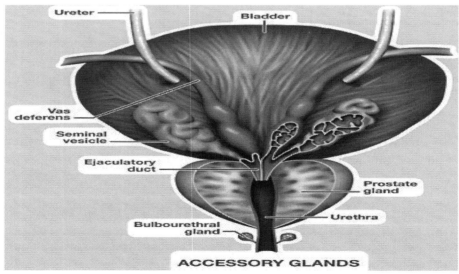

Ureter

Bladder

Vas deferens

Seminal vesicle

Ejaculatory duct

Prostate gland

Urethra

Bulbourethral gland

ACCESSORY GLANDS

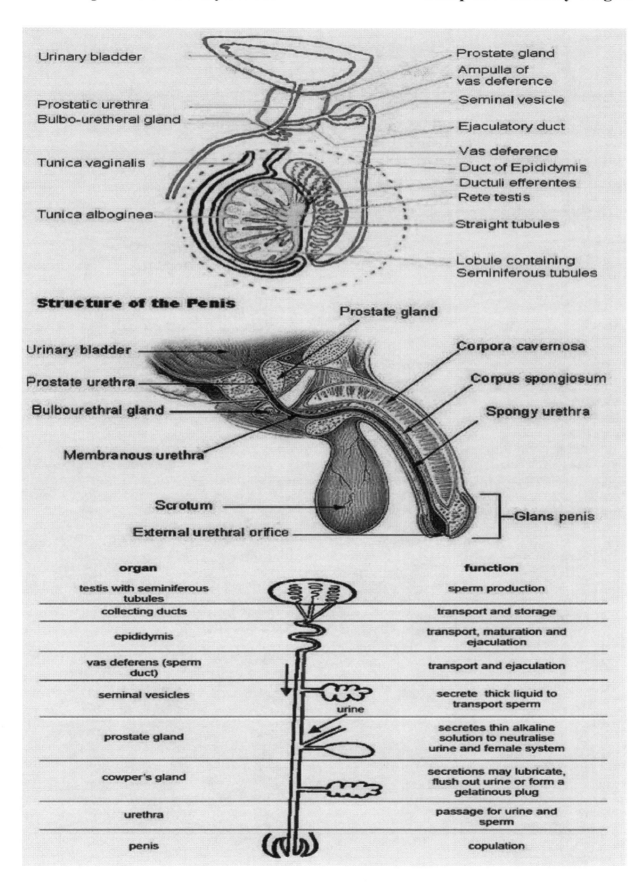

Structure of the Penis

organ	function
testis with seminiferous tubules	sperm production
collecting ducts	transport and storage
epididymis	transport, maturation and ejaculation
vas deferens (sperm duct)	transport and ejaculation
seminal vesicles	secrete thick liquid to transport sperm
prostate gland	secretes thin alkaline solution to neutralise urine and female system
cowper's gland	secretions may lubricate, flush out urine or form a gelatinous plug
urethra	passage for urine and sperm
penis	copulation

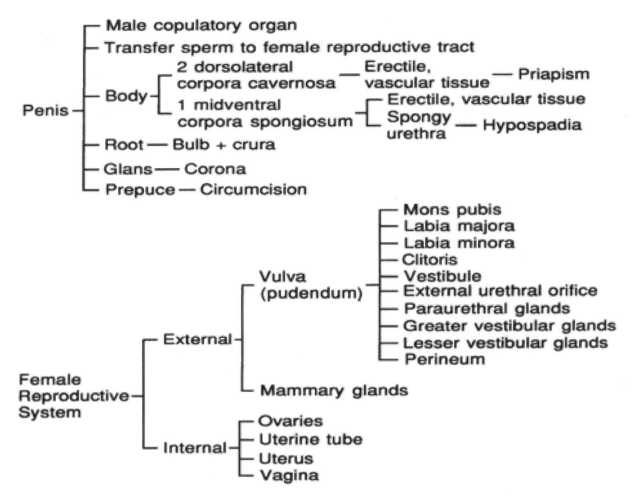

- Penis
  - Male copulatory organ
  - Transfer sperm to female reproductive tract
  - Body
    - 2 dorsolateral corpora cavernosa — Erectile, vascular tissue — Priapism
    - 1 midventral corpora spongiosum
      - Erectile, vascular tissue
      - Spongy urethra — Hypospadia
  - Root — Bulb + crura
  - Glans — Corona
  - Prepuce — Circumcision

- Female Reproductive System
  - External
    - Vulva (pudendum)
      - Mons pubis
      - Labia majora
      - Labia minora
      - Clitoris
      - Vestibule
      - External urethral orifice
      - Paraurethral glands
      - Greater vestibular glands
      - Lesser vestibular glands
      - Perineum
    - Mammary glands
  - Internal
    - Ovaries
    - Uterine tube
    - Uterus
    - Vagina

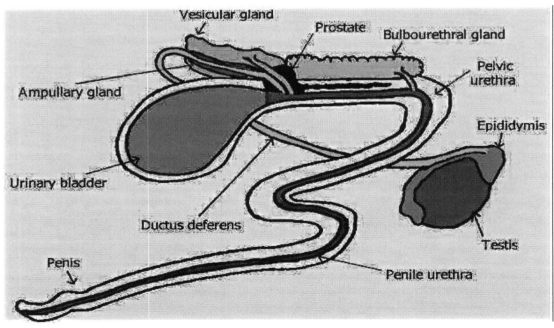

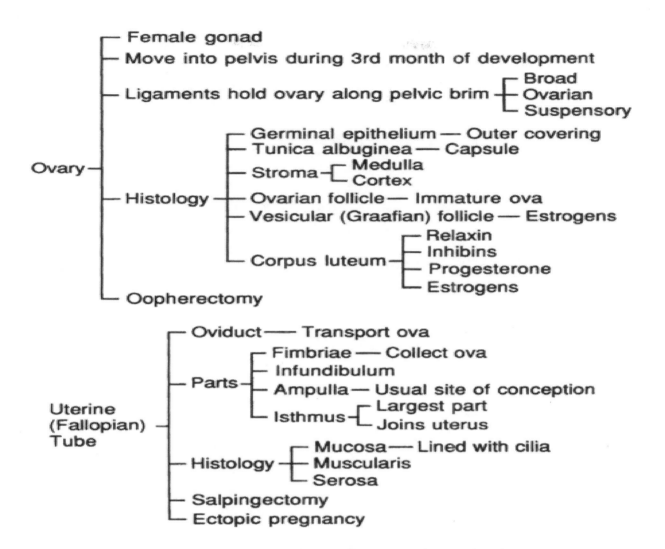

- Ovary
  - Female gonad
  - Move into pelvis during 3rd month of development
  - Ligaments hold ovary along pelvic brim
    - Broad
    - Ovarian
    - Suspensory
  - Histology
    - Germinal epithelium — Outer covering
    - Tunica albuginea — Capsule
    - Stroma
      - Medulla
      - Cortex
    - Ovarian follicle — Immature ova
    - Vesicular (Graafian) follicle — Estrogens
    - Corpus luteum
      - Relaxin
      - Inhibins
      - Progesterone
      - Estrogens
  - Oopherectomy

- Uterine (Fallopian) Tube
  - Oviduct — Transport ova
  - Parts
    - Fimbriae — Collect ova
    - Infundibulum
    - Ampulla — Usual site of conception
    - Isthmus
      - Largest part
      - Joins uterus
  - Histology
    - Mucosa — Lined with cilia
    - Muscularis
    - Serosa
  - Salpingectomy
  - Ectopic pregnancy

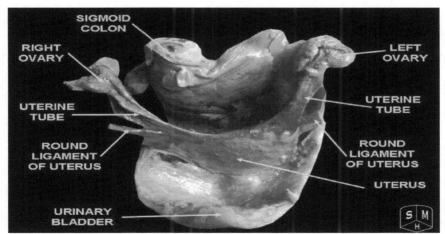

SIGMOID COLON
RIGHT OVARY
LEFT OVARY
UTERINE TUBE
UTERINE TUBE
ROUND LIGAMENT OF UTERUS
ROUND LIGAMENT OF UTERUS
UTERUS
URINARY BLADDER

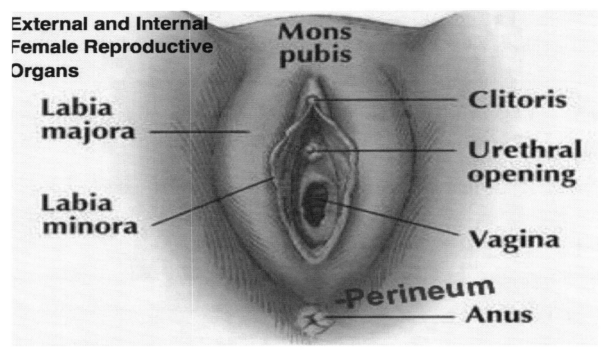

External and Internal Female Reproductive Organs

- Mons pubis
- Clitoris
- Urethral opening
- Labia majora
- Labia minora
- Vagina
- Perineum
- Anus

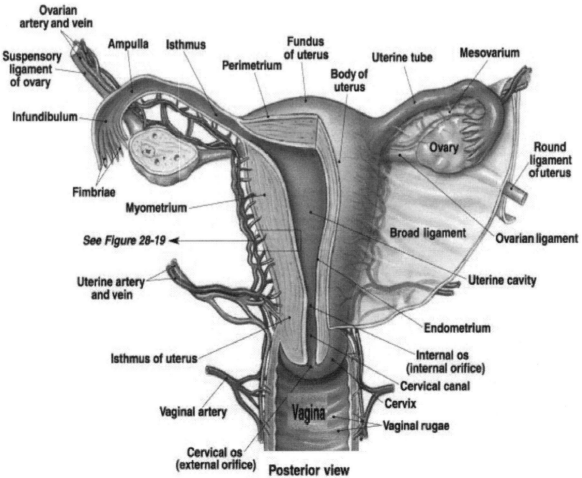

- Ovarian artery and vein
- Suspensory ligament of ovary
- Infundibulum
- Ampulla
- Isthmus
- Perimetrium
- Fundus of uterus
- Body of uterus
- Uterine tube
- Mesovarium
- Ovary
- Round ligament of uterus
- Fimbriae
- Myometrium
- See Figure 28-19
- Broad ligament
- Ovarian ligament
- Uterine cavity
- Uterine artery and vein
- Endometrium
- Isthmus of uterus
- Internal os (internal orifice)
- Cervical canal
- Cervix
- Vaginal artery
- Vagina
- Vaginal rugae
- Cervical os (external orifice)
- Posterior view

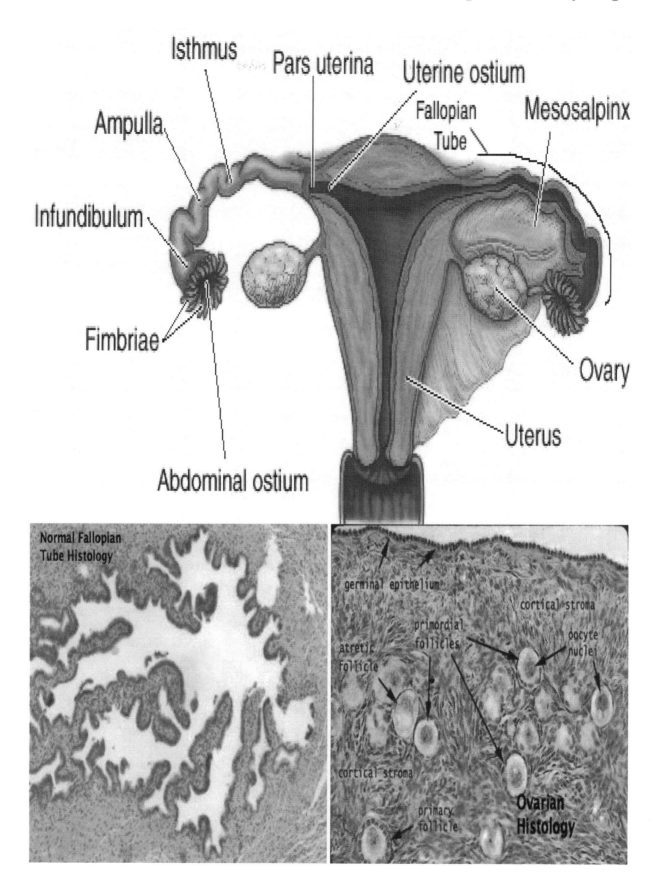

Isthmus

Pars uterina

Uterine ostium

Ampulla

Fallopian Tube

Mesosalpinx

Infundibulum

Fimbriae

Abdominal ostium

Ovary

Uterus

Normal Fallopian Tube Histology

germinal epithelium

cortical stroma

primordial follicles

atretic follicle

oocyte nuclei

cortical stroma

primary follicle

Ovarian Histology

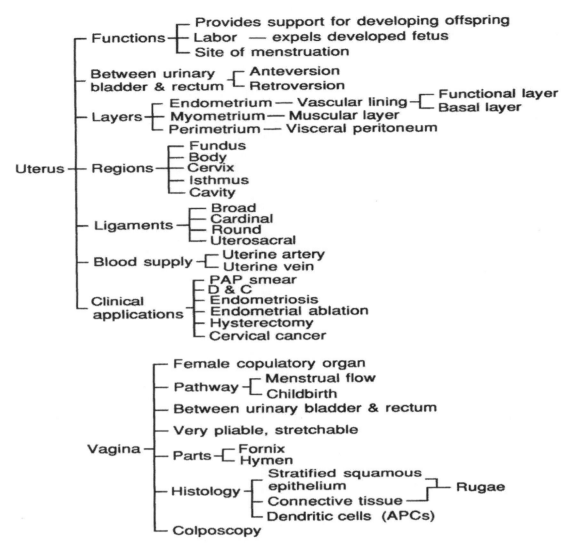

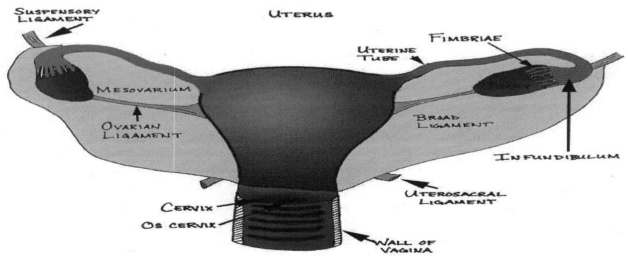

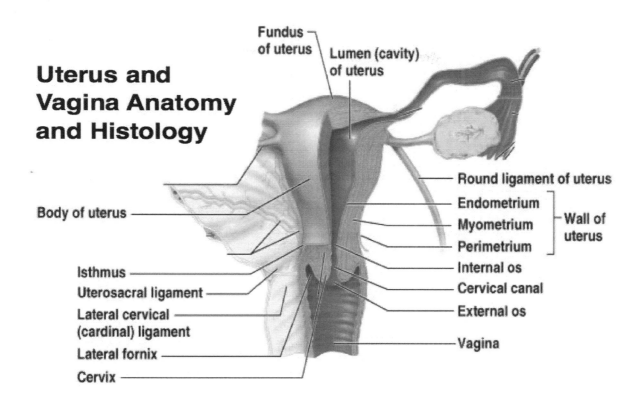

Uterus and Vagina Anatomy and Histology

Fundus of uterus

Lumen (cavity) of uterus

Body of uterus

Isthmus

Uterosacral ligament

Lateral cervical (cardinal) ligament

Lateral fornix

Cervix

Round ligament of uterus

Endometrium

Myometrium

Perimetrium

Wall of uterus

Internal os

Cervical canal

External os

Vagina

Uterus Histology

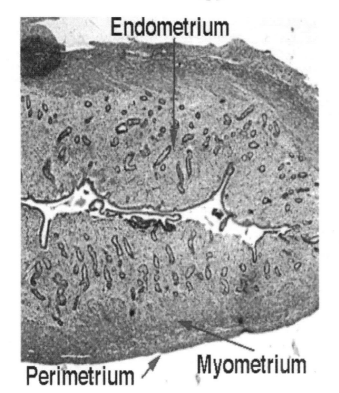

Endometrium

Perimetrium

Myometrium

Vagina

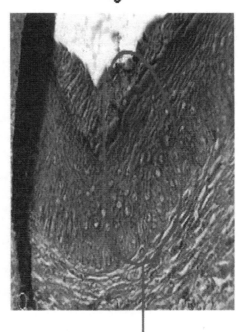

Stratified Squamous Epithelium

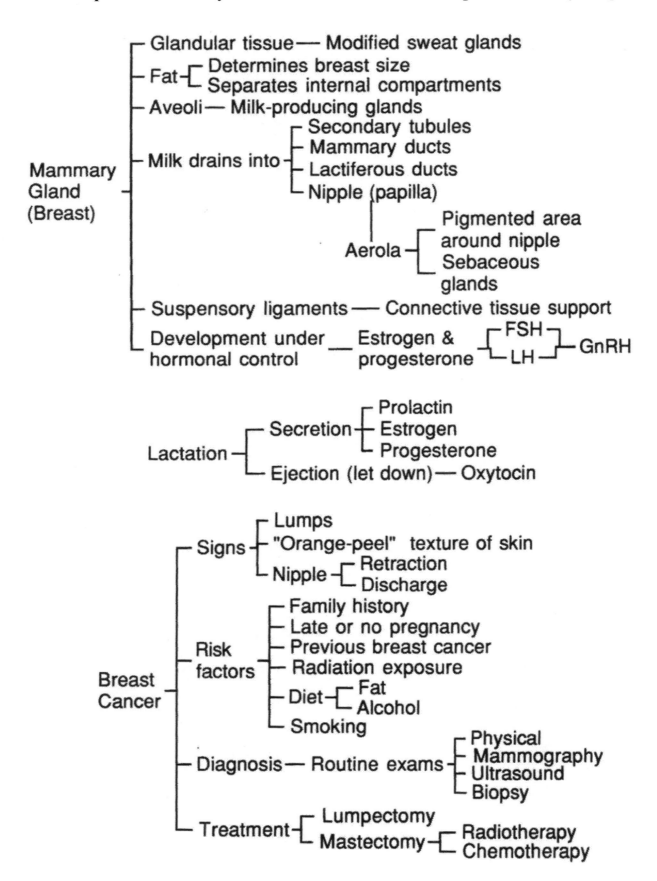

Mammary Gland (Breast)
- Glandular tissue — Modified sweat glands
- Fat
  - Determines breast size
  - Separates internal compartments
- Aveoli — Milk-producing glands
- Milk drains into
  - Secondary tubules
  - Mammary ducts
  - Lactiferous ducts
  - Nipple (papilla)
    - Aerola
      - Pigmented area around nipple
      - Sebaceous glands
- Suspensory ligaments — Connective tissue support
- Development under hormonal control — Estrogen & progesterone — FSH / LH — GnRH

Lactation
- Secretion
  - Prolactin
  - Estrogen
  - Progesterone
- Ejection (let down) — Oxytocin

Breast Cancer
- Signs
  - Lumps
  - "Orange-peel" texture of skin
  - Nipple
    - Retraction
    - Discharge
- Risk factors
  - Family history
  - Late or no pregnancy
  - Previous breast cancer
  - Radiation exposure
  - Diet
    - Fat
    - Alcohol
  - Smoking
- Diagnosis — Routine exams
  - Physical
  - Mammography
  - Ultrasound
  - Biopsy
- Treatment
  - Lumpectomy
  - Mastectomy
    - Radiotherapy
    - Chemotherapy

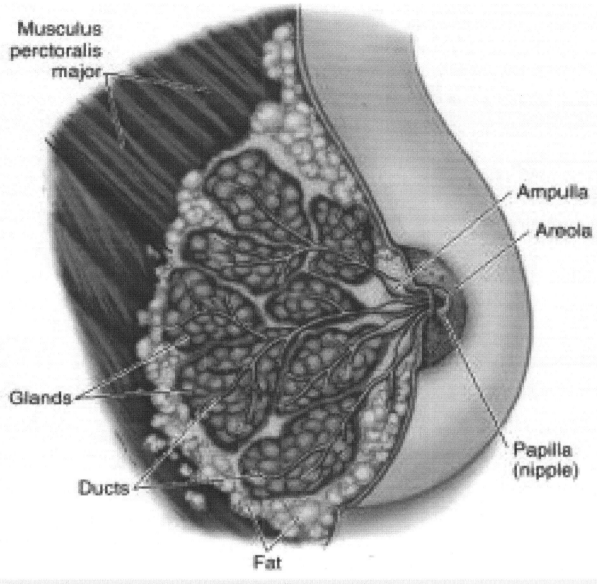

Musculus perctoralis major

Ampulla

Areola

Glands

Papilla (nipple)

Ducts

Fat

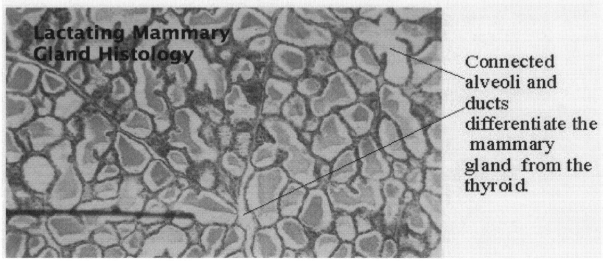

Lactating Mammary Gland Histology

Connected alveoli and ducts differentiate the mammary gland from the thyroid.

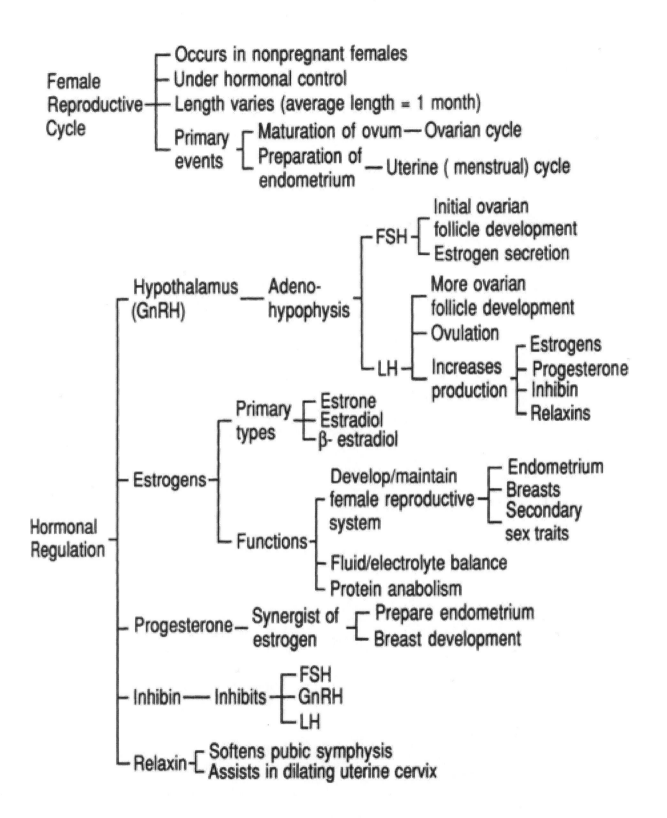

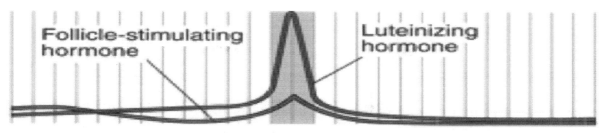

Pituitary Hormone Cycle

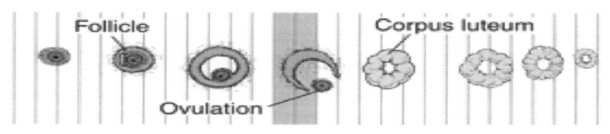

Ovarian Cycle

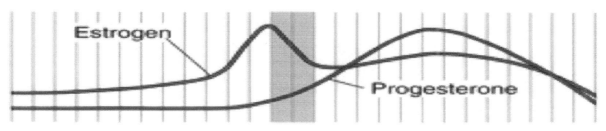

Sex Hormone Cycle

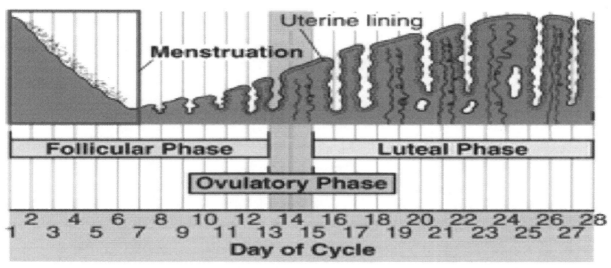

Endometrial Cycle

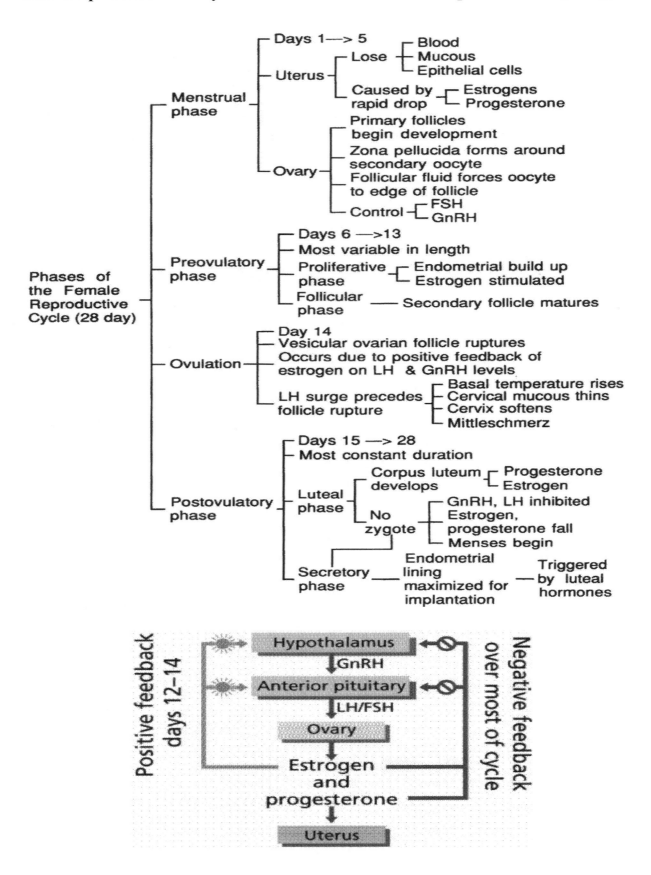

Phases of the Female Reproductive Cycle (28 day)

Menstrual phase
- Days 1—>5
- Uterus
  - Lose
    - Blood
    - Mucous
    - Epithelial cells
  - Caused by rapid drop
    - Estrogens
    - Progesterone
- Ovary
  - Primary follicles begin development
  - Zona pellucida forms around secondary oocyte
  - Follicular fluid forces oocyte to edge of follicle
  - Control
    - FSH
    - GnRH

Preovulatory phase
- Days 6 —>13
- Most variable in length
- Proliferative phase
  - Endometrial build up
  - Estrogen stimulated
- Follicular phase
  - Secondary follicle matures

Ovulation
- Day 14
- Vesicular ovarian follicle ruptures
- Occurs due to positive feedback of estrogen on LH & GnRH levels
- LH surge precedes follicle rupture
  - Basal temperature rises
  - Cervical mucous thins
  - Cervix softens
  - Mittleschmerz

Postovulatory phase
- Days 15 —> 28
- Most constant duration
- Luteal phase
  - Corpus luteum develops
    - Progesterone
    - Estrogen
  - No zygote
    - GnRH, LH inhibited
    - Estrogen, progesterone fall
    - Menses begin
- Secretory phase
  - Endometrial lining maximized for implantation
  - Triggered by luteal hormones

Positive feedback days 12–14

Negative feedback over most of cycle

Hypothalamus
↓ GnRH
Anterior pituitary
↓ LH/FSH
Ovary

Estrogen and progesterone

Uterus

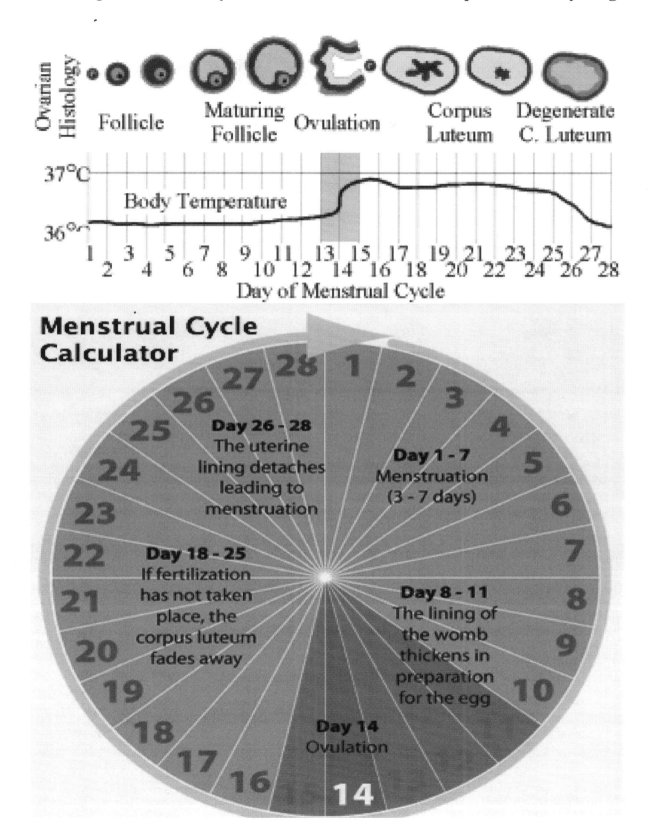

Ovarian Histology

Follicle   Maturing Follicle   Ovulation   Corpus Luteum   Degenerate C. Luteum

37°C

Body Temperature

36°C

1 2 3 4 5 6 7 8 9 10 11 12 13 14 15 16 17 18 19 20 21 22 23 24 25 26 27 28

Day of Menstrual Cycle

Menstrual Cycle Calculator

Day 26 - 28
The uterine lining detaches leading to menstruation

Day 1 - 7
Menstruation (3 - 7 days)

Day 18 - 25
If fertilization has not taken place, the corpus luteum fades away

Day 8 - 11
The lining of the womb thickens in preparation for the egg

Day 14
Ovulation

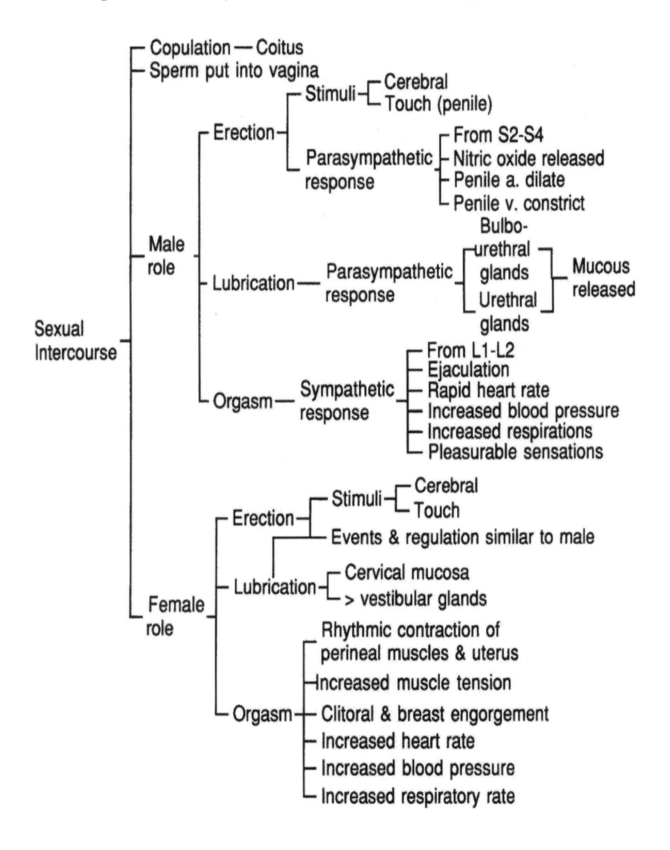

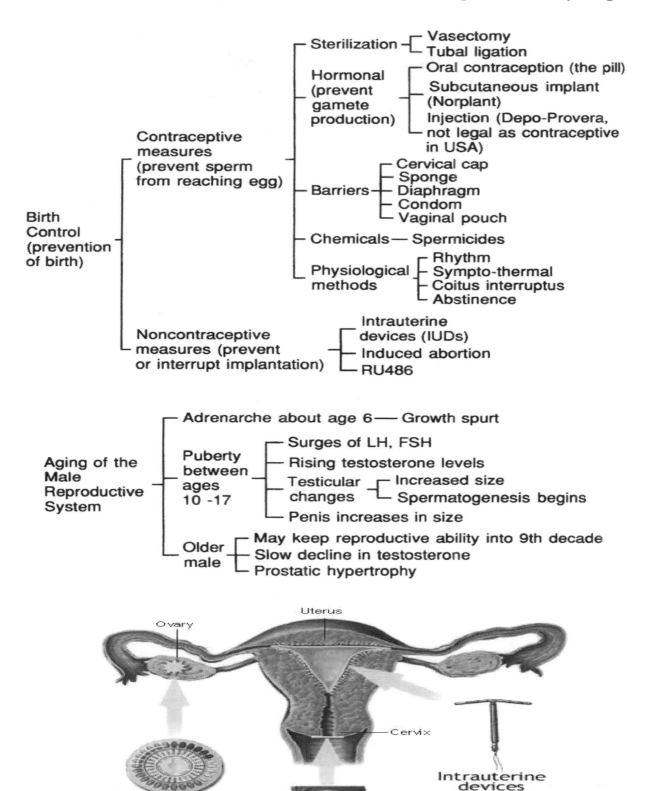

Birth Control (prevention of birth)
- Contraceptive measures (prevent sperm from reaching egg)
  - Sterilization
    - Vasectomy
    - Tubal ligation
  - Hormonal (prevent gamete production)
    - Oral contraception (the pill)
    - Subcutaneous implant (Norplant)
    - Injection (Depo-Provera, not legal as contraceptive in USA)
  - Barriers
    - Cervical cap
    - Sponge
    - Diaphragm
    - Condom
    - Vaginal pouch
  - Chemicals — Spermicides
  - Physiological methods
    - Rhythm
    - Sympto-thermal
    - Coitus interruptus
    - Abstinence
- Noncontraceptive measures (prevent or interrupt implantation)
  - Intrauterine devices (IUDs)
  - Induced abortion
  - RU486

Aging of the Male Reproductive System
- Adrenarche about age 6 — Growth spurt
- Puberty between ages 10 -17
  - Surges of LH, FSH
  - Rising testosterone levels
  - Testicular changes
    - Increased size
    - Spermatogenesis begins
  - Penis increases in size
- Older male
  - May keep reproductive ability into 9th decade
  - Slow decline in testosterone
  - Prostatic hypertrophy

Ovary
Uterus
Cervix
Intrauterine devices
Oral contraceptives
CONDOM
Barrier devices

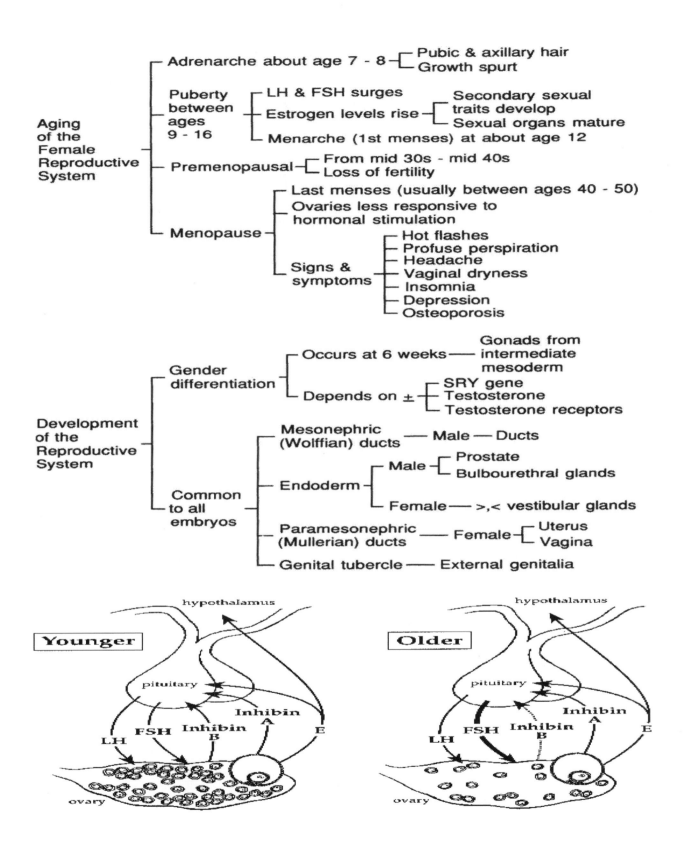

Aging of the Female Reproductive System
- Adrenarche about age 7 - 8
  - Pubic & axillary hair
  - Growth spurt
- Puberty between ages 9 - 16
  - LH & FSH surges
  - Estrogen levels rise
    - Secondary sexual traits develop
    - Sexual organs mature
  - Menarche (1st menses) at about age 12
- Premenopausal
  - From mid 30s - mid 40s
  - Loss of fertility
- Menopause
  - Last menses (usually between ages 40 - 50)
  - Ovaries less responsive to hormonal stimulation
  - Signs & symptoms
    - Hot flashes
    - Profuse perspiration
    - Headache
    - Vaginal dryness
    - Insomnia
    - Depression
    - Osteoporosis

Development of the Reproductive System
- Gender differentiation
  - Occurs at 6 weeks — Gonads from intermediate mesoderm
  - Depends on ±
    - SRY gene
    - Testosterone
    - Testosterone receptors
- Common to all embryos
  - Mesonephric (Wolffian) ducts — Male — Ducts
  - Endoderm
    - Male
      - Prostate
      - Bulbourethral glands
    - Female — >,< vestibular glands
  - Paramesonephric (Mullerian) ducts — Female
    - Uterus
    - Vagina
  - Genital tubercle —— External genitalia

Younger

Older

hypothalamus

pituitary

LH   FSH   Inhibin B   Inhibin A   E

ovary

The development of the external genitalia in the male and female

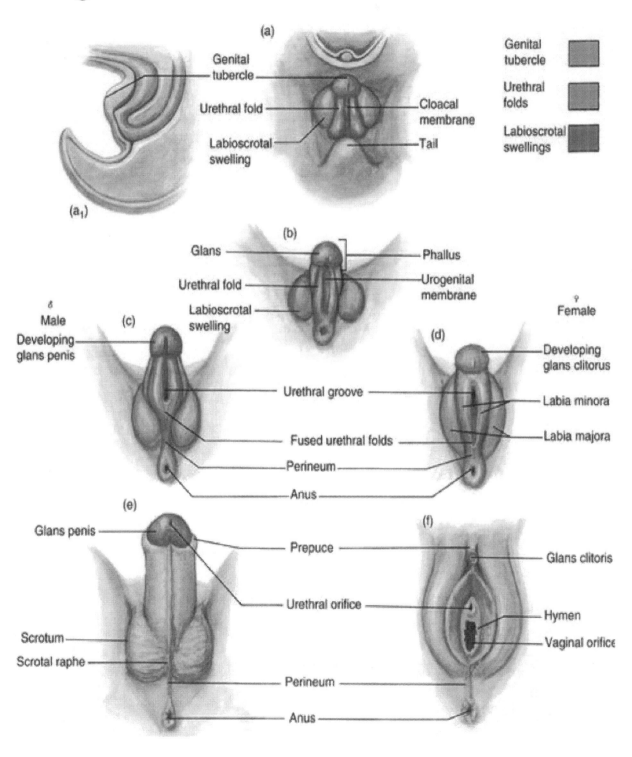

Sexually Transmitted Diseases (STDs)
- Venereal diseases (VD)
- Spread by sexual contact
- Incidence can be reduced by use of "safer" sexual practices
  - Condoms
  - Spermicides
- Includes
  - Gonorrhea (clap)
  - Syphillis
  - Genital herpes
  - Chlamydia
  - Trichomoniasis
  - Genital warts
  - AIDS

Gonorrhea (clap)
- Infectious bacterial disease — Neisseria gonorrhoeae
- Most frequent among 15-24 year olds
- Attacks mucous membranes
  - Urogenital
  - Rectal
  - Ocular
- Signs & symptoms
  - Inflammation
    - Pus
    - Painful urination
  - Female may be asymptomatic
    - Sterility
    - Peritonitis
  - May cause infant blindness — Silver nitrate
- Treatment — Antibiotics (ceftriaxone)

Chlamydia
- Infectious bacterial disease — Chlamydia trachomatis
- Male — Urethritis — Most signs mimic UTI
- Female
  - Urethritis
  - Spreads to reproductive tract
  - Increases risk of ectopic pregnancy
- Fetus — Blindness
- Treatment — Antibiotics
  - Tetracycline
  - Doxycycline

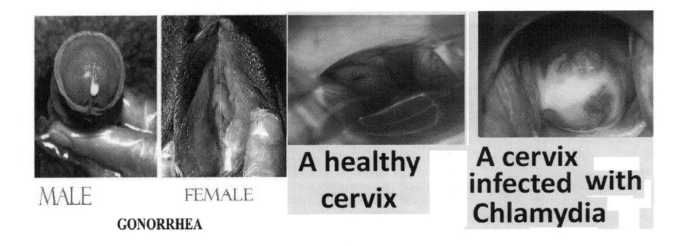

MALE   FEMALE   A healthy cervix   A cervix infected with Chlamydia

GONORRHEA

Syphillis
- Infectious bacterial disease — _Treponema pallidum_
- Most frequent among 20-39 year olds
- Transmitted
  - Sexual intercourse
  - Placenta
- Stages
  - Primary
    - Last 5-6 weeks
    - Chancre sore
  - Secondary
    - Occurs 1.5 - 6 months later
    - Lasts 1-3 months
    - Rash
    - Fever
    - Musculoskeletal aches
    - Not infectious
  - Latent — No observed symptoms
  - Tertiary
    - Organ degeneration
    - Nervous system — Neurosyphilis
- Fetal infection — Devasting effects — Fetal immune system not yet competent
- Treatment — Antibiotics

Genital Herpes
- Infectious viral disease — Herpes simplex (II)
- Sexually transmitted
- Can't be cured
  - Virus remains along neuron even when no symptoms are present
  - Recurrent disease
- Signs & symptoms
  - Genital blisters
  - Fever, chills
  - Flu-like symptoms
  - Lymphadenopathy
- Treatment
  - Acyclovir
  - Inter Vir-A
  - Hydrocortisone

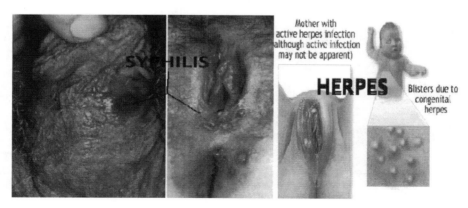

SYPHILIS

HERPES

Mother with active herpes infection (although active infection may not be apparent)

Blisters due to congenital herpes

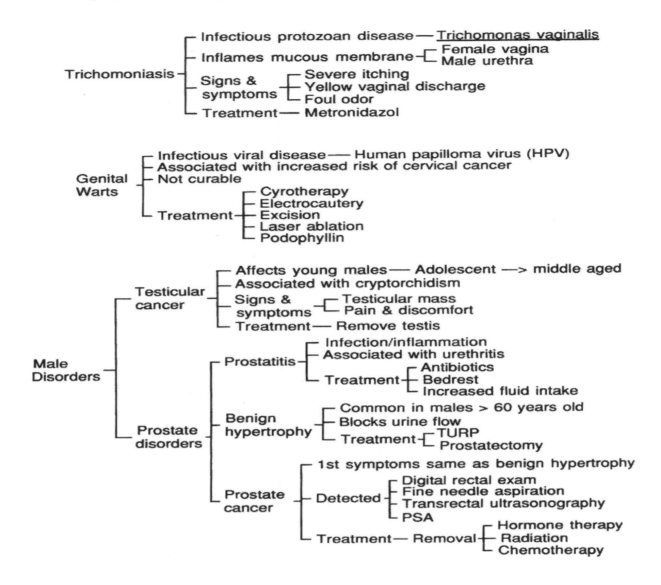

Trichomoniasis
- Infectious protozoan disease —— <u>Trichomonas vaginalis</u>
- Inflames mucous membrane
  - Female vagina
  - Male urethra
- Signs & symptoms
  - Severe itching
  - Yellow vaginal discharge
  - Foul odor
- Treatment —— Metronidazol

Genital Warts
- Infectious viral disease —— Human papilloma virus (HPV)
- Associated with increased risk of cervical cancer
- Not curable
- Treatment
  - Cyrotherapy
  - Electrocautery
  - Excision
  - Laser ablation
  - Podophyllin

Male Disorders
- Testicular cancer
  - Affects young males —— Adolescent ——> middle aged
  - Associated with cryptorchidism
  - Signs & symptoms
    - Testicular mass
    - Pain & discomfort
  - Treatment —— Remove testis
- Prostate disorders
  - Prostatitis
    - Infection/inflammation
    - Associated with urethritis
    - Treatment
      - Antibiotics
      - Bedrest
      - Increased fluid intake
  - Benign hypertrophy
    - Common in males > 60 years old
    - Blocks urine flow
    - Treatment
      - TURP
      - Prostatectomy
  - Prostate cancer
    - 1st symptoms same as benign hypertrophy
    - Detected
      - Digital rectal exam
      - Fine needle aspiration
      - Transrectal ultrasonography
      - PSA
    - Treatment —— Removal
      - Hormone therapy
      - Radiation
      - Chemotherapy

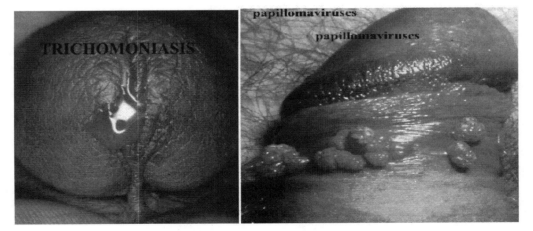

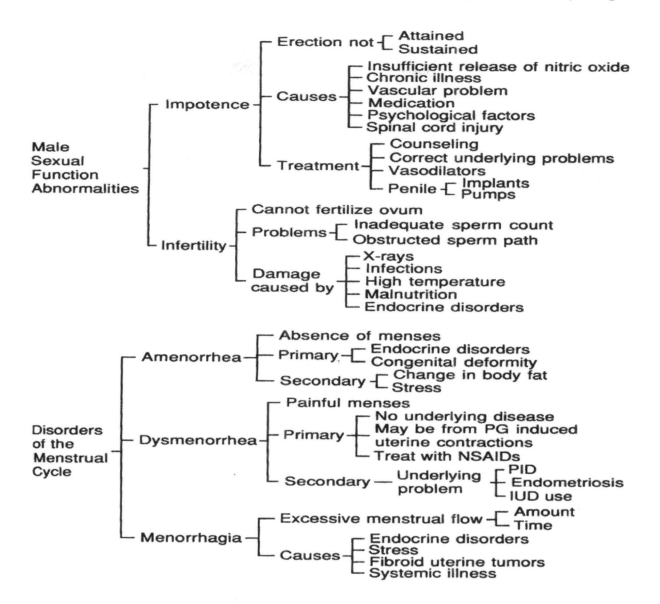

- Male Sexual Function Abnormalities
  - Impotence
    - Erection not
      - Attained
      - Sustained
    - Causes
      - Insufficient release of nitric oxide
      - Chronic illness
      - Vascular problem
      - Medication
      - Psychological factors
      - Spinal cord injury
    - Treatment
      - Counseling
      - Correct underlying problems
      - Vasodilators
      - Penile
        - Implants
        - Pumps
  - Infertility
    - Cannot fertilize ovum
    - Problems
      - Inadequate sperm count
      - Obstructed sperm path
    - Damage caused by
      - X-rays
      - Infections
      - High temperature
      - Malnutrition
      - Endocrine disorders

- Disorders of the Menstrual Cycle
  - Amenorrhea
    - Absence of menses
    - Primary
      - Endocrine disorders
      - Congenital deformity
    - Secondary
      - Change in body fat
      - Stress
  - Dysmenorrhea
    - Painful menses
    - Primary
      - No underlying disease
      - May be from PG induced uterine contractions
      - Treat with NSAIDs
    - Secondary — Underlying problem
      - PID
      - Endometriosis
      - IUD use
  - Menorrhagia
    - Excessive menstrual flow
      - Amount
      - Time
    - Causes
      - Endocrine disorders
      - Stress
      - Fibroid uterine tumors
      - Systemic illness

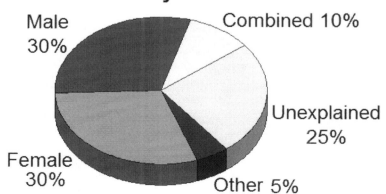

Infertility causes

Male 30%
Combined 10%
Unexplained 25%
Other 5%
Female 30%

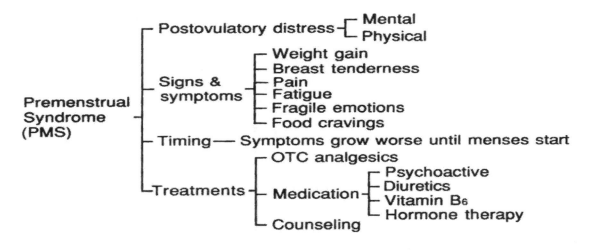

Premenstrual Syndrome (PMS)
- Postovulatory distress
  - Mental
  - Physical
- Signs & symptoms
  - Weight gain
  - Breast tenderness
  - Pain
  - Fatigue
  - Fragile emotions
  - Food cravings
- Timing — Symptoms grow worse until menses start
- Treatments
  - OTC analgesics
  - Medication
    - Psychoactive
    - Diuretics
    - Vitamin B_6
    - Hormone therapy
  - Counseling

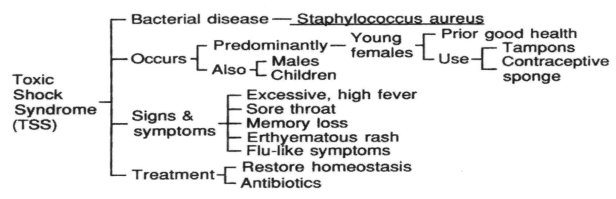

Toxic Shock Syndrome (TSS)
- Bacterial disease — _Staphylococcus aureus_
- Occurs
  - Predominantly — Young females
    - Prior good health
    - Use
      - Tampons
      - Contraceptive sponge
  - Also
    - Males
    - Children
- Signs & symptoms
  - Excessive, high fever
  - Sore throat
  - Memory loss
  - Erthyematous rash
  - Flu-like symptoms
- Treatment
  - Restore homeostasis
  - Antibiotics

Ovarian Cysts
- Fluid containing sacs within ovary
- Occur
  - Elderly females
  - Menstruating females

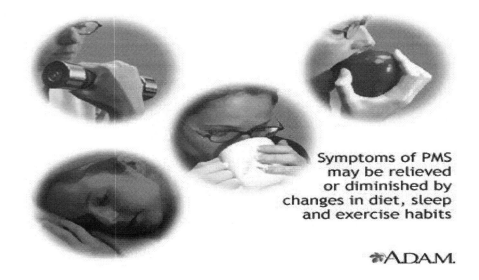

Symptoms of PMS may be relieved or diminished by changes in diet, sleep and exercise habits

✱A.D.A.M.

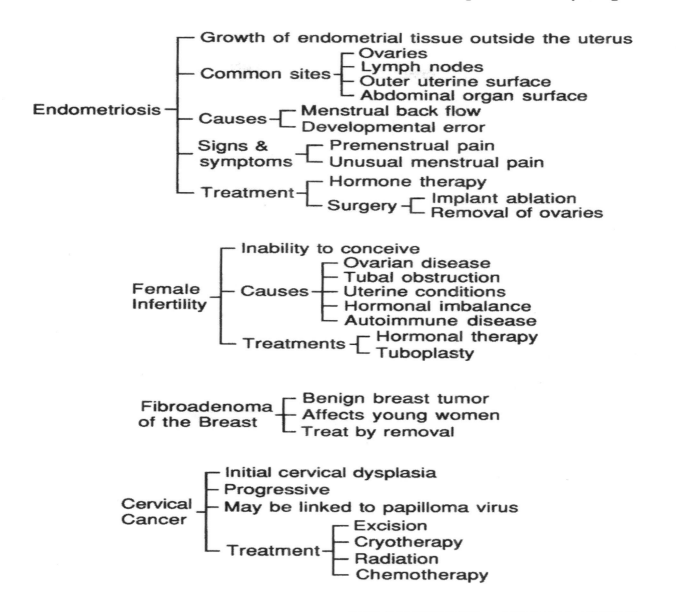

Endometriosis
- Growth of endometrial tissue outside the uterus
- Common sites
  - Ovaries
  - Lymph nodes
  - Outer uterine surface
  - Abdominal organ surface
- Causes
  - Menstrual back flow
  - Developmental error
- Signs & symptoms
  - Premenstrual pain
  - Unusual menstrual pain
- Treatment
  - Hormone therapy
  - Surgery
    - Implant ablation
    - Removal of ovaries

Female Infertility
- Inability to conceive
- Causes
  - Ovarian disease
  - Tubal obstruction
  - Uterine conditions
  - Hormonal imbalance
  - Autoimmune disease
- Treatments
  - Hormonal therapy
  - Tuboplasty

Fibroadenoma of the Breast
- Benign breast tumor
- Affects young women
- Treat by removal

Cervical Cancer
- Initial cervical dysplasia
- Progressive
- May be linked to papilloma virus
- Treatment
  - Excision
  - Cryotherapy
  - Radiation
  - Chemotherapy

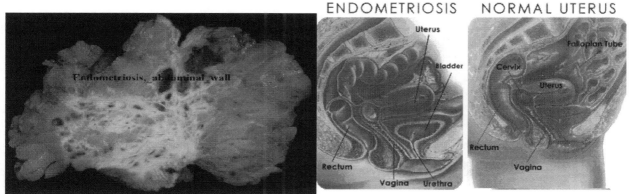

Endometriosis, abdominal wall

ENDOMETRIOSIS

Uterus

Bladder

Rectum

Vagina   Urethra

NORMAL UTERUS

Fallopian Tube

Cervix

Uterus

Rectum

Vagina

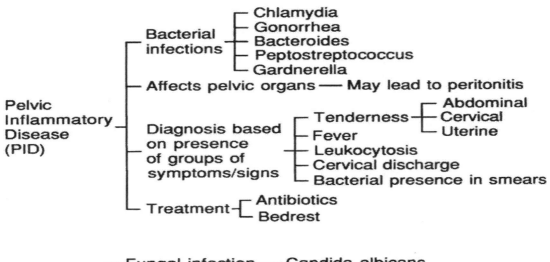

Pelvic Inflammatory Disease (PID)
- Bacterial infections
  - Chlamydia
  - Gonorrhea
  - Bacteroides
  - Peptostreptococcus
  - Gardnerella
- Affects pelvic organs — May lead to peritonitis
- Diagnosis based on presence of groups of symptoms/signs
  - Tenderness
    - Abdominal
    - Cervical
    - Uterine
  - Fever
  - Leukocytosis
  - Cervical discharge
  - Bacterial presence in smears
- Treatment
  - Antibiotics
  - Bedrest

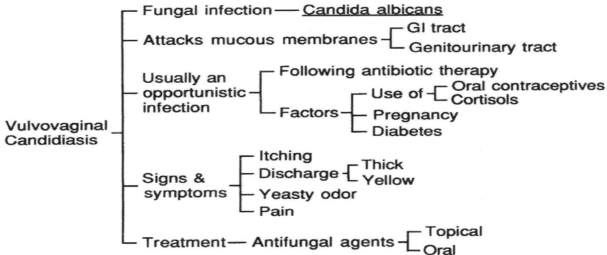

Vulvovaginal Candidiasis
- Fungal infection — Candida albicans
- Attacks mucous membranes
  - GI tract
  - Genitourinary tract
- Usually an opportunistic infection
  - Following antibiotic therapy
  - Factors
    - Use of
      - Oral contraceptives
      - Cortisols
    - Pregnancy
    - Diabetes
- Signs & symptoms
  - Itching
  - Discharge
    - Thick
    - Yellow
  - Yeasty odor
  - Pain
- Treatment — Antifungal agents
  - Topical
  - Oral

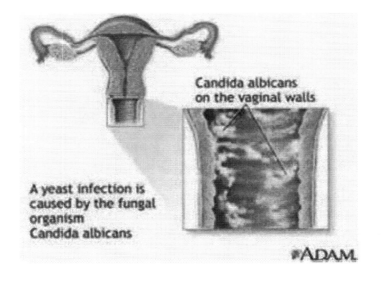

Candida albicans on the vaginal walls

A yeast infection is caused by the fungal organism Candida albicans

#ADAM.

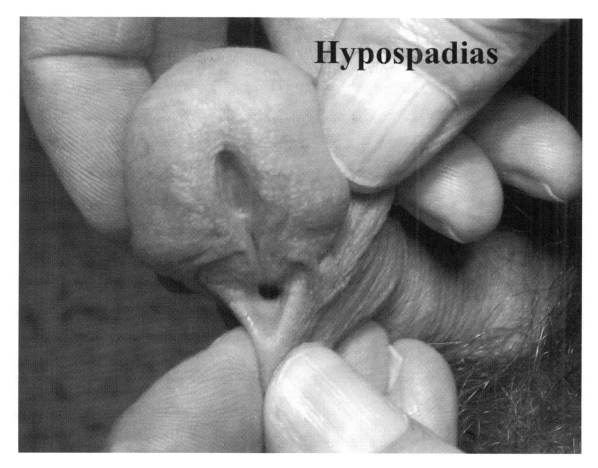

Hypospadias

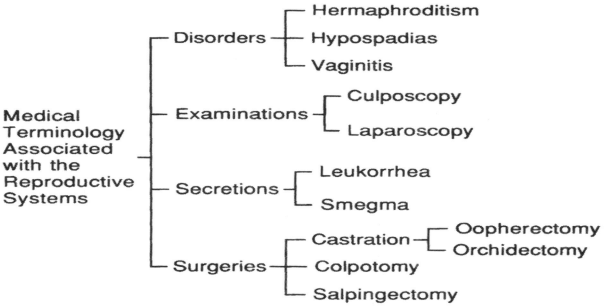

Medical
Terminology
Associated
with the
Reproductive
Systems

- Disorders
  - Hermaphroditism
  - Hypospadias
  - Vaginitis
- Examinations
  - Culposcopy
  - Laparoscopy
- Secretions
  - Leukorrhea
  - Smegma
- Surgeries
  - Castration
    - Oopherectomy
    - Orchidectomy
  - Colpotomy
  - Salpingectomy

CHAPTER TWENTY NINE

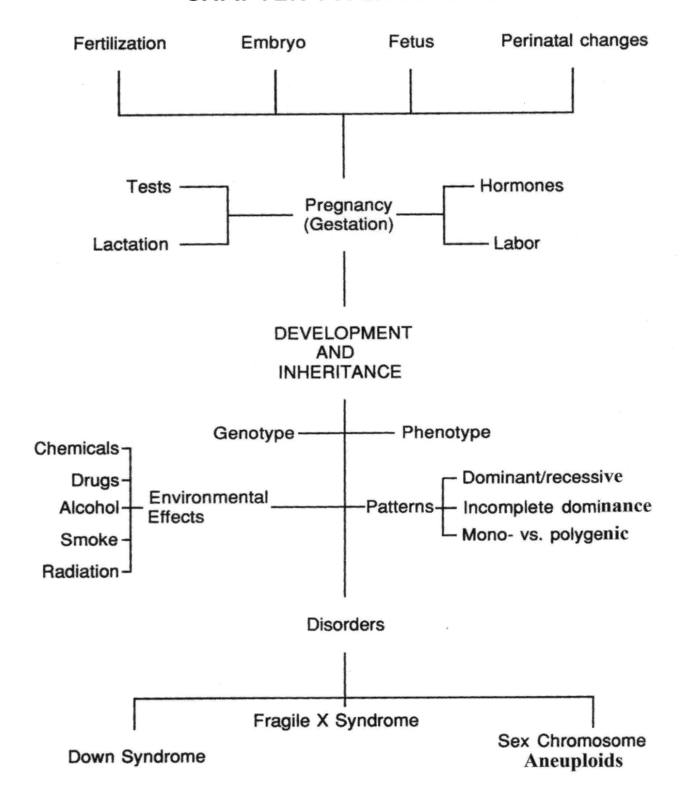

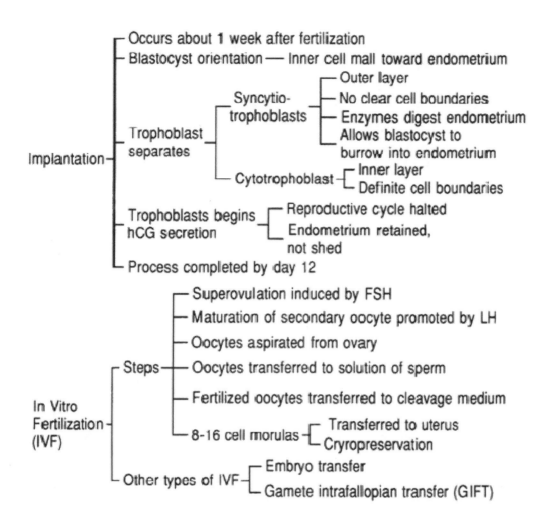

Implantation
- Occurs about 1 week after fertilization
- Blastocyst orientation — Inner cell mall toward endometrium
- Trophoblast separates
  - Syncytio-trophoblasts
    - Outer layer
    - No clear cell boundaries
    - Enzymes digest endometrium
    - Allows blastocyst to burrow into endometrium
  - Cytotrophoblast
    - Inner layer
    - Definite cell boundaries
- Trophoblasts begins hCG secretion
  - Reproductive cycle halted
  - Endometrium retained, not shed
- Process completed by day 12

In Vitro Fertilization (IVF)
- Steps
  - Superovulation induced by FSH
  - Maturation of secondary oocyte promoted by LH
  - Oocytes aspirated from ovary
  - Oocytes transferred to solution of sperm
  - Fertilized oocytes transferred to cleavage medium
  - 8-16 cell morulas
    - Transferred to uterus
    - Cryropreservation
- Other types of IVF
  - Embryo transfer
  - Gamete intrafallopian transfer (GIFT)

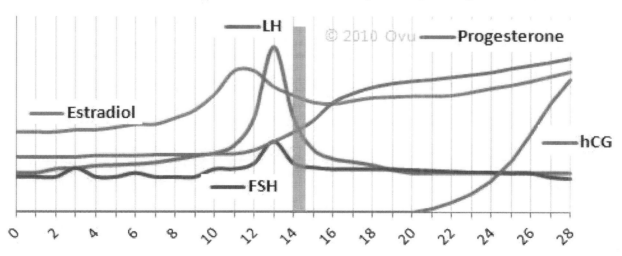

Menstrual cycle and conception, days 1-28

© 2010 Ovu

LH
Progesterone
Estradiol
FSH
hCG

0 2 4 6 8 10 12 14 16 18 20 22 24 26 28

Fertilization in humans. The sperm and ovum unite through fertilization, creating a zygote that (over the course of 8-9 days) will implant in the uterine wall, where it will reside over the course of 9 months.

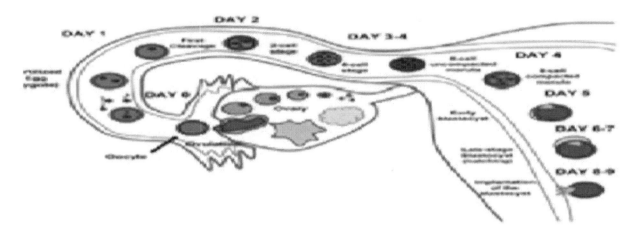

Implantation, Gastrulation and Embryo Development

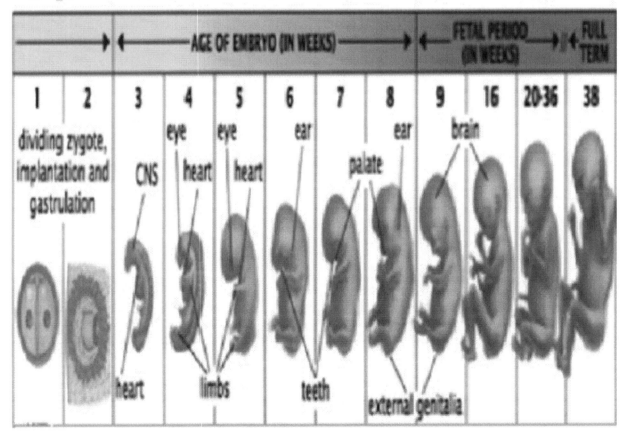

Implantation

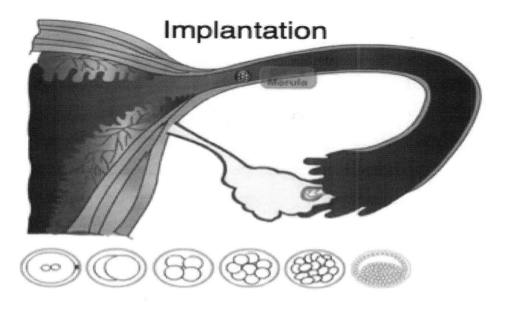

With tubal movement the embryo is transported.

Development of the Embryo: Week 1

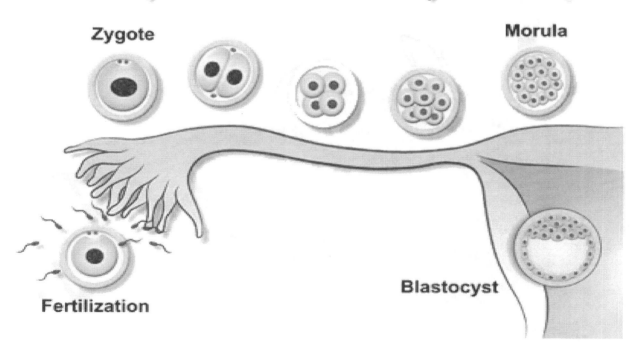

Zygote

Morula

Fertilization

Blastocyst

In Vitro Fertilization

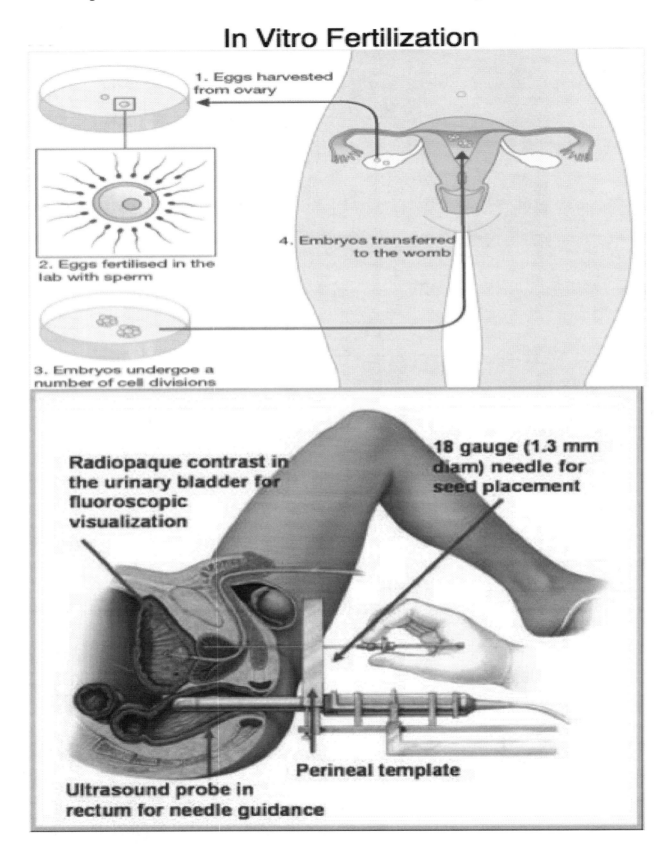

1. Eggs harvested from ovary

2. Eggs fertilised in the lab with sperm

3. Embryos undergoe a number of cell divisions

4. Embryos transferred to the womb

Radiopaque contrast in the urinary bladder for fluoroscopic visualization

18 gauge (1.3 mm diam) needle for seed placement

Perineal template

Ultrasound probe in rectum for needle guidance

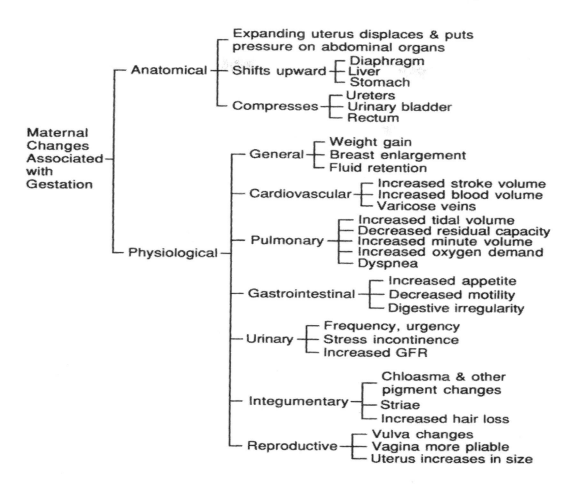

- Maternal Changes Associated with Gestation
  - Anatomical
    - Expanding uterus displaces & puts pressure on abdominal organs
    - Shifts upward
      - Diaphragm
      - Liver
      - Stomach
    - Compresses
      - Ureters
      - Urinary bladder
      - Rectum
  - Physiological
    - General
      - Weight gain
      - Breast enlargement
      - Fluid retention
    - Cardiovascular
      - Increased stroke volume
      - Increased blood volume
      - Varicose veins
    - Pulmonary
      - Increased tidal volume
      - Decreased residual capacity
      - Increased minute volume
      - Increased oxygen demand
      - Dyspnea
    - Gastrointestinal
      - Increased appetite
      - Decreased motility
      - Digestive irregularity
    - Urinary
      - Frequency, urgency
      - Stress incontinence
      - Increased GFR
    - Integumentary
      - Chloasma & other pigment changes
      - Striae
      - Increased hair loss
    - Reproductive
      - Vulva changes
      - Vagina more pliable
      - Uterus increases in size

Maternal Changes Associated with Gestation

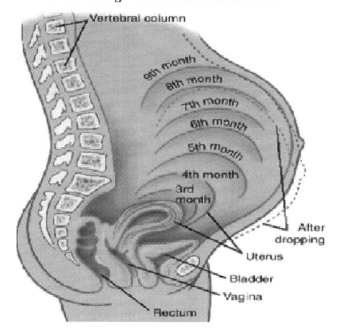

Vertebral column

9th month
8th month
7th month
6th month
5th month
4th month
3rd month

After dropping

Uterus

Bladder

Vagina

Rectum

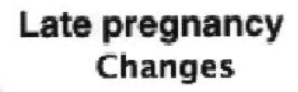

Late pregnancy
Changes

The breasts and uterus grow, adding weight to the front of the body.

Abdominal muscles stretch as the baby grows.

Nerves may be pressed as the baby grows or shifts position.

Pelvic ligaments and joints loosen and become strained.

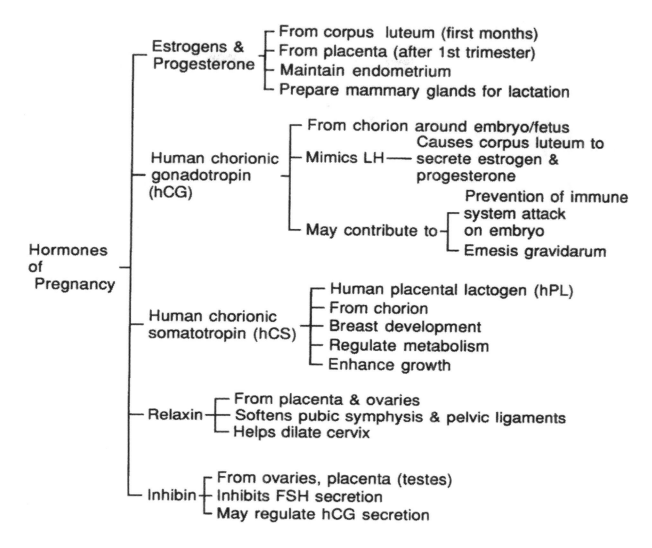

Hormones of Pregnancy

- Estrogens & Progesterone
  - From corpus luteum (first months)
  - From placenta (after 1st trimester)
  - Maintain endometrium
  - Prepare mammary glands for lactation
- Human chorionic gonadotropin (hCG)
  - From chorion around embryo/fetus
  - Mimics LH — Causes corpus luteum to secrete estrogen & progesterone
  - May contribute to
    - Prevention of immune system attack on embryo
    - Emesis gravidarum
- Human chorionic somatotropin (hCS)
  - Human placental lactogen (hPL)
  - From chorion
  - Breast development
  - Regulate metabolism
  - Enhance growth
- Relaxin
  - From placenta & ovaries
  - Softens pubic symphysis & pelvic ligaments
  - Helps dilate cervix
- Inhibin
  - From ovaries, placenta (testes)
  - Inhibits FSH secretion
  - May regulate hCG secretion

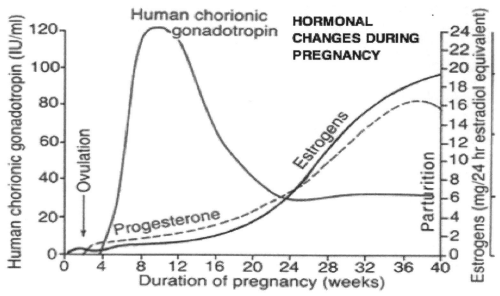

HORMONAL CHANGES DURING PREGNANCY

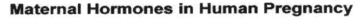

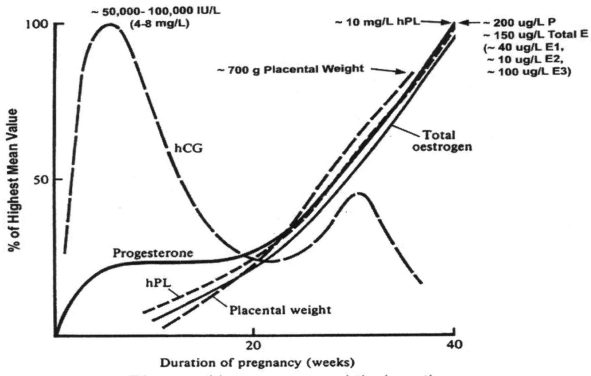

Maternal Hormones in Human Pregnancy

Placental hormones and their actions

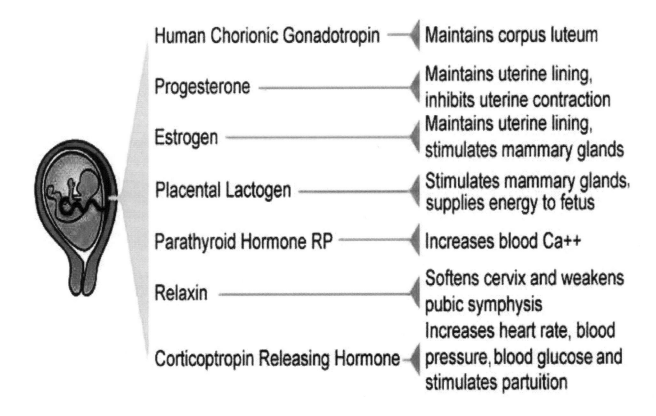

Hormone	Action
Human Chorionic Gonadotropin	Maintains corpus luteum
Progesterone	Maintains uterine lining, inhibits uterine contraction
Estrogen	Maintains uterine lining, stimulates mammary glands
Placental Lactogen	Stimulates mammary glands, supplies energy to fetus
Parathyroid Hormone RP	Increases blood Ca++
Relaxin	Softens cervix and weakens pubic symphysis
Corticoptropin Releasing Hormone	Increases heart rate, blood pressure, blood glucose and stimulates partuition

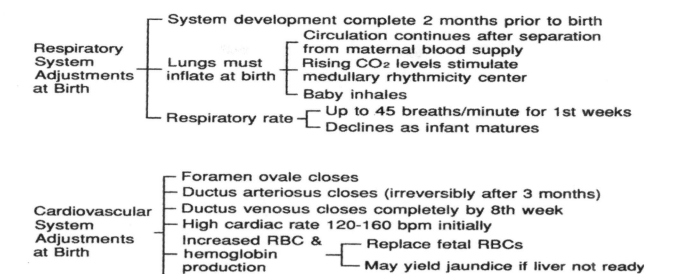

Respiratory System Adjustments at Birth
- System development complete 2 months prior to birth
- Lungs must inflate at birth
  - Circulation continues after separation from maternal blood supply
  - Rising CO_2 levels stimulate medullary rhythmicity center
  - Baby inhales
- Respiratory rate
  - Up to 45 breaths/minute for 1st weeks
  - Declines as infant matures

Cardiovascular System Adjustments at Birth
- Foramen ovale closes
- Ductus arteriosus closes (irreversibly after 3 months)
- Ductus venosus closes completely by 8th week
- High cardiac rate 120-160 bpm initially
- Increased RBC & hemoglobin production
  - Replace fetal RBCs
  - May yield jaundice if liver not ready
- Initially high WBC count —— Drops during 1st week

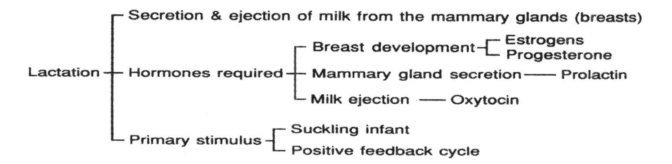

Lactation
- Secretion & ejection of milk from the mammary glands (breasts)
- Hormones required
  - Breast development
    - Estrogens
    - Progesterone
  - Mammary gland secretion —— Prolactin
  - Milk ejection —— Oxytocin
- Primary stimulus
  - Suckling infant
  - Positive feedback cycle

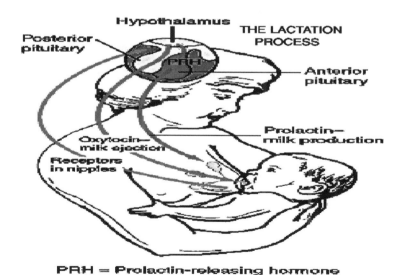

THE LACTATION PROCESS

Hypothalamus
Posterior pituitary
PRH
Anterior pituitary
Oxytocin— milk ejection
Prolactin— milk production
Receptors in nipples

PRH = Prolactin-releasing hormone

Physiologic Changes In Pregnancy

Cardiovascular	Increased cardiac output
	Increased blood volume
	Increased resting heart rate
	Decreased peripheral resistance
	Decreased blood pressure (second trimester)
Pulmonary	Increased respiratory rate
	Decreased functional residual capacity
	Increased tidal volume
	Increased minute ventilation
	Respiratory alkalosis
Gastrointestinal	Decreased gastric motility
	Decreased esophageal sphincter tone
Musculoskeletal	Increased ligament laxity

Maternal Respiratory Changes

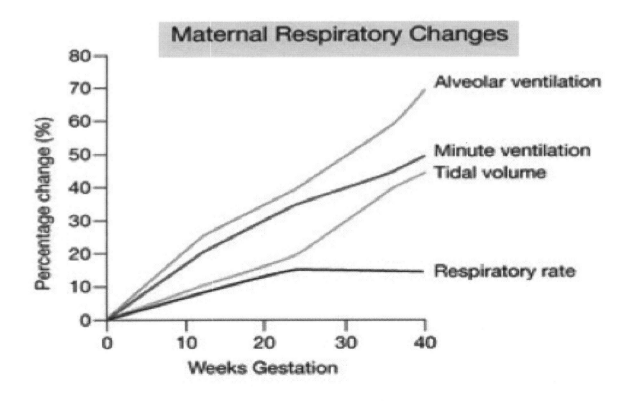

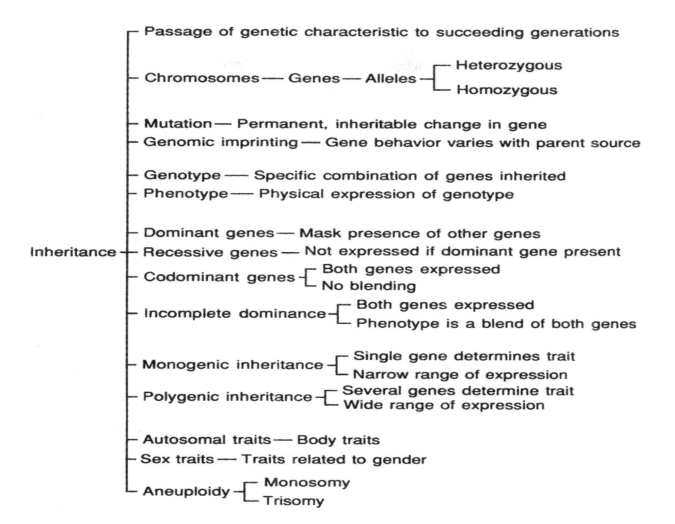

Inheritance
- Passage of genetic characteristic to succeeding generations
- Chromosomes — Genes — Alleles
  - Heterozygous
  - Homozygous
- Mutation — Permanent, inheritable change in gene
- Genomic imprinting — Gene behavior varies with parent source
- Genotype — Specific combination of genes inherited
- Phenotype — Physical expression of genotype
- Dominant genes — Mask presence of other genes
- Recessive genes — Not expressed if dominant gene present
- Codominant genes
  - Both genes expressed
  - No blending
- Incomplete dominance
  - Both genes expressed
  - Phenotype is a blend of both genes
- Monogenic inheritance
  - Single gene determines trait
  - Narrow range of expression
- Polygenic inheritance
  - Several genes determine trait
  - Wide range of expression
- Autosomal traits — Body traits
- Sex traits — Traits related to gender
- Aneuploidy
  - Monosomy
  - Trisomy

Normal Process of Meosis

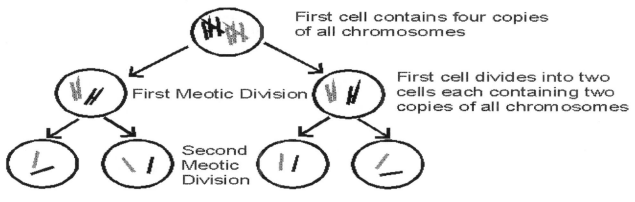

First cell contains four copies of all chromosomes

First Meotic Division — First cell divides into two cells each containing two copies of all chromosomes

Second Meotic Division

Cells divide again to form four cells each containing one copy of all chromosomes

Dominant and Recessive mutations

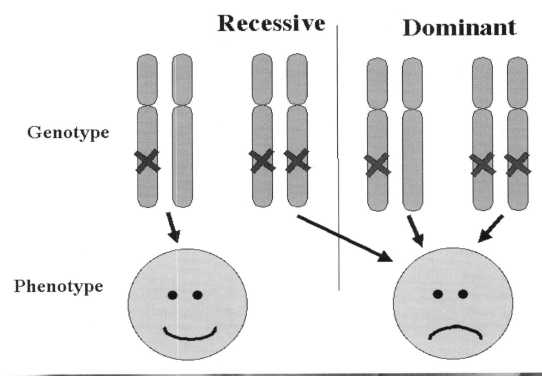

Recessive   **Dominant**

Genotype

Phenotype

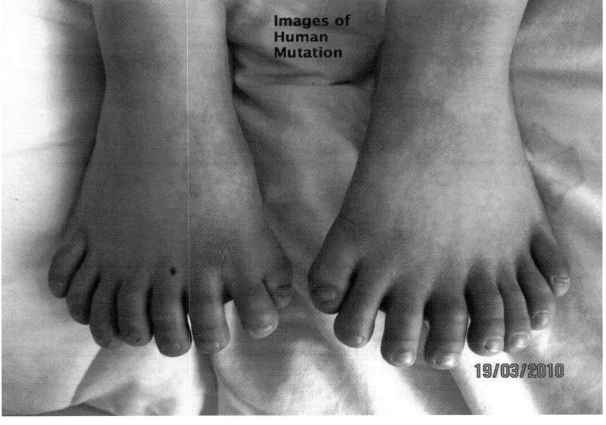

Images of
Human
Mutation

19/03/2010

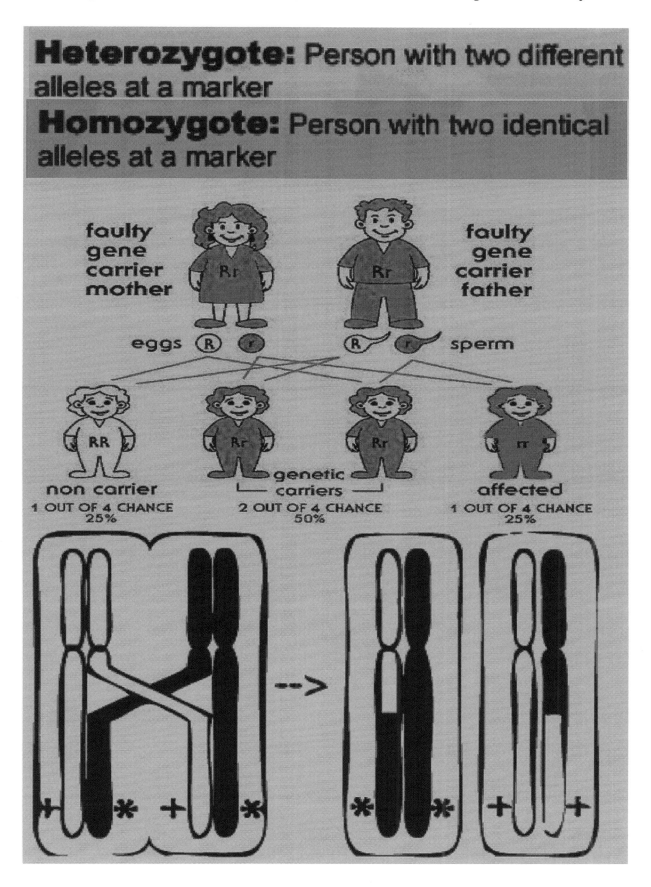

Inheritance of Cystic Fibrosis (CF)

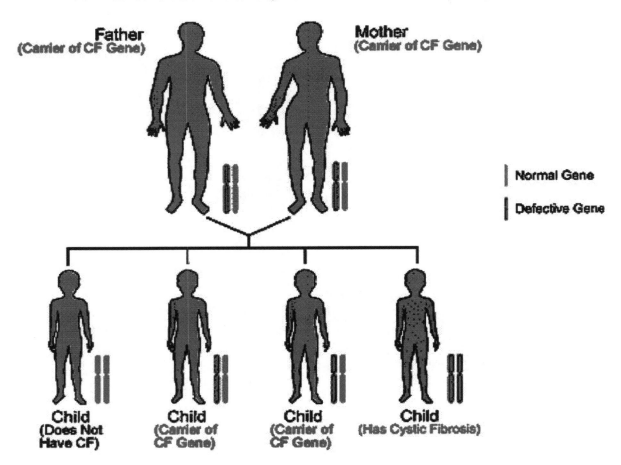

INHERITANCE OF EYE COLOR

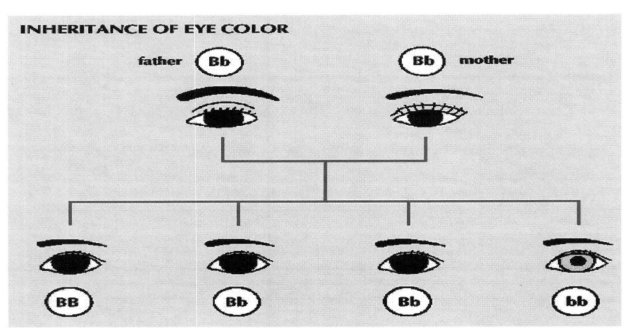

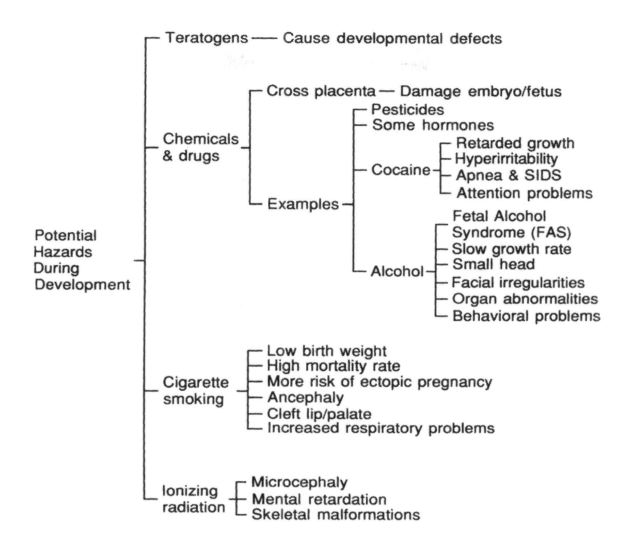

Potential Hazards During Development
- Teratogens —— Cause developmental defects
- Chemicals & drugs
  - Cross placenta — Damage embryo/fetus
  - Examples
    - Pesticides
    - Some hormones
    - Cocaine
      - Retarded growth
      - Hyperirritability
      - Apnea & SIDS
      - Attention problems
    - Alcohol
      - Fetal Alcohol Syndrome (FAS)
      - Slow growth rate
      - Small head
      - Facial irregularities
      - Organ abnormalities
      - Behavioral problems
- Cigarette smoking
  - Low birth weight
  - High mortality rate
  - More risk of ectopic pregnancy
  - Ancephaly
  - Cleft lip/palate
  - Increased respiratory problems
- Ionizing radiation
  - Microcephaly
  - Mental retardation
  - Skeletal malformations

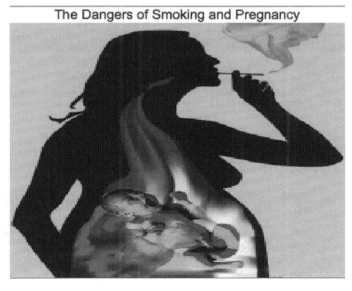

The Dangers of Smoking and Pregnancy

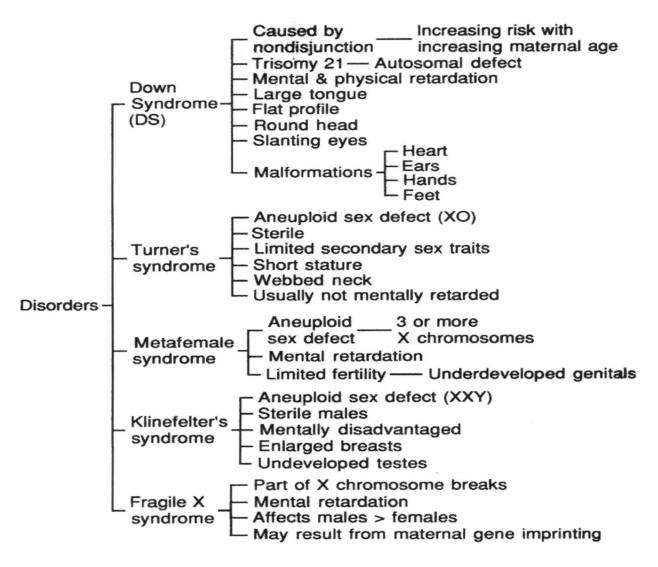

Disorders

- Down Syndrome (DS)
  - Caused by nondisjunction —— Increasing risk with increasing maternal age
  - Trisomy 21 — Autosomal defect
  - Mental & physical retardation
  - Large tongue
  - Flat profile
  - Round head
  - Slanting eyes
  - Malformations
    - Heart
    - Ears
    - Hands
    - Feet

- Turner's syndrome
  - Aneuploid sex defect (XO)
  - Sterile
  - Limited secondary sex traits
  - Short stature
  - Webbed neck
  - Usually not mentally retarded

- Metafemale syndrome
  - Aneuploid sex defect —— 3 or more X chromosomes
  - Mental retardation
  - Limited fertility —— Underdeveloped genitals

- Klinefelter's syndrome
  - Aneuploid sex defect (XXY)
  - Sterile males
  - Mentally disadvantaged
  - Enlarged breasts
  - Undeveloped testes

- Fragile X syndrome
  - Part of X chromosome breaks
  - Mental retardation
  - Affects males > females
  - May result from maternal gene imprinting

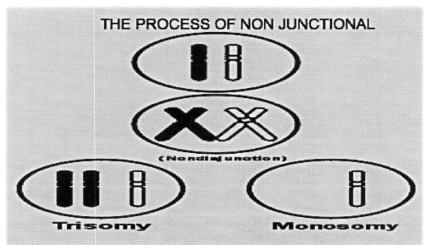

THE PROCESS OF NON JUNCTIONAL

(Nondisjunction)

Trisomy   Monosomy

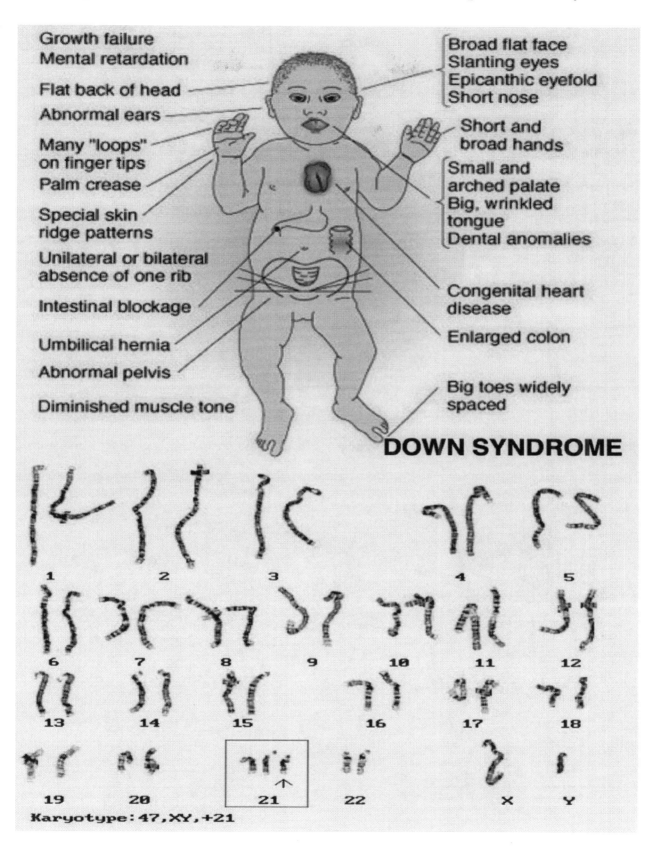

Growth failure
Mental retardation

Flat back of head

Abnormal ears

Many "loops"
on finger tips

Palm crease

Special skin
ridge patterns

Unilateral or bilateral
absence of one rib

Intestinal blockage

Umbilical hernia

Abnormal pelvis

Diminished muscle tone

Broad flat face
Slanting eyes
Epicanthic eyefold
Short nose

Short and
broad hands

Small and
arched palate
Big, wrinkled
tongue
Dental anomalies

Congenital heart
disease

Enlarged colon

Big toes widely
spaced

DOWN SYNDROME

1 2 3 4 5
6 7 8 9 10 11 12
13 14 15 16 17 18
19 20 21 22 X Y

Karyotype: 47,XY,+21

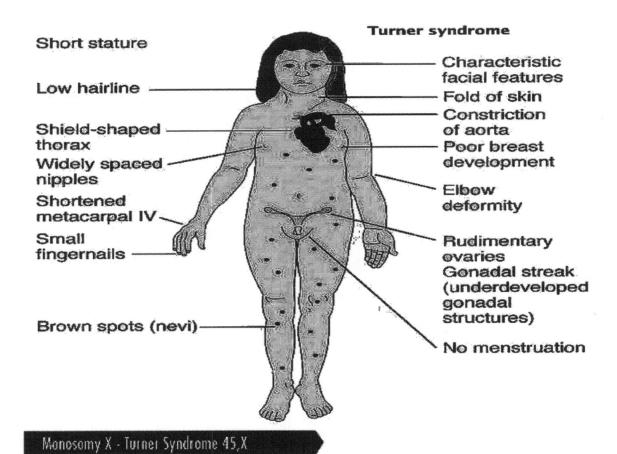

Turner syndrome

Short stature

Low hairline

Shield-shaped thorax

Widely spaced nipples

Shortened metacarpal IV

Small fingernails

Brown spots (nevi)

Characteristic facial features

Fold of skin

Constriction of aorta

Poor breast development

Elbow deformity

Rudimentary ovaries

Gonadal streak (underdeveloped gonadal structures)

No menstruation

Monosomy X - Turner Syndrome 45,X

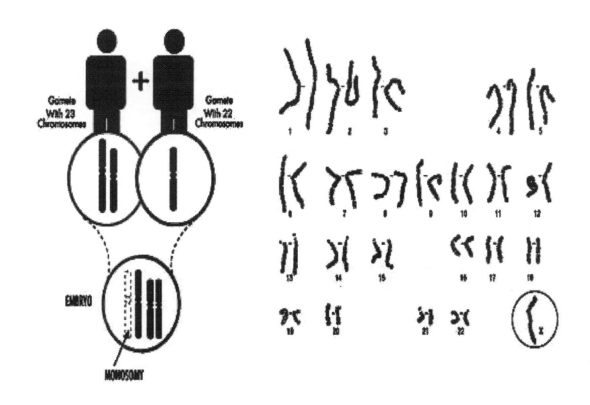

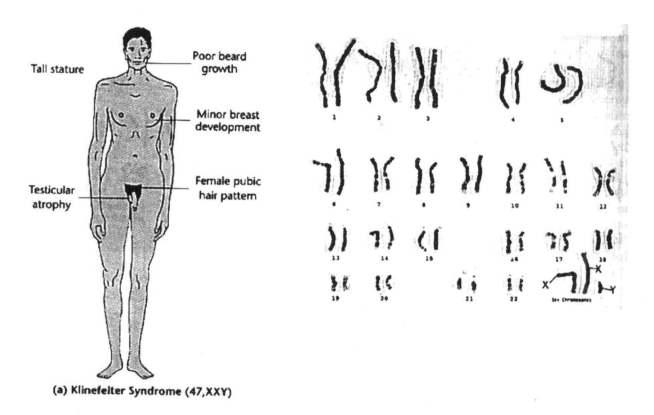

(a) Klinefelter Syndrome (47,XXY)

Fragile X Syndrome

☞ **Most common inherited form of mental retardation (1/1000 males)**

☞ **Due to unstable CGG repeat at Xq27**

☞ **All full mutations derive from a premutation (56-200 repeats)**

☞ **Expansion from pre- to full mutation only occurs through <u>female</u> meiosis**

☞ **Severity of disease correlates with # of CGG repeats**

References

1. Principles Of Anatomy And Physiology Tortora-Grabowski, Ninth Edition
2. Principles Of Anatomy & Physiology 13th Edition Gerard J. Tortora; Bergen community college & Bryan Derrickson; Valencia community college, John Wiley & Sons, Inc.
3. Concept Maps In Anatomy And Physiology To Accompany Erzouki's Medical Physiology
4. Erzouki's Medical Physiology Volume I, II & III 2010
5. Practical Physiology Handout By Hashim Khalil. Erzouki M.D. Ph.D. & Wassan H, Jassim M.B.Ch.B, Msc.
6. Al-Mustansiriya College Of Medicine Physiology Laboratory Manual
7. Human Anatomy And Physiology, Laboratory Manual By Elaine N. Marieb, R. N., Ph. D. Holyoke Community College Eighth Edition
8. Human Anatomy And Physiology, By Elaine N. Marieb, R. N., Ph. D. Holyoke Community College Second Edition
9. Sylvia S. Madre: Understanding Human Anatomy & Physiology, Fifth Edition The McGraw Hill Companies, 2004.
10. Anatomy & Physiology By Frederic H. Martini Ph. D. First Edition
11. Sites And Mechanisms Responsible For The Cardiovascular effects Of Cocaine, Dr. Hashim Khalil Erzouki, , Georgetown University Washington, D.C. Ph D. Thesis in Physiology, April 18, 1991.
12. Textbook Of Medical Physiology, Eleventh Edition By Arthur C. Guyton, M.D And John E. Hall, Ph.D. 2003.University Of Mississippi Medical Center Jackson, Mississippi
13. Manual Of Practical Physiology, Syrian International Private University For Science And Technology, College Of Medicine, By Dr Hisham S. Ibrahim Alnuaimy M. Sc Physiology Second Edition 2008-2009.
14. Lymphocyte Apoptosis In Normal Menstruating Females, By Dr Wassan Hassan Jassim M.B.Ch.B, Msc. Physiology, Thesis At Al-Nahrain University, College Of Medicines, Baghdad, Iraq, 2004-2006.
15. Sylvia S. Madre: Understanding Human Anatomy & Physiology, Fifth Edition The McGraw Hill Companies, 2004.
16. Oxfords Handbook Of Clinical Medicine, Sixth Edition
17. Human Physiology, Fourth Edition, By Rodney Rhoades, Ph. D
18. Brain Facts: A Primer On The Brain And Nervous System The Society For Neuroscience
19. Goldman: Cecil Medicine, 23rd Ed. Copyright © 2007 Saunders, An Imprint Of Elsevier
20. Clinical Anesthesia, 5th Edition Editors: Bearish, Paul G.; Cullen, Bruce F.; Stoelting, Robert K. Copyright ©2006 Lippincott Williams & Wilkins
21. Human Physiology By Stuart Ira Fox — Twelfth Edition

22. Handbook Of Eating Disorders Edited By J. Treasure, U. Schmidt And E. Van Furth. Second Edition
23. Atlas of Human Anatomy for the Artist Stephen Rogers Peck Oxford University Press
24. Hole's Human Anatomy and Physiology 11th Edition
25. Acid-Base, Fluids, And Electrolytes Made Ridiculously Simple By Richard A. Preston, M.D, M.B.A, Department Of Medicine University Of Miami School Of Medicine
26. Anatomy & Physiology: The Unity Of Form And Function 5th Edition By Kenneth S. Saladin Georgia College and State University
27. Applied Physiology In Intensive Care Medicine M. R. Pinsky · L. Brochard · J. Mancebo · G. Hedenstierna (Eds.) Second Edition
28. Mayo Clinic Gastroenterology And Hepatology Board Review
29. Third Edition Editor Stephen C. Hauser, MD Co-Editors Darrell S. Pardi, MD John J. Poterucha, MD
30. Ganong's Review Of Medical Physiology, Twenty-Third Edition Copyright © 2010 By The McGraw-Hill Companies
31. Harrison's: Principles Of Internal Medicine Eighteenth Edition Harrison's Is A Trademark Of The Mcgraw-Hill Companies, Inc.
32. Pathophysiology Of Disease: An Introduction To Clinical Medicine, 5th Edition, Authors: Mcphee, Stephen J.; Ganong, William F.
33. Clinical Anatomy Made Ridiculously Simple By Stephen Goldberg, M. D. University Of Miami School Of Medicine Miami, Florida
34. Clinical Biochemistry Made Ridiculously Simple By Stephen Goldberg, M. D. University Of Miami School Of Medicine Miami, Florida
35. Clinical Neuro-Anatomy Made Ridiculously Simple By Stephen Goldberg, M. D. University Of Miami School Of Medicine Miami, Florida
36. Clinical Pharmacology Made Ridiculously Simple By Jim Olson, M.D Ph. D. University Of Washington Seattle, Wa
37. Concept Maps In Physiology By Hashim Khalil Erzouki, M. D., Ph. D. September 2010
38. Davidson's Principles And Practice Of Medicine, Twenty-First Edition 2010
39. Exercise Physiology For Health, Fitness, And Performance Third Edition By Sharon A. Plowman Northern Illinois University & Denise L. Smith Skidmore College
40. Human Physiology From Cells To Systems By Lauralee Sherwood Seventh Edition, Department Of Physiology And Pharmacology School Of Medicine West Virginia University
41. Hutchison's Clinical Methods - An Integrated Approach To Clinical Practice, 22nd Edition
42. Marieb Human Anatomy And Physiology
43. Medical Physiology Principles For Clinical Medicine Fourth Edition By Rodney A. Rhoades, Ph.D. And David R. Bell, Ph.D. Indiana University School Of Medicine Indiana
44. Mood Disorders A Handbook Of Science And Practice By Mick Power University Of Edinburgh And Royal Edinburgh Hospital
45. Pathophysiology - Concepts Of Altered Health States 7th Edition - Carol Mattson Porth
46. Practicing Neurology What You Need To Know, What You Need To Do Second Edition By Rahman Pourmand MD, Department Of Neurology, Stony Brook University Hospital, Stony Brook, NY

Anatomy & Physiology   **Review & Guide**

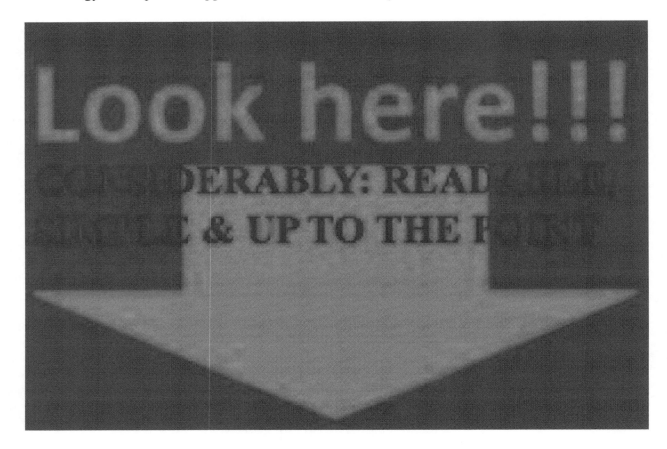

CONSIDERABLY READABLE, SIMPLE & UP TO THE POINT

Anatomy & Physiology   **Review & Guide**

Anatomy Physiology Made Incredibly Clear Useful & Readable

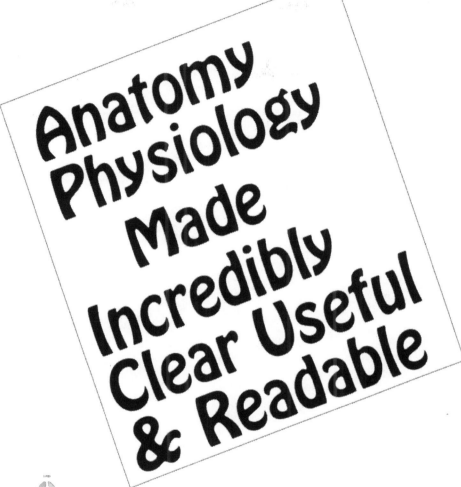

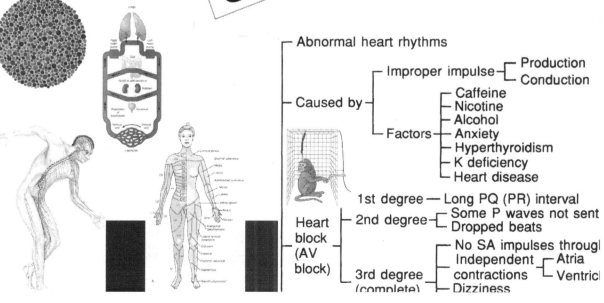

- Abnormal heart rhythms
- Caused by
  - Improper impulse
    - Production
    - Conduction
  - Factors
    - Caffeine
    - Nicotine
    - Alcohol
    - Anxiety
    - Hyperthyroidism
    - K deficiency
    - Heart disease

- Heart block (AV block)
  - 1st degree — Long PQ (PR) interval
  - 2nd degree
    - Some P waves not sent
    - Dropped beats
  - 3rd degree (complete)
    - No SA impulses througl
    - Independent contractions
      - Atria
      - Ventricl
    - Dizziness

Anatomy & Physiology   **Review & Guide**

Made in the USA
Middletown, DE
20 June 2023

32455973R00347